public health

Administration and practice

public
health

Administration and practice

John J. Hanlon, M.S., M.D., M.P.H.

Professor, School of Public Health, San Diego State University;
formerly Assistant Surgeon General, U.S. Public Health Service;
Director, Community Health Services, Philadelphia;
Commissioner of Health, Detroit and Wayne County

George E. Pickett, M.D., M.P.H.

Professor, School of Public Health,
University of Alabama in Birmingham;
formerly Director of Health, West Virginia;
Director of Health and Welfare, San Mateo County;
Commissioner of Health, Detroit and Wayne County

EIGHTH EDITION

with 23 illustrations

TIMES MIRROR/MOSBY
COLLEGE PUBLISHING

ST. LOUIS • TORONTO • SANTA CLARA   1984

Editor: Nancy K. Roberson
Editing supervisor: Lin Dempsey
Manuscript editor: Diane Ackermann
Design: Jeanne Bush
Production: Carolyn Biby

EIGHTH EDITION

Copyright © 1984 by Times Mirror/Mosby College Publishing
A division of The C.V. Mosby Company
11830 Westline Industrial Drive
St. Louis, Missouri 63146

Previous editions copyrighted 1950, 1955, 1960, 1964, 1969, 1974, 1979

Printed in the United States of America

Library of Congress Cataloging in Publication Data

Hanlon, John J. (John Joseph), 1912-
    Public health.

    Includes index.
    1. Public health. 2. Public health administration.
I. Pickett, George E. II. Title. [DNLM: 1. Public
health administration. WA 525 H241p]
RA425.H29 1984   362.1'068   82-24981
ISBN 0-8016-2061-9

GW/VH/VH 9 8 7 6 5   02/C/233

To our families

Preface

When the first edition of this book appeared about 35 years ago, public health was both very different and very much the same as it is now. Health departments seemed to fit the classic model of physician, nurse, and sanitarian, and Emerson's prescription for what health departments should be doing was generally acceptable. There were not many useful textbooks for students who were studying the organization and management of health services, and none of them seemed to pay sufficient attention to the history and values of public health.

From a historical perspective, it is now apparent that organizations were neither as simple nor as homogeneous in their design as had been imagined. Many progressive health departments had developed extensive programs to provide primary care to high-risk population groups, and others had forged creative coalitions with other community organizations to solve complex problems, often of a uniquely local nature. By 1983, atypical arrangements have become the norm. In most states, public health agencies are intricately intertwined with many other agencies, both public and private not-for-profit organizations, to enable them to fulfill the role of what has come to be known as "the governmental presence in health." The problems involved in providing medical care, particularly to the medically indigent, have become very complex, as have the problems of the environment. The existing and potential solutions to these problems are remarkably diverse. Many of the problems, particularly those involving the cost of medical care and our increasingly toxic environment, are not presently solvable. The pace of change has increased steadily since this book first appeared, and that has naturally shaped its contents.

The first three parts of the book, which attempt to describe the history of public health and its bases in sociology, economics, philosophy, and government, have remained the same in their theses, although there have been numerous amendments to those theses as well as an accumulation of important new data, which provide more insight into the nature of the problems and the efficacy of the social instruments designed to deal with them. There have been dramatic changes in both the geography and the age distribution of the world's population—changes that have emerged much more rapidly than anyone might have imagined just 10 years ago.

The epidemiology chapter has been completely rewritten in an attempt to show the relevance of epidemiology to problem solving in the development and management of public health services. There are by now many excellent textbooks that effectively present epidemiologic concepts, the epidemiology of chronic and infectious diseases, and the epidemiology of social and behavioral diseases. It is apparent that epidemiology will play a larger role in determining health policy in the United States over the next decade. Similarly, the chapter on health education has been broadened to encompass recent developments in health promotion and disease prevention.

The chapters on the environment reflect the rapid changes that have occurred both in the priorities assigned to air and water pollution and toxicology and hazardous wastes as well as in the organization and management of services at the state and local level. Many of the systems that had been developed during the earlier part of this century are now showing signs of obsolescence. Water and sewage treatment plants built as recently as the 1960s have begun to fail as costs have risen and maintenance has decreased. Recent studies have shown that a disturbing number of the nation's public water supply systems do not provide the safe product the community has a right to expect. While these "old" problems have reappeared as current and continuing problems, requiring skillful design and economic analysis by trained public health engineers, other issues have emerged that suggest that the continued assault of humans on their environment has begun to have global effects. There is justifiable concern that the buildup of chemical effects in the stratosphere as well as on the surface of the earth may cause major changes in the nature of plant and animal life in the not-too-distant future.

Part VI divides problems into Maternal and Child Health, School and Adolescent Health, and Aging. Although the distinctions may be somewhat artificial from a physiologic point of view, they represent distinct areas of programmatic emphasis and social concern. The health problems of the elderly have become particularly acute both because of the rapid increase in the cost of medical care and because the number of people over the age of 75 is increasing more rapidly than was anticipated less than 10 years ago. As late as 1977 and 1978, the classic demographic projections had shown the older age groups moving through the sequential 5-year periods and accounting for about 11% of the population, but by 1980 it was apparent that a remarkable decline in the cardiovascular disease death rate was occurring in the older age groups and that their life span was extending beyond age 65 at a surprising rate. More recent demographic projections indicate a very different shape to the population curve than had been anticipated, with major consequences for the social security system, the organization of public health services, and the provision of primary care throughout the United States.

Major changes have begun to occur in the field of behavioral health as well. The nation has begun to realize that violence in its many forms is a major public health problem. New voluntary health organizations have been formed that have made important inroads on legislation affecting drunk driving and highway safety—the major cause of death and disability among young people. Risk-taking behavior by adolescents has come under closer scrutiny by qualified sociologists, epidemiologists, and pediatricians, and many health departments have begun to develop adolescent health service programs.

Other personal health service programs are changing as well. Nursing continues to evolve as a potential source of primary care, and the nature of dental health services has changed dramatically with the significant decrease in dental caries. Dental health research continues to produce rich dividends, and it seems likely that the nature of dental practice will change considerably over the next decade. This may provide valuable insight into the nature of the problems that will occur as the traditional role of the medical profession changes in the face of more effective preventive interventions by nonphysician health professionals.

As both the boundaries of public health and its interrelationships with other spheres of interest have expanded, this book and the work of its authors must change. The field of practice is more complex now than it was 3 decades ago, and so is the body of knowledge available to those who choose public health as a career and as a way of life. We are indebted to our colleagues, our families, and our students who have helped us immeasurably in our efforts to understand the changing world of public health and its place in the collection of human priorities.

JOHN J. HANLON
GEORGE E. PICKETT

Contents

public
health

Administration and practice

PART ONE

Roots of public health

Before embarking on the main purpose of this book, it is well to consider the origins and meaning of the present-day public health movement. These introductory chapters are presented in the belief that an acquaintance with the history of society, its health problems, and its attempts to solve them may contribute to greater understanding and professional satisfaction.

CHAPTER 1

Philosophy and purpose of public health

Philosophy is able to fancy everything different from what it is.
It sees the familiar as strange, and the strange as familiar.

William James

PUBLIC HEALTH AS A PROFESSION

Throughout the world there are now large numbers of people from many professions engaged in the field commonly referred to as public health. Typically they may be fairly characterized as unusually idealistic and dedicated with a strong sense of social responsibility that transcends such barriers as race, religion, or nationalism. Perhaps the reason is their conviction that in this field more than others one can find an opportunity to serve humanity and to help to adapt it and nature to mutual advantage rather than to submit helplessly to the vagaries of chance. But what can be accomplished in the face of superstition, ignorance, public apathy, political interference, and inadequate resources? Is their idealism justified? One is reminded of a statement by the Irish parliamentarian Edmund Burke (1729-1797) in the face of repeated criticism: "Those who carry on great public schemes must be proof against the most fatiguing delays, the most mortifying disappointments, the most shocking insults, and what is worst of all, the presumptuous judgments of the ignorant." Sir Henry Cole once showed this statement to his close friend public health pioneer Edwin Chadwick and commented that Chadwick should have it pinned to his sleeve as an epigraph.

An essential point to be made is that despite all handicaps, spectacular successes of far-reaching consequences have been achieved during an amazingly brief historical period. At the time of Cole's comment to Chadwick in the midnineteenth century, the average age at death in large English cities was only 36 years for the gentry, 22 years for tradespeople, and 16 years for the laboring class! More than half of the children of the working class and a fifth of the children of the gentry died before their fifth birthday. Since then, the average life expectancy at birth has increased in the United States and several other countries to well over 70 years, and the death rate before the fifth birthday has decreased about 95%.

The late Milton J. Rosenau justified patience on the basis that the recorded history of civilization encompasses relatively few generations. Only 3,500 years have passed since the time of Moses; and if the average length of a generation has been about 35 years, there have been only about 100 generations from Moses to us. When one considers that most of those generations contributed little to the knowledge and social advancement of mankind, there remain perhaps a scant dozen, most of them in the immediate past, that have accounted for most of social and scientific progress.

Public health necessarily has been closely identified with medicine. The practice of medicine is commonly regarded as one of the oldest professions. Yet modern medicine is hardly more than a century old. Indeed, it has been said that not until 1910 did the average patient in the United States have a fifty-fifty chance of being diagnosed correctly.[1] Effective treatment was something else again. Now medical knowledge and techniques become outdated with accelerating rapidity. Similarly, the public health movement, although presaged by occasional and sporadic earlier glimmerings, dates back only about a century. It also is important to realize that these developments have not occurred by themselves. They have been intimately related in conception and development to a broad and multifaceted philosophic and social revolution that has had as its driving force a growing appreciation of the innate value and dignity of mankind. These developments have been a critical part of a broad spectrum of social reforms that includes public education, public welfare, racial and sexual equity, the rights of labor, the humane care of the mentally ill, and penal management, to mention only a few.

These relationships have prompted Beauchamp[2] to conclude that "while many forces influenced the development of public health, the historic dream of public health that preventable death and disability ought to be minimized is a dream of social justice." The logical conclusion is that public health must really be regarded as an ethical enterprise, an agent of social change, not just for the sake of change but to make possible the achievement of the improved lot of mankind. For much of its history, public health has striven for this goal through professional application of scientific and technical knowledge. Dubos[3] has pointed out that changes in the human environment require new adaptive responses that if inadequate result in ill health and other consequences. Changes, hence the need for adaptation, are constantly occurring, since both we and our environment are dynamic, not static. New factors are introduced into the human environment not only by technical innovations as well as geologic or climatic changes but also by the ever evolving human wants, habits, and aspirations. Perhaps the greatest challenge results from the fact that although science may provide solutions to problems inherited from the past, it seldom if ever can do the same for specific problems of the future—it simply does not know what they will be. Public health workers, therefore, must always be ready to contend with the unknown problems of the future. They must think and be ready to act prospectively, in contrast with those in therapeutic professions who think and act on a retrospective basis. This often places public health workers in a difficult position, since so many other professions and most public officials are unaccustomed to this point of view. As stated by Draper and associates[4]:

. . . public health not only involves, it actually *demands* confrontation with received wisdom and the established

powers. All this is not to say, however, that being controversial is a *sufficient* qualification for being effective today in public health, but it certainly seems to be a *necessary* qualification. But if persuasion and sometimes open conflict are not occurring, we should realize that we have lost a "public health movement."

DEFINITIONS OF PUBLIC HEALTH

There have been many attempts to define public health. Chronologically, these definitions present a word picture of the evolution of the field. Early definitions were limited essentially to sanitary measures invoked against nuisances and health hazards with which the individual was powerless to cope and which, when present in one individual, could adversely affect others. Thus initially insanitation and later communicability were the criteria followed in deciding whether a problem fell within the purview of public health. With the great bacteriologic and immunologic discoveries of the late nineteenth and early twentieth centuries and the subsequent development of techniques for their application, the concept of prevention of disease in the individual was added. Public health then came to be regarded as as integration of sanitary science and medical science. As will be discussed later, it has more recently come to be regarded as a social science.

In 1920 Winslow,[5] a strong advocate of this broader viewpoint, enunciated what became the best known and most widely accepted definition of public health and its relationship to other fields. For analytic purposes it is presented here in the following manner:

Public Health is the Science and Art of (1) preventing disease, (2) prolonging life, and (3) promoting health and efficiency through organized community effort for
   (a) the sanitation of the environment,
   (b) the control of communicable infections,
   (c) the education of the individual in personal hygiene,
   (d) the organization of medical and nursing services for the early diagnosis and preventive treatment of disease, and
   (e) the development of the social machinery to insure everyone a standard of living adequate for the maintenance of health,
so organizing these benefits as to enable every citizen to realize his birthright of health and longevity.

Even today, Winslow's definition appears timely and comprehensive. It allows inclusion of almost everything in the fields of social evolution and service as they relate to health and well-being. In addition, it provides a concise summary, not only of public health and its administration, but also of its historic development and present-day and probable future trends.

From a somewhat different viewpoint, one of us (J.J.H.) has considered the multifaceted relationships of health and public health in the following terms:

Health is a state of total effective physiologic and psychologic functioning; it has both a relative and an absolute meaning, varying through time and space, both in the individual and in the group; it is the result of the combination of many forces, intrinsic and extrinsic, inherited and contrived, individual and collective, private and public, medical, environmental, and social; and it is conditioned by culture, economy, law, and government.

Accordingly,

Public health is dedicated to the common attainment of the highest level of physical, mental, and social well-being and longevity consistent with available knowledge and resources at a given time and place. It holds this goal as its contribution to the most effective total development and life of the individual and society.

Another widely known definition appears in the Constitution of the World Health Organization:

Health is a state of complete physical, mental and social well-being and not merely the absence of disease or infirmity.

This is not so much a definition as a statement of goals.

It is evident from these definitions that there has occurred a gradual extension of the horizons of public health. In conformance with the advances of medical and scientific knowledge and keeping pace with social and political progress, public health work has expanded from its original concern with gross environmental insanitation to, in sequence of addition, sanitary engineering, preventive physical medical science, preventive mental medical science, the positive or promotive as well as social and behavioral aspects of personal and community medicine, and more recently, the promotion and assurance of comprehensive health services for all.

The inevitable and continuous extension of the boundaries of public health was clearly recognized a third of a century ago by Mountin,[6] who stated:

The progressive nature of public health makes any restricted definition of the functions and responsibilities of health departments difficult. More than that—there is a real danger in attempting to narrow down a moving or growing thing. To tie public health to the concepts that answered our needs 50 years ago, or even a decade ago,

can only hamstring our contribution to society in the future.

This perceptive statement still remains valid.

THERAPEUTIC MEDICINE, PREVENTIVE MEDICINE, AND PUBLIC HEALTH

A short discussion about the distinctions between therapeutic medicine, preventive medicine, and public health is appropriate. To a major extent, the practice of medicine has been concerned with diagnosis and treatment of damage already done—the realignment of a broken limb, the healing or removal of a diseased organ, or the readjustment of an unsettled mind. The nature of the problems necessitates an individualized approach that is important in its own right. Preventive medicine goes a step further, but its primary goal is still partially the prevention of disease in the individual. Thus it consists of four areas of action:

1. The prevention by biologic means of certain diseases such as specific communicable and deficiency diseases
2. The prevention of some of the consequences of preventable or curable chronic diseases, such as syphilis, tuberculosis, cancer, diabetes, and hypertension
3. The minimization of some of the consequences of nonpreventable and noncurable diseases, such as many genetic conditions
4. The motivation of improved health in individuals by changed life-styles that minimize the potential impact of behavioral and other health hazards

Because of the increasing possible applications of preventive concepts to the early diagnosis and treatment of incipient or established diseases, preventive medicine should be regarded as a component of good clinical medical practice. As a result of the increased teaching of community and family medicine, the development of comprehensive medicine, and the continuity of care, there is a growing tendency by private physicians to incorporate preventive medicine into their practices.

It is possible to go further, however, and encourage the development of constructive and promotive health in which the center of interest is still the individual but now as a social or community integer, a member of a family and of a social group. Health workers must not be content with the mere preservation of a person's health but must strive for the development of its maximum potentials. It is notable that in Winslow's definition, the emphasis in public health has changed from the physical environment, or sanitation, to preventive medicine and, more recently, back to the individual and the environment but now in terms of the individual's relationship with the complex social and physical environment.

This change has brought a more mature realization on the part of both organized medicine and public health workers that each is an adjunct to and a partner of the other and that both exist to serve society.

It would be preferable, of course, if medical practitioners served in a total sense—as personal or family health counselor, therapist, and provider of all preventive and health education and promotive services. To be able to do so, however, would require some philosophic reorientation, some reorganization, more time, and a more extensive use of allied health personnel as well as automated and electronic technology. A method increasingly used is personal health hazard appraisal or risk assessment. This useful tool of prospective medicine is discussed in Chapter 18 in relation to health maintenance. Its wide acceptance and use will probably depend on effective cooperative efforts of public health organizations, schools of medicine, practitioners of medicine, educational institutions, and insurance and similar companies. Already it serves as a basis for the national health program of Canada.[7]

From what has been said earlier, it is evident that public health goes a step further than therapeutic or even preventive medicine. Its patient is the entire community or indeed the world, and its armamentarium is more extensive than those of the other fields. Gershenson[8] summarizes the difference well in saying:

Public health provides a framework to deal with social illness, to alter the ecology, to make constructive use of all the necessary disciplines. The hierarchial medical model had its time and place: it is dysfunctional in dealing with social illness.

The various shifts in personal opportunity, social attitude, and medical practice that have occurred over the years have led inevitably to a reevaluation of the meaning and purpose of health. Until recently, many people have pursued health as an ultimate goal in itself. Increasingly, however, it is realized that health has value only to the extent that it promotes efficiency and makes possible a satisfactory total living experience. After all, it is the quality of life that is meaningful, not merely the quantity. Health in and of itself is of little if any use. Its true value lies in worthwhile activities made possible by virtue of it. Futhermore, it is erroneous to think of complete and lasting health as attainable or even desirable. Dubos[9] used this as the theme of his provocative book, *Mirage of Health*. He emphasized that health and happiness, so long regarded as absolute and permanent values supposedly achieved by some in the golden ages of the past and still sought after in our time, appear to be illusions. To be otherwise is unnatural because, as he indicated, complete freedom from disease, stress, frustration, and struggle is incompatible with the process of living and evolution. In this vein, he mused:

Life is an adventure in a world where nothing is static, where unpredictable and ill-understood events constitute dangers that must be overcome, often blindly and at great cost; where man himself, like the sorcerer's apprentice, has set in motion forces that are potentially destructive and may someday escape his control. Every manifestation of existence is a response to stimuli and challenges, each of which constitutes a threat if not adequately dealt with. The very process of living is a continual interplay between the individual and his environment, often taking the form of a struggle resulting in injury or disease.

He concluded wryly that "complete and lasting freedom from disease is but a dream remembered from imaginings of a Garden of Eden designed for the welfare of man."

SCOPE OF PUBLIC HEALTH

During recent years, the perimeters of public health concern have been expanding rapidly. Whereas not long ago many would limit public health matters to general sanitation and the control of infectious disease, today all aspects of Winslow's famous definition are not only included but even surpassed. With reference to man's environment, public health workers now think in the broadest possible terms—the total ecologic relationship between man and the environment of which he is a part. As for personal health services, health agencies are already deeply involved, not only in problems of distribution and quality of health personnel and facilities, but also in the assurance of adequate comprehensive health care for all. This is evidenced by a spectacular increase in significant legislative actions and programs during recent years.

In general, public health is concerned with three broad areas: (1) health service systems, (2) health behavior and motivation, and (3) environmental hazards. More specifically, public health activities appear to fall into the following seven categories:

1. Activities that must be conducted on a community basis
   a. Supervision of community food, water, and milk supplies as well as medications, household products, toys, and recreational equipment
   b. Insect, rodent, and other vector control
   c. Environmental pollution control, including atmospheric, soil, and aquatic pollution control; prevention of radiation hazards; and noise abatement
2. Activities designed for prevention of illness, disability, or premature death from
   a. Communicable diseases, including parasitic infestations
   b. Dietary deficiencies or excesses
   c. Behavioral disorders, including alcoholism, drug habituation, narcotic addiction, certain aspects of delinquency, and suicide
   d. Mental illness, including mental retardation
   e. Allergic manifestations and their community sources
   f. Acute and chronic noncommunicable respiratory diseases
   g. Neoplastic diseases
   h. Cardiac and cerebrovascular diseases
   i. Metabolic diseases
   j. Certain hereditary or genetic conditions
   k. Occupational diseases
   l. Home, vehicular, and industrial accidents
   m. Dental disorders, including dental caries and periodontal disease
   n. Certain risks of maternity, growth, and development
3. Activities related to comprehensive health care
   a. Promotion of development, availability and quality of health, personnel, facilities, and services in the broadest sense
   b. Operation of programs for early detection of disease
   c. Promotion and sometimes operation of emergency medical service systems
   d. Promotion and sometimes operation of treatment centers, varying from disease-specialty clinics to comprehensive health centers
   e. Facilitation of and participation in pregraduate and continuing health professional and paraprofessional education
4. Activities concerned with collection, preservation, analysis, and use of vital records
5. Public education and motivation in personal and community health
6. Comprehensive health planning and evaluation
7. Research—scientific, technical, and administrative

Obviously many public health agencies do not find it possible or necessary to engage in all of these activities. In each case it is desirable to determine local needs, wishes, resources, and capabilities and to adapt the program of the community to them. Various administrative and planning tools exist to aid in accomplishing this. Several of these are considered in the chapter on planning and evaluation.

It must be realized that public health agencies cannot and should not attempt to carry out the foregoing activities by themselves. To be successful and acceptable requires that most if not all of them be done in cooperative partnership with many other agencies, organizations, professions, and community groups.

HEALTH AND GOVERNMENT

Some object to the concept that the protection and promotion of the public's health is an appropriate concern of government. Social and political philosophy did not always encourage this concept. The Roman Empire was notable for its concern for the protection and enhancement of the health and well-being of its own people. During most of history, however, the prevailing attitude has been to regard any such action as unnecessary and dangerous pampering of the masses. Indeed, this was one of the basic points made by Malthus[10]—that not only should the genetically and otherwise inferior be allowed to die according to nature's plan but the conditions of the poor should not be improved lest they lose a sense of responsibility and moral restraint.

Subsequently, lack of positive action was also justified on the basis of unwarranted and improper interference on the part of government in the private rights of the individual. Beck-Storrs[11] describes the dilemma in her discussion of the beginning of public health legislation in England in the late nineteenth century against a background of liberalism and individualism. She points to the conflict between the concept of public health and the prevailing idea of freedom of the individual:

> It suddenly dawned upon Englishmen that the modern apostles of health challenged the tradition of local government. They thought that they were called upon to make a decision between two evils, namely, either to let disorder and disease continue as before, or to suffer the monster of a civilized state.

She points out that public health threatened the Englishman's "right to be dirty" if he were so inclined. The affluent and the legislators, in the face of widespread communicable disease, were willing to agree to certain changes to protect themselves, but they did not want to go too far. The recommendations of The Royal Sanitary Commission, which was established in 1869, required the services of inspectors—but how could their authority be limited? To control the spread of infectious diseases, a system of compulsory notification would be necessary. Rules would have to be enforced for slum clearance. Minimum specifications for low-cost housing for workers were likely to force landlords and landowners to spend more money than they had intended. According to Beck-Storrs:

> Here for the first time in the modern period, arose the problem of state supported welfare measures which threatened to interfere with the economic activities of private citizens. And this happened at a time when economic liberalism was believed to be the principle reason for the prosperity of the 19th century.

To the extent possible, the government of England attempted to present the desired changes in a positive context—rights rather than restrictions, protections rather than prohibitions. Thus the state was empowered to ensure that a man was no more likely to have his well poisoned through the neglect of his neighbor than he was to be robbed with impunity. Health inspectors were given the responsibility of surveillance over drainage and sewerage systems, water supplies, bathhouses, and wash-houses as well as health conditions in workshops, mines, and bakeshops. Under the existing circumstances, the inspectors were natural targets of a public highly sensitive to its freedoms. Success depended on their training and tact and also on whether the instinctive resentment against such invasions of a person's private affairs could be overcome. The Royal Sanitary Commission, anticipating this reaction, therefore recommended "employment of only well-trained men, capable of administering on a national level the measures instituted by the proposed central authority." It may be worth observing parenthetically that this recommendation is as valid now and in America as it was in England at the time it was made.

In the developing United States attitudes were if anything even more individualistic. As Roemer[12] has pointed out, the Western world's negative attitude toward government has deep roots, especially in America, where the colonists revolted against a domineering British monarchy. One result was the explicit limitation placed on the central government in the Constitution and the absence of Constitutional reference to health as either a personal right or a governmental responsibility. Roemer also emphasizes that the medical profession, having much earlier achieved independence from feudal landlords and religious authority in Europe, was doubly suspicious of governmental interference. As a result, as Shryock[13] has reasoned, medicine had little tangible impact on American society before 1875. Indeed, this held true into the early twentieth century.[14] More recently, however, medicine and related fields, by either their presence or their absence, have had an increasingly significant influence on the problems, nature, and even survival of society. This, no government can afford to ignore.

In his book *Government in Public Health*, Mustard[15] analyzed the situation in more colorful but effective terms:

> Public health service at any given time and place represents, in a way, the confluence of two streams in human progress. First there is the fairly clear and clean, but somewhat cold, trickle that filters down through the very fine sands of science; and second, there is the somewhat muddy flow of varying temperature that gushes intermittently from the rich but unpatrolled sociopolitical pastures. Taking their rise as they do in such entirely different sources, it is not astonishing that these tributaries do not completely or smoothly mix on their conjunction; nor need one be discouraged because there are eddies and backwashes, flotsam and froth. It is a powerful stream and one that will continue to flow.

Few now question health as a human right and its protection as a governmental responsibility. Thus the Director General of the World Health Organization stated that " . . . social justice demands that all citizens of the world should reach an acceptable level of health that permits them to lead socially and economically productive lives.[16]

Hence it is frustrating to observe the cautious and somewhat tortuous approach of an inherently individualistic United States to the inevitable formulation and implementation of a comprehensive health care program for all of its people.

There are numerous reasons for governmental action in public health. Many public health activities can be carried out only by group or community action. This is particularly true in urban and suburban areas, which are so characteristic of the increasingly concentrated industrialized societies. Sanitary water systems and sewage disposal facilities are obvious examples; so too, however, is the organization of quality comprehensive health care. Many necessary health activities must have an authoritative and legal base such as is available only to government. Isolation and quarantine regulations and many aspects of environmental health work are obvious examples. Some other activities such as the collection and analysis of vital records can be carried out only through a well-organized, well-staffed, stable, and continuing governmental agency. The most important organizing force is government, which passes, enforces, and finances health legislation that in the final analysis determines the content and pattern of health services and protection for all of the people. It is the only mechanism that can do this in the total sense. However, as Kruse[17] has indicated, "This concentration of political, economic, and social power, with its vast organization, is at the expense of the individual. . . . He surrenders liberty for opportunity and security."

HEALTH AND ECONOMICS

Even cursory thought and observation leads to an implicit relationship between health and economics. This relationship has been the subject of numerous published papers by individuals in economics as well as in human services. The American Public Health Association and the World Health Organization have each issued policy statements on poverty as a prime source of ill health and premature death. Brenner[18] has carried out and published a series of provocative studies that show the relationship between periods of economic recession and increases in miscarriages, stillbirths, prematurity, infant deaths, depression, alcohol consumption, suicide, admissions to mental institutions, and cardiovascular and cerebrovascular disease. Since the goals and methods of public health are quite different from those of clinical medicine, the bases of measurement are not the same. Public health work is not fundamentally concerned with the diagnosis and repair of damage already done. Rather, it focuses on the prevention of damage in the first place as well as the promotion of positive health. Furthermore, while living is expensive, illness is even more so, and it should be possible to demonstrate that preventive and promotive health activities offer a sound financial investment to the individual and to society.

Most intelligent people appreciate the reduction in human suffering that has resulted from the public health movement. It must be realized, however, that the further removed one is by time and space from the threat of personal suffering the less consideration is likely to be given to it. Success in public health work tends to mask its value. Therefore, it is appropriate for public health workers to pay increasing attention to the costs and benefits of public health programs.[19]

As indicated elsewhere, the costs of all services have persistently increased. Proportionately speaking, the expenditure for public health services represents an area of considerable expansion. This has caused some to point to public health programs as an added economic burden to the taxpayer. It is important to point out and to demonstrate that an increased sum of money spent wisely for health services represents not an increase but actually an eventual decrease in the net bill for personal and community welfare and protection. The construction and maintenance costs of public water purification and sewage disposal plants are admittedly great. The costs, however, do not represent a net addition to the taxpayers' economic burden. Their absence would cost a greater sum for individual facilities, for increased medical care, and for lost earnings resulting from the illnesses that would not be prevented. Single or repeated outbreaks of typhoid fever, for example, would cost a community much more in the long run than would installation of engineering and other measures designed for their prevention. A sound financial policy for public health services therefore must take into consideration not only the humanitarian and social gains but also the economic advantages to be derived therefrom. The problem then is to make the public conscious of costs that in any case are certain to occur either as hidden individual expenditures or as socially beneficial public appropriations. Public health is one of the best forms of social and economic insurance.

Beyond the inevitability of these expenditures there is the added factor of the economic value of the lives made possible or continued by public health endeavors. To many, the thought of placing a monetary value on human life may seem distasteful. Essentially, reactions to life and death are based on emotion and sentiment, and ordinarily people deliberately avoid any thought of an economic or cost-value label on a human being. Yet to be realistic, it must be admitted that life does have a monetary value. The death of a parent brings to society as a whole as well as to the particular family involved an economic as well as a sentimental loss that is real and irreparable. This may manifest itself in a lowered standard of living for the family, the necessity of public financial aid, or the loss of a trained worker. Furthermore, governmental recognition is given to the value of a life, and one seldom hears objections to the concept of income tax exemptions.

In addressing himself to this question, Fuchs[19] makes several telling observations:

What, then, is the justification for such an inquiry? The principle one is the fact that the question of the contribution of health services is being asked and answered every day. It is being asked and answered implicitly every time consumers, hospitals, universities, business firms, foundations, government agencies and legislative bodies make decisions concerning the volume and composition of health services, present and future. If economists can help to rationalize and make more explicit the decision making process, can provide useful definitions, concepts and analytic tools, and can develop appropriate bodies of data and summary measures, they will be making their own contribution to health and to the economy.

In the same vein it must be recognized that whereas members of appropriating bodies may be humane and sympathetic, collectively they must be analytic and practical. As a result, it is becoming more difficult to sell public health programs, especially on the basis of sentimentality or intangibles. This was illustrated in June 1980 when the Secretary of Health and Human Services announced that the Medicare program would no longer pay for heart transplant operations, which cost about $100,000. The Secretary commented, "I don't like the idea of assessing the value of a human life. At the same time we have to find out what the costs are. We have to ask, 'Will we buy this or will we buy something else?'"[21] Similar comments have been made with reference to kidney dialysis and kidney transplants, the treatment of acute leukemia, the use of interferon, and an ever growing number of other types of medical care. It is obvious therefore that the public health worker increasingly must be in a position to validate proposals and actions in economic terms. This was emphasized by an expert group at a World Health Organization Seminar on Health Economics[22]:

. . . a knowledge of the applications of economics to the administration of public health enables health planners to hold their own in discussions with other planners, with planning commissions, and with key government departments such as finance ministries.

It is unfortunate that so many results of public health programs, although of great social value, are largely of an intangible nature, for example, diseases and deaths prevented, problems avoided, and the like. This makes it all the more imperative that health program planning and evaluative procedures have incorporated in them from the beginning a consideration not only of economic costs but also of the anticipated economic return. Such cost-benefit as well as risk-benefit data can be of inestimable value both in obtaining public understanding and support and in budgetary presentations.

In attempting to do so, however, one is immediately confronted with two fundamental problems: (1) problems of definition—What is health? What is incapacitation? etc.—and (2) problems of measurement—How does one measure something that is not there? What base line can one use? The seriousness of these problems varies with time, place, and circumstance, as indicated by Linnenberg.[23] He points out that if a community or nation has a high incidence of a disease, which existing knowledge and methods systemically applied can quickly bring under control, it is possible to make an advance estimate not only of the cost of the methods but also of the likely benefits in terms of worker time not lost and treatment costs avoided. But, he adds, drama of this sort stems only from a sudden breakthrough, as in the case of a new effective vaccine, or from an area being widely afflicted with a serious and especially an economically detrimental disease, such as malaria or yaws, which is anachronistic from the standpoint of modern medicine and which can be brought under control quickly, even though little or nothing is done about other health problems. Our difficulty, he concludes, is that such classic simplicity is absent from most public health work in this country, where public health achievement has progressed so far that our health problems are not so much the yes or no kind as the more or less kind.

As far as countries in general are concerned, the World Health Organization has found the following among the obstacles to adequate quantification: (1) the widespread inadequacy of health and demographic statistics, (2) common exclusive reliance on input rather than output indicators, (3) the lack of an adequate measure of development of national welfare, and (4) the tendency of scientific disciplines to proceed in isolation from political science, economics, and sociology in studies that require a comprehensive approach.[24]

ECONOMIC VALUE OF LIFE

Many have tried to evaluate human life and to price its economic worth. One of the earliest attempts was that of Sir William Petty (1623-1687), who originated many ideas later used by the political economist Adam Smith in *Wealth of Nations* and other works. Petty[25] derived his estimate as follows:

Suppose the People of England be Six Millions in number, that their Expense at £7 per head be 42 Millions: Suppose also that the Rent of the Lands be 8 Millions, and the yearly profit of all the Personal Estate by 8 Millions more; it must needs follow that the Labour of the People must have supplied the remaining 26 Millions that which multiplied by 20 (the Mass of Mankind being worth 20 years purchase as well as land) makes 520 Millions as the value of the whole people; which number divided by 6 Millions makes about £80 the value of each Head of Man, Woman and Child and of adult Persons Twice as much; from whence we may learn to compute the loss we have sustained by the Plague, by the Slaughter of Men in War and by sending them abroad into the Service of Foreign Princes.

In 1876 Sir William Farr[26] made more scientific computations using the life-table technique, which by that time had been developed. Subsequently this approach was applied more extensively and effectively by Dublin and his associates.[27] More recently this "human capital" approach has been improved and refined by a series of analysts* prominent among whom are Fein,[28] Mushkin and Collings,[29] Weisbrod,[30] Klarman,[31] Rice and Cooper,[32] Hartunian and associates,[33] and Landefeld and Seskin.[34] Landefeld and Seskin, in addition to broadening the methodology by adding the concept of "willingness-to-pay" (or in some situations one might add, "willingness-to-act"), have presented a brief review of the nature of the contributions of the others to whom reference has been made. Reference should also be made to a special issue of *Public Health Reports:* "The Cost of Disease and Illness in the United States in the Year 2000,"[35] and to a report of the National Academy of Sciences, Institute of Medicine: *Costs of Environment-related Health Effects.*[36]

As an analogy, the human body may be considered similar to a machine. Its proper function depends on various physical and biochemical components. It might be compared to an internal combustion engine with limbs in place of pistons and the endocrine system acting as the carburetor. Superimposed is the supervisory function of the human mind. In like manner, the human body may be regarded as an economic unit brought into existence for measurable, potential, productive purposes.

A machine must pass through several phases before it is ready to be of productive value. First, it must be built, which presupposes the existence of a factory in which it will be installed. Its construction therefore involves from the start a considerable capital outlay for factory site, labor, and tools. On completion, the machine must be prepared for use or function. This involves a series of installation expenditures for inspection and checking, for transfer to the site where it is to function, and for lubrication, tune-up, and other preparations. After this, it is ready to become productive; and the extent and efficiency of its usefulness depend on its original quality or lack of structural defects, the cor-

*Each of these has published a number of articles and in some cases books on the subject. The specific references made here are to especially significant contributions.

rectness of its installation, and the manner in which it is routinely cared for while in use. It must be carefully and repeatedly lubricated, fed the proper fuel, inspected, overhauled, and repaired. Its ultimate economic value can be determined only after the costs of construction, installation, and preparatory expenditure and effort are deducted from the gross value of its productivity.

It is the hope of the manufacturer that his machine will continue to function with relative efficiency at least long enough to produce sufficient items for sale to offset all of the debits incurred by the capital investment and the installation and maintenance costs. In other words, from the moment the machine is purchased the curve of the cumulative investment in it continues to rise, and the curve of cumulative productive value lags for a considerable period. It is not until these two curves cross that the manufacturer can breathe easily and begin to reap a net benefit from the use of the machine. If any untoward circumstances develop before the two curves cross, the manufacturer will suffer a loss.

Many things may go wrong after purchase. The machine may have been defective, it may have been damaged during transportation and installation, or it may have worn out prematurely as a result of improper use or care. These are only a few of the undesirable potentialities the manufacturer must constantly guard against. Even after the two curves cross, all is not necessarily clear sailing, because the longer the machine is used the greater is the tendency for parts to wear out and for maintenance and repair costs to increase. Sooner or later a time is reached when these costs become greater than the value of the items produced, and the two curves cross again. Continued use is no longer economically profitable. The machine has now passed into the phase of obsolescence.

If one sets aside for the moment the very real but unmeasurable social and spiritual values of human life, there are some similarities with the foregoing analogy. With humans and their societies, however, there are many complex variables to be considered in approximating the average value of future earnings to be applied to the ultimate economic value of life. Time, place, and economic conditions are critically important. Related to these are varying labor force participation rates, variations in salaries

for different age groups, whether the value of a housewife's services are included, continued but varied extensions of life expectancies, social programs that provide substitutes for earned income, and many other factors. Illness or other difficulties that may affect not only the individual but also those close to him or her can also alter productivity. Table 1-1 presents some of the chief items that contribute to the debit and credit columns of a human life.

If one considers some but by no means all of these

TABLE 1-1. Factors in the socioeconomic value of human life— summary

Capital cost*
  1. Economic incapacitation of mother
  2. Risk of death to mother
  3. Risk of injury to mother with immediate or subsequent effect on her economic value
  4. Immediate costs of childbearing
  5. Risk of infant death
  6. Risk of infant illness or injury
  7. Interest on capital investment

Installation cost†
  1. Shelter, clothing and food
  2. Value of time mother devotes to child care
  3. Education—family and community contribution
  4. Medical and dental care and health protection
  5. Recreation and transportation
  6. Insurance
  7. Sundries and incidentals
  8. Risk of death during first 18 years
  9. Risk of disability during first 18 years
  10. Interest on installation costs

Period of productivity‡
  Credit
  1. Earning potential
  2. Interest on earnings
  3. Noneconomic potential
  Debit
  1. Risk of disability during productive period
  2. Medical costs
  3. Risk of premature death
  4. Risk of becoming substandard or antisocial
  5. Interest on debit items

*The investment that society has in each infant by the time it is born.
†The investment that society has in each individual at 18 years of age.
‡The return that society can expect from its investment, with the risks involved during this period.

factors, the 1980 cost of raising a child successfully to the age of 18 years in the United States and then financing him or her through a public college has been estimated at about $85,000. This figure considers only direct costs. If the "lost" earnings of a mother who chooses to remain at home to raise her children instead of gainfully working are added, the total cost varies from about $100,000 for low-income families to about $140,000 for middle-income families. Costs are greater for urban than for nonurban families and are lowest in the north central states and highest in the western states.[37] These very general variations indicate again the complexity of the problems encountered in attempts to quantify life from an economic or any other viewpoint. Both the philosophic difficulty and the need for some practical approach have been stated succinctly by Muller:[38]

Observation of society shows that there is no one mode of valuing life or of comparing the social worth of a year in the lives of two different individuals. A pecuniary standard is adopted whenever reference to comparative productivity loss is used as a guide to health policy, and this is in tune with the workings of institutions in which money talks—i.e., markets. Yet this standard is biased by social discrimination factors influencing productivity and earnings of different race, age, and sex categories.

ECONOMIC VALUE OF HEALTH PROGRAMS

The increasing use of cost-benefit analysis has by now provided many examples of the economic justification of public health programs. About a half century ago, an appropriation for an intensive diphtheria immunization program in New York City was shown to result in savings of more than $500,000. About the same time and in the same city, a $500,000 appropriation for an antipneumonia program saved at least $5 million annually. Also at that time in Detroit a special appropriation of $1 million for an early case-finding program against tuberculosis resulted in savings of over $5 million each year. A more recent example is found in an analysis[39] of the benefits from a widespread measles vaccination program in the United States in the 1960s. The reduction of deaths, of cases of mental retardation, and of hospital and medical care needs, as well as days lost from school or work, resulted in a 5-year saving of about $423 million (Table 1-2).

The economic validity of automobile seat belt installation and use has been estimated at more than $1,000 saved for each dollar invested.[40] Similarly a cost-benefit ratio of over $5 for each dollar invested has been shown for air pollution control.[41] On a larger scale, Mushkin[42] calculated that the value in 1960 of the products attributable to workers added to the labor force in the United States as a result of the reduction of death rates since 1900 was the equivalent of $820 billion. Consider also only a few of the causes of death against which public health measures have played a major role (Table 1-3). For practical purposes, two thirds of them have been eradicated in the United States, and the others have been very greatly reduced. Considered as a whole, if the 1900 rates still applied in 1976, they would have killed about twice as many people (3,727,301) as they actually did (1,892,879). If even a conservative dollar value were placed on the 1,834,422 who did not die, the net national saving would be enor-

TABLE 1-2. Summary statement of savings because of immunization against measles

Type of savings	1963-1965	1966-1968	Total
Health and resource			
Cases averted	1,140,000	8,590,000	9,730,000
Lives saved	114	859	973
Cases of retardation averted	380	2,864	3,244
Hospital days saved	65,000	490,000	555,000
Workdays saved	189,000	1,435,000	1,624,000
Schooldays saved	3,775,000	28,450,000	32,225,000
Economic			
Economic benefits	$63,192,000	$468,351,000	$531,543,000
Costs of immunizing persons	43,500,000	64,800,000	108,300,000
Net economic savings	19,692,000	403,551,000	423,243,000

Roots of public
health

TABLE 1-3. Estimated saving in lives during 1976 as a result of public health measures taken against certain diseases, United States*

Causes of death	Death rates†		Deaths		Lives saved
	1900	1976	Theoretic	Observed	
All causes	1,719.1	884.5	3,727,301	1,892,879	1,834,422
Infant mortality	99.9‡	16.0	315,024	50,525	264,499
Tuberculosis	194.4	1.6	421,492	3,333	418,159
Syphilis and its sequelae	17.7‡	0.1	38,377	272	38,105
Typhoid and paratyphoid	31.3	0.0	67,864	3	67,861
Dysentery	12.0	0.1	26,018	62	25,956
Diarrhea and enteritis	139.9	1.1	303,327	2,010	301,317
Smallpox	0.3	0.0	650	0	650
Measles	13.3	0.0	28,837	20	28,817
Diphtheria	40.3	0.0	87,377	5	87,372
Pertussis	12.2	0.0	26,452	8	26,444
Scarlet fever and streptococcal sore throat	9.6	0.0	20,814	15	20,799
Malaria	6.2	0.0	13,443	4	13,439

*Population 1976 = 214,000,000.
†Per 100,000 population, except infant mortality, which is per 1,000 live births.
‡1915 rates.

mous—and certainly much more than had been expended on control measures.

The previous discussion deals with past successes. Consider in addition the potential savings in lives and money that could be made now and in the future if it were possible to apply all existing knowledge to the total current picture of sickness and death in the United States. The results arrived at are staggering. Slee,[43] for example, considered the problem of the thousands of deaths that occur every year in the United States that could be prevented if existing medical and scientific knowledge were effectively used. For each cause of death he estimated the potential percentage of reduction attainable at that time (1947), indicating for each the major factors that would contribute to the reduction. His estimates have been modified to bring them up to date (Table 1-4). Each of the theoretic percentage reductions was then applied to the number of deaths that were attributable during 1976 to each particular cause of death (Table 1-5).

The difference between the resulting figures and the number of deaths that actually occurred indicates a total potential saving at the present time of almost 610,000 lives per year. This saving, if it had been effected, would have reduced the crude death rate in the United States in 1976 by 32%, from 8.9 to 5.9 per 1,000 population. That this is not a fantastic concept is given testimony by the fact that some American communities and several nations have actually reduced their rates close to that level. If the lives that could theoretically be saved are distributed appropriately by age groups, it is seen that benefits are possible at every point in the lifespan. The greatest savings, however, would occur in the adolescent and young adult age groups, in which death involves the greatest possible economic loss. If this analysis were to be pursued further by applying estimated monetary values to each of the 610,000 deaths potentially preventable, the magnitude of the economic loss entailed would indeed be great.

Such an accomplishment is obviously the stuff of dreams and wishes. The reality is indicated by the extensive analysis of the cost of disease and illness by the Public Services Laboratory of Georgetown University.[35] The charge to those involved in the analysis was to project the economic cost of illness in the United States in the year 2000. To the extent that dollar expenditures applied

TABLE 1-4. Postulated percentage reductions in deaths, by cause, if all available knowledge were used*

Cause of death	Reduction (%)	Suggested action
Typhoid and paratyphoid	100	Environmental measures
		Immunization
		Epidemiologic control
Meningococcal infections	100	Control of epidemics
		Adequate and early chemotherapy
		Antibiotics
Streptococcal infections	100	Chemotherapy
		Antibiotics
		Antitoxin
Pertussis	100	Early and thorough immunization
		Hyperimmune serum, chemotherapy, and antibiotics for secondary infections
Diphtheria	100	Early immunization and adequate antitoxin
Tuberculosis—all forms	100	Intensive early case finding
		Hospitalization and treatment
		Adequate diet and housing
Dysenteries	100	Environmental control
		Chemotherapy
Malaria	100	Environmental control
		Chemotherapy
Syphilis	100	Intensive early case finding
		Treatment
		Epidemiologic control
Measles	100	Immunization
		Chemotherapy
		Antibiotics
Poliomyelitis	100	Immunization
Neoplasms	50	Early cancer detection and treatment centers
		Best possible physician and surgeon
		Chemotherapy
		Radiation therapy
		Surgery
		Environmental controls
		Elimination of smoking
Rheumatic fever	95	Best possible physician
		Prophylactic antibiotics
Diabetes mellitus	60	Best possible physician
		Intensive early case finding
		Diet
		Insulin
		Applied genetics

*Where chemotherapy and/or antibiotics have been listed as the explanations for the reductions in deaths, objection on the basis of the development of drug-resistant organisms will no doubt be raised. Gains possible today might be much less in a few years. It is believed that research will be able to remain one or two drugs, at least, ahead of the organisms.
With the one exception (all other causes), no variation of effectiveness of therapy and other control measures with age of the individual has been postulated. Since any scheme of correction would probably have been as liable to criticism as no correction, the latter course was followed. *Continued.*

TABLE 1-4. Postulated percentage reductions in deaths, by cause, if all available knowledge were used—cont'd

Cause of death	Reduction (%)	Suggested action
Diseases of thyroid gland	100	Best possible physician Newer drugs Surgery Iodization of all salt
Nutritional diseases	100	Adequate diet Diagnosis and treatment
Alcoholism and addictions	25	Psychiatry Nutritional therapy Sociology Education
Intracranial vascular lesions	10	Best possible physician Antihypertensive drugs and diet Anticoagulants Avoidance of infections Antibiotics
Diseases of the heart	10	Best possible physician Surgery
Pneumonia, broncho-	75	Chemotherapy Antibiotics
Pneumonia, lobar	90	Chemotherapy Antibiotics
Pneumonia, unspecified	75	Chemotherapy Antibiotics
Influenza	85	Immunization Chemotherapy and antibiotics for complications
Peptic ulcer—stomach and duodenum	50	Psychiatry Best possible physician
Diarrhea, enteritis, etc.	95	Environmental controls Chemotherapy Antibiotics
Appendicitis	100	Surgery Chemotherapy Antibiotics
Hernia, intestinal obstruction	95	Best possible physician and surgeon
Cirrhosis of the liver	25	Newer nutritional knowledge
Biliary calculi	25	Best possible physician and surgeon
Nephritis and nephrosis	25	Chemotherapy Antibiotics Best possible physician
Diseases of the prostate	50	Best possible physician and surgeon
Complications of pregnancy	87	Complete elimination of deaths from toxemia and sepsis, and reduction of deaths from hemorrhage by 50%
Congenital malformations	10	Diet during pregnancy Avoidance of viral infections and chemical carcinogens Surgery
Premature births	70	Adequate prenatal care and diet
Suicide	50	Psychiatry Sociology
Homicide	50	Psychiatry Sociology, including gun control
Accidents—motor vehicle	50	Education Psychiatry Engineering

TABLE 1-4. Postulated percentage reductions in deaths, by cause, if all available knowledge were used—cont'd

Cause of death	Reduction (%)	Suggested action
Accidents—motor vehicle—cont'd		Traffic planning and control
		Safety measures
Accidents—other	50	Education
		Psychiatry
		Safety measures
		Engineering
All other causes	50	Better medical care (except for under 1 year, where deaths from congenital debility, birth injury, and others peculiar to the first year of life could be reduced by 75%), genetic counseling, family planning, adequate prenatal care and diet, and adequate care during first year of life

TABLE 1-5. Theoretic savings of lives, United States, 1976, had all available knowledge been effectively applied

Cause of death	Total deaths 1976	Theoretic reduction (%)	Theoretic deaths	Theoretic saving
Meningococcal infections	1,630	100		1,630
Tuberculosis—all forms	3,290	100		3,290
Syphilis	250	100		250
Other infective and parasitic diseases	3,630	80	726	2,904
Neoplasms	374,780	50	187,390	187,390
Diabetes mellitus	35,090	60	14,036	21,054
Cerebrovascular diseases	189,000	10	170,100	18,900
Diseases of the heart	726,700	10	654,030	72,670
Hypertension	6,060	70	1,818	4,242
Pneumonia and influenza	62,980	90	6,298	56,682
Bronchitis, emphysema, asthma	24,610	25	18,457	6,153
Peptic ulcer—stomach and duodenum	6,260	50	3,130	3,130
Diarrhea, enteritis, etc.	2,000	95	100	1,900
Hernia, intestinal obstruction	5,940	95	297	5,643
Cirrhosis of the liver	31,130	25	23,347	7,783
Biliary calculi, etc.	2,690	25	2,017	673
Nephritis and nephrosis	8,830	25	6,622	2,208
Diseases of the prostate	1,190	50	595	595
Congenital malformations	13,780	10	12,402	1,378
Conditions of early infancy	24,870	70	7,461	17,409
Suicide	25,200	50	12,600	12,600
Homicide	18,970	50	9,485	9,485
Accidents—motor vehicle	45,800	50	22,900	22,900
Accidents—other	54,630	50	27,315	27,315
All other causes	242,690	50	121,345	121,345
TOTALS	1,912,000	31	1,302,471	609,529

Population 1976	214,000,000			
Death rate (per 1,000 population)	8.9			
Percentage reduction of death rate (actual to theoretic)				32%

TABLE 1-6. Total costs of illness in year 2000, in billions of 1975 dollars and year 2000 dollars*

Mortality indicators	Indirect costs			Direct	Total costs
	Mortality	Morbidity	Total		
	Year 2000 dollars				
Mortality: single year loss	$ 21.5	$ 336.1	$ 387.6	$1,013.6	$1,401.2
Mortality: present value of future earnings loss discounted at 10 percent	356.4	366.1	722.5	1,013.6	1,736.1
Mortality: present value of future earnings loss discounted at 2.5 percent	715.2	366.1	1,081.3	1,013.6	2,094.9
	1975 dollars				
Mortality: single year loss	$ 5.2	$ 89.5	$ 94.7	$ 416.4	$ 511.1
Mortality: present value of future earnings loss discounted at 10 percent	87.2	89.5	176.7	416.4	593.1
Mortality: present value of future earnings loss discounted at 2.5 percent	174.9	89.5	264.4	416.4	680.8

From Mushkin, S.J., and others: Public Health Rep. **93:**493, Sept.-Oct. 1978.
*Assuming constant labor force participation rates and including household values. Direct costs deflated by the medical care price index and indirect costs deflated by an index of average earnings. Productivity increase of 2 percent assumed.

throughout reflect the relative extent of specific disease categories, their findings as shown in Table 1-6 are germane to the subject at hand.

They note that gains are considered in their projections, that is, certain declines in death rates, an increase in the available work force, and a reduction in disability and in work time loss caused by illness. It is pointed out that "the gain in economic resources through the prevention or cure of diseases and postponement of death to an old age takes the form of added numbers of workers and added work time."[35]

Again, however, it must be emphasized that such studies, valuable as they are, deal specifically with the economics of health and disease and not their human aspects. The latter was vividly described by Hilbert[44] in closing his Presidential Address to the American Public Health Association.

The mother in an environment harboring a dying infant, a wayward son, a prematurely aging husband, and a house falling into shambles thinks not in terms of epidemiological justifications or bacteriological samples proudly presented in tabular form. She thinks of happi-

ness never quite attained, satisfaction never fully gained, frustrations never totally banished, poverty never surmounted, needs never fulfilled, and of health never fully realized. When preventive public health with all its ramifications extends its imagination to the creation of a new dimension that reaches into the hearts and lives of all mankind, then may come the hope that this preventive health cathedral may attain completion.

PUBLIC HEALTH AND NATURAL SELECTION

One other aspect of public health merits passing consideration. One sometimes encounters objection to public health on the basis that it promotes the survival and propagation of the biologically or genetically unfit at the expense of the fit and to the ultimate detriment of the human species. Advocates of this view claim that public health activities interfere with or negate the forces of natural biologic selection, which in a coldly impersonal manner supposedly weeds out "the lame, the halt, and the blind" as well as "protoplasm of poor genetic quality." Thus referring to public health as unnatural, Huxley[45] called it the very essence of the myth of progress. Bowes[46] concluded that whereas modern public health measures will continue to make life comfortable during the few remaining generations of Western civilization, a few "good old-fashioned epidemics" such as the Black Death might be desirable because they tend to wipe out many mental and physical weaklings who at present are coddled through life. Other examples among many that could be cited are those of a sociologist,[47] on the one hand, and a physician,[48] on the other, who point to the public health efforts that protect the unfit while more desirable human specimens are sent off to war.

One may ask, however, how the "fit" (whoever they may be) can survive if disease is allowed to run rampant among the "unfit." It is true that uncontrolled disease tends to eliminate those who appear to be weak or inferior according to some standards. Those who are chronically tired, hungry, cold, or aged are indeed more likely to succumb. In most instances, however, uncontrolled disease strikes blindly, producing a variety of diseases in all components of a society. Disease and death have often entered palaces and mansions through the back door. A normal or gifted infant may be disastrously affected by disease. Generally speaking, the use of the terms *unfit, undesirable,* or *inferior* represent psychologic blind spots or social labels based on subjective biases and judgments.

The societal risk involved in uncontrolled disease is strikingly illustrated at Stratford-on-Avon. At that cultural shrine is a church register with the record of birth of William Shakespeare. Several lines above may be seen the entry "juli 11, 1564. Oliverus Gume—hic incipit pestis [here began the plague]." During the year 1564, that little village suffered 242 deaths from plague. This probably represented one third to one half of the population. During the upswing of the epidemic, there was born a helpless infant who easily could have been one of those affected but who by chance alone was spared, subsequently to give us some of civilization's greatest cultural treasures. If he had become infected and died, would that infant have been considered unfit or inferior?

The question arises therefore—who are the fit and the unfit? Observation indicates that the definition varies with time and place. Steinmetz was a congenital cripple; Toulouse-Lautrec was afflicted with hereditary osteochondritis fragilitas; Mozart, Chopin, and many other great figures in the arts and sciences died at early ages from tuberculosis;

and Schumann and numerous other notable persons died from typhoid fever. Would anyone dare label these and thousands like them unfit? Americans can least afford to point the finger. Most citizens of the United States of America are descendants of persons who by one standard or another would have been considered undesirable or unfit. The reasons have varied—religious, ethnic, economic, social, political, and cultural—whatever reason has been most expedient to those in power at the moment.

Although some individuals or even groups admittedly may suffer from physical or other handicaps, it is false reasoning to suppose that they are necessarily stigmatized for all time or places. The Bantu people, from whom so many American blacks descended, carried the gene for sickle cell anemia. This was unfortunate. Yet that same gene also provided resistance to malaria, enabling the Bantu to survive when others did not. No health worker would deny that the profession makes it possible for many to live who otherwise would die. These beneficiaries and their progeny have lived; and although much yet needs to be done, they have prospered. Each Olympic tournament sees new records of physical prowess. The descendants of immigrants are taller and of greater physical stamina than their forebears or their counterparts in their countries of origin. This is not meant to deny the need to apply the increasing knowledge of genetics in personal and marital counseling. However, one cannot help but ponder the potential magnitude of the benefits that would accrue to the human race from a truly vigorous application of present knowledge. Rosenau had this in mind when he wrote concerning preventive medicine and public health:

It dreams of a time when there shall be enough for all, and every man shall bear his share of labor in accordance with his ability, and every man shall possess sufficient for the needs of his body and the demands of health. These things he shall have as a matter of justice and not of charity. It dreams of a time when there shall be no unnecessary suffering and no premature deaths; when the welfare of the people shall be our highest concern; when humanity and mercy shall replace greed and selfishness; and it dreams that all these things will be accomplished through the wisdom of man. It dreams of these things, not with the hope that we, individually, may participate in them, but with the joy that we may aid in their coming to those who shall live after us. When young men have vision the dreams of old men come true.

Some people may dismiss this as impractical idealism. But the achievement of the greatest success and satisfaction in a social field such as public health demands a full share of idealism. As a final word of caution, however, it must be realized that idealism and pragmatism are not necessarily immiscible, as are oil and water. In fact, their admixture is sorely needed now more than ever before in this incredibly rapidly evolving age. The prefacing statement by Lowell[49] in his book *Conflicts of Principle* is as timely and pertinent now and to the present public health purpose as when he wrote it half a century ago:

People often call some men idealists and other practical folks as if mankind were by natural inclination so divided into these two groups that an idealist cannot be practical or a man of affairs have a lofty purpose whereas in fact no man approaches perfection who does not combine both qualities in a high degree. Without either he is defective in spirit and unscientific in method; the idealist because he does not strive to make his theory accurate, that is consonant with the facts; the so-called practical man if he acts upon the impulse of the occasion without the guidance of an enduring principle of conduct. Hence both lack true wisdom, the idealist more culpably for he should be diligent in thought and seek all the light he can obtain. It is useful to repeat that many men have *light* enough to be visionary, but only he who *clearly sees* can *behold* a vision.

REFERENCES

1. Blumgart, H.L.: Caring for the patient, N. Engl. J. Med. **270:**449, Feb. 27, 1964.
2. Beauchamp, P.E.: Public health as social justice, Inquiry **13:**3, March 1976.
3. Dubos, R.: The dreams of reason, New York, 1961, Columbia University Press.
4. Draper, P., Best, G., and Dennis, J.: Health and wealth, R. Soc. Health J. **97:**121, June 1977.
5. Winslow, C.-E.A.: The untilled field of public health, Mod. Med. **2:**183, March 1920.
6. Mountin, J.W.: The health department's dilemma, Public Health Rep. **67:**223, March 1952.
7. A new perspective on the health of Canadians, Ottawa, 1974, Ministry of National Health and Welfare.
8. Gershenson, C.P.: Child maltreatment, family stress, and ecological insult, Am. J. Public Health **67:**602, July 1977.
9. Dubos, R.J.: Mirage of health, Garden City, N.Y., 1960, Doubleday & Co., Inc.
10. Malthus, T.R.: An essay on the principle of population as it affects the future improvement of society, London, 1798. Reprint, London, 1926, Royal Economic Society.
11. Beck-Storrs, A.: Public health and government control, Soc. Stud. **45:**211, Oct. 1954.
12. Roemer, M.I.: The influence of government on American medicine, Oslo, 1962, Gyldendal Norsk Forlag.
13. Shryock, R.H.: The interplay of social and internal factors in the history of modern medicine, Sci. Month. **76:**221, April 1953.
14. Shryock, R.H.: Medicine and society in America: 1660-1860, Ithaca, N.Y., 1960, Cornell University Press.
15. Mustard, H.S.: Government in public health, New York, 1945, Commonwealth Fund.
16. Mahler, H.: Health for all, WHO Chron. **31:**491, Dec. 1977.
17. Kruse, H.D.: The great bane, Bull. N.Y. Acad. Med. **42:**2, Feb. 1966.
18. Brenner, M.H.: Estimating the social costs of national economic policy: implications for mental and physical health, and criminal aggression, Report to the Congressional Research Service of the Library of Congress and the Joint Economic Committee of Congress, Washington, D.C., 1976, U.S. Government Printing Office.
19. Abel-Smith, B.: Poverty, development, and health policy, Public Health Papers No. 69, Geneva, 1978, World Health Organization.
20. Fuchs, V.R.: The contribution of health services to the American economy, Milbank Mem. Fund Q. **44:**65, Oct. 1966.
21. Schwartz, H.: How much is a life worth? Wall St. J., Sept. 15, 1980.
22. Health economics, Public Health Papers No. 64, Geneva, 1975, World Health Organization.
23. Linnenberg, C.C.: How shall we measure economic benefits from public health services? In Economic benefits from public health services, PHS Pub. No. 1178, Washington, D.C., 1964, U.S. Government Printing Office.
24. Interrelationships between health programmes and socio-economic development, Public Health Papers No. 49, Geneva, 1973, World Health Organization.
25. Petty, Sir W.: Political arithmetic or a discourse concerning the extent and value of lands, people, buildings, etc., ed. 3, London, 1699, Robert Clavel.
26. Farr, W.: Contribution to the 39th annual report of the registrar general of births, marriages, and deaths for England and Wales, 1876.
27. Dublin, L.I., Lotka, A.J., and Spiegelman, M.: The money value of a man, ed. 2, New York, 1946, The Ronald Press Co.
28. Fein, R.: Economics of mental illness, New York, 1958, Basic Books.

29. Mushkin, S.J., and Collings, F.A.: Economic costs of disease and injury, Public Health Rep. **74:**795, Sept. 1959.

30. Weisbrod, B.A.: Economics of public health, Philadelphia, 1961, University of Pennsylvania Press.

31. Klarman, H.: Syphilis control programs. In Dorfman, R., editor, Measuring benefits of government investments, Washington, D.C., 1965, The Brookings Institute.

32. Rice, D.P., and Cooper, B.S.: The economic value of human life, Am. J. Public Health, **57:**1954, Nov. 1967.

33. Hartunian, N.S., Smart, C.N., and Thompson, M.S.: The incidence and economic costs of cancer, motor vehicle injuries, coronary heart disease and stroke: a comparative analysis, Am. J. Public Health **70:**1249, Dec. 1980.

34. Landefeld, J.S., and Seskin, E.P.: The economic value of life: linking theory to practice, Am. J. Public Health, **72:**555, June 1982.

35. Mushkin, S.J., and others: The cost of disease and illness in the United States in the year 2000, Public Health Rep. **93:**493, Sept.-Oct. 1978.

36. National Academy of Sciences, Institute of Medicine: Costs of environment-related health effects, Washington, D.C., 1980, National Academy Press.

37. Espenshade, T.J.: The value and cost of children, Washington, D.C., 1980, Population Reference Bureau.

38. Muller, C.F.: Economic costs of illness and health policy, Am. J. Public Health **70:**1245, Dec. 1980.

39. Axnick, N.W., Shavell, S.M., and Witte, J.J.: Benefits due to immunization against measles, Public Health Rep. **84:**673, Aug. 1969.

40. Gross, R.N.: Cost benefit analysis of health service, Ann. Am. Acad. Polit. Soc. Sci. **339:**89, Jan. 1972.

41. Brennen, A.J.: Environmental health: a look at the cost of air pollution, J. Sch. Health, **43:**300, May 1973.

42. Mushkin, S.: Health programs and economic development. In Proceedings of Southern Regional Legislative Seminar on State Health Problems, Atlanta, 1969, Council of State Governments.

43. Slee, V.N.: Public health and old people, Unpublished study, School of Public Health, University of Michigan, June 1947.

44. Hilbert, M.S.: Prevention, Am. J. Public Health **67:**353, April 1977.

45. Huxley, A.: Brave new world, Life **25:**63, Sept. 20, 1948.

46. Bowes, G.K.: Epidemic disease: past, present, and future, J. R. San. Inst. **66:**174, July 1946.

47. Gillette, J.M.: Perspective of public health in the United States, Sci. Month. **53:**235, Sept. 1941.

48. Johnson, A.S.: Medicine's responsibility in the propagation of poor protoplasm, N. Engl. J. Med. **238:**715, May 27, 1948.

49. Lowell, A.L.: Conflicts of principle, Cambridge, Mass., 1932, Harvard University Press.

CHAPTER 2

Historical perspectives

Those who forget the past are doomed to repeat it.

George Santayana

A LOOK AT THE PAST

Although the primary purpose of this book is to consider the various administrative factors involved in the practice of public health, it is also important to consider its genesis. This is not merely to pay tribute to those who went before, although Osler[4] once claimed it to be a sign of a dry age when the great men of the past are held in light esteem. Beyond this, historical review provides insight into the social significance of current events. Many circumstances and events of the past help to explain some present-day problems and trends that otherwise might be puzzling. As mentioned in the preceding chapter, as with all other constructive social movements, numerous difficulties have been encountered in the field of public health; superstition, public apathy, political interference, and inadequate funds and personnel are only a few. Sometimes shortsighted individuals criticize past and present public health practices in terms of these factors or because progress seems too slow. Appreciation of the origins of different social structures and of the public health movement may provide better perspective and greater understanding of the relative importance of these factors and the reason why they still exert some influence. This is not meant to condone or encourage complacency, but merely to point out that sound planning for the future is best accomplished by honest evaluation and understanding of the past and present.

For two extensive and scholarly presentations of this subject, see *A History of Public Health* by Rosen[1] and *The History of American Epidemiology* by Top.[2] For other references, see Hanlon and others.[3]

PRIMITIVE SOCIETIES

Little is known about the prehistoric origins of either personal or community hygiene. Some hints may be gleaned, however, from a study of tribal customs and rules of contemporary primitive groups. With few exceptions they have a certain amount of group and community hygienic sense usually derived from experience with survival. Rules against the fouling of family or tribal environments are almost universal. Many have taboos against the use of the upstream side of the camp site for excretory purposes. Burial of excreta is not uncommon. However, this practice is sometimes based on superstition rather than sanitary concepts. Many groups have elaborate provisions for disposal of the dead. Almost all primitive people recognize the existence of disease and engage in forms of voodoo or tribal dancing (psychosomatic medicine), temporary banishment (isolation and quarantine), or smoke and noise (fumigation) to drive away the evil spirits of disease. One is reminded, however, that as recently as the end of the nineteenth century, the practice of burning pitch and firing cannons was used to combat yellow fever in some American communities.

CLASSICAL CULTURES

Archeologic evidence and other records show that Minoans, 3000-1430 BC, and Myceneans, 1430-1150 BC, built drainage systems, water closets, and water-flushing systems. Herodotus wrote that Egyptians of about 1000 BC were the healthiest of all civilized people. They had a considerable sense of personal cleanliness, possessed numerous pharmaceutic preparations, and constructed earth closets and public drainage pipes. The Hebrews extended Egyptian hygienic thought and formulated in Leviticus, about 1500 BC, what is probably the world's first written hygienic code. It dealt with a wide variety of personal and community responsibilities, including cleanliness of the body, protection against the spread of contagious diseases, isolation of lepers, disinfection of dwellings after illness, sanitation of campsites, disposal of excreta and refuse, protection of water and food supplies, and the hygiene of maternity.

The Athenian civilization circa 1000-400 BC, is of interest for two reasons. It was there that personal hygiene was developed to a degree never previously approached. Much concern was given to personal cleanliness, exercise, and dietetics in addition to environmental sanitation. A point of interest, however, is that, in contrast with present-day public health thought, the weak, ill, and crippled were ignored and sometimes destroyed. It is important to realize that this was essentially a culture of a minority of nobles, and the benefits of the culture were not available to the majority who were poor farmers or slaves.

The Roman component of the classical civilization that succeeded Athens is well-known for its administrative and engineering achievements. At its zenith it had laws for the registration of citizens and slaves; for a periodic census; for the prevention of nuisances; for inspection and removal of dilapidated buildings; for the elimination of dangerous animals and foul smells; for the destruction of unsound goods; for the supervision of weights and measures; for the supervision of public bars, taverns, and houses of prostitution; and for the regulation of building construction. A supply of good and cheap grain was assured to the population. Numerous public sanitary services were provided. Many streets were paved, and some even had gutters and were drained by a network of underground conduits. Provision was made for the cleaning and repair of streets and for the removal of garbage and rubbish. Public baths were constructed and extensively used. An adequate and relatively safe public water supply was made available by the construction of magnificent aqueducts and tunnels. It is of interest to note that several of the aqueducts and subsurface drains (cloacae) constructed by the Romans are still in use, having been incorporated into the present-day water and sewerage systems of Rome and other cities.

The Roman civilization, like that of Athens, rested on a majority of poor farmers and especially enormous numbers of slaves obtained by military conquest. When the limits of conquest were reached and the supply of new lands and slaves diminished, the civilization weakened, and the vaunted legions were disastrously defeated by Gothic hordes in AD 378 at Adrianople. This led to the beginning of Western civilization based on quite different concepts of society, religion, government, economics, agriculture, and technology. These changes were so drastic, however, that a transitional period was inevitable.

THE MIDDLE AGES

The transitional period, which lasted from about AD 500 to 1500, is especially interesting from a hygienic and epidemiologic viewpoint. Classical ideology was dualistic and believed that full spirituality could be achieved only by freeing the spirit from the body and from the material world. It regarded the world and the flesh as evil. The Western philosophy that eventually developed is pluralistic. As Quigley[5] described it, "Western ideology believes that the material is good and the spiritual is better but they are not opposed to each other since the material world is necessary for the achievement of the spiritual world." In other words, after all, God made the body as well as the spirit! It took time for such philosophies to spread and become accepted. Therefore there was a period from the final collapse of the Roman Empire about AD 500 to the early part of the tenth century that has been somewhat unfairly called the Dark Ages. One of its characteristics was a reaction against anything reminiscent of the Roman Empire. Many people, especially early monks and anchorites, believed that the Athenians and Romans, despite their dualism, pampered the body to the detriment of the soul. Therefore they preached the belittlement of worldly things. This became known as "mortification of the flesh."

So intense was the reaction that it even included a significant change in attitude toward sanitation and personal hygiene. It was considered immoral to view even one's own body; therefore people seldom bathed and wore notoriously dirty garments. This is said by some to have been partly responsible for the eventual widespread use of perfume in this period. Diets in general were apparently poor and consisted of badly prepared or preserved foods. This gave rise to the widespread use of spices and the search for trade routes to obtain them. Sanitation was ignored. Refuse and body wastes were allowed to accumulate in and around dwellings. Slops were thrown onto the roads or streets, hence the famous cry, *gardez l'eau*. These and other unsalubrious customs carried over even into relatively recent times, as depicted so well by Hogarth's prints of life in eighteenth-century England.

However, as time passed, some significant medical and hygienic developments occurred. Generally they were reactions to the disastrous effects of an uncontrolled nature or the fruits of ill-conceived habits and customs. Terrifying pandemics of disease occurred that were among the most intense experiences in the history of mankind. During the seventh century a new religion, Islam, appeared. It attracted many followers in Africa, the Near East, Asia, and to some extent the Balkans and the Iberian peninsula. As with Judaism, it placed great emphasis on cleanliness.

However, after the death of Mohammed, it became a religious custom to make a pilgrimage, or hajj, to Mecca, the place of the prophet's birth about AD 570. During each great hajj, among the many thousands who converged on the small city were some from far-off Asia, including India, which was and still is the endemic center of cholera. Cholera naturally spread rapidly throughout the thousands of pilgrims, who disseminated it along their homeward routes of travel and throughout their respective homelands. Thus each hajj was almost invariably followed by a pandemic of cholera.

Complicating this, beginning in AD 1095, were the hordes of Christian crusaders to the Middle East from all parts of Europe whose wanderings inevitably resulted in periodic seeding of the European continent with the vibrio of cholera as well as other agents of disease. The vibrio prospered in a gradually urbanizing Europe, whence centuries later it was transferred to America by the invading settlers. During the period from 1830 to about 1880, cholera repeatedly reentered America, spreading along the water routes and accompanying the prospectors to the gold fields of California. At one time or another, most settlements were affected by cholera, often resulting in the death of one third to one half of the population. It is of more than incidental interest that a resurgence of cholera has been occurring in recent years.

During the early Dark Ages, leprosy spread probably from Egypt to Asia Minor and eventually throughout Europe, compounded by the Crusades and other great migrations. It apparently was a far more acute and disfiguring disease than is presently observed in most of the western world, and because of the terror to which it gave rise, laws were passed to regulate the conduct and movement of those afflicted. In many places lepers were declared civilly dead and were banished from human communities. They were compelled to wear identifying clothes and to warn of their presence by means of a horn, bell, or clapper and by crying the word *unclean*. This had a twofold result: it was an effective isolation measure, and it usually brought about a relatively rapid death from hunger and exposure as well as from lack of treatment and care. These measures, inhuman as they were, almost eradicated leprosy in Europe (but by no means in the world) by the sixteenth century and may be regarded as an early, although unplanned, victory in epidemiology.

The Black Death

No sooner had leprosy passed its zenith and begun to decline than an even deadlier menace appeared in the form of bubonic plague. Its spread is illustrative of a momentous ecologic phenomenon. The origin of the source was the vast plain of central Asia. The four biologic factors were the *Yersinia pestis,* which infected fleas, which lived on and infected *marmosets* and *man.* The men who were infected were Mongols whose traditional life was that of nomadic herdsmen. Their leader, Chingis Khan, lived at a tent capital, Karakorum. In 1219 he gathered an army that was rapidly mobile by means of fast ponies and began a vast sweep of conquest that eventually included western Asia, the Middle East, Egypt, the Balkans, and eastern and central Europe.[6] With them they brought the *Yersinia pestis,* which had been transferred to them from the marmoset. Conditions of living compounded by the chaos of conquest then resulted in the transfer from infected humans to the rodents, predominantly rats, in the areas conquered.

From then on the spread of plague was rapid and repetitive, compounded by other military activities, crusades, dislocated populations, and trade. Probably nothing ever came so close to exterminating the human species. During the 1340s more than 13 million people died from the disease in China. India was almost depopulated. Tartary, Mesopotamia, Syria, and Armenia were said to be covered by dead bodies. At its peak, Aleppo lost about 500 people and Cairo, from 10,000 to 15,000 people daily. In Gaza 22,000 people and most of the animals were carried off within 6 weeks. Cyprus was depopulated, and ships without crews were often seen in the Mediterranean and in the North Sea, drifting aimlessly and spreading plague when they drifted ashore. It was reported to Pope Clement VI that half the population of the known world had died. The figure given was about 43 million. The total mortality from the Black Death is thought to have been over 60 million.[7] Europe, particularly during 1348, was devastated. Florence lost 60,000 people, Venice 100,000, Marseilles 16,000 in 1 month, Sien 70,000, Paris 50,000, St. Denys 14,000, Strasbourg 9,000, and Vienna 1,200 daily. In many places in France only 2 out of 20 survived.

In Avignon, where 60,000 people died, the Pope consecrated the Rhone river so bodies might be thrown into it without delay, since the churchyard was full. In Vienna, burial in churchyards or churches was prohibited; the dead were arranged in layers by thousands in six large pits outside the city. (In a main square in Vienna can be seen an elaborate monument commemorating the end of the great epidemic.) Crossing the channel, the Black Death destroyed half the population of medieval England and at least 100,000 in London alone.

Altogether it is estimated that Europe's tribute to plague in the midfourteenth century was about 25 million, and this one horrifying visitation was just a beginning. Plague continued to ebb and flow like a tide, periodically sweeping over the European continent. For example, in London in 1603 over one sixth of the population died, in 1625 another sixth, and in 1665 about one fifth. During 1790 Marseilles and Toulon lost 91,000 people; in 1743 Messina lost 70,000; and in 1759 about 70,000 died on the island of Cyprus. It must also be realized that great as these figures are, they are proportionately enormous in relation to the populations of those times.

Out of these terrifying experiences and despite the view of divine or cosmic causation of disease, certain groping attempts were made to forestall the apparent inevitability of epidemic disaster. In 1348 the great trading port of Venice banned entry of infected or suspected ships and travelers. In 1377 at Ragusa (present-day Dubrovnik) it was ruled that travelers from plague areas stop at designated places outside the port and remain free of disease for 2 months before being allowed to enter. Historically this represents the first quarantine measure, although it involved a 2-month interval rather than the literal 40 days. This procedure is of particular interest in that it implied a vague realization of the existence of an incubation period for a communicable disease. Six years later, in 1383, Marseilles passed the first actual quarantine law and erected the first quarantine station. These are historic landmarks in public health administration and epidemiology, but unfortunately their effectiveness was impaired by the fact that although great attention was paid to humans, the role of the rat and the flea had not yet been discerned.

Other diseases

Some mention, even if necessarily inadequate, should be made of the rapid dissemination of syphilis throughout Europe and the Near East after the discovery of America, where it is commonly thought to have originated. Some measure of its incidence and seriousness is indicated by its vernacular name, "the great pox," which was used to distinguish it from smallpox, now considered serious enough. Incidentally, it is curious that little historic reference is made to the other diseases that are known to have existed with incidences far exceeding any now occurring, for example, diphtheria, the streptococcal infections, the dysenteries, typhoid, typhus, and others. The most probable reason is that in the first place, people undoubtedly became accustomed to their inevitable endemicity and accepted them as part of the routine risk of life, and in the second place, they were so dramatically overshadowed by the tremendous impact of the great periodic pandemic killers as to merit relatively little mention in the historic writings of the times. In summary, therefore, the people of Europe emerged from the Middle Ages and in fact came all the way to recent times with little substantial comprehension of any principles of public health other than those of crude, inhumane, and inefficient isolation and quarantine.

RENAISSANCE AND REASON

In a period marked by expanding trade and population movement and concentration, the risks presented by disease were necessarily magnified. The great pandemics of the Middle Ages therefore must have caused considerable social and political frustrations that could lead only to attitudes of fatalism and general disregard for the welfare of individuals. In this regard Hecker[7] commented:

The mind of nations is deeply affected by the destructive conflict of the powers of nature, and . . . great disasters lead to striking changes in general civilization. For all that exists in man, whether good or evil, is rendered conspicuous by the presence of great danger. His inmost feelings are aroused—the thought of self-preservation masters his spirit—self denial is put to severe proof, and wherever darkness and barbarism prevail, there the affrighted mortal flies to the idols of his superstition, and all laws, human and divine, are criminally molested.

The way of life of a people likewise has a significant effect on their state of health or illness. In this respect Erasmus wrote to Cardinal Wolsey's physician describing the average English household of the sixteenth century:

As to floors, they are usually made with clay, covered with rushes that grow in the fens and which are so seldom removed that the lower parts remains sometimes for twenty years and has in it a collection of spittle, vomit, urine of dogs and humans, beer, scraps of fish and other filthiness not to be named.

Winslow,[8] in his precis of the modern public health movement, points out how long it has taken the human race to improve such conditions, presenting examples as disgusting as the preceding from England in 1842 and New York City in 1865. Indeed, even now in many parts of the world, circumstances such as these may be seen.

Gradually some began to doubt the teleologic origin of disease as a punishment for sin. It might be noted, however, that this stigma has only recently been removed from cancer, leprosy, and tuberculosis. Indeed, venereal infection is still considered by many as punishment for immorality. By the end of the Middle Ages, several diseases had been differentiated. Among them were leprosy, influenza, ophthalmia, trachoma, scabies, impetigo, erysipelas (St. Anthony's fire), anthrax, plague, consumption, syphilis (the great pox), smallpox, diphtheria and scarlet fever (considered as one), and typhus and typhoid fever (also considered together).

The people of Europe emerged from this stunted period of history slowly and cautiously and began

to open their eyes and think as free individuals. An increasing number of outstanding thinkers appeared, among whom were Montaigne, Paracelsus, Galileo, Spinoza, Bacon, and Descartes, to mention a few. Each in his own way hammered at the bars that imprisoned the minds and bodies of men. Their combined efforts resulted in remarkable subsequent accomplishments, especially in the late eighteenth century and throughout the nineteenth century. The concepts of the innate dignity and the rights of humankind began to be emphasized more and more. The search for scientific truth was at last advocated for its own sake.

THE EIGHTEENTH AND NINETEENTH CENTURIES
The plight of children

Meanwhile, other changes were occurring. Among them were the development of nationalism, imperialism, and industrialization, with their tragic and degrading concomitants. The false gods of power and profit were placed on even higher pedestals, and individual liberties, labors, and lives were sacrificed on a scale probably unprecedented since the building of the pyramids. As an example, in one of the most shameful actions in history there came about in England a legally condoned practice of apprentice slavery, whereby pauper children were indentured to owners of mines and factories. The socially accepted pattern was for parishes to assume responsibility for orphans and pauper children. This responsibility was met at first by paying private "nurses" for taking the infants and younger children into their homes for a few years and putting them out to work as apprentices when they grew older. Partly because of the increasing numbers and partly as a remedy for frequent abuse of young children, parish workhouses began to be established in the late seventeenth and early eighteenth centuries as a substitute for parish nurses.

Theoretically the workhouses were intended to provide some training for the children, but this was kept at a minimum and was largely concerned with inculcating the ideals of obediance, labor, industry, virtue, and religion. As George[9] surmises, it was hoped that the workhouses would "cure a very bad practice in parish officers, who to save expence, are apt to ruin children by putting them out as early as they can to any sorry master that will take them, without any concern for their education and welfare."

In her authoritative review of life in England in

the eighteenth century, George presents a picture of these methods and ideals in practice by describing the London Workhouse in Bishopsgate Street in 1708:

> . . . thirty or forty children were put under the charge of one nurse in a ward, they lay two together in bunks arranged round the walls in two tiers, "boarded and set one above the other . . . a flock bed, a pair of sheets, two blankets and a rugg to each." Prayers and breakfast were from 6:30 to 7. At 7 the children were set to work, twenty under a mistress, "to spin wool and flax, knit stockings, to make new their linnen, cloathes, shooes, mark, etc." This work went on till 6 PM with an interval from 12 to 1 for "dinner and play." Twenty children were called away at a time for an hour a day to be taught reading, some also writing. Some children, we are told, "earn a halfpenny, some a penny, and some fourpence a day." At twelve, thirteen or fourteen, they were apprenticed, being given, at the master's choice, either a "good ordinary suit of cloaths or 20s, in money."

When children reached the age of apprenticeship, their lot became infinitely worse. A writer on the Poor Laws in 1738 said the following:

> A most unhappy practice prevails in most places to apprentice poor children, no matter to what master. Provided he lives out of the parish, if the child serves the first forty days we are rid of him for ever. The master may be a tiger in cruelty, he may beat, abuse, strip naked, starve or do what he will to the poor innocent lad, few people take much notice, and the officers who put him out the least of anybody. . . . The greatest part of those who now take poor apprentices are the most indigent and dishonest, in a word, the very dregs of the poor of England, by whom it is the fate of many a poor child, not only to be half-starved and sometimes bred up in no trade, but to be forced to thieve and steal for his master, and so is brought up for the gallows into the bargain. . . .

Children apprenticed to chimney sweepers fared among the worst. In 1767 Hanway, a leading reformer of the period, described the miseries of their neglect and ill-treatment, of their being forced up chimneys at the risk of being burnt or suffocated, and of their being forced to beg and steal by their masters. "Chimney-sweepers," he says, "ought to breed their own children to the business, then perhaps they will wash, clothe and feed them. As it is they do neither, and these poor black urchins have no protectors and are treated worse than a humane person would treat a dog." In apprenticing children in large groups, it was usual to require that for every 30 normal children, one idiot must be accepted. The unfortunate children, forced to work from 15 to 18 hours a day (sometimes literally chained to their machines), fed a minimum of food scarcely fit for consumption, and housed under the most crowded and filthy conditions, usually were released from their sufferings and abuse by early death.

As mentioned in Chapter 1, in 1842 Edwin Chadwick pointed out that more than one half of the children of the working classes died before their fifth birthday and that in cities such as Liverpool the average ages at death of the various social classes were 36 years for the gentry, 22 years for tradesmen, and 16 years for laborers.[10]

Sanitary conditions

During this period the condition of the streets of most European cities became deplorable, caused in part by nightmen and scavengers emptying their carts in the streets instead of the places assigned for the purpose. The accumulated filth of the eighteenth-century house was in many cases simply thrown from the doors or windows.

> Although eighteenth-century London was incredibly dirtier, more dilapidated and more closely-built than it afterwards became, was there no compensation in its greater compactness, the absence of straggling suburbs, the ease with which people could take country walks? This is at least doubtful. The roads round London were neither very attractive nor very safe. The land adjoining them was watered with drains and thickly sprinkled by laystalls and refuse heaps. Hogs were kept in large numbers on the outskirts and fed on the garbage of the town. A chain of smoking brick-kilns surrounded a great part of London and in the brick-fields vagrants lived and slept, cooking their food at the kilns. It is true that there was an improvement as the century went on. In 1706 it was said of the highways, tho they are mended every summer, yet everybody knows that for a mile or two about this City, the same and the ditches hard by are commonly so full of nastiness and stinking dirt, that oftentimes many persons who have occasion to go in or come out of town, are forced to stop their noses to avoid the ill-smell occasioned by it.[9]

These conditions under which so many people lived and worked had dire results. Smallpox, cholera, typhoid, tuberculosis, and many other diseases reached exceedingly high endemic levels, and the contamination of streams became so bad as to prompt the statement in Parliament in 1859: "India is in revolt and the Thames stinks." Southwood

Smith pointed out at the time that the annual slaughter in England and Wales from typhus and typhoid fevers was double the number of lives lost by the allied armies in the battle of Waterloo. With reference to smallpox, it has been estimated that in eighteenth-century Europe, as many as 1 person in 10 died from smallpox, half of them children. Annual death rates varied from 1% or 2% to as high as 33%. An unpocked face was rare, since about 95% of Europeans who survived had had smallpox.

These conditions were not confined to England, and they concerned the inheritors of the age of reason in many lands. Increasingly liberal views of the nature and role of man were expressed and broadcasted, especially by philosophers and writers such as Smith, Hume, Bentham, and Mill in England; Montesquieu, Voltaire, Diderot, and Rousseau in France, and Jefferson, Franklin, Dickinson, and Samuel Adams in the American colonies. In a very real sense, the broader concerns of these men and others like them constructed the political and social platform on which it was possible to promote and develop sanitary reforms and other measures for the protection of the public health.

ENGLISH SANITARY REFORMS

Concern with the economic consequences of existing social and sanitary conditions began to appear, providing leaders in sanitary reform with forceful arguments. Thus Chadwick[10] reported the following:

This depressing effect of adverse sanitary circumstances on the labouring strength of the population, and on its duration, is to be viewed with the greatest concern, as it is a depressing effect on that which most distinguishes the British people, and which it were truism to say constitutes the chief strength of the nation—the bodily strength of the individuals of the labouring class. The greater portion of the wealth of the nation is derived from the labour obtained by the application of this strength, and it is only those who have had practically the means of comparing it with that of the population of other countries who are aware how far the labouring population of this country is naturally distinguished above others. . . . The more closely the subject of the evils affecting the sanitary condition of the labouring population is investigated, the more widely do their effects appear to be ramified. The pecuniary cost of noxious agencies is measured by data within the province of the actuary, by the charges attendant on the reduced duration of life, and the reduc-

tion of the periods of working ability or production by sickness. The cost would include also much of the public charge of attendant vice and crime, which come within the province of the police, as well as the destitution which comes within the province of the administrators of relief. Of the pecuniary effects, including the cost of maintenance during the preventible sickness, any estimate approximating to exactness could only be obtained by very great labour, which does not appear to be necessary.

Public health went unrecognized in a legal sense in England until 1837, when the first sanitary legislation was enacted. It established a National Vaccination Board and appropriated 2,000 Pounds for its support. As a result, a few vaccination stations were set up in the city of London. This modest beginning was followed in 1842 by Edwin Chadwick's momentous *Report on an Inquiry into the Sanitary Conditions of the Labouring Population of Great Britain,* one result of which was the establishment in 1848 of a General Board of Health for England. Significantly, the same year saw the appointment as first medical officer of health for London, of John Simon, who 7 years later was to assume that office for the nation as a whole.

Improvements rapidly followed. Advances in sanitation and hygiene did not go forward alone. Legislation was passed concerning factory management; child welfare; care of the aged; the mentally ill, and the infirm; education; and many other phases of social reform. It was not long before the horrors of previous conditions were forgotten and the standards of order, decency, and sanitation began to be taken for granted.

. . . pride was based on real achievements, which had an undoubted effect on the health of the town, and in which London was a pioneer among large cities. The foot-pavements, the lamps, the water-supply, the fire-plugs, the new sewers, defective enough by later standards, were admired by all. . . . Beneath the pavements are vast subterranean sewers arched over to convey away the waste water which in other cities is so noisome above ground, and at a less depth are buried wooden pipes that supply every house plentifully with water, conducted by leaden pipes into kitchens or cellars, three times a week for the trifling expense of three shillings per quarter. . . . The intelligent foreigner cannot fail to take notice of these useful particulars which are almost peculiar to London.[10]

The seeds of sanitary and social reform spread rapidly to other large urban centers of England. However, benefits to the smaller towns and rural areas was slower. As early as 1830, Chadwick had recommended the employment of local sanitary officers, including medical personnel, for adequate coverage of the nation. His proposals originally met with considerable opposition, some of which continued even when he demonstrated the economic soundness of the costs incurred.

ENGLISH INFLUENCE ON AMERICA

Conditions and developments in Great Britain may seem to have been unduly stressed. However, any discussion of backgrounds must necessarily emphasize those extraterritorial developments that have exerted the greatest influence on North America. It is true that many advances had been made elsewhere, notably in the Low Countries, in Germany, and on the Scandinavian peninsula. By mid-nineteenth century, France had long since embarked on significant studies and activities relating to public health and sanitation, and many scientific papers were being published. The establishment of the *Annales d'Hygiene Publique* gives testimony to this. The work of the Belgian Quételet was already widely known, and Pettenkofer in Munich and Virchow in Berlin already had far-reaching influences.

Nevertheless, the early intimate ties—social, economic, and otherwise—between the North American continent and Great Britain made events in the latter of particular significance to the former. The relationship was aptly described in 1876 by Bowditch,[11] first president of the Massachusetts State Board of Health:

But by far the greatest influence has been exerted upon us in America by England, who, by her unbounded pecuniary sacrifices and steady improvement in her legislation, and her able writers, has far outstripped any country in the world in the direction of State Preventive Medicine. . . . The consummate skill in the discovery, removal, and prevention of whatever may be prejudicial to the public health, shown under the admirable direction of Mr. Simon, late Medical Officer of England's Privy Council, by his corps of trained inspectors is wholly unequalled at the present day, and unprecedented, I suspect, in all past time in any country on the globe.

Although scientific research may have progressed further in some other countries, the application of the new knowledge, especially in terms of administrative organization and procedure, occurred more rapidly and more successfully in England than elsewhere. Since administrative organization depends to a considerable degree on legal procedure, it is noteworthy that America, from the beginning followed the pattern set by English law. Thus when the time came for American commu-

nities to pass sanitary ordinances, they did so in the tradition of the English common law.

COLONIAL AMERICA

Transferring attention to the developing North American continent, certain public health problems were recognized early by the colonists. They had good reason for being conscious of the threat of disease. Many of the early settlements had been completely obliterated by epidemic diseases, particularly smallpox. Among these were the colonies at Jamestown and probably the colony at Roanoke Island. On the other hand, it was ironically probably because of disease that colonial powers were able to establish footholds in the Western Hemisphere. The settlers of the Massachusetts Bay Colony, for example, came to a territory in which the natives were by no means peaceful. Yet by the time the Pilgrims landed at Plymouth, the hostile natives of the surrounding countryside had been all but eliminated, apparently by smallpox introduced by the Cabot and Gosnold expeditions. Smallpox also appears to have played some role in the weakening and eventual conquest of the Aztec Empire. In this instance it is known to have been introduced by a servant of Narvaez, who joined Cortez in 1520.[12] It has been estimated that during the early periods of colonization of Central and North America, the Indian population was decimated by diseases introduced by the invaders, whether peaceful or otherwise.[13] In the Caribbean and the southern colonies in North America, smallpox as well as yaws, yellow fever, and malaria were spread by the slave trade with ill-fated consequences.[14]

The registration of vital events is essential to sound, efficient public health awareness and practice. It is of interest that its recording was an early concern of the New England colonists. As early as 1639, an act was passed by the Massachusetts colony ordering that each birth and death be recorded. Subsequent acts outlined the necessary administrative responsibilities and procedures. Not only was the information made available locally but copies had to be made by the town clerks and transmitted to the clerks of the county courts. The law also specified fees and penalties. Similar laws were enacted at about the same time by the Plymouth colony.[15]

Most of the early activities of a public health na-

ture in America were concerned with gross insanitation and attempts to prevent the entrance of exotic diseases. For example, as early as 1647 the
Massachusetts Bay Colony passed a regulation to
prevent pollution of Boston Harbor. Between 1692
and 1708 Boston, Salem, and Charleston passed
acts dealing with nuisances and trades offensive or
dangerous to the public health. In 1701 Massachusetts passed laws for the isolation of smallpox
patients and for ship quarantine, to be used whenever necessary. The difficulty with such measures
was that no continuing organization or even committee existed to assure ready recognition of undesirable situations or noncompliance with the requirements of the enacted legislation.

In the century during which the American colonies drew together and eventually formed a federation of states, little progress of a public health
nature was made. Recognition must be given,
however, to at least one notable person of the period.
The multifaceted Dr. Benjamin Rush wrote that
political institutions, economic organization, and
disease were so interrelated that any general social change produced accompanying changes in
health.[16] Regretfully there are still many today who
seem unable to grasp this simple concept. After the
American Revolution the threat of various dieseases,
particularly yellow fever, which caused the aban-
donment of the national capital in Philadelphia, led
to widespread interest in the development of legislation for the establishment of permanent boards
of health. Permissive legislation of this type was
passed in 1797 by the states of New York and Massachusetts, followed in 1805 by Connecticut. There
is some controversy over the establishment of the
first permanent local *board* of health. Boston is
commonly said to have organized the first in 1799,
with Paul Revere as its chairman. However, this
has been contested by the cities of Petersburg, Va.,
(1780), Philadelphia, (1794), New York, (1796),
and Baltimore (1793). As an example of function,
by the end of the eighteenth century New York City,
with a population of 75,000 had formed a public
health committee concerned with the "quality of
the water supplies, construction of common sewers,
drainage of marshes, interment of the dead, plant-
ing of trees and healthy vegetables, habitation of
damp cellars, and the construction of a masonry
wall along the water front."

THE NINETEENTH CENTURY IN AMERICA

Between 1800 and 1850, while the United States
expanded greatly in size and population, public
health activities remained essentially stationary.
Threats to public health and welfare and the resulting incidence of disease, however, did not.
Many epidemics, especially of smallpox, yellow fever, cholera, typhoid, and typhus, repeatedly entered and swept over the land. Tuberculosis and
malaria reached high levels of endemicity. In Massachusetts in 1850, for example, the tuberculosis
death rate was over 300 per 100,000 population;
the infant mortality was about 200 per 1,000 live
births; and smallpox, scarlet fever, and typhoid
were leading causes of deaths. As a result, by 1850
the average life expectancy in Boston and most of
the other older cities in the United States was less
than that in London, which was then the object
of criticism. The American social scene was the
subject of scathing comments by visitors from
abroad who were impressed with the crudity and
"barbarism" of life in the United States and the
generally unkempt appearance of its communities.
As so often has happened, improvements in sanitation and public health were delayed by lack of
progress in other fields. Thus the British hygienist
Newsholme[17] described this period of American social history as follows:

> The rapid growth of cities tended to out run the forces
> of law and order and to smother under the weight of
> numbers any attempts at civic reform. Before public
> health measures could be adopted or enforced, other more
> pressing problems had to be solved. An effective police
> force, the first requisite of community life, did not make
> its appearance in the Atlantic seaboard cities until 1853,
> and satisfactory fire prevention came even later. Protec-
> tion against the dirt and filth of human aggregation, which
> threatened the life of every man, woman, and child, had
> to wait upon the adequate enforcement of law and order.

The inadequacies of the times were reflected in
the low quality of medical care. Professional teaching facilities were few and inadequate. Many "physicians" were self-designated and itinerant. The
prestige of the medical profession was at its lowest
ebb, and its ranks were disorganized and split by
the development of numerous healing philosophies
and cults. Kramer[18] summarized the situation:
"The doctors were victims of their own want of
knowledge, of the absence of adequate medical
standards and of a chaotic educational system."
Healing agents used included not only empiric
remedies left over from medieval Europe but, in

addition, many newly discovered "remedies" often borrowed from the American aborigines. This state of therapeutic affairs led Holmes[19] to remark that "if the whole materia medica as now used, could be sunk to the bottom of the sea, it would be all the better for mankind—and all the worse for the fishes."

The Shattuck report[20]

American public health in midnineteenth century is most notable for the extraordinary *Report of the Sanitary Commission of Massachusetts*. Its author, Lemuel Shattuck (1793-1859), a most unusual man, led the diversified life of teacher, historian, book dealer, sociologist, statistician, and finally, legislator in the state assembly. Although a layman, he had keen interest in sanitary reform as a result of gathering and tabulating the vital statistics of Boston. Because of his persistent complaints regarding the lack of sanitary progress, he was appointed chairman of a legislative committee for the study of health and sanitary problems in the commonwealth. From this committee and essentially from Shattuck's pen came the report. With remarkable insight and foresight, it included a detailed consideration not only of the present and future public health needs of Massachusetts but also of its component parts and of the nation as a whole. This most remarkable of all American public health documents, if published today, in many respects would still be ahead of its time.

The content of the Sanitary Commission report may be appreciated when it is realized that when it was written, there were no national or state public health programs, and such local health agencies as existed were still embryonic. Medical practice in general was far from scientific; facilities for medical training were few and in a most confused state; and provisions for nurses' training were entirely lacking. Almost a half century was to pass before the spectacular era of Pasteur, Koch, and the other contributors to the golden age of bacteriology.

Among the many recommendations made by Shattuck a century and a third ago were those for the establishment of state and local boards of health; a system of sanitary police or inspectors; the collection and analysis of vital statics; a routine system for exchanging data and information; sanitation programs for towns and buildings; studies on the health of schoolchildren; studies on tuberculosis; the control of alcoholism; the supervision of mental disease; the sanitary supervision and study of problems of immigrants; the erection of model tenements, public bathhouses, and washhouses; the control of smoke nuisances; the control of food adulteration; the exposure of nostrums; the preaching of health from pulpits; the establishment of nurses' training schools; the teaching of sanitary science in medical schools; and the inclusion of preventive medicine in clinical practice, with routine physical examinations and family records of illness.

Unfortunately, although the report presented the principal concepts and modes of action that would ultimately form the basis of much of today's public health practice, its importance was not appreciated for nearly a quarter of a century. One of the earliest appraisals of it was given in 1876 by Bowditch,[11] first president of the State Board of Health of Massachusetts, in an address before the International Medical Congress at Philadelphia:

The report fell flat from the printer's hand. It remained almost unnoticed by the community or by the profession for many years, and its recommendations were ignored. Finally, in 1869, a State Board of Health of laymen and physicians, exactly as Mr. Shattuck recommended, was established by Massachusetts. Dr. Derby, its first secretary, looked to this admirable document as his inspiration and support. In giving this high honor to Mr. Shattuck, I do not wish to forget or to undervalue the many and persistent efforts made by a few physicians, among whom stands pre-eminent Dr. Edward Jarvis, and occasionally by the Massachusetts Medical Society, in urging the State authorities to inaugurate and to sustain the ideas avowed by Mr. Shattuck. But there is no doubt that he, as a layman, quietly working, did more towards bringing Massachusetts to correct views on this subject than all other agencies whatsoever. Of Mr. Edwin Chadwick, I need say nothing. You all know him. Fortunately for himself, he has lived to see rich fruits from his labors. That was not granted to Mr. Shattuck.

The comparison of Shattuck, the American, and Chadwick, the Englishman, is of more than passing interest. Some lessons may be learned by comparing the effects of the work of the two men. Shattuck's report consisted essentially of straightforward, unembellished, unillustrated statements of fact, followed by specific and detailed recommendations. This contrasted with Chadwick's report, which included many vivid descriptions of the appalling conditions that existed. The latter caused an immediate emotional response on the part of all who read or heard of the report. One wonders if Shattuck's report might have had a more immediate effect had it provided readers with mental images of existing conditions for contrast with further mental images of desirable conditions attainable. On the other hand, although Chadwick's report brought about a prompt reaction that resulted in the establishment of a General Board of Health in 1848, the response was not long lasting. Chadwick's over-enthusiasm and impatience demanded immediate action, for which the British people were not yet ready.[21] Much antagonism and resistance developed, which resulted in the demise of the General Board of Health after only 4 years of existence. This reversal caused an unfortunate delay in the ultimate development of a sound national health program in Great Britain. The reports of Chadwick and Shatuck therefore, remarkable as they were, provide examples of administrative failure, one because of underpromotion and the other because of overpromotion.

DEVELOPMENT OF OFFICIAL HEALTH AGENCIES IN THE UNITED STATES

Official public health action occurs on four levels: local, state, national, and international. It is not surprising, however, that in the United States it began on the local, and specifically on the urban, level since it is there that people and their problems are concentrated. Originally, communities followed the path of self-determination, but as they grew and spread and as social and economic intercourse increased, urban-rural boundaries became less meaningful. Subsequently, essentially the same change in relationship became true among the states. As a result, although each political level has its own public health structure, no one of them is by any means completely independent of the others. To the contrary and increasingly, there occurred a melding of local public health functions and responsibilities with those of the state and in turn of state functions and responsibilities with those of the federal government.

Local health departments

The first half of the nineteenth century saw a gradual trend toward the more or less full-time employment of persons to serve as the functional agents of local boards of health, which now were

increasing in number. This represented the first step in the formation of full-time local health *departments*. Some of the earliest were established in Baltimore (1798), Charleston, S.C., (1815), Philadelphia, (1818), Providence (1832), Cambridge (1846), New York City (1866), Chicago (1867), Louisville (1870), Indianapolis (1872), and Boston (1873). The last illustrates the lag, in this instance three quarters of a century, that often occurs between the formation of local boards of health and the establishment of functional agencies. As might be expected, the initial activities of these early health departments were determined by current epidemiologic theories that placed particular emphasis on the elimination of sanitary nuisances. For example, at the midpoint of the nineteenth century the population of New York City had reached 300,000. Its board of health was concerned only with crowded living conditions, dirty streets, and the regulations of public baths, slaughterhouses, and pigsties.

Public health organization on the rural level developed under somewhat different circumstances and much later than in urban areas. In 1910-1911 one of a series of severe typhoid fever epidemics occurred in Yakima County, Wash. Because it was uncontrolled by local authorities, L.L. Lumsden of the U.S.Public Health Service was requested to bring it under control. Lumsden not only solved the particular epidemiologic problem but also suggested ways of preventing its recurrence. One strong recommendation he made was the establishment of a full-time staff to deal with all public health matters.

Meanwhile, the Rockefeller Sanitary Commission,[22] which had been active in hookworm control in the southeastern United States and in Central and South America, concluded that no single disease or sanitary or public health problem could be successfully attacked without concurrent efforts aimed at all phases of public health. As a result, it also recommended the establishment of local full-time public health staffs. Thus there occurred the coincidence of the same idea at almost the same moment at two different places for two different but related reasons, resulting in the establishment of the first full-time county health departments in Guilford County, N.C. in June 1911 and in Yakima County, Wash., in July 1911.* The basic soundness

---

*Some difference of opinion exists with regard to priority: many contend that Jefferson County, Ky., was the first in 1908.

of the principle is indicated by the subsequent growth of local health units, which now serve most of the population of the nation.

State health departments

Repeated outbreaks of yellow fever and other epidemic diseases caused Louisiana in 1855 to establish a commission to deal with quarantine matters in the port of New Orleans. Some therefore claim priority for Louisiana in the establishment of a state board of health. However, in terms of the more usual concept of the general functions of a state board of health Massachusetts, despite its delayed response to Shattuck's recommendations, is generally considered to have established the first true state board of health under the Act of 1869.*

The board shall take cognizance of the interests of health and life among the citizens of this Commonwealth. They shall make sanitary investigations and inquiries in respect to the people, the causes of disease, and especially of epidemics, and the sources of mortality and the effects of localities, employments, conditions and circumstances on the public health; and they shall gather such information in respect to these matters as they may deem proper, for diffusion among the people.

In determining policy at early meetings, the board, under the leadership of Bowditch, concerned itself with public and professional education in hygiene, various aspects of housing, investigations of various diseases and measures for their prevention, methods of slaughtering, the sale of poisons, and conditions of the poor. It decided also to send a circular letter to local boards of health to inquire about their powers and duties and to collect for publication the number and prevailing causes of deaths in the most populous cities and towns in the state. The board requested each community to designate a physician to act as correspondent. It has been observed[23] that this correspondence was the beginning of productive cooperation between state and local health authorities. In 1878 the Massachusetts Department of Health merged with the Department of Lunacy and Charity because of political pressure and a desire for "economy." As a result, matters dealing with public health were effectively submerged by the weight of the other two interests. Eventually, however, this situation was reversed, and a sound program was made possible by reestablishment of the health agency as an entity. It is interesting to note that the second state

health department was established 1 year after the one in Massachusetts on the opposite side of the continent, in California. By the end of the nineteenth century, 38 other states had followed suit, to be joined during the early decades of the twentieth century by the remainder.

National health agencies

*The Marine Hospital Service.** To consider the history and development of the Public Health Service, the most important federal health agency, it is necessary to return to the year 1798. The United States of America had just come into existence. Although still largely undeveloped, it was already vigorous and enterprising, one manifestation of which was its expanding maritime trade. Sailing ships for world commerce were coming down the ways at an ever-increasing rate, and the merchant marine was becoming one of the nation's most important resources.

The farmer of Virginia and the tradesman of Boston had firm roots in their respective communities, which they supported through taxes. The merchant seaman on the other hand, led a precarious existence somewhat resembling that of the itinerant or vagabond. Often he had neither a permanent abode nor a permanent route. His ship was the closest substitute for a home, and his ship might be in New York harbor one week, in Charleston the next, and in Liverpool within a month. Despite this, he too was an American citizen and deserved whatever security and assistance his nation could provide its citizens. For a period, however, things did not work out that way. Like anyone, the sailor was subject to injury or illness. In fact, because of the unusual hazards of his occupation, he was subject to greater than average risk. Furthermore he was underpaid, and whatever he received at the end of the journey was more often than not quickly removed from him in the taverns and brothels that thrived in the vicinity of the wharves. As a result, he usually found it difficult or impossible to obtain or pay for whatever medical or hospital care he needed. Because he paid no local or state taxes and generally was not a member in good standing of whatever port city he happened to be in when ill, responsibility

---

*Act of 1869, General Court of Massachusetts.

*For a detailed account of the history of the agencies discussed in this section see *The United States Public Health Service, 1798-1950.*[24]

for him was usually avoided by the local authorities.

The young American Congress quickly became aware of this problem, and the first bill introduced at the first session of the first Congress addressed it. Because of several circumstances, however, a Marine Hospital Service Act was not passed until June 1798. It authorized the President to appoint physicians in each port to furnish medical and hospital care for sick and disabled seamen. Twenty cents a month was deducted from the pay of each man; the money was collected from the paymasters by the customs officers of the Treasury Department. Since the money was placed in the custody of the Treasury Department, there came about the anomalous situation whereby until 1935 most federal public health services were carried out under the aegis of the Treasury Department. The small sum of 20 cents a month is of particular interest in that it actually represented the first prepaid comprehensive medical and hospital insurance plan in the world, under the administrative supervision of what eventually became a public health agency. In 1884 the monthly deduction was discontinued and replaced by a tonnage tax, which is still collected but now goes into the general Treasury, from which the Public Health Service hospitals and outpatient clinics are supported through appropriations.

At first, physicians who served the plan were also engaged in the private practice of medicine, but before long the need became so great that physicians were employed full time. Originally, sailors who needed hospital care were placed in whatever public or private hospitals existed at the ports. However, as in the case of physicians, the demand for hospital services soon became so great that within 2 years (1800) the first marine hospital was constructed at Norfolk, Va. This was followed by similar hospitals throughout the country, at first at certain seaports and later at a number of places along inland waterways.

It is interesting that a medical director or supervising surgeon for the Public Health Service was not appointed until 1870. Compensation was a salary of $2,000 plus travel expenses. This developed eventually into the position of Surgeon General.

The Port Quarantine Act. The growing concern of the federal and state governments with the introduction of epidemic diseases led to the passage in 1878 of the first port quarantine act. At that time, entrance into the country was limited to its ports, which represented the nation's first line of defense against epidemic diseases. Since the incidence of these diseases was invariably greater at ports, the physicians of the Marine Hospital Service had more opportunity to become knowledgeable about them. In addition, since epidemics usually began at and frequently spread from ports, states developed the custom of asking and authorizing federally employed Marine Hospital Service physicians to aid in the control of local outbreaks. It was logical therefore to assign responsibility for port quarantine activities to the Marine Hospital Service. Much later, this was extended to international airports.

The law of 1878 embodies another important feature in authorizing the investigation of the origin and causes of epidemic diseases, especially yellow fever and cholera, and the best methods of preventing their introduction and spread. With little delay, control measures were initiated at ports of origin. Marine Hospital Service physicians were attached to the U.S. consular service in major foreign ports, and a system of reporting communicable disease through the consular service was put into effect. In 1890 domestic quarantine was added to provide interstate control of communicable disease. This was an immediate outgrowth of another particularly devastating epidemic of yellow fever that entered at New Orleans and spread throughout the Mississippi Valley. Between the time of the Louisiana Purchase in 1803 and the beginning of the twentieth century, New Orleans experienced no fewer than 37 severe epidemics of yellow fever in addition to constantly recurring outbreaks of cholera, plague, and smallpox.

In 1890 Congress gave the Marine Hospital Service authority to inspect all immigrants. This was intended first to bar "lunatics and others unable to care for themselves," but the following year "persons suffering from loathsome and contagious diseases" were added. In that year Congress also provided quasi-military status for the personnel of the Marine Hospital Service, who were given commissions and uniforms.

The National Quarantine Conventions. At this point one should turn back a few years to the mid-nineteenth century. Those concerned with public health in America felt a need for closer, more effective contact to solve problems of mutual concern. Because of the efforts especially of Wilson Jewell, the health officer of Philadelphia who had recently attended the Conference Sanitaire in Paris in 1851-1852, a series of National Quarantine Conventions was called.[25] The first, a 3-day meeting, was held in Philadelphia in 1857. The 54 members in attendance discussed many subjects of common interest, including prevention of the introduction of epidemic diseases such as typhus, cholera, and yellow fever; port quarantine; the importance of stagnant and putrid bilge water; putrescible matters; filthy bedding; baggage and clothing of immigrant passengers; and air that has been confined. It was recommended that immigrants not previously protected against smallpox be vaccinated. The second convention, held in Baltimore in 1858, was noteworthy for proposals for a uniform system of quarantine laws and the organization of a Committee on Internal Hygiene or the Sanitary Arrangement of Cities. In these days, when much is made of multidisciplinary and consumer representation, it is interesting to note that one half of those who attended the second convention were not physicians. Two more conventions were held, in New York, in 1859 and in Boston in 1860, when the outbreak of the American Civil War precluded further meetings.

The American Public Health Association.[26] The seed planted by the quarantine convention did not die. On April 18, 1872, after the termination of the war, 10 men, including Elisha Harris and Stephen Smith, met informally in New York City to reactivate interest in national meetings for the consideration of public health matters. Meeting again at Long Branch, N.J., in September with several additional representatives, they chose a name, adopted a constitution, and elected Dr. Stephen Smith first president of the American Public Health Association. In a later discussion of the early days Smith[27] said, "The American Public Health Association had its origin in that natural desire which thinkers and workers in the same fields, whether of business or philanthropy, or the administration of civil trusts, have for mutual council, advice and cooperation."

Since the National Quarantine Conventions were necessarily concerned primarily with quarantine matters, the formation of the American Public Health Association represented a considerable advance in that the scope of interest was greatly broadened. This was reflected in its earliest meetings, wherein were presented papers on many aspects of sanitation, the transmission and prevention of diseases, quarantine, longevity, hospital hygiene, and other diverse subjects. Through its more than a century of existence, the American Public Health Association has served its members and the public well, providing a common fount of knowledge, information, and advocacy for the improvement of health.

The National Board of Health: its birth and death. An early concern of both the quarantine conventions and the American Public Health Association was the need for a national board of health. Smillie[28] described the circumstances that led to the ultimate formation of such a national board, its controversial 4 years' existence, and its painful, premature death from politically inspired financial starvation. Meetings were held in Washington in 1875 and attended by representatives of many state and city health departments for the purpose of considering plans for the formation of a federal health organization. The meetings degenerated into a jurisdictional dispute involving the army, the navy, and the Marine Hospital Service, the three existing federal agencies that already provided certain services in this field. In 1878 a devastating epidemic of yellow fever swept over much of the country. Since the disease was known to have entered through the port of New Orleans, the Louisiana authorities were charged with laxity. As a result, not only the army and the Marine Hospital Service but also the American Public Health Association sponsored legislation for a national health department. The bill proposed by the American Public Health Association was finally passed by Congress in 1879. It transferred from the Marine Hospital Service all health duties and powers, including maritime quarantine. The act created a board of presidental appointees consisting of seven physicians and representatives from the army, the navy, the Marine Hospital Service, and the Department of Justice. About 2½ months later another act was passed that gave the board extensive quarantine powers and authorized an appropriation of $500,000 for its work. This second act included an unfortunate clause that limited the powers to 4 years, requiring reenactment of the bill for the work to continue.

The membership of the first board was notable; included were J.L. Cabell, J.S. Billings, J.T. Turner, P.H. Bailhoche, S.M. Bemiss, H.I. Bowditch, R.W. Mitchell, Stephen Smith, S.F. Phillips, and T.S. Verdi. The 4 years of life of the National Board of Health were marked by an ambitious and efficient program of studies and services marred by the persistent and vociferous opposition of Joseph Jones, secretary of the Louisiana Board of Health, who objected to the presence of "Federal agents and spies." Jones seized every opportunity to belittle and misrepresent the activities of the National Board of Health. Intent as he was on destroying the new organization, he was saved the trouble by John Hamilton, the Surgeon General of the Marine Hospital Service. Hamilton, although professionally inept, possessed considerable political astuteness. He realized that the National Board of Health would pass out of existence unless the law of 1879 was reenacted in 1883 and that in such an event its powers and functions would revert to the Marine Hospital Service. Accordingly, he worked quietly and effectively to prevent reenactment, charging misuse of funds, extravagance, and incompetence.

From the beginning, one of the members of the board, Stephen Smith, had favored conferring all national public health duties and powers on the National Board of Health but incorporating into it the officers, staff, and activities of the Marine Hospital Service and any other agencies concerned with public health matters. Smillie[28] analyzed the situation in the following terms:

He foresaw that Congress would lose interest in the National Board of Health, but would continue to support a service agency that had full-time career officers and was incorporated as an integral part of national government machinery.

In retrospect we realize that Stephen Smith was right. The unwieldy board of experts, each living in a different community and attempting to carry out administrative duties, with no cohesion, no real unity of opinion and no central authority, was an impossible administrative machine. A centrally guided service, such as actually developed, had unity and purpose, but unfortunately lacked intelligent leadership. The public health policies for a great nation for many years were determined solely by the opinions—sometimes the whims and personal prejudices—of a single individual. It would have been a much better plan in Dr. Stephen Smith's half-formulated plan on 1883 could have been carried out, thus salvaging the really important features of the National Board of Health and incorporating in it a service agency with a full-time personnel, an esprit de corps, and a strong central administrative machine. The members of the Board of Health selected by the President of the United States

because they were public health experts, should have been continued as a Board of Health and should have served as a permanent policy-forming body, advising and aiding their administrative officer. The Marine Hospital Service was the most logical existing national agency with which to vest this national public health function. The Surgeon General should have been made the executive officer of the board, and all actual administrative responsibility should have been centered in him. It was a great opportunity to have organized a close-knit, effective National Health Service, but there was no single man who had the vision or the power to solve this simple problem.

These events are of particular interest in view of recent pressures to establish a separate cabinet-level Department of Health.

The Public Health Service. In 1902, recognizing that the responsibilities of the Marine Hospital Service had been greatly broadened, Congress renamed it the Public Health and Marine Hospital Service and gave it a definite form of organization under the direction of a Surgeon General. The reorganization act was of further significance in that for the first time the Surgeon General was authorized and directed to call an annual conference of all state and territorial health officers. In 1912 the service was renamed the U.S. Public Health Service.

From this point on the Public Health Service grew rapidly under the impetus of an increasingly complex society, several great wars and national emergencies, and economic depressions. In 1917 the National Leprosarium at Carville, La., was established. In the same year the service became responsible for the physical and mental examination of all arriving aliens. The year 1917 was also noteworthy for a congressional appropriation of $25,000 to the Public Health Service for studies and demonstrations in rural health work in cooperation with states. This modest appropriation represented the beginning of a new administrative approach in federal-state public health relationships. In 1918, because of problems brought to public awareness by involvement in World War I, a Division of Venereal Diseases was created, with power to cooperate with state departments of health for the control and prevention of these diseases. In 1929 a Narcotics Division, later expanded to the Division of Mental Hygiene, was created with hospital facilities at Lexington, Ky., and Fort Worth, Tex., for the confinement and treatment of narcotic addicts.

The Social Security Act. The 1930s were years of great social ferment. In 1935 the Social Security

Act was passed. It set in motion many developments of far-reaching consequence. Title VI of the act, which related to the Public Health Service, was written "for the purpose of assisting states, counties, health districts, and other policital subdivisions of the states in establishing and maintaining adequate public health service, including the training of personnel for state and local health work. . . ." Associated with the act was an appropriation that made possible grants-in-aid to the states and territories according to budgets submitted to and approved by the Surgeon General. This created the difficult administrative problem of determining an equitable basis on which to distribute grant-in-aid funds. Although subject to frequent adaptation, an attempt was, and is, made in general to allocate these funds on the basis of four factors: (1) population, (2) public health problems, (3) economic need, and (4) training of public health personnel. This allocation of funds has been of educational value for state legislators, since many grants-in-aid must be matched by state and local appropriations. Results were rapidly forthcoming. Within 1 year after funds were first made available, not only was there a great increase in the number of new local health departments but in addition many states began to strengthen and expand their health programs significantly. In 1938 a second Federal Venereal Disease Control Act was passed, designed to promote the investigation and control of venereal diseases and to provide funds for assistance to state and local health agencies in establishing and maintaining adequate programs. One significant result was the breaking of a long-standing "silence barrier" concerning these diseases by Surgeon General Parran.

In 1939, as part of President Roosevelt's program for the reorganization and consolidation of federal services, a Federal Security Agency (now the Department of Health and Human Services) was created for the purpose of bringing together many of the health, welfare, and educational services of the federal government. After 141 years, only 9 year less than the life of the nation itself, the Public Health Service left the anachronistic administrative jurisdiction of the Treasury Department. At that time the service had the following 8 divisions, each under an assistant surgeon general:

> Division of Scientific Research (including the National Institute of Health and the National Cancer Institute)

> Division of Domestic Quarantine (including State Relations)
> Division of Foreign and Insular Quarantine
> Division of Sanitary Reports and Statistics
> Division of Marine Hospitals and Relief
> Division of Mental Hygiene
> Division of Venereal Disease Control
> Division of Personnel and Accounts

Meanwhile many other developments of consequence occurred. In 1946, at the end of World War II, Congress passed the Hospital Services and Construction (Hill-Burton) Act, which gave the Public Health Service administrative responsibility for a nationwide program of hospital and health center construction. This marked the first major attempt to redevelop health institutions. For many years thereafter, Congress appropriated substantial amounts of monies for this purpose. State or local funds had to match federal contributions by one to two thirds. In 1954 Congress extended the program to permit federal assistance in the construction of other types of health facilities as well as hospitals and health centers. Included were general hospitals, mental hospitals, tuberculosis hospitals, chronic disease hospitals, public health centers, diagnostic and treatment centers, rehabilitation facilities, nursing homes, state health laboratories, and nurse training facilities. The construction need is now considered essentially met, and a shift is underway toward a program of low-interest loans for improvement and modernization.

Research: the National Institutes of Health. The research activities of the Public Health Service date back to 1887, when a one-room Laboratory of Hygiene was established in the Marine Hospital on Staten Island. Initially this laboratory was devoted to bacteriologic studies of returning seamen. It grew slowly to become the National Hygienic Laboratory, later renamed the National Institute of Health in Bethesda, Md., about 10 miles from Washington. From these humble beginnings developed the greatest public health and medical research center in the world. Fortunately, from the start it was developed with great skill, imagination, and foresight. Originally organized by three divisions of chemistry, zoology, and pharmacology, the National Institute of Health's functions were expanded in 1912 by an act that authorized it to "study and investigate the diseases of man and conditions influencing the origin and spread thereof including sanitation and sewage, and the pollution directly or indirectly of navigable streams and lakes of the United States and may from time to time issue information in the form of publications for the use of the public." Under consistently able direction, it attracted and developed a steady stream of outstanding investigators, including Carter, Sternberg, Rosenau, Goldberger, Frost, Leake, Armstrong, Stiles, Lumsden, Francis, Spencer, Maxcy, and Dyer, to name only a few. The contributions of these men and their coworkers caused William H. Welch to state publicly that there was no research institute in the world that was making such distinguished contributions to basic research in biology, medicine, and public health. Testimony to this is provided by the fact that through 1976, the research of 66 Nobel laureates throughout the world have been financed by the National Institutes of Health. Included are several members of its staff.

In 1937 Congress indicated its concern over a rapidly growing health problem by passing the National Cancer Act, which provided for the establishment of a National Cancer Institute for research into the causes, diagnosis, and treatment of cancer; for assistance of public and private agencies involved with the problem; and for the promotion of the most effective methods of prevention and treatment of the disease. In subsequent years public and congressional concern led to the establishment of a series of additional institutes for heart, lung, and blood disorders; microbiology, experimental biology, and medicine (these three later joined to address allergic and infectious diseases); dental research; mental health (now a separate entity, the Alcoholism, Drug Abuse, and Mental Health Administration); neurologic diseases and blindness (later separated into the Eye Institute and the Institute of Neurological and Communicative Disorders and Stroke); arthritis and metabolic and digestive diseases; general medical sciences; child health and human development; and environmental health sciences. Partway through this development it was recognized that the specialized institutes should be interrelated, so in 1948 the overall name was pluralized to become the National Institutes of Health. It now constitutes the greatest health and disease research complex in the world, supporting research not only within its many walls but also in many

universities and other pertinent organizations in the United States and other nations.

To accelerate research and its confirmation and final application, the Public Health Service in 1953 completed and opened the National Clinical Center on the grounds of the National Institutes of Health in Bethesda, Md. This is a research hospital of almost 600 beds, with twice as much space for laboratories as for patient care. When a problem is selected, the methods of approach are determined by a research team, which may include scientists from more than one institute and from other research organizations. Special provisions are made so that outstanding laboratory scientists and research physicians from other institutions in the United States or abroad may work in the center for periods ranging from a few months to a year or more on problems of their own choosing.

To return for a moment of 1956, another significant event was the transfer of the U.S. Army Medical Library to the Public Health Service and its later development into a greatly expanded National Library of Medicine on the grounds of the National Institutes of Health. In 1968 the library became a constituent of the institutes complex. An innovative activity at the library has been the development of the computer-based MEDLARS (Medical Literature Analysis and Retrieval System), which is a computerized bibliographic service to assist users in the library itself or in selected medical centers in the nation as well as abroad by means of satellites in obtaining prompt bibliographies and abstracts of material pertinent to their subject of interest. The service is increasingly important because of the inability of conventional methods to keep current with the tremendous growth of medical literature.

To further meet these needs there also was developed the National Center for Biomedical Communications (named after the late Senator Lister Hill) and a National Medical Audiovisual Center. In 1968, recognizing the importance of international collaboration, Congress established the Fogarty International Center for Advanced Study in the Health Sciences as part of the National Institutes of Health. Here, leading scholars in the health field from any part of the world may study and carry out investigations in residence.

Mention should be made of several other important post-World War II additions to the Public Health Service. One was the development of the National Office of Vital Statistics, later renamed the National Center for Health Statistics. It provides a vast amount of detailed data concerning health, illness, injuries, and death.

The Center(s) for Disease Control. Of great significance was the establishment during World War II of the Communicable Disease Center in Atlanta, Ga., This renowned institution, now known as the National Centers for Disease Control, has grown to become not only one of the world's great epidemiologic centers but also an outstanding training center for various types of health personnel and a leading center for health communications and educational methods. In 1954 the Taft Sanitary Engineering Center was established in Cincinnati as a focus for research and training in environmental health. In 1966 this institution and the responsibility for water pollution control were transferred to a new Federal Water Pollution Administration in the Department of Interior and subsequently in 1971, in company with most of the other environmental programs of the Public Health Service, to a new Environmental Protection Agency. In 1971 a National Center for Toxicological Research was established at Pine Bluff, Ark., under the direction of the Food and Drug Administration, which by this time had become part of the Public Health Service.

Legislation. Congressional interest in health has not been limited to research. During recent years, Congress has shown increasing concern about the prompt application of acquired knowledge for the well-being of the people. The Eighty-ninth Congress was especially notable in this regard. It had the distinction of being known as the most "health minded" Congress in the history of the nation.[29] An astounding number of legislative acts passed by it and subsequent Congresses, if wisely used, will completely recast the nature, structure, and effectiveness of public health, medical care, and social security in the United States. Forgotson[30] has observed,

The deep and long-term significance of the 1965 federal health legislation . . . lies in the changing role of government in the direction of widening the responsibility of the public sector (as exemplified by the Medicare amendments) and in developing new patterns of medical service and continuing education (as exemplified by the Regional Medical Programs). The introduction of systems engineering and operations analysis into the total health endeavor will permit the development of sound priorities, effective controls, and improved administration. Comprehensive legislation covering every facet of resources and services make 1965 the turning point in health legislation.

The cumulative effect of the foregoing developments has been a remarkable growth in the size and usefulness of the health component of the Department of Health and Human Service. This growth may be illustrated in terms of expenditures. In 1900 the budget of the Marine Hospital Service was about $1.4 million. In 1950 the budget of the Public Health Service was almost $120 million; by 1960 it was about $300 million; and by 1980 it had reached more than $8 billion.

In summary, it is fair to state that through the years since 1798, great responsibilities have been placed on the Public Health Service. It is fortunately appropriate to state that throughout its long history the service has met its responsibilities and opportunities as a governmental agency remarkably well, as is readily evident from its admirable record. It is probable that no one in the nation passes a day without being affected beneficially by this agency's efforts in some way.

The Children's Bureau. The conception, establishment, development, and fate of this specialized agency provides a valuable case study for students of public administration. Although on the surface it is concerned with matters of noncontroversial nature, the bureau from its inception was a principal in many disputes and the target of several administrative and ideologic struggles.

The idea of a separate Children's Bureau was first suggested to President Theodore Roosevelt. As pointed out by Julia Lathrop,[31] who served as the first chief of the bureau from 1912 to 1921, it was no coincidence that "this bureau was first urged by women who have lived long in settlements and who by that experience have learned to know as well as any person in the country certain aspects of dumb misery which they desired through some governmental agency to make articulate and intelligible."

Support came promptly from the National Consumers League, the National Child Labor Committee, and many national women's organizations and church groups. Arguing for a center of research and information concerning the welfare of mothers and children, they maintained an active lobby and pressure group in Washington until their goal was ultimately obtained. An effective argument was that the federal government had already set a precedent by establishing centers of research and information in other fields relating to national resources and that it might well become similarly concerned with its most important resource, the mothers and children of the nation. Between 1906 and 1912 many bills concerned with the establishment of a Children's Bureau were introduced, and extensive hearings were held. Both Presidents Theodore Roosevelt and Taft supported the movement, which incurred little opposition. Eventually Congress was spurred to final action and passed a measure* sponsored by Senator Borah on April 9, 1912.

One reason for delay was controversy over the placement of the bureau in the federal govenmental structure. The three possibilities suggested were the Bureau of Labor and the Bureau of the Census, both in the then Department of Commerce and Labor, and the Bureau of Education in the Department of the Interior. It is significant that the U.S. Public Health Service, then in the Treasury Department, was not considered, apparently because of the submergence of the health aspects by the broader social welfare aspects of the proposed bureau. The failure on the part of the Public Health Service to concern itself with the problem at the time was to lay the groundwork for subsequent controversies over administrative jurisdiction and organization.

The act that established the Children's Bureau placed it in the Department of Commerce and Labor. When this department was divided the next year, the bureau was retained by the Department of Labor. The act directed that the "said Bureau shall investigate and report . . . upon all matters pertaining to the welfare of children and child life, among all classes of people, and shall especially investigate the questions of infant mortality, the birth rate, orphanages, juvenile courts, desertions, dangerous occupations, accidents, and diseases of children, employment, legislation affecting children in the several states and territories." Although originally given authority merely to *investigate* and *report,* the Children's Bureau trained a highly technical staff of experts who rapidly gained in experience. The bureau thus became the natural agency to be entrusted with new programs dealing with problems of maternal and child welfare. During the early years of its existence, the bureau, in accord

*37 Stat. 79, 737, 1912.

with Congressional direction, followed a path of extensive and fruitful scientific research and dissemination of information. Many studies were made of the effect of income, housing, employment, and other factors on the infant and maternal mortality rates. These studies led to the White House Conferences on child health, the first of which was held in 1919. Meanwhile, evidence gathered in some of the investigations was used by the National Child Labor Committee in obtaining the passage of the Federal Child-Labor Law in 1915. This law, with the Children's Bureau designated as the administering agency, was effective from 1917 to 1918, when it was declared unconstitutional by the Supreme Court.

Study of maternal and infant care problems of rural areas led to the introduction of proposed national legislation to encourage the establishment of maternal and child welfare programs by means of grants-in-aid to the states. The Children's Bureau, designated in the bills as the administering and supervising agency, quickly found itself the subject of attacks from several quarters. It was argued that the adoption of the Sheppard-Towner Bill would provide an entering wedge for socialized medicine, that is would centralize power in the hands of federal bureaucrats, and that personal, family, and states' rights would be violated. The American Medical Association, the Anti-Suffragists, the Sentinels of the Republic, and several other organizations arrayed themselves in opposition.

During the hearings a controversy that had begun to smolder between the Public Health Service and the Children's Bureau broke through. Some of the opponents of the bill were willing to compromise by favoring administration by the Public Health Service. The decision depended on whether the chief concern of the bill was with health or with general child welfare. Congress, deciding on the broader viewpoint, retained the Children's Bureau as the administering agency when final approval was given in 1921. One authority[32] has pointed out that unquestionably the bureau was able to maintain its position "by right of discovery and occupation and that the Public Health Service had been derelict in not promoting this type of work with sufficient vigor to maintain its belated claim to jurisdiction." This conclusion merits careful reading by present-day public health administrators. When a new health program is proposed, one of the first concerns is with the agency of administration; and the proposing or initiating agency usually is favored.

The Sheppard-Towner Act established a pattern for maternal and child health programs throughout the country. It provided federal grants-in-aid assistance to states to attack problems of maternal and infant welfare and mortality. The states were given authority to initiate and administer their own plans subject to approval by a Federal Board of Maternity and Infant Hygiene, consisting of the Chief of the Children's Bureau, the Surgeon General of the Public Health Service, and the Commissioner of Education. Before the passage of the act, 32 states had established divisions or bureaus of child hygiene. During the following 2 years an additional 15 states developed programs of this nature. Although it is difficult to prove, the Children's Bureau is generally given major credit for the increased interest and action.

The original act provided for a 5-year program. In 1926 a bill was introduced for an extension of the act to 7 years. This provided opponents with another opportunity for attack. The 2-year extension that was granted signaled the end of the program. The importance of the federal aid was well illustrated by the fact that after expiration of the program, 35 states decreased appropriations, 9 states eliminated appropriations, and only 5 states reported increases for maternal and child health programs.

With the adoption of the Social Security Act in 1935 the Children's Bureau not only regained its lost functions but added to them. Under Title V, Part 4, of the Social Security Act, the Children's Bureau was given responsibility for the administration of programs dealing with maternal and child health, crippled children, and child welfare services. To implement these ends, the bureau was allotted an annual budget of $8.17 million for grants-in-aid exclusive of administrative costs. In 1939 this sum was increased to $11 million and in 1946 to $22 million. Within 10 months after the grants-in-aid became available, all of the 48 states, the District of Columbia, and the then territories of Alaska and Hawaii submitted requests and plans for approval. In this way state maternal and child health programs received a much needed financial transfusion.

Through time there has been ample evidence of the success of the pioneering and stimulating efforts of the Children's Bureau. Thus in 1940 federal contributions accounted for 48% of the total sum spent for maternal and child health activities; since then, state and local governments have assumed increasing proportions of the costs.

With the entrance of the United States into World War II and the subsequent draft of a large proportion of the male population, many wives, expectant mothers, and infants found themselves in somewhat precarious economic positions. This was reflected in their inability to pay for private obstetric and medical care. The Children's Bureau made Congress aware of the problem; and as a result, an Act for the Emergency Maternity and Infant Care for the Wives and Children of Servicemen was passed. The Children's Bureau was designated as the administering agency. Once again the factor of prior interest and occupation decided the issue of administrative jurisdiction. The Children's Bureau had attempted, to the best of its ability and using some of its grants-in-aid funds, to do what it could to alleviate the situation. Congress decided to take action by means of supplementing the grants-in-aid funds of the bureau. As a result, a series of appropriation acts was passed, involving a total of more than $130 million. The use of these sums made possible the provision of much needed obstetric care for about 1.2 million expectant mothers and pediatric care for about 200,000 infants. It is of interest that the Children's Bureau quickly made the services as comprehenisve as possible within the limits of the legislation. Another significant result was that the staffs of the Children's Bureau and of many state health departments obtained valuable experience in health care administration.

The Children's Bureau continued to expand its leadership in many fields, including audiology, perinatal mortality, prematurity, rheumatic fever, epilepsy, cerebral palsy, mental retardation, juvenile delinquency, nutrition of growth and development, problems of children of migratory workers, and childrens dentistry.[33] It shared significantly in the momentous legislative advances of the mid-1960s. Because of increased awareness and concern about the relatively high rate of perinatal mortality as well as premature births, handicapping conditions, and mental retardation, Congress passed the Maternal and Child Health and Mental Retardation Planning Amendments of 1963. This law authorized project grants to meet up to 75% of the costs of projects to provide comprehensive maternity care for high-risk mothers in low-income families and to provide care for their children. Two years later in 1965, when Section 532 of Title V, Part 4, of the Social Security Act was amended, provision was made for the development of high-quality comprehensive health services for children and youth.

The combined objective of these two pieces of legislation was to reduce maternal, infant, and child morbidity by assisting communities to organize and use their services and resources to maximum efficiency. For improved maternal and infant care, funds were used for the establishment of prenatal and postpartum clinics, hospitalization, medical salaries or fees, salaries of public health nurses, health education, and various other services. The Social Security Amendments of 1965 made possible some major departures from traditional public health services. Comprehensiveness and continuity of care were stressed. There was no separation of preventive and promotive health services from treatment and rehabilitation, nor were services limited to particular illness categories. All health problems of the children involved were covered by the program, either by direct services or by referral to appropriate resources. Medical, dental, and emotional health problems were all included, and since particular emphasis was placed on children of families often unaccustomed to seeking care, outreach casefinding was provided. These two programs were especially needed in areas where there were many people of low incomes and where there were likely to be few practitioners of medicine and dentistry, a situation common to city slums. These efforts attempted to bring convenient, well-organized, comprehensive health services to those who needed them the most and obtained them the least. In the process, health agencies in many cities developed new, interesting, and effective working relationships with medical schools and other organizations in their jurisdictions. Furthermore, wherever programs were subsequently developed under the aegis of the Economic Opportunity Act to assist the socioeconomically disadvantaged, attempts were made to coordinate them with the maternal and child health programs.

Despite these valiant efforts, those in a position to watch noted that the Bureau's identity was being whittled away. Early in 1963, soon after its fiftieth anniversary, the Children's Bureau became part of a new Welfare Administration in the Department of Health, Education, and Welfare. Subseqently, in August 1967 it became part of another new major unit in the department, the Social and Rehabilitation Service, which also included the functions of the former Welfare Administration, the Vocational Rehabilitation Administration, the Administration on Aging, and the Mental Retardation Division of the Public Health Service. This new agency was designed to join under single leadership both the income-support programs for those in need and the social service and rehabilitation programs required by many individuals and families. Eventually, in 1973 the health functions of the Children's Bureau were split off to form the Maternal and Child Health Program of the present Bureau of Community Health Services in the Health Resources and Services Administration of the Public Health Service.

The Food and Drug Administration. The first efforts of the federal government to bring about control and supervision of the quality of foods were in 1879 when a bill was introduced in Congress to prohibit the adulteration of food and drink. This and several subsequent efforts came to naught, and 27 years passed before successful action was achieved. The present Food and Drug Administration grew out of a unique combination of efforts.[34] The major roles were played by a dedicated and determined public servant, Dr. Harvey Wiley of the Bureau of Chemistry of the Department of Agriculture; several concerned professional societies, notably the American Medical Association and the American Pharmaceutical Association; two widely read popular magazines, the Ladies Home Journal and Colliers; and a well-known crusading writer, Upton Sinclair. The greatest share of the credit for the ultimate success of the difficult pure food and drug movement goes to Wiley for his tireless campaigning and to Sinclair for his famous book, *The Jungle*. The book became an overnight best seller, was translated into 47 languages, and made its socialist author a wealthy man.[35] Despite great opposition from lobbies representing the canning industry, drug and whiskey interests, and those who manufactured and sold a vast array of proprietary medicines, bills were introduced and finally passed by Congress; and on June 30, 1906, the Pure Food and Drugs Act was signed into law by President Theodore Roosevelt.

The legislation resulted in the establishment of

a program to supervise and control the circumstances of manufacture, labeling, and sale of food. The responsibility was given to the Bureau of Chemistry of the Department of Agriculture, with Dr. Wiley in charge. Subsequent acts greatly broadened the program to include not only food, meat, and dairy products but also pharmaceuticals, cosmetics, toys, and numerous household products and appliances. In 1927 the Secretary of Agriculture recommended the establishment of a Food and Drug Administration to administer all of the accumulating responsibilities. As time passed, it became increasingly obvious that the legislation needed updating. As a result, on June 25, 1938, President Franklin Roosevelt signed the present Federal Food, Drug, and Cosmetic Act. Two years later the agency was transferred from the Department of Agriculture to the Federal Security Agency (now the Department of Health and Human Services) as an integral unit. Subsequently, in 1968 it was made one of the basic components of the Public Health Service.

SUMMARY

There appear to have been three critical turning points in the history and development of public health in the United States. It is interesting that they have been about 50 years, or two generations, apart: the 1860s, when the Shattuck Report began to exert an influence; the 1910s, when the groundwork was laid for so much of the public health development since; and the 1960s, when public health really began to broaden its horizons and abandon the barrier between it and medical care and when Congress decided to make undreamed-of accomplishments possible. It would appear that public health has now come of age.

REFERENCES

1. Rosen, G.: A history of public health, New York, 1958, MD Publications, Inc.
2. Top, F.H.: The history of American epidemiology, St. Louis, 1952, The C.V. Mosby Co.
3. Hanlon, J., Rogers, F., and Rosen, G.: A bookshelf on the history and philosophy of public health, Am. J. Public Health **50:**445, April 1960.
4. Osler, W.: The functions of a state faculty, Maryland Med. J. **37:**73, May 1897.
5. Quigley, C.: The evolution of civilizations, Indianapolis, 1979, Liberty Fund, Inc.
6. Chambers, J.: The devil's horsemen: the Mongol invasion of Europe, New York, 1979, Athenum Publishers.
7. Hecker, I.F.: The epidemics of the Middle Ages, Philadelphia, 1837, Haswell, Barrington & Haswell.
8. Winslow, C.-E.A.: The evolution and significance of the modern public health campaign, New Haven, 1923, Yale University Press.
9. George, M.D.: London life in the XVIIIth century, New York, 1925, Alfred A, Knopf.
10. Richardson, B.W.: The health of nations, a review of the works of Edwin Chadwick, vol. 2, London, 1887, Longmans, Green & Co.
11. Bowditch, H.I.: Address on hygiene and preventive medicine. Transactions of the International Medical Congress, Philadelphia, 1876.
12. Prescott, W.H.: History of the conquest of Mexico, New York, 1936, Random House, Inc.
13. Woodward, S.B.: The story of smallpox in Massachusetts, N. Engl. J. Med. **206:**1181, June 9, 1932.
14. Marr, J.: Merchants of death: the role of the slave trade in the transmission of disease from Africa to the Americas, Pharos, Winter 1982, p. 31.
15. Chadwick, H.D.: The diseases of the inhabitants of the commonwealth, N. Engl. J. Med. **216:**8, June 10, 1937.
16. Rosen, G.: Benjamin Rush on health and the American revolution, Am. J. Public Health **66:**397, April 1976.
17. Newsholme, A., Sir: The ministry of health, London, 1925, G.P. Putnam's Sons, Ltd.
18. Kramer, H.D.: The beginnings of the public health movement in the United States, Bull. Hist. Med. **21:**369, 1947.
19. Holmes, O.W.: Writings, IX, medical essays, Boston, 1891, Houghton Mifflin Co.
20. Shattuck, L., and others: Report of the Sanitary Commission of Massachusetts: 1850 (Dutton & Wentworth, State Printers, Boston, 1850), Cambridge, 1948, Harvard University Press.
21. Beck-Storrs, A.: Public health and government control, Soc. Stud. **45:**211, Oct. 1954.
22. Boccaccio, M.: Ground itch and dew poison: the Rockefeller Sanitary Commission, 1909-1914. J. Hist Med. **27:**30, Jan. 1972.
23. Patterson, R.S., and Baker, M.C.: Seventy-five years of public health in Massachusetts, Am. J. Public Health **34:**1271, Dec. 1944.
24. Williams, R.C.: The United States Public Health Service 1798-1950, Washington, D.C., 1951, Commissioned Officers Association of the United States Public Health Service.
25. Cavins, H.M.: The National Quarantine and Sanitary Conventions of 1857 to 1860 and the beginnings of the American Public Health Association, Bull. Hist. Med. **13:**404, April 1943.
26. Bernstein, N.R.: APHA, the first one hundred years,

Washington, D.C., 1972, American Public Health Association.

27. Smith, S.: Historical sketch of the American Public Health Association, Public Health **5:**7, 1889.

28. Smillie, W.G.: The National Board of Health, 1879-1883, Am. J. Public Health **33:**925, Aug. 1943.

29. Rusk, H.: Congress and medicine, The New York Times, Nov. 20, 1965.

30. Forgotson, E.: 1965: The turning point in public health law—1966 reflections, Am. J. Public Health **57:**934, June 1967.

31. Lathrop, J.C.: Children's Bureau, Am. J. Sociol. **18:**318, Nov. 1912.

32. Key, V.O.: The administration of federal grants to states, Chicago, 1937, Public Administration Service.

33. Eliot, M.M.: The Children's Bureau, fifty years of public responsibility for action in behalf of children, Am. J. Public Health **52:**576, April 1962.

34. Janssen, W.F.: Food and Drug Administration: 75 years later, Public Health Rep. **96:**487, Nov.-Dec. 1981.

35. Kantor, A.F.: Upton Sinclair and the Pure Food and Drugs Act of 1906, Am. J. Public Health **66:**1202, Dec. 1976.

CHAPTER 3

Culture, behavior, and health

Why do you laugh? Change but the name, and the story is told of you.

Horace
Satires, I.

THE HUMAN FACTOR

Each of us tends to view his or her interests as of paramount significance. There is some danger therefore that health workers may consider their professional goals as ends in themselves and the activities required for their achievement as necessarily of primary interest to society. If they do, disappointment and disillusionment are inevitable. This is particularly true if goals have been determined arbitrarily and activities planned and carried out by "experts," who themselves are necessarily biased, without concern for the needs, ideas, and wishes of the group to be served. The group or public may look on the goals and activities quite differently. Furthermore, for reasons of pride, cohesion, or even survival, the group may be forced into the psychologic position of objection or resistance.

Actually, although health is a common need and the effort to attain it represents a common drive, it is of secondary rather than primary importance. Even primitive man is concerned with the achievement of a total or integrated way of life. Because of the complexity of its ingredients, this is not easy to define. Some distinctions are possible, however, especially through study of certain situations such as primitive societies and societies under stress. In such circumstances it soon becomes clear that although people and their societies are subject to many needs, urges, or drives, only a few of these are primary or basic (i.e., the need for food, for shelter, and for sexual expression or propagation). As for many other goals, of which health is only one, most individuals and society in general are interested only to the extent that they make possible the achievement of related goals, especially those that are primary in nature. As this is written, much

of the world is confronted by a complex of economic problems that is exerting limitations on both national and individual expenditures for many important things including health. In the United States, almost half of the families surveyed said they were spending less on essential health care and health products to cope with inflation. Among minority families the figure was 60%, and for single parent families it was 72%. Twelve percent of families said they were less concerned about health than they were a few years earlier.[1]

Comfort, the absence of pain, and well-being are relative terms. Thus in societies where the majority acquire malaria or trachoma, these conditions tend to be regarded as part of the normal pattern of life and are adapted to as well as possible. Under such circumstances ill health tends to be considered as the presence of any condition that is unusual or beyond these. Furthermore, one must recognize the intimate and meaningful relationships in many cultures of individuals in the present with those in the past, as well as with the many natural forces around them. As a consequence, disease may be regarded not so much as something to be controlled or cured but as something to be understood and acknowledged as part of the plan of life and nature. As Kaufman[2] has written, "The totality of the organism and its adaptiveness . . . can be placed in a frame of reference which is truly psychobiological Psychogenesis, ontogenesis and ecology, each with its proper weight and each unique for the particular individual involved, remain the bases for understanding the functioning of the individual in health and disease."

This is put into another dimension by Dreitzel,[3] who indicates that since there is no objective definition of illness, one must ask in whose interest and for what purpose "illness" is defined by different social classes and ethnic and religious groups. Generally illness tends to be defined by patients as any impairment of their physical well-being that conforms with what society tends to accept as "being sick." Merely to feel unwell does not suffice if the individual is not seriously disabled for work or social interaction. "Only then," Dreitzel concludes, "does unwell become socially accepted and the role of the patient is granted, entitling the afflicted to attention, care and protection."

Earlier it was said that humans will strive for food, shelter, and sexual expression in the absence of complete health, but they will not strive for complete health in the absence of the others. A few examples may help to place the desire for health in its proper perspective. A man and woman stranded on an island will ordinarily seek to assure themselves of food, shelter, and sexual satisfaction before giving attention to other needs. In most instances they will seek to satisfy these three needs or urges in the order given because of the differing critical intervals involved. Furthermore, they will do so in the face of actual or potential threats to their health or safety. Thus if the only source of food or of materials for shelter is in or near an insalubrious spot, they will still seek them out. Later, perhaps, they may seek out a more desirable alternative.

With regard to sexual expression and health, the venereal diseases could probably be eradicated by universal abstinence from sexual intercourse. The chances of this being followed are obviously nil because when faced with a choice between the two, the risk of infection would be accepted by the majority. This example is more than theoretical, since the suggestion has been made on more than one occasion to individuals or special groups to no avail.

An example of health being relegated to a secondary position for economic reasons was encountered in relation to technical assistance activities in malaria control in North Africa. In certain areas the date is the basic element in the food supply and economy. Despite the recognized relief from malaria, spraying was opposed in some communities because the insecticide DDT killed not only the malaria-transmitting *Anopheles* but also the species of fly that carried pollen from the male to the female

date palm. To assure both desirable ends, modifications in control techniques had to be developed. By like token, economic objections to environmental control of air, water, and soil pollution are also notoriously common.

Sometimes public health or medical deterrents to death may be regarded as undesirable. This may come as a shock to those accustomed to regarding health and the preservation of life as universally desired goals. When conditions for life and survival are difficult and especially when disease and premature death are common, the social attitude toward death may differ from one's own. In some cultures, death of infants or the aged is not necessarily a grievous event. The infant does not yet have a fully developed personality and may be regarded as an added economic burden to the family. The child's timely removal may mean more food and other things for the rest of the family and less suffering and misery for itself in the long run. This is sometimes evidenced in funeral ceremonies in societies with high death rates.

The difference between the funeral of a productive adult and that of a very young child or of an elderly person is striking. In the former there usually is genuine regret shown by the mourners. The adult has been around long enough to be known by others as a personality. Beyond this, the death is recognized as the economic loss of a producer for the family and the group. In funerals of elderly persons there is again genuine regret, but not as much as in the former case. True, the elderly individual's personality is well-known and familiar in the local scene. However, they have served their social and economic purpose by working, by producing offspring, and by transmitting the mores of the group. They now have become an economic and even a social burden that has to be supported. Furthermore, they are now entitled to their well-earned release to the rewards and security of the hereafter. In the case of infants and young children, the difference may be even greater. Many are not named until their first birthday. In the case of death there may be relatively little mourning. The funeral procession may appear bright and, in some cultures, even rather joyous. Songs may be sung, bands may play, and when the small body is finally removed, there may be a social event, with feasting, drinking, dancing, visiting, and other forms of social interaction. Even in more sophisticated societies, gradations of these differences in attitudes may be observed. Suffice to point to the often expressed ameliorating comment that a deceased child was "pure of heart" and hence much more likely to achieve everlasting happiness.

In his review of life in England and western Europe between 1500 and 1800, Stone[4] described the callous and even cruel attitudes toward children that coincide with the foregoing. Infants (below the age of 2 years) were regarded as scarcely human, "smelly, noisy little creatures, driven by instinct, not reason, incapable of communicating except at the animal level and with only the most precarious hold on life." It was logical not to be particularly concerned about them, and very few were. After all, it was easy enough to get more of them at no cost, unlike livestock, which had a clear economic value. Stone points to the lack of emotional response to the death of children. He found ". . . no evidence of the purchase of mourning—not even an armband—on the death of very small children in the sixteenth, seventeenth and early eighteenth centuries, nor of parental attendance at the funeral." Even if the infant survived, there was little subsequent contact between them and their parents because of the common practice by all classes of society of "fostering out" the young children to live with and usually work for other families. Fortunately these destructive attitudes began to change to some extent during the nineteenth century.

Finally, attention is directed to certain societies in which to be ill and suffering is to be considered saintly or godlike. In addition, there are groups or cultures in which it is believed that to become ill and die during a religious pilgrimage assured reward in the hereafter.

The foregoing is not intended to belittle or discourage efforts toward the improvement of public health. Rather, the purpose is to point out that health is a relative concept, that its definition and value vary from one place to another, and that even over time in a given society it is only one facet of the total concern and welfare of the individual and the society. As such it is in constant competition with all other factors of greater or lesser importance to the individual and the society. It is important to realize this because, as Koos[5] has pointed out, "What we can expect a community to provide, and its members to accept, in the way of health activities must therefore be viewed in a framework which is peculiar to that community. This in no way prevents the establishing of uniform goals or standards for health, but it does mean that community efforts directed toward better health are necessarily custom-built."

SOCIAL ANALYSIS

Each of us is many things. First, we are individuals, a composite or compromise of various strengths and weaknesses, interests and prejudices, abilities and failings. But as some philosophers have claimed, perhaps there is no such thing as a true individual. Each of us is the most recent product of a series of generations and environments. Beyond being individuals we are members of families and, beyond that, members of varying numbers and types of social groups with shared and common needs and interests—complexes of interrelated families, the guild, the village, the clan, eventually agglutinating to form various types of cultural and national entities.

Human beings everywhere are members of groups. To varying degrees they are dependent on one another for sustenance, education, inspiration, economic welfare, entertainment, and many other needs. The individual needs the group, but not necessarily only a particular group, or always the same group, or the same group for all needs. The same conditions also apply to the group's need for the individual. Although the bonds that link the individual to the group must be strong if they are to be of value, they are not necessarily fixed. They may be and in fact often are broken or transferred. Accordingly, individuals are seldom found to be members of only one group. Different groups serve different purposes. Although this is less apparent in primitive societies, even there individuals have multigroup attachments—to the family, to a larger kinship group, to a totem group, and to a maturation cult or secret society as well as to the tribe. In more highly developed societies the plurality of group membership is more evident. In addition to the family, there is the school, the church, the social club, the athletic club, the business and professional associations, and many others.

The question arises whether all of these groups are necessary and important or whether, for health promotional purposes or other reasons, it is possible to successfully approach and influence all individuals through one group. Stated otherwise, is it possible to focus all of our interests on one all-important group? Is it possible to have one group that would satisfy all needs? Clearly the answer is found in reality. Innumerable groups exist because people develop them to meet their various and varying needs. An individual requires a social complex of many different groups to obtain sufficient significant or fruitful relationships that will satisfy the various facets of the personality and interests. Repeated attempts have been and continue to be made to relate the complete allegiance of people to one single supergroup, for example, the state. So far in the long run such attempts have failed, and it would appear that all future attempts will experience the same fate. Life devoted exclusively to one group is necessarily extremely narrow and self-limiting. "The man who can live wtihout society," said Aristotle, "is either a beast or a god. But the man who can live exclusively for the state, if indeed such a being exists, is either a tyrant or a slave."

Granted that it is our nature to identify with various groups, how does this affect our behavior and our receptivity to ideas? Important in this regard is that our behavior as individuals is usually different from our behavior as members of a group or of society, and that social or group behavior varies from group to group. Furthermore, when a point of common concern or mutual interest exists and can be adequately identified, widely differing groups may join forces and with regard to that particular interest jointly behave differently from the way each group behaves alone. This does not mean that any one group forfeits its identity. As Skinner[6] has pointed out, "Social behavior arises because one organism is important to another as part of its environment. A first step, therefore, is an analysis of the social environment and of any special features it may possess."

Since the intention here is social analysis for the purpose of community or social organization for public health improvement, it is important to distinguish and identify groups that may be of significance toward that end. There are three general categories of identifiable groups of which we should be constantly aware. They are important because community organization for health cannot be carried on apart from the social worlds in which people for whom it is designed live. Furthermore, community organization cannot ignore the strength of factors that create distinctive values regarding health and that place them high or low in the hierarchy of values that are an essential part of life.

The first of these groups provides for *ethnic identification.* This is represented by racial, nationality, and often religious groups, each with its own prescriptions, prohibitions, and ideals, any one of which may be of significance in relation to health and sickness.

A second category is related to *ethos identification,* that is, bonds that identify individuals as belonging to the same ethical, economic, or social group. Often this is coincident with a neighborhood. The economic, educational, or moral nature of the group may determine the extent or manner of participation in activities designed for the improvement of public health.

Finally, there is the *family,* which usually represents the most powerful example of social cohesion. To ignore the predominant influence of the family in the development or conduct of a public health program usually guarantees failure. The pertinence of Koos'[5] remarks in this regard justifies their repetition here:

We may well question the logic of industry or school-centered programs that ignore the importance of the family as a "conditioner of attitudes," and which may send the individual back into his family to face conflicting ideologies about health and its value. This is not a plea to abandon school- or industry-centered programs; it is to point out that such programs can work effectively only if they send the individual back to his family prepared to adjust differences that may have been engendered; to make him, in effect, a health organizer in his own small family world. If the individual is not so prepared . . . the cost in tensions and frustrations can outweigh any small good the program may have accomplished.

SOCIETY AND CULTURE

In a discussion such as this, it is important to distinguish between society—the subject matter of sociology—and culture—the subject matter of social or cultural anthropology. A society is any community of individuals drawn together by a common bond of nearness and interaction, that is, a group of people who act together in general for the achievement of certain common goals. A society has both quantitative and qualitative characteristics. Thus it is possible to count and measure the number of individuals who constitute a society. One of the qualitative characteristics is its culture or the manner in which the group as a unit tends to think, feel, believe, and react to stimuli;—in other words, its basis for behavior. As Kluckhohn[7] described it,

"A culture refers to the distinctive ways of life of such a group of people . . . a culture constitutes a storehouse of the pooled learning of the group." Simmons and Wolff[8] in turn said that "culture sets the stage, ascribes the parts, and defines the terms whereby society's drama is enacted". On the other hand, one may consider society the instrument, the mechanism, and the organization that provides the environment for a culture to develop, grow, and manifest itself.

Every society has its own distinctive culture, and since there are innumerable societies in each community, in each country, and on each continent, there are therefore innumerable cultures, each differing to a greater or lesser degree from all of the others. The study of these cultures, their components, and their relationships with each other is the subject matter of cultural anthropology, the purpose of which is to aid us in understanding ourselves. Kluckhohn graphically stated, "Anthropology holds up a great mirror to man, and lets him look at himself in his infinite variety." Somewhat the same views have been focused on the health field by Brownlee.[9] According to her, health workers everywhere "need to gain a more complete understanding of both the visible and invisible elements of their own culture, and the culture of the community around them . . . if they are to provide a program that really meets the needs of the community."

Throughout the entire course of human history, every member of our species was born into some sort of culture. Some cultures were primitive, simple, and crude, whereas others were complex and highly developed. Some dwindled and died, whereas others flourished and grew. All of them, however, regardless of their degree of complexity or simplicity, developed techniques, religious beliefs, social systems, and art forms. Every child born and reared in a particular group culture is certain to be influenced more by it than by anything in his entire life. "As a matter of fact," according to White,[10] "his culture will determine how he will think, feel and act. It will determine what language he will speak, what clothes if any he will wear, what gods he will believe in, and how he will marry, select and prepare his foods, treat the sick, and dispose of the dead. What else could one do but react to the culture that surrounds him from birth to death?"

This behavioral determining effect of culture on the individual and the importance of understanding it was emphasized by Benedict.[11]

. . . The life history of the individual is first and foremost an accommodation to the patterns and standards traditionally handed down in his community. From the moment of his birth the customs into which he is born shape his experience and behaviour. By the time he can talk, he is the little creature of his culture, and by the time he is grown and able to take part in its activities, its habits are his habits, its beliefs his beliefs, its impossibilities his impossibilities. Every child that is born into his group will share them with him, and no child born into one on the opposite side of the globe can ever achieve the thousandth part. There is no social problem it is more incumbent upon us to understand than this of the role of custom. Until we are intelligent as to its laws and varieties, the main complicating facts of human life must remain unintelligible.

Also according to Benedict:

The study of different cultures has another important bearing upon present-day thought and behaviour. Modern existence has thrown many civilizations into close contact, and at the moment, the overwhelming response to this situation is nationalism and racial snobbery. There has never been a time when civilization stood more in need of individuals who are genuinely culture-conscious, who can see objectively the socially conditioned behaviour of other peoples, without fear and recrimination.

The importance of culture and the contribution that an awareness of cultural anthropology may make to public health programs have become somewhat more evident to those who have worked in countries other than their own and in the field of international health. They have come to realize, with Carothers,[12] that "the visitor to foreign lands is always most impressed by the general peculiarities of peoples, whereas in his homeland . . . he notices only the individual divergencies." This is a very significant choice of words! It is important to call attention, however, to the often overlooked fact that it is unnecessary to visit foreign or exotic lands to encounter different cultures. It is fundamental that the domestic health worker realize that he too has been born into and has grown up in a particular culture, received his training in possibly still another culture, and in the conduct of his work must deal with additional different cultures in his own community.

It is well to realize that, as Oliver Wendell Holmes so aptly remarked, "The people in every town feel that the axis of the earth passes through its main street." That is why so many tribal and national names, when traced to their origins, are found to mean "the human beings," "the real or principal people," or similar accolades. As Gittler[13] discovered, "The Greenland Eskimo believes that Europeans have been sent to Greenland to learn virtue and good manners from him. Their highest form of praise of an outsider is that he is or soon will be as good as a Greenlander." Exactly the same statement has been made with regard to some immigrants to the United States. It is unnecessary to go to the ends of the earth to find other cultures; we can find them, must understand them, and must live and work with them in our own communities.

In this connection, sound action in a field such as public health requires careful evaluation of circumstances and situations. It is important therefore to recognize that the evaluations of public health workers are colored by their own cultural background.

According to Benedict[11]:

The truth of the matter is that the possible human institutions and motives are legion, on every plane of cultural simplicity or complexity, and that wisdom consists in a greatly increased tolerance toward their divergencies. No man can thoroughly participate in any culture unless he has been brought up and has lived according to its forms, but he can grant to other cultures the same significance to their participants which he recognizes in his own.

What is the purpose of culture? All cultural traits, habits, prejudices, and the like are based essentially on a mixture of conscious and subconscious urges for individuals and group survival and perpetuation. As Kluckhohn[7] has indicated, "Any cultural practice must be functional, or it will disappear before long; that is, it must somehow contribute to the survival of the society or to the adjustment of the individual." Every society has developed institutions and methods of behavior to safeguard and perpetuate the practices and beliefs that its members consider the most important and valuable. In every society, social arrangements or organizations have been developed over long periods of time on the basis of proved group experience to meet life's basic needs. Programs such as public health necessarily involve the introduction of new, strange, and often upsetting practices and changes in these arrangements into the culture of the society. If such

programs are to be constructive rather than disruptive forces, the social structure and the traditional cultural way of life of the community must be taken into account and used.

Not only are the accepted value systems of a culture deeply ingrained but disadvantaged people adhere particularly strongly to their attitudes and beliefs. This is to be expected, since people, who for a long time have been accustomed to crowded living conditions, low economic status, discrimination, and philosophic systems that serve to make life difficult, regard change with misgivings and suspicion (see also *The Ordeal of Change* by Hoffer[14]). Their greatest fear is that things might get worse, and to them, on the basis of their experience, change often implies that very possibility. One is reminded of Plautus' maxim "Keep what you have; the known evil is best."

Advantageous incentives to change and demonstrations of the value of new ideas, techniques, or actions are necessary to overcome the natural reluctance of people to change their ways and to overcome their fear of the possible risks involved in following new practices. They need to have proved to them in one way or another that the suggestions will make possible genuine and lasting improvements in their standard of living. Furthermore, they need to be assisted in their attempts to implement the suggestions made and to integrate them with the rest of their cultural pattern. A public health program must demonstrate to people that the continued improvement in their welfare and level of living is its true purpose. It is insufficient merely to enunciate general principles or objectives of health as if they were the end and to think of the people involved merely as a means to that end. Instead, people must be able to see clearly and unequivocally that the public health activity or program is one that attacks problems not merely in terms of improved community health in the abstract but in terms of all the needs of people with much the same aspirations the world over for their families and for their neighbors.

One aspect of culture that is easily overlooked is that it is much more than a collection of customs; it is a *system* of customs, each one more or less related to the others in a meaningful fashion. A culture has structure as well as content; it is not like a haphazard pile of bricks. This provides a clue to the reason for the tenacity with which societies hold on to their customs. Each one is like a gear in a transmission system, important and necessary for the total function and directly or indirectly related to all of the other gears. As it is impossible to remove a gear from a transmission system and still have the system function without an adequate substitute, so it is impossible to remove a custom from a culture without providing an equally satisfactory or better substitute. This is what Robert Ruark had in mind when he gave the title *Something of Value* to his book about the plight of the natives of late-colonial Kenya.* If the analogy is pursued further, the end result of a transmission system is the product of its component gears, not merely their sum. Similarly a total culture is the product of its component parts or customs—not merely the sum—and if any one basic part is destroyed or reaches zero, the entire culture collapses.

Benedict[11] once narrated a significant and touching anecdote in this regard. She told of her conversations with a chief of the Californian Digger Indians who had been "civilized" and integrated to a greater or lesser degree with Western civilization. He told her of life in earlier times, of the ceremonies, the agriculture, the tribal economy, and of how each of these and other customs were so meaningful to the tribe: "In those days," he said, "his people had eaten 'the health of the desert' and knew nothing of the insides of butchershops." It was such innovations that had degraded his people in the latter days. Then one day he added: "In the beginning God gave to every people a cup, a cup of clay, and from this cup they drank their life. They all dipped in the water, but their cups were different. Our cup is broken now. It has passed away."

In discussing the social disorganization that occurred in the little Guatemalan town of Tiquisate from an ill-conceived experiment in agricultural productive efficiency, Hoyt[15] warned:

The potential economic effects of increasing production cannot be abstracted from the actual psychosocial effects; and it is possible, if we are not careful, that the disorganization accompanying the latter may be greater than the constructive services of the former.

According to her:

If Tiquisate is an outstanding example of productive efficiency, it is also an outstanding example of social disorganization, even to the extent that the latter threatens the former. This is evidenced by a great deal of drunkenness and prostitution—which the people themselves de-

*Ruark, R., Something of value, Garden City, N.Y., 1955, Doubleday & Co., Inc.

plore—by lax family relations, and by strong social antagonisms. . . . Although new values appeared, they did not take the place of the old; neither did they furnish a framework within which the psychic aspects of the people's old life could find their place and get the necessary response.

Some years ago, a similar phenomenon was observed on the island of Bali. The government of the then new nation Indonesia, of which Bali is a part, wanting to take its rightful place in the modern society of nations, apparently deplored any custom that might cause other nations to consider it backward or primitive. It therefore passed a law that required the women of Bali to cover their breasts. According to observers who had lived there for some time, there soon came about a noticeable change in the attitude of Balinese males toward female breasts and toward women, and it is significant that within a brief time after that law was passed prostitution appeared on the island. That a causal relationship actually existed is not possible to determine. The circumstances and timing, however, give one some reason to wonder.

In summary to this point, all human beings are members of societies, each with its own culture consisting of a complex mosaic of interrelated customs. These customs have developed through the ages as a result of group experience in the struggle for survival and for a reasonably satisfactory life. Accordingly, people relinquish customs reluctantly, and it is well that they do; each custom has stood the test of time, and it or a truly adequate substitute is fundamental to the continued existence of the society. The great contribution of cultural anthropology to the conduct of programs in a field such as public health is to constantly identify and point out the importance of cultural patterns of the groups or societies that constitute a community or a nation. Social evolution inevitably disturbs cultural patterns, but that is one price of progress. However, cultural patterns need not and should not be disturbed more deeply or more rapidly than the people involved are able to tolerate and adapt to. This principle should underlie all of the actions of the public health worker.

EFFECT OF CULTURAL FACTORS ON HEALTH

With the foregoing in mind, one may expect that many if not all cultural patterns bear some relationships to the degree of health of a people and the extent to which they will accommodate themselves or be receptive to efforts that might be made to improve their state of health. It is not intended at this point to consider the desirable or positive effects of certain cultural patterns on health or the even more obvious contributions of sound public health measures in general to cultural development. Instead some examples will be given of cultural patterns that may have a disadvantageous effect on the health of a people.

There are many reasons for ill health, only a few of which will be discussed. One easily recognized reason is ignorance or lack of knowledge about the factors involved in the. causation of illness and death. During a period when the infant mortality for the city of Detroit was rapidly declining, several districts were not sharing in the improvement. Analysis indicated that they were populated predominantly by individuals of a particular mid-European nationality. Study of their cultural attitudes indicated a considerable family attachment to the infant as well as a typically neat and clean household environment. However, further inquiry brought out that traditionally infants were taken off the breast at a very early age and fed adult foods, often directly from the family table. Further study indicated a high incidence of death caused by severe digestive disturbances and intestinal infections. It was necessary over a period of several years to bring to bear the efforts of a special public health nursing program, assisted by appropriate nutritional and pediatric consultation. In addition to this instance, there are groups in which it is the custom for mothers to prechew solid foods for their babies and young children, not realizing the bacteriologic risk in their attempt to carry out what seems to them a logical procedure.

Frequently, economic factors are cultural reasons for ill health. In some places certain methods of earning a living have resulted in high incidence of pulmonic and other diseases. The use of human feces for fertilizer and the inherent health risks involved are well known and need not be dwelt on. There are many societies in which cattle excrement is one of the most valuable commodities because of its use as fertilizer, as fuel, or as a binder in making mud walls.'

Bogue and Habashy[16] have described the attitude of the Egyptian villager toward his animals and its effect on attempts to improve health conditions:

The fellah has his own habits and traditions which have come down with his long heritage. Many of these habits are good but many contribute to bad health because of lack of experience or ignorance of their effect. The poorest farmers keep their cattle and other animals in the same house they live in themselves. . . . In attempting to get at the basis of such a peculiar habit in this modern time, many approaches were made by the social workers. One old man explained it to a health educator simply that "We like our animals and want them where we can see them at night. . . . They are our wealth. They are our most prized possessions on which we depend for our very food and livelihood." Such a realistic answer causes social maneuverers to stop and think before making a casual suggestion to move them to a shed.

Although on the surface this may seem bizarre, one is reminded of the presence in many homes in our own societies of all sorts of animal pets, some of which are none too clean, others transmitters of specific diseases such as psittacosis, and to many of which humans may become allergic. Despite all of this, they are maintained on a sentimental or a companionship basis.

Some years ago an example of misguided effort and of the effect of economic limitation was observed in several communities in Java. Apparently some time previously an effective promotional program on the merits of brushing teeth had been carried out. Imported toothpaste, however, was beyond the economic capacity of many of the people. Nevertheless, it was common to see individuals with toothbrushes in their pockets stop to brush their teeth in the many canals that then ran through many streets. Since these were actually open sewers used for bathing, laundering—and for brushing teeth—the risk-benefit aspects were questionable.

Conflict of desirable health practices with other cultural values that may be considered more important is another reason for the development or perpetuation of health problems. Few things are as important to people as their religious beliefs. If it is customary to avoid a certain type of food such as animal protein, individuals will tend to do so even if an adequate nonanimal substitute is unavailable. Similarly, although many realize that certain traditional pilgrimages mean sickness and death for some people, nothing can deter them from the tremendous cultural drive to participate in the event. Modesty or moral values are factors of considerable import to most people. There have been periods in history and there are still cultures where to see the naked body, even one's own or that of one's child, is considered immodest and immoral. In such instances personal cleanliness and hygiene may be inadequate. The type of clothing customarily worn is part of the culture of a people and often has been developed in conformance with the environment. Sometimes, however, clothing acts as a deterrent to cleanliness and health and as a spreader of disease. The barracan, worn by many people in North Africa, is a very practical garment for protection from the environment. However, in some places with scarce water and soap, a common use of the long loose sleeves to wipe one's eyes, nose, and mouth and those of children makes it a factor in the spread of disease, particularly trachoma, which is so prevalent in that area.

An example of a cultural value, this time the wish for fertility, that supersedes not only health but even convenience, is described by Bogue and Habashy[16]:

I recall being told in Egypt of a wealthy landowner who had dug good wells, out of which his fellaheens could obtain clear and pure drinking water. After some three days' use of this safe water, the fellaheens returned to drinking the polluted water of the Nile. On inquiring into their reasons, the landowner was told that the people preferred the Nile water, that it was obviously better because the Nile made the fields fertile and would therefore make the people fertile.

One might speculate on the possible value of an explanation of the relationship between the river water and the ground water through subterranean diffusion as well as evaporation and precipitation. In addition, it might have been possible to point to families of desirable size who used water from a well rather than from the river.

Examples of cultural values as deterrents to health are by no means limited to less developed areas of the world. A provocative example is described in a study by Croog and Richards.[17] A high proportion of men who survived heart attacks stopped smoking. The actual threat to their lives and their physicians' advice apparently caused a significant behavioral change. In general, however, little change occurred in the smoking habits of their wives despite their witness to the threats to the health and lives of their husbands. With reference to another health problem, the sexual revolution has resulted in a willingness by American women to be examined for possible cancer of the cervix. Unfortunately, the same cannot be said with regard to digital or instrumental examinations for detection of colorectal cancer. Even in otherwise educated and sophisticated societies, there still remain some taboos regarding the excretory function.

EFFECT OF CULTURE ON HEALTH PROGRAMS

From the examples given, it is evident that public health programs are frequently hampered by failure to inquire into or understand customs that the members of a group consider important. It is a rare public health worker who can truthfully claim unqualified success of every program undertaken. Most have had the experience of meticulously planning a program, bringing to bear all technical knowledge available, only to be thwarted or disillusioned by an apathetic or resistant public. Often the reason is human behavior or motivation.

There are many barriers to public health success. One of the most common is inadequate communication. Public health workers frequently think that since they understand what they are thinking and saying, everyone else does. Komaroff[18] has presented a number of the communication barriers that may be encountered. They vary from antagonistic and negative individuals who practically refuse to hear, much less react, to those who are agreeably affirmative whether or not they comprehend. The latter unfortunately invalidate many surveys and health programs in the southwestern United States and in health assistance efforts in Latin America. Many people of Spanish-American heritage tend to answer "yes" to questions either because they want to please the questioner, because they have learned from unpleasant experience that is is generally safer to do so,[19,20] or because they do not have confidence in the questioner and his or her promises (for further information see *Hispanic culture and health care* by Martinez[21]).

Even within one's own communities or among age groups, language differences may serve as a communication barrier. Particularly in larger communities there are sizable groups whose ability to speak and understand the official national language is limited. More than one patient has received inappropriate diagnosis or treatment in a hospital, clinic, or health center because he and his examiner could not communicate. Any irony of such situations is that the more educated of the two is the least likely to admit to his handicap or failing. Even where the same language is ostensibly spoken, there may easily be differences in interpretations of what is said. There are also such factors as regionalism and provincialism; many words and phrases in a language may have different meanings in different sections of a country, not to mention the varying accents that those who speak them may use. Note, for example, the use of the word *country* in the preceding sentence. It is intended to imply *nation*, but in some places it connotes *rurality*.

An interesting and valuable lesson on communication as a barrier was encountered in connection with a health education program in Bolivia. Few of the rural people could read, so the use of educational films along with other techniques was indicated. At first, films on health that had been produced for use in the United States were shown. As would be expected, they meant little if anything to those who saw them. The people, their clothes, houses, foods, behavior, and in fact everything in the pictures were strange and foreign to the viewers. The medical and hospital environments presented conditions much too advanced to be of any practical use or applicability to the local situation. Then several health agencies in the United States had cartoon-type health education films made. These were better in that the characters shown had a more or less universal appeal. However, they were first used with English sound tracks, followed sometimes by verbal explanations in the native language. But the crucial moment of maximum impact had passed, and the chief result had still been entertainment. After this the films were made with Spanish sound tracks, since that was the official language of the country. Now they became useful as health education films in some areas, notably in a few of the larger cities. However, they were still incomprehensible to the majority of the people who needed them the most because they were Indians, many of whom did not understand Spanish. Therefore the sound tracks were translated into the two most common native languages of the Andes. Now the films really meant something to the people, and they began to respond. Incidentally, they were said to have been the first films with speech in the Quechua language of the Incas and the even more ancient language of the Aymara. One must add, however, that the scenes and figures projected were still not really familiar to those watching.

Differences in cultural patterns may negate carefully planned and well-intentioned public health endeavors. For example, the manner in which people relieve themselves may vary. Many American-type privies have gone unused for failure to realize that some people by tradition are "sitters," whereas others are "squatters." Actually it is unimportant for its public health purpose whether a privy has a seat or whether the squatting method is used. Even when privies are adopted and used, culture-based problems may arise. Thus in privies designed for rural Burmese, the use of convenient, inexpensive local materials seemed logical. However, it was overlooked that in rural Burma, as in many other places, paper is scarce. Of even more consequence was the failure to learn that by custom, pieces of bamboo were used for the same purpose as paper in the Western toilet. As a result, before long the bamboo superstructure of the privies tended to have a rather moth-eaten appearance, and the privy pit became clogged with pieces of bamboo. A provocative conversation, through an interpreter, with a rural Thai is also recalled. He said, in effect, "You Americans are strange. Before you came here, if I felt like relieving myself, I found a quiet spot in the open with gentle breezes and often a pleasant vista. Then you came and convinced me that this material that comes from me is dangerous, so I and others should stay as far away from it as possible. Then the next thing you told me was that I should dig a hole, and not only I, but many other people, should concentrate this dangerous material in that hole. So now I have even closer contact not only with my own but everyone else's, and in a dark, smelly place with no view at that." Which of us was the more logical?

Traditionally in many cultures, the removal of any material from the body is regarded with suspicion. Sebai[22] narrates an excellent example in relation to the institution of health programs among Bedouins in a rural area of western Saudi Arabia. Various blood tests were needed for clinical and laboratory diagnosis. Promptly the people showed great reluctance to the drawing of blood, especially from children. The loss of blood meant loss of power and strength. Rumors spread that the health workers who drank tea instead of polluted water were using "the power in the blood" by adding it to their tea. The health workers were also suspected of selling the blood to the blood bank in Mecca. It was also thought that the children's blood was being analyzed to select them for the army when they came of age. In contrast to such views, the same people expect health workers to treat them with injections that "go directly to the blood."

People will seek to attain and maintain health provided there are no conflicting cultural forces. Even in sophisticated societies people may react in what they know are illogical or ill-advised ways because of deep-seated folkways or cultural behaviorisms of which they are sometimes not even aware. Here, too, behavioral science may be of assistance to the public health worker, either through analysis of a situation or by explanation of the same or similar problems in simpler or more primitive societies. For example, why do some people resist hospitalization? It may be that their group customarily regards a hospital as a place to go to die. This idea was common in many immigrants to the United States and persisted into their next generation. In addition, behavioral scientists have found that a common if not universal cultural trait is a strong feeling of identification with the land or, in a nonrural situation, at least with the home. Remote in the history of the human species, but in many places still, is the feeling that when one dies it should be at home, that the spirit will reside in the place where one dies, and that the spirit's place is with the family. To some people death away from home means that the spirit must wander homeless and will be in an unfavorable position from which to intercede with the gods on behalf of the family who remains behind.

Another common reason for resistance to hospitalization is reaction against its tendencies to break down the cultural sense of responsibility for a family member in distress. In addition to pride, this may be based on the concept that the individual is continuous with his family unit. Still another reason may be an unwillingness to admit that one is sick, weak, or inadequate. This is closely related to one reason for resistance to surgery, that is, shame or a feeling of resultant incompleteness. This is emphasized particularly if by custom much importance is placed on the part removed, such as a breast, the uterus, or the testes. Again, one does not have to leave the domestic scene to observe this. Closely related to the concept of continuity of the individual with the land is the fear that the excised part or, in the case of obstetrics, the placenta or the dead fetus will not be destroyed or will be separated in space from the environment of the rest of the body or from the family. In some primitive societies, of course, it is believed that the excised part, if not

destroyed, may be used as a fetish. But then, one need only regard the relics in some western religions to find a cultural basis for such beliefs.

In obstetrics and gynecology innumerable taboos or cultural barriers are encountered. One reason is hinted at in a study of Yap culture by Schneider.[23] Yap women believe their genitals to be the source of power over their husbands. Since sex organs enable one to secure and keep a husband and to raise a family, they constitute one's personal secrets, which must not be revealed to female rivals. Yap women never allow other women to see their genitals; therefore attempts to use native female attendants in delivery rooms met with resistance. The substitution of nonindigenous female attendants proved somewhat more acceptable. Although women, they were alien to the native system of power and sex competition. A husband may see his wife's secrets, but she knows that no self-respecting Yap husband would allow any man, including an obstetrician, to see and manipulate his wife's secret parts. The wife herself does not believe that exposure before any man is as undesirable as exposure before another woman, but she is constrained by the knowledge that she would be violating her husband's personal rights if she allowed the former. A solution was found in the compromise of using nonnative female attendants and postponement of the mechanics of antisepsis and delivery by the physician until after anesthetization.

This leads logically to consideration of difficulties encountered in regard to nursing in many parts of the world. In many cultures the position of women is still subservient, and in some cultures women are not even allowed to be seen or to move about freely. Under such circumstances it is difficult to develop much-needed nurse training programs. In some other cultures a woman who would touch, cleanse, or come in contact with the discharges or internal parts of other people is customarily held in extremely low regard. In such circumstances it is difficult to elevate nursing to the status of a useful, esteemed profession, since among other things only the poorest, least educated, and least dependable women are free to engage in the activities necessary. Among some cultures, it is feared that to be touched by or given food by a female nurse might bring impotence, illness, or even death if she were menstruating.

Spectacular curative measures are more readily accepted than preventive measures. This is true in the United States and Western Europe as well as elsewhere. The degree to which this is true varies significantly among social groups. For example, Helsing and Comstock[24] found that in Maryland the use of automobile seat belts was much lower among women, those with lesser education and lower income, and infrequent church attenders. Enigmatically, among young adults, marriage increased the use of seat belts by women but decreased their use by men. In most parts of the world, therefore, it is impractical to disassociate promotive and preventive measures from those that are curative. Erasmus[25] has pointed to the difference in reception and support of the campaigns against yaws carried on by the Institute of Inter-American Affairs in collaboration with the governments of Colombia and Ecuador in contrast with measures to prevent intestinal parasitism. The results of the treatment of yaws with antibiotics were rapid and dramatic, and even the native healers readily admitted that the modern medicine was much more effective than their own herbal and magical treatments. By contrast, many looked on the symptoms of intestinal parasitism in a young child as a manifestation of the "evil eye," outside the realm of scientific medicine. Since the conditions under which they lived and their failure to understand the rationale of the suggested measures made obvious rapid improvement impossible, the measures were not successfully adopted.

Summarizing his findings, Erasmus concludes:

... Needs created by the process of specialization and the desire for increased production and profit actually seem the easiest for technicians from another culture or subculture to meet. The solution is often largely technical, fewer cultural barriers to a common understanding are presented, and the perception and feeling of needs are more easily shared by the innovators and the people.

However, when change is being attempted in a field not directly related to increased production in a cash economy, in other words not directly in terms of profits, the difficulties increase. In the field of public health, for example, the innovator may consider it highly desirable to introduce basic disease prevention measures into an underdeveloped area. But the folk still subscribed to an age-old system of beliefs about the cause, prevention, and treatment of disease, a system so different that the preventive measures of the innovator were meaningless.

Lacking an understanding of the modern concepts of the etiology of disease and consequently the reasons for modern methods of prevention, they may feel no need to adopt the prescribed changes. Thus, despite the fact that they feel a general need for assistance in combating the ailments common among them, they may fail to perceive the need for the specific measures proposed and may actively resist them.

Public health workers, particularly the medical component, should always realize that often they are in competition with ancient folklore, superstitions, and erroneous but well-accepted ideas, even in modern societies. The practice of the healing arts is the oldest specialized activity known and one of the few, along with the priesthood (with which it is closely allied), that appears to be a universal characteristic of all cultures. Despite this, the phrase "world's oldest profession" is commonly applied to a rather different activity. Yet as Murdock[26] has pointed out:

Prostitution, historically, is a relatively recent phenomenon. I have personally read accounts of many hundreds of primitive societies, and in not a single one of them is genuine prostitution reported. Many of them exhibit forms of such behavior that we would regard as exceedingly lax, but such laxity does not take the specific form of prostitution except in the so-called "higher" civilizations. . . . Specialized occupations are exceedingly few in the simpler societies, and with a single exception, none occurs more than sporadically. This exception is the medical profession. Specialized practitioners of the healing art are found, to the best of my knowledge, in every known society, however primitive. The "medicine man," in one form or another, is universal and hence must be regarded as the oldest professional specialist.

If this is true, medical and public health programs would appear to have an advantage over other types of social programs, provided they are designed to make possible ease of adequate transference from the old way to the new. The need to recognize the existence and acceptance of the old ways must be emphasized. If medical and public health measures have an advantage over the other social measures, it is also true that the medicine man, the *curandero,* and the medical superstitions and folkways have an advantage over the new and strange ideas of modern medicine and public health, especially if promoted by outsiders.

In all instances, from primitive societies in the most underdeveloped areas to groups in sophisticated western communities, there appears to exist an interesting dichotomous attitude toward illness and what might be done about them. The continued extensive use of patent medicines, the enormous amount of self-medication, and the extent to which various types of charlatans, faith healers, and pseudophysicians are consulted by sophisticated, otherwise intelligent people provide testimony to this.[27] Documentation is provided by a study[28] showing that millions of consumers base important health decisions on the idea that almost any treatment may be beneficial. Faith in this approach is reinforced by psychosomatic effects and unaided recovery. Forty-two percent of the persons interviewed would not be convinced by almost unanimous expert opinion that a hypothetic "cancer cure" was worthless. Only 45% thought such a medicine should be banned by law. (The recent laetrile controversy also illustrates this point.[29]) Three fourths of the public believe that extra vitamins provide more pep and energy, the most common of the misconceptions investigated in the survey. Although their disorders had never been diagnosed by a physician, 12% of those interviewed reported that they had arthritis or rheumatism, asthma, allergies, hemorrhoids, heart trouble, high blood pressure, or diabetes. Twelve percent of the sample also indicated that they would self-medicate—without seeing a doctor—for longer than 2 weeks for such ailments as a sore throat, cough, sleeplessness, or upset stomach. Twenty-six percent had used nutritional supplements, expecting specific observable benefits, without a physician's advice. About 2% of the persons indicated that they did something every day or nearly every day to help with bowel movement and that they were not following a physician's advice. More than a third believed in various erroneous concepts of weight control, the most common being that sweating is a means of substantially losing weight. Other popular items were nonprescription appetite depressants, massage, and the latest published diets. One of the most interesting findings was that older people are generally less likely than young people to make irrational decisions on health problems and are more skeptical about efficacy claims for drugstore remedies.

It may be of value to explore the background of these tendencies in less complex circumstances. In connection with a 10-year evaluation of the cooperative health programs of the Institute of Inter-American Affairs, Foster[30] studied the distinction between folk illnesses and those recognized by medical science. He found that certain diseases are recognized as not responsive to treatment methods

of *curanderos* but curable or preventable by the scientific physician. On the other hand, there are illnesses that are considered best treated by home remedies or with the aid of *curanderos,* that is, illnesses that are believed to be not understood by scientific physicians and the very existence of which they may deny. These illnesses, which may be referred to as "folk diseases," are particularly those considered to be of magical or psychic origin. "If an illness is diagnosed, for example, as 'evil eye,' obviously it is poor judgment to take the patient for treatment to a person who denies the existence of the disease."

Sometimes the illness is actually admitted and recognized by a scientific physician. Even then, if individuals of the culture involved, on the basis of past experience and social custom, regard the condition a result of magical or psychologic etiology, they will tend to rule out the potential usefulness of the scientific physician—and it must be remembered that it is the patient who makes the decision as to whom to ask for assistance. Attempts have been made to measure the practical effect of the distinction between "folk diseases" and "doctor's diseases." Surveys conducted in Chile, Ecuador, Columbia, and elsewhere indicated that conditions customarily thought to be caused by the "evil eye," bad air, fright, shock, or other magical or psychic causes, about which most people believed modern physicians were ignorant, were almost universally treated at home with folk remedies or by a *curandero.* This, of course, often prejudiced chances of ultimate recovery, since often the symptoms were misleading and related to serious illnesses. On the other hand, certain clear-cut conditions such as anemia, appendicitis, hernia, meningitis, pneumonia, smallpox, typhoid, and the like generally but not invariably were considered to be within the province of a scientific physician.

Interestingly, a study conducted by Banks and Keller[31] in metropolitan Columbus, Ohio, elicited a surprisingly similar picture. A representative sample of households was presented with a list of 29 symptoms and asked to rate them in terms of the following:

1. I would handle it myself because it is not very serious.
2. If it got worse or kept on I would go to a doctor.

3. I would see a doctor and have him check it out.
4. I would go to Emergency.

In general, symptoms such as bleeding, palpable lumps, frequent vomiting, urinary difficulties, or chest pain tended to be placed in the third or fourth category, whereas sore throat, overweight, poor appetite, frequent headaches or colds, nervousness, joint pains or stiffness, or dizziness were usually placed in the first or second category.

Despite this, it is tempting for those who have experienced only modern scientific thought to belittle or ignore practitioners of folk medicine as if they were completely unworthy of consideration. The illogic of this has been expressed by Elkins[32] on the basis of his work in Australia.

Aboriginal medicine men are far from being rogues, charlatans or ignoramuses. They are men of high degrees . . . men who have undergone tests and have taken degrees in the secrets of life much beyond that which ordinary men have a chance to learn. This training involves steps which imply a discipline, mental effort, courage and perseverance. In addition, they are men of respected, and often of outstanding personality. Thus, they are of immense social significance, with the health of the group depending largely on faith in their powers. Furthermore, the various psychic powers attributed to them must not be readily dismissed as mere "make-believe," for many of them have specialized in the workings of the human mind and in the influence of mind on mind, and mind on body. And, what is more, they are deeply convinced of their powers, so much so, that as long as they observe the customary discipline of their "order," their professional status and practice continues to be a source of faith and healing power to both themselves and their fellows.

In reference again to the Latin American scene, Foster's[30] analysis of the relationship between the scientific physician and the curandero is of particular pertinence and merits quoting at length. His observations may be applied to our domestic scene with adequate provision for differences in degree and type of social camouflage.

The conflict between folk medicine and scientific medicine is summed up in the persons of the physician and curandero. Each represents the highest achievement in his field. The attitudes of the people of Latin America towards each, therefore, are pertinent to this study. Unfortunately, the physician frequently comes off second best. This is due in part to the inherent nature of the situation, and in part to native suspicion of individuals in other social classes, particularly those above them.

The curandero operates under conditions that are relatively more favorable than those of the physician, from the point of view of impressing the patient with concrete results and apparent success. He treats folk illnesses, the symptoms of which often are so ill-defined that he cannot help but succeed in alleviating them. If the vague physiological symptoms identified with the illness persist or reappear after the cure, the curandero can always say that the case has become complicated and requires another series of cures or a different cure, or that a new and different illness has attacked the patient. Also, most curanderos do not claim to cure all illnesses, and in many cases can even recommend that a patient consult a physician. These factors establish the curanderos in the minds of the folk as fair, open-minded individuals willing to admit their limitations. Finally, the curandero's diagnostic techniques do not require elaborate and exhaustive questioning of the patient as to symptoms, case history, and the like. He has certain magical or automatic devices which he applies to specific situations, and the answers follow almost like clockwork. Moreover, there are many cases reported by field observers in which a physician failed to cure an individual and a curandero had apparently genuine success

The physician enjoys few of these advantages. His diagnosis is seldom cut and dried, he cannot guarantee quick results, and he seldom enjoys the faith and confidence accorded the curandero because he is from a social class instinctively distrusted by the majority of his patients. Moreover, the physician seldom admits that a curandero can cure things which he is incapable of treating, and this is interpreted as meaning that he conceitedly and selfishly believes himself to be the sole repository of medical knowledge—a point of view which the villager is loath to accept.

Criticisms of physicians and their professional methods are rife among the patients of the lower class, and such criticisms are usually based on a complete lack of comprehension of medicine, its methods, and its limitations. Several patients pointed out that physicians asked them questions about their symptoms, which showed that the physicians were not as smart as they thought they were. A good curandero doesn't have to ask questions, so why should a man who pretends to know a great deal more have to do so? Another patient scornfully pointed out that a President of Colombia died "even though he had 50 physicians at his bedside." The implication was that if 50 physicians could not keep a man from dying, a single doctor in a short interview was almost worse than worthless.

A final handicap of the physician is the general tendency of the people to exhaust home remedies and the arts of the curandero before appealing to the physician. The physician, therefore, gets many cases too late to effect a cure and many others which are simply incurable.

Hence, the failures of folk medicine as well as those of his own profession are heaped upon his shoulders.

The consequences of the foregoing have been sharpened by Dreitzel,[3] who after briefly describing the development of medicine from primitive superstition through the enlightenment to the success of modern science, nevertheless makes the observation that at least 50% of patients suffer from "functional disturbances." He concludes therefore:

Necessary as it is in combination with what one might call an ecological view, the scientist's perspective in medicine has become a serious impediment to a deeper understanding of the nature of health and illness in modern society *if* exclusively applied to diagnosis and treatment. And this still holds true for the overwhelming majority of medical practitioners in America in spite of the mental health movement, and in spite of much research effort in the sociology of medicine.

It must be admitted that there are many points of value in folk medicine. In a sense, one might consider modern scientific medicine as a natural outgrowth, extension, or elaboration of folk medicine, thereby representing scientific folk medicine. The number of effective drugs that have originated in folk medicine is impressive: quinine, rauwolfia, mescaline, chaulmoogra, opium, coca, curare, and many laxatives and emetics, to mention only a few. As for physical techniques, one might mention massage, baths, sweating treatments, surgery, and even inoculation. In the field of mental health and psychotherapy, a great deal can be learned from the practitioner of simple folk medicine.[33] Increased recognition of these facts, augmented by the significant number of western health and medical professionals who by now have had work experience in the developing areas of the world, has led to a new look at traditional medicine and its practitioners. This has occurred especially in relation to mental health and psychosomatic ailments. Two other factors have contributed to this change in attitude—first, the realization that there will never be sufficient scientifically trained personnel to serve the almost overwhelming needs of most of the world's people and, second, the great influx of Latin Americans, Asians, and Africans into the United States and many of the nations of Western Europe. Numerous training programs have been developed throughout the world to extend the knowledge and ability of traditional health workers so that they may constitute extensive cadres of "first-line" health auxiliaries. Fundamental to this

movement is assurance of adequate supervisory and consultative "backstopping" as well as periodic refresher sessions.[34]

It is interesting that although knowledge of the causative agents may be lacking, certain illnesses traditionally have been considered communicable, and it was believed that those who suffered from them should be kept apart from the other members of society. Beyond this it is commonly believed that individuals subject to certain debilitating illnesses are in a weakened condition and that visitors may unintentionally harm them by their strong "humors." Therefore, aside from possible communicability, isolation is carried out for the patient's own good. It is worthy of note that the attitude of public health workers toward the value of isolation has shifted substantially to this point of view. Where concern exists with regard to the evil effects of *aire*, strong humors, or similar folk influences, it may be possible to take advantage of this, since whatever the reasoning, an essentially hygienic practice is followed—one that can be made use of by physicians and nurses in the treatment and prevention of spread of communicable diseases. Physicians need not express an opinion on the potential dangers of *aire*. They can simply say that visitors are undesirable for the patient's sake, and the patient's family will probably follow the recommendation, even though physicians are thinking in terms of contagion and the family in terms of magic.

In most instances it is probably ill advised to ignore patients' ideas about their illness and the relationship of established folkways to it. Foster[35] has warned, "The common tendency on the part of doctors and nurses to ignore, if not to ridicule, folk concepts of illness, probably reduces their effectiveness. . . ." He illustrates this with several instances in which modern physicians and especially nurses wisely listen to patients' complaints and to their ideas of magical and metaphysical relationships thereto, then follow up by relating their suggestions for modern scientific treatment to those familiar, accepted ideas. This accomplishes several things. It raises the physician and nurse in the patient's estimation, since not only did they not belittle the patient's valued ideas and folk traditions, but they actually exhibited some interest and understanding of them. From this starting point there develops a rapport and a greater understanding and receptivity

by the patient of scientific medicine and its practitioners. This is one of the most important ways
that erroneous folk practices may eventually be
adapted or dropped and more effective and suitable
scientific practices substituted.

A sense of fatalism presents one of the most difficult obstacles to the health worker. It exists in
varying degrees and forms throughout the world;
Kismet, Che sarà sarà, God's wish, the will of Al-
lah—the terms are many. Often illness is considered a form of divine punishment or retribution for
some real or imagined transgression. Sebai[22] gives
an example from his work with desert Bedouin. They
believe in two main causes of disease: (1) super-
natural power, (God, jinn, or evil eye) and (2) physical agents (cold, heat, or fatigue). Although multiple causation is the pattern, God is the primary
cause of all disease. Among those surveyed, about
50% attributed mental illness to God, who orders a
jinn to enter the body of a person who is frightened
or is walking alone at night. Occasional danger may
result from fatalistic beliefs, as evidenced by an
incident in Srinagar, India in the early 1970s.
Health workers attempting to vaccinate against
cholera were locked in their dispensary by a crowd
shouting, "Disease is God's punishment." They
threatened to burn alive the health workers, who
were finally rescued by police.[36]

Sometimes professional individuals tend to make
a fetish of terminology. After all, words and titles
are of little consequence. The fundamental concept
and effective action are what is important.

An experience by one of us (J.J.H.) suggests a
way to meet situations such as those described. The
locale was a county in a southeastern state, the
county seat of which was the headquarters of a
fundamentalist religious group. This religious
group not only refused to recognize the germ causation of some diseases but even refused to admit
the reality of illness of any kind. If there was something the matter with an individual, he was not
sick—rather, God was displeased with him or with
something in the environment, and when God became happy again, the individual would recover.
Meanwhile, of course, he might die from an otherwise preventable condition. These ideas were deeply ingrained in the religious beliefs of these people.
It was obviously futile to try to convince them otherwise. In terms of their religious tenets, in which

they had absolute faith, they were certain they were
right, and after all, they were entitled to whatever
religious beliefs they wished. Nevertheless, this
posed a serious problem not only with regard to
their welfare but also with regard to the welfare of
everyone with whom they had contact.

Actually it worked out reasonably well. As health
officer, I made a sincere effort to become friendly
with the elderly bishop who was head of the church.
He was a good and sincere man. He believed that
he and his people were doing the right thing. Why
deny it? One day I casually said to him: "Bishop,
you and I may disagree on a philosophic basis about
certain things. We do, however, have one important
common interest—we are both honestly interested
in the well-being of your people and of all people.
Furthermore, we also have an important point of
agreement. We each recognize that at certain times
something undesirable happens to people. Let us
not argue about what causes that something to happen. After all, the cause is incidental to the effect.
If you want to say that it is displeasure on the part
of God, that is all right with me. On the other hand,
if I happen to think that it is a bacterium, it can do
no harm for me to think so. But let us, you and I,
work together in doing something about the result."
After that there was no more difficulty. If isolation
of an infectious person was necessary, it was done
on the basis of preventing contact of the general
public with influences that had displeased God. If
immunization was indicated, it was on the basis of
injecting God-inspired material to help keep away
unknown, displeasing factors that might harm people. If drugs and medicines were prescribed, it was
on the basis of giving materials to assist in driving
out or removing from the body the things that had
displeased the Lord.

How does the foregoing tie together? One may
gain a clue if one accepts the idea that the goal as
health workers must be to make desirable personal
and community health practices an accepted part
of the way of life and culture of people. This cannot
occur spontaneously, and it cannot be done merely
by destroying what the health worker thinks are
erroneous customs. It requires careful planning
and often much patience. Workers in public health
must recognize the inadequacy of doing things *to*
or even *for* people. The best way is to do things
with people, and to do so the public health worker
must understand as thoroughly as possible the cultural factors that make themselves and others believe and act the way they do and tailor suggestions

and programs as much as is practical to the accepted general cultural pattern of the group. The public health worker should constantly relate to something familiar, something most people already know, do, and accept. In addition, we as health workers must recognize that our own communities, sophisticated as they may appear on the surface, consist of numerous societies and numerous cultures. We must recognize that so-called sophistication may merely substitute city ways for folkways and that many of our customs are fundamentally the same as those found elsewhere, having merely been transferred, transformed, or adapted to a new environment or set of social conditions.

EFFECT OF HEALTH ACTIVITIES ON CULTURAL PATTERNS

Discussion to this point has centered on the effect of cultural patterns on health and on public health activities. Brief consideration of the reverse relationship would seem in order. If public health programs successfully improve the physical and mental health of a people, invariably there follow complex, far-reaching effects on most other phases of the culture of the people. Thus if workers become healthier and more alert mentally, their ingenuity and inventiveness tend to increase. To the extent that they may produce more and better mechanical aids to their labors, they then find it not only possible to produce more but they do it more easily and in less time. This makes possible a shorter average workday. With more leisure, people tend to engage more in the pursuit of various cultural activities (i.e., recreation, study, reading, and the fine arts), and because of an increased standard of living, they have more money for such activities.

A measurable effect of public health activities is a decrease in the number of deaths and an increase in the average life expectancy. Thus in the United States since the beginning of the twentieth century, infant death rates have been lowered from about 200 per 1,000 live births to 11.7 per 1,000 in 1981. This means that instead of every fifth baby dying, less than every fiftieth baby now dies. During the same period, the average life expectancy at birth has been raised from about 49 years to about 74 years of age. The social consequences of such a rapid effect of public health activities are many and far reaching. There are more mouths for families and the nation to feed, greater housing needs, and more recreation facilities and other civic and social activities needed. Offsetting these are the de-

creased needs for school facilities, baby foods, and pediatricians, as zero population growth is approached as a result of family planning. At the same time, many more facilities are needed for the larger number of older citizens. On the other hand, it also means that less money is needed for the care of preventable illnesses, much less family worry and sadness, a changed attitude toward illness and death, and healthier children who in a short time become more alert, better informed, and capable citizens and workers. One might generalize by saying that in many or all such situations, rapidly improved health conditions tend to result first in increased social pressures and problems, followed by greatly multiplied social benefits.

The development of healthier people therefore sets off a chain of events that results in general in the improvement of national culture and in an improved standard of living for everyone. More people become available to work in offices, businesses, farm lands, and factories, and because on the average they are healthier than their parents and grandparents, they can produce more. This means an increase in the individual share of the material things of life. At the same time, attitudes toward marriage and family life are strongly affected by the results of public health measures. To approach this negatively, if death rates are high in general and if maternal mortality rates are high in particular, family structure must be adapted accordingly. The husband and children must accept the possibility of having several wives and mothers. For the woman, childbirth is surrounded by fear and superstition. Because of the frequency of deaths of mothers, the position of older surviving female relatives is more important in the total family picture than in the present typical American situation. Also, because of high infant and child mortality, husbands, public opinion, and nature conspire to keep the woman pregnant much of the time. One might say further that the generally pregnant wife results in the most significant accentuation of the double standard. The husband tends toward more promiscuous relationships, which tend to be accepted more readily by society. This in turn incidentally invites a greater prevalence of venereal diseases.

Interestingly, some of the same manifestations of cultural change have occurred among many young people of both sexes as a result of recent technologic and scientific advances in combination with increased affluence, mobility, and population concentration, to all of which improved public health has contributed. In many places some consequences have included significant changes in attitude toward family, religion, schools, property, interpersonal relations, morals, and other social institutions.

Lowered infant mortality and maternal mortality rates, on the other hand, tend eventually to bring about a pattern of smaller families that, in some respects at least, have stronger immediate family bonds. In present-day American society this has had a considerable effect on the size of houses and even their architecture and on the use that is made of the home. A social complication has resulted, however, from the concurrent lengthening of life and the increasing number of elderly individuals. This, in relation to a change in social attitude or interpretation of family constituency and responsibility and to the change that has occurred in the size and design of the modern small home, has left many, especially grandparents and other elderly persons, with little or no home base. The development of such an unfortunate type of social problem results inevitably in a social reaction. This is evident in the increasing literature and social legislation dealing with the older or senior citizens' needs for medical care, housing, and other necessities.

Successful public health programs may bring about a great change in attitude toward previously deep-seated "health" customs. The wearing of charms of all types is a common practice in this and many other countries. Usually they are not readily relinquished. Because of the success of the antiyaws program of the Institute of Inter-American Affairs during the 1950s, it became necessary to place boxes at the treatment and health centers as receptacles for the charms and fetishes that some of the now convinced patients discarded in large numbers.

One should always be conscious of the delicate balance in which a society operates. This applies particularly to activities in a field such as public health that may have prompt and far-reaching influences. Whereas it is axiomatic that progress in one cultural direction inevitably results in progress in other aspects of a culture, it is equally true that the artificial stimulation of great sudden advancements in one phase of a culture alone may bring about at least a temporary social difficulty, if not even chaos. Thus workers in public health may actually be wielding a two-edged sword if they suddenly, rapidly, and exclusively apply all of the present public health knowledge to a situation. If this is done without consideration of family planning and the basic social needs of the additional people, there is real danger of causing irreparable distortion and harm to a culture or a society. There may develop increased food problems, social and economic imbalance, and political unrest, to mention only a few potential results. Public health workers need not be pessimistic about this, however. The important thing is to realize the potentialities and implications and to emphasize the great importance of public health workers working in cooperation with agriculturists, educators, political scientists, social workers, behavioral scientists, and many others.

THE IMPACT OF ENVIRONMENT ON HUMAN BEHAVIOR

Even a cursory consideration indicates a direct relationship between undesirable living circumstances and various types of social and health problems. This is especially evident in urban situations where sheer numbers and crowding accentuate such problems. The numerous social difficulties of urban areas are commonly concentrated in slum or substandard neighborhoods. People tend to be crowded together in profitable subsistence living space. Little or no consideration is given to amenities. Often, and through no accident, industry is located nearby—close to a supply of labor eager for employment. The crowding of buildings, the generally narrow streets, the absence of open recreational areas, and the smoke of factories limit considerably the amount of sunshine and fresh air. Cleanliness and sanitation are difficult to maintain. Death or injury is invited by narrow, traffic-laden streets, rickety abandoned structures, and poorly planned flammable dwellings. Both education and nutrition also tend to be substandard and combine with insanitation and overcrowding to maintain a high incidence of illness. Lack of privacy encourages immorality and is conducive to a lowering of self-respect. Bars and taverns are plentiful. These and other psychologic insults to the developing child and adolescent breed attitudes of hopelessness, constant frustration, cynicism, resentment, and explosive pent-up hostility. Responsibility and initiative appear pointless, and what often seem to be the only roads open to self-expression and escape are socially undesirable. Reactions of rebellion, such as destructiveness or crime, or of defeat, such as addictions or prostitution, tend to occur. It is perhaps not coincidental that the word for town dweller *(pagani)* had the etymologic root that it does. A subsequent chapter on aggression and violence presents some aspects of the problem in greater detail.

These relationships have been repeatedly and conclusively shown to exist. Much of the writings of Southwood Smith and Chadwick discussed this subject. Earlier, in 1828, Villermé, one of the originators of social statistics, presented to the French Academy of Medicine a memoir comparing the death rates of the rich and the poor. The classic studies by Sydenstricker[37] during the early 1930s in the United States showed about 20% of the land area of several metropolitan areas to be of a substandard, blighted, or slum quality. These areas, aside from factories, included the living quarters of a third of the populations of those cities. However, they accounted for 35% of the fires, 50% of the disease in general, 65% of the tuberculosis cases, 55% of the juvenile delinquents, and 50% of the arrests. Although they contributed only 6% of the tax revenue of the cities, they required 45% of the cities' expenditures.

That this was not limited to the past is evidenced by a recent study by the Sacramento City Planning Commission[38] of the city's substandard housing area, where most of the unemployed live. Although this area contained only 20% of the population, it accounted for 42% of adult crime, 36% of juvenile delinquency, 26% of fires, and 76% of cases of tuberculosis. It required 25% of the city's fire protection, 41% of the city's police protection, and 50% of the city's health services. On the other hand, it contributed only 12% of the city's taxes. It was estimated that an average person taken off welfare rolls and placed in a steady job would contribute $10,000 to the gross national product, pay $300 in state and local taxes, increase purchasing power for goods and services by $3,400, relieve the government of welfare or support payments of $1,308 a year, and reduce unemployment costs and the need for other community services.

With specific reference to the relationship of general environment to disease and death, a considerable body of data has now accumulated. This has been especially true for the general death rate, infant and maternal mortality, tuberculosis and pneumonic infections, and malnutrition. Even differences in the prevalence of chronic diseases have been demonstrated.

Actually this is an increasingly complex question in a rapidly changing society. Thus Stockwell,[39] in his comparative studies of Hartford, Conn., and Providence, R.I., found that the extent of association was not the same for all components of socioeconomic status, nor did all aspects of mortality show similar associations with the same components of socioeconomic status. He suggests that "the failure to realize this may lie behind much of the disagreement pertaining to the nature and extent of the relationship between socioeconomic status and mortality in the United States today." Whereas studies in the past indicated a marked inverse relationship between socioeconomic status and all aspects of mortality, present evidence is much less conclusive. An additional precaution is brought out by Chilman,[40] who points out that although most studies of this nature relate to cities, actually socioeconomic disadvantage is more consequential in rural circumstances.

If one looks for them, relationships may be found between factors in the social environment, and almost all diseases. Their significance varies with both the particular group of individuals and their social environment, and with particular diseases. In the case of diseases such as tuberculosis, silicosis, or gastric ulcer, the relationship may be readily evident, whereas in others it may be somewhat obscure. The number of social factors potentially related to disease is undoubtedly legion. Furthermore, they are of several different types and affect health in a number of different ways—some directly, some indirectly. Certain factors such as tendencies to develop certain mental conditions, physical malformations, or blood dyscrasias are sometimes inherent in the members of the group. Other factors such as exposure to siliceous dust or to fumes are related to occupation. Factors such as overcrowding or proximity to brothels are dangerous because they are conducive to exposure. Still others such as certain dietary habits or infant feeding customs are related to cultural factors.

Admittedly, it is difficult to determine direct cause-and-effect relationships between poor housing and ill health. Nevertheless, the consistency of their occurrence together cannot be ignored. As Pond[41] has reasoned:

A cautious and critical analysis of available data relating to the effects of housing on health leads to but one conclusion: one cannot state that substandard housing alone begets ill health. However, no reasonable student of the subject has yet stated that bad housing is compatible with good health. In the absence of irrefutable proof that housing has no ill effect on health, it may reasonably be hypothesized that good housing promotes the attainment of good health.

In their stimulating discussion of social science in medicine, Simmons and Wolff[8] present the interplay of several aspects of man and his social and physical environment in an unusually descriptive manner well worth repeating:

. . . as an organism man is borne along by his physical environment, but he is also buffeted about by some of its elements. As a member of society, he is supported and reinforced by some fellow agents, while he may be frustrated, handicapped, or even vanquished by others. Similarly, as a personality, he is both a product of his culture and a potential victim of its compelling or conflicting norms and codes.

Anyone may be carried along comfortably in his milieu for a while, only to be torn down miserably after a time as these various environmental components of his life converge and impinge upon him. During long stretches of time, harmful and helpful forces may blend and balance, permitting his a workable and safe equilibrium amid many minor fluctuations. What is most important for us to realize, however, is the possibility that the scales may be *tipped* critically at a particular time by a clustering of forces from any one area, or from a combination of the triad of environmental pressures, and that, for the individual, a landslide of ill effects is started.

The following is a possible classification of some of the many group and social factors that may be related to disease. It is admittedly general and is presented merely to illustrate the variety and to provoke consideration of others:

   I. Factors in the members of the group
      A. Inherent characteristics
         1. Group susceptibility
         2. Genetic tendencies
      B. Cultural characteristics
         1. Racial, ethnic, or religious customs
         2. Agricultural customs and methods
         3. Dietary habits or customs
         4. Educational limitations
         5. Linguistic barriers
         6. Traditional family size
         7. Relative status of races, tribes, or nationalities
         8. Relative status of sexes
         9. Relative status of age groups
       10. Relative importance of the family in total social life
  II. Factors in the activities of the group
      A. Political
         1. Stability
         2. Quality
         3. Honesty
         4. Foresight of leadership
      B. Occupation and income
         1. Types of occupation
         2. Level and stability of personal income
         3. Trade unionism
      C. Economy
         1. Basis
         2. Stability
         3. Trade
      D. Leisure behavioral pattern
         1. Active or passive
         2. Social or antisocial
         3. Solitary or group
         4. Physical risks
      E. Mobility
         1. Travel
         2. Migration
      F. Traditional household habits
      G. Traditional purposes of the household
 III. Factors in the environment of the group
      A. Geologic and climatic
         1. Severity of winters and summers
         2. Amount of rainfall and available water
         3. Topography
         4. Drainage
         5. Nature of subsoil
         6. Mineral content of soil
         7. Degree of geographic isolation
      B. General environment
         1. Atmospheric pollution
         2. Soil and water pollution
         3. Amount of arable land available
         4. Proximity to detrimental factors (railroads, highways, industries, brothels, bars, fire hazards)
         5. Availability of recreation areas and facilities

C. Home environment
1. Size (persons per room)
2. State of repair
3. Type of structure
4. Sanitary facilities
5. Natural and artificial light
6. Ventilation

Consideration of these social and environmental influences emphasizes the importance of regarding public health work for what it really is—an applied social science through which is brought to bear appropriate medical, engineering, nursing, educational, and many other disciplines. It is only by considering the social and environmental conditions under which people live, sleep, work, recreate, procreate, and rear their young that health workers can hope to understand and control disease in the most complete sense. It is only in this way that they can eventually grasp the meaning of total health.

ROLE OF SOCIAL SCIENTISTS IN HEALTH

Much of what has been presented in this chapter is material usually neglected in the education of health personnel. The intent here has been twofold: (1) to provide a taste of some of the most interesting and pertinent aspects of the subject and (2) to familiarize health workers with the existence and potential contributions of social scientists to health-related activities. While the term *social scientist* actually includes a somewhat broad spectrum of professions, reference at this point is made particularly to social psychologists, behavioral scientists, and cultural anthropologists. The relationships that such specialists may have with health workers and their activities are varied. Kelman[53] has described these as being of four types of situations. The first and most usual is essentially basic research in that it focuses on the processes involved in the functioning and change of social and cultural systems. What are the cultural ideologies, attitudes, values, and institutions that determine the possibility of social change in a society? A second role is to provide support to an action program by developing some of the necessary tools—selection devices, feedback questionnaires, and the like—for planning, action, and evaluation. The third type of role involves active participation in the development and implementation of the action program; in other words, to participate in determining the course of the program. A fourth type of role is to assess the effects and implications of new policies or action

programs. As Kelman summarizes, these four types of roles represent a gradient of degree of independence or actual involvement of the social scientist in relation to the program of social change.

In other words, social scientists can study cultural characteristics and differences and provide expert advice and consultation when programs or changes are contemplated. They can also provide warnings when those working in public health appear to be in danger of serious error because of misunderstanding of the motivations of individuals and groups. Finally, if public health workers do find themselves in inexplicable difficulty, the social scientist, by virtue of a somewhat different way of looking at things, may be able to find out why and to point to a way out of the dilemma.

On the basis of his extensive review of technical assistance programs in health, Foster[35] developed a list of factors to be considered by health workers engaged in social change, as indeed they all are. He warned that it was merely suggestive and illustrative and not a definitive catalogue. It does, however, provide a useful checklist and a fitting conclusion to this chapter.

Although it is desirable to know as much about a culture as possible, there are obviously strict limitations as to what can be known. Social scientists have barely made a beginning in the formidable task of describing the elements of the cultures of the world and interpreting their significance. It must be assumed that for any given program there are certain categories of information about the culture in which the work is to be carried out which are of primary importance, and others that are of lesser importance. A "trial run" in compiling a list of primary classes of data for public health programs gives the following picture.

Folk medicine and native curing practices. The importance of this has been discussed at some length above and need not be commented on further at this point.

Economics, particularly incomes and costs of living. Since in the final analysis the success of public health programs rests upon major changes in the habits of people with respect to diet, housing, clothing, agriculture, and the like, knowledge of the economic potential of an area is paramount.

Social organization of families. A bride often lives in her husband's home, under the domination of her mother-in-law. There are cases in which pregnant women failed to follow, or had difficulty in following, health center recommendations because these conflicted with what the mother-in-law thought was best.

Men and women who live together are frequently not legally married. Under such circumstances, a man is less likely to recognize obligations to his companion and their children, and it is therefore more difficult to persuade him to come to the health center for venereal or other treatment. Recognition of these and similar problems makes the responses of patients more intelligible.

Education and literacy and comprehension. Ability to comprehend the real nature of health and disease, to profit by health education, and to understand and follow the physician's instructions depends on the education and literacy of the people.

Political organization. Local conditions under which physicians and other staff members are appointed, the local attitude toward nepotism, bureaucratic rules which govern operations, and the like, are factors which will affect public health programs. In one country, for example, a large health center, not yet placed in operation, was seriously threatened by the conflicting interests of the state governor, the local nurses' union, and other bureaucratic factors.

Religion. A basic analysis of religious tenets is not essential, but some parts of the religious philosophy of the people should be known. Are there any beliefs which hinder or directly conflict with proposed programs? Is death, for example, at any age considered a welcome relief from a world of suffering? Are there food taboos based on religious sanction which should be taken into consideration in planning diets?

Basic value system. What are the goals, aspirations, fundamental values, and major cultural premises, consciously or unconsciously accepted, which give validity to the lives of the people in question? What is the practical significance, for example, of a fatalistic approach to life and death? What part does prestige play in determining customary behavior patterns of the people? Is male vanity and ego a factor to consider? What are the ideas of bodily modesty? What are the types of stimuli and appeal to which people respond most readily?

Other types of data. Planners and administrators of public health programs should also have at hand such information as credit facilities and money usages, labor division within the family, time utilization, working and eating schedules, cooking and dietary practices, and the importance of alcoholism.

Categories of culture in which precise knowledge would appear to be of lesser importance include agriculture, fishing, and other primary productive occupations, industrial techniques (except as working conditions may affect health), trade and commerce, religious fiestas and church observances, wedding ceremonies, burial customs, and music and folk tales.

REFERENCES

1. News item: people cutting back on health care, Nations' Health, June 1979, p. 2.
2. Kaufman, K.: Psychiatry: why "medical" or "social" models? Arch. Gen. Psychiatry 17:347, Sept. 1967.
3. Drietzel, H.P.: The social organization of health, New York, 1971, Macmillan, Inc.
4. Stone, L.: The family, sex, and marriage in England 1500-1800, New York, 1977, Harper & Row, Publishers, Inc.
5. Koos, E.L.: New concepts in community organization for health, Am. J. Public Health 43:466, April 1953.
6. Skinner, B.F.: Science and human behavior, New York, 1953, Macmillan, Inc.
7. Kluckhohn, C.: Mirror for man: the relation of anthropology to modern life, New York, 1949, Whittlesey House.
8. Simmons, L.W., and Wolff, H.G.: Social science in medicine, New York, 1954, Russell Sage Foundation.
9. Brownlee, A.T.: Community, culture, and care: a cross-cultural guide for health workers, St. Louis, 1978, The C.V. Mosby Co.
10. White, L.A.: Man's control over civilization, an anthropocentric illusion, Sci. Month. 66:238, March 1948.
11. Benedict, R.: Patterns of culture, New York, 1934, The New American Library of World Literature, Inc.
12. Carothers, J.C.: The African mind in health and disease, WHO Monogr. Ser. No. 17, 1953.
13. Gittler, J.B.: Man and his prejudices, Sci. Month. 69:44, July 1949.
14. Hoffer, E.: The ordeal of change, New York, 1964, Harper Colophon Books.
15. Hoyt, E.E.: Tiquisate: a call for a science of human affairs, Sci. Month. 72:114, Feb. 1951.
16. Bogue, R., and Habashy, A.: Health education pilot project in three villages in Egypt, 1955. Unnumbered Publication of World Health Organization Regional Office, Alexandria.
17. Croog, S.H., and Richards, N.P.: Health beliefs and smoking patterns in heart patients and their wives, Am. J. Public Health 67:921, Oct. 1977.
18. Komaroff, A.L.: The practitioner and the compliant patient, Am. J. Public Health 66:833, Sept. 1976.
19. Aday, L.A., Chiu, G.Y., and Anderson, R.: Methodological issues in health care surveys of the Spanish heritage population, Am. J. Public Health 70:367, April 1980.
20. Berkanovic, E.: The effect of inadequate language translation on Hispanics' responses to health surveys, Am. J. Public Health 70:1273, Dec. 1980.
21. Martinez, R.A.: Hispanic culture and health care: fact, fiction, folklore, St. Louis, 1978, The C.V. Mosby Co.
22. Sebai, Z.A.: The health of the family in a changing Saudi Arabia, Jedda, 1981, Tihama Publishers.
23. Schneider, D.M.: In Paul, B.D.: Health, culture, and

community, New York, 1955, Russel Sage Foundation.

24. Helsing, K.J., and Comstock, G.W.: What kinds of people do not use seat belts? Am. J. Public Health **67:**1043, Nov. 1977.

25. Erasmus, C.J.: An anthropologist views technical assistance, Sci. Month. **78:**148, March 1954.

26. Murdock, G.P.: Anthropology and its contribution to public health, Am. J. Public Health **42:**8, April 1952.

27. Dusseau, J.L.: Dr. Donald Duck: The quack in practice, Pharos, July, 1977, p. 17.

28. National Analysts, Inc.: A study of health practices and opinions, Springfield, Va., 1972, National Technical Information Service.

29. Lerner, I.J.: Laetrile, a lesson in cancer quackery, CA **31:**91, Mar.-April 1981.

30. Foster, G.M.: Use of anthropological methods and data in planning and operations, Public Health Rep. **68:**853, Sept. 1953.

31. Banks, F.R., and Keller, M.D.: Symptom experience and health action, Med. Care **9:**498, Nov.-Dec. 1971.

32. Elkins, A.: Aboriginal men of high degree, Sydney, 1944, Australasian Publishing Co., Ltd.

33. Traditional medicine (special issue), World Health, Nov. 1977.

34. Bannerman, R.H.: Traditional medicine in modern health care, World Health Forum **3**(1):8, 1982.

35. Foster, G.M.: A cross-cultural anthropological analysis of a technical aid program, Washington, D.C., 1951, Smithsonian Institution.

36. News item, Hospital Tribune, April 22, 1974.

37. Sydenstricker, E.: Health and environment, New York, 1933, McGraw-Hill Book Co.

38. Osborne, P.B.: The war that business must win, New York, 1970, McGraw-Hill Book Co.

39. Stockwell, E.G.: A critical examination of the relationship between socioeconomic status and mortality, Am. J. Public Health **53:**956, June 1963.

40. Chilman, C.S.: Growing up poor. SRS Pub. No. 109, Washington, D.C., 1969, U.S. Department of Health, Education, and Welfare.

41. Pond, M.A.: How does housing affect health? Am. J. Public Health **61:**667, May 1946.

42. Kelman, H.C.: Roles of behavioral scientist in policy-oriented research. In Coelho, G.V., and Rubinstein, E.A., editors: Social change and human behavior, DHEW Pub. No. (HSM) 72-9122, Washington, D.C., 1972, U.S. Government Printing Office.

CHAPTER 4

World health: problems and programs

The twentieth century will be remembered chiefly, not as an age of political conflicts and astonishing technical inventions, but as an age in which human society dared to think of the health of the whole human race as a practical objective.

Arnold Toynbee

HEALTH: A GLOBAL ISSUE

The ultimate measure of a nation is the supportable number and quality of its people. All else—including agricultural, mineral, industrial, and economic potential—is of value only to the extent and manner in which it may be related to people. The quantitative measure of a people is the population, especially the number of persons able to produce goods or children. This, of course, should be closely balanced with resources, present and future, of the nation and the world of which it is a part. An important qualitative measure of a people is the degree of illness or health and the rates of survival or death. Four factors influence the growth or decline of a nation's population: the numbers of births, deaths, immigrants, and emigrants. The first two are of major social, economic, political, public health, and medical importance to every nation. Beyond this, their relationship to similar factors in other countries, especially those nearby, is important. It is fundamental, therefore, to any consideration of international problems or relationships that there be an adequate fund of accurate statistical data relating to the number of persons in each nation as well as the rates and manner in which they are born, live, and die. Unfortunately this is not commonly available. The student of international health problems is confronted at the outset by gross inadequacies in this respect and is forced to think, plan, and function to a considerable degree on the basis of impressions, estimates, and generalizations.

It is not the purpose here to evaluate the completeness, accuracy, or comprehensiveness of various national or international vital statistics. However, it should be recognized that understandably the most complex, industrialized, and highly developed countries have the most exact and adequate vital data, whereas the least developed and youngest nations, and unfortunately many of those with the most outstanding health problems, tend to have the least satisfactory information about their people. One might generalize that population enumeration and birth and death registration are relatively good in the countries of northern and western Europe, parts of central and southern Europe, the British Isles, North America, Australia, New Zealand, and Japan. Conversely, they are less accurate (to varying degrees, of course) in most countries of Central and South America, parts of eastern and southern Europe, and most of Africa, the Middle East, and Asia.

GENERAL OBSERVATIONS

Despite these limitations, there is sufficient information to indicate considerable variation among countries with regard to the fertility, health, and longevity of their populations. For detailed information the reader is referred to the various statistical and epidemiologic reports of the World Health Organization.[1] In evaluating these variations, one must realize that many biologic, environmental, and social factors are involved. Thus climate, the nature of the soil, food consumption and habits, physical inheritance, folk customs, superstitions, and habits of work or exercise may affect the fertility, health, and mortality experiences of populations. Beyond these there are, of course, the influences of public health personnel, facilities, medical and nursing services, housing standards, and occupational conditions. In the broadest sense, economics, agronomy, education, and national political policy are probably the most important factors.

The key factor in determining the size of a population is the extent to which it can reproduce and maintain or increase itself.* Various methods have been devised to measure this, the most common of which is the birthrate. In general, an inverse relationship appears to exist between the birthrate and the degree of development or complexity of a nation. Thus the greater the degree of industrial and scientific progress, urbanization, and elevation of the standard of living, the more the birthrate tends to be depressed. There are, of course, several exceptions to this generalization. Nevertheless, birthrates have declined rather consistently in Western Europe and the British Isles, North America, and Japan. By contrast, birthrates have tended to fall more slowly or to increase in the countries of Asia, Africa, and Central and South America.

The birthrate in itself is neither a true measure of human fertility nor indicative of the extent to which the number of births is sufficient to maintain or to increase the population of a nation. Because of this, additional indices such as the rate of natural increase and fertility rates have been devised. The rate of natural increase is simply the annual excess of births over deaths per 1,000 population. In general this rate is highest in the countries of Africa, the Middle East, Asia, southeastern Europe, and parts of Central and South America and is lowest in northern and western Europe and North America.

Even this rate of numerical excess of births over deaths, however, is not a conclusive indication of the ability of a country's population to reproduce itself. A particular country at a given time may have an extremely large excess of births over deaths, yet its birthrate, especially when determined in relation to the number of persons of childbearing age, may not be high enough to maintain the present population eventually. This can occur when a country has a temporarily high proportion of young adults

as a result of immigration or as a result of a mass delayed reproductive action, such as occurs during a period of warfare followed by the return home of large numbers of young men. As a result of such circumstances, the birthrate temporarily may be much higher than the death rate, but the gross number of births may not be large enough to maintain such a favorable age distribution permanently. There results eventually a population with a relatively high proportion of older persons and a concomitant fall of the birthrate, even below the level of the death rate.

As a result of these influences, it is fair to expect not only continued variations in population numbers, rates of increase, and density but also significant accentuation of the differences in these factors among the nations and regions of the world[2] (Table 4-1). North America, the United Kingdom, Japan, the USSR, and western Europe will probably experience stabilized or even decreasing populations unless net reproductive rates increase, death rates decrease even more than they have, or major immigrations occur. Most of Asia, Africa, the Middle East, and Central and South America, on the other hand, appear destined to experience great, dangerous, and unsupportable increases in population if present fertility rates continue. In addition, barring the influence of other factors, these increases will be greatly magnified as death rates decline. There are many factors that might change or even reverse these trends. Important among them are improved education and standards of living combined with prompt and energetic sustained family planning programs.

The crude death rate is one of the most common and convenient indices of the state of health of a community or nation. On the world scene, despite inadequate information, it is readily observed that in general the highest death rates occur in the countries of Africa, the Middle East, Asia, and parts of Central and South America as well as in a few southern and eastern European nations. Significantly lower death rates are experienced by western Europe, the USSR, the British Isles, Australia, New Zealand, North America, Japan, and a few countries in South America. It is immediately apparent that the national or regional variations in death rate essentially parallel the variations in birthrate.

Progress in combating preventable disease and

*The problem of overpopulation is considered in detail in Chapter 5. Concern here is with its relation to health and illness.

Roots of public
health

reducing mortality has been closely related to the widespread application of advances in medical, physical, and chemical sciences. This has occurred to the greatest extent in the western European countries and in North America, the most highly industrialized and urbanized areas in the world. To the extent to which this has been accomplished in the lesser developed countries, it has been largely because of assistance from outside—from some of the more developed nations and from international agencies and foundations, which in turn are supported largely by the more developed nations. One may generalize, therefore, that death rates are lower in the more highly developed countries and higher in the more underdeveloped countries. Similarly, death rates tend to be lower in the more urbanized and industrial countries and higher in the more rural and predominantly agricultural countries.

Although this relationship appears to apply to many specific death rates, it is by no means universally true. Certainly the relationship applies to the infant death rate and maternal mortality, as it also applies to the specific rates of death from almost all of the communicable diseases that can be controlled by public health, sanitation, and immunization methods. One outstanding group of exceptions, however, does exist. Death rates for the degenerative diseases of middle and later life, such as cancer, hypertension, and the like, are generally much higher in the economically more advantaged and industrially and scientifically advanced countries of western Europe, the USSR, the British Isles, North America, Australia, New Zealand, and Japan. This apparent difference is undoubtedly because of the higher proportion of persons who reach later life as a result of public health measures and also to more accurate cause-of-death reporting in the more advanced countries.

In addition to birthrates and death rates, but as a function of the latter, average expectation of life should be considered briefly. The average life expectancy varies considerably among the different nations of the world, from a low of about 39 years in Ethiopia to a high of about 76 years in Japan. As would be expected from the preceding consideration of death rates, the average life expectancy is much greater in Western Europe, the USSR, the British Isles, North America, Australia, New Zealand, and Japan than it is in most of the rest of the world. There are, however, several exceptions to this general picture.[3]

TABLE 4-1. Health and related socioeconomic indicators

Index	Least developed countries	Other developing countries	Developed countries
Number of countries	31	89	37
Total population (millions)	283	3,001	1,131
Infant mortality rate (per 1000 live born)	160	94	19
Life expectancy (years)	45	60	72
% infants with birth weight of 2500 g or more	70%	83%	93%
% population with access to safe water supply	31%	41%	100%
Adult literacy rate	28%	55%	98%
GNP per capita	US$ 170	US$ 520	US$ 6,230
Per capita public expenditure on health	US$ 1.7	US$ 6.5	US$ 244
Public expenditure on health as % of GNP	1.0%	1.2%	3.9%
Population per doctor	17,000	2,700	520
Population per nurse	6,500	1,500	220
Population per health worker (any type, including traditional birth attendant)	2,400	500	130

From WHO Chron. **35:**223, June 1981.
NOTE: Figures in the table are weighted averages based on estimates for 1980 or for the latest year for which data are available.

The differences among countries and regions are significant at all age levels but appear to diminish consistently as older ages are approached. The obvious conclusion, substantiated by age-specific death rates, is that the greatest risk to life in the lesser developed and less advantaged areas are experienced by infants and young children. In the poorer less developed nations, up to one half of infants die, and deaths of children between 1 and 5 years of age are 12 to 15 times greater than in the developed nations. Survivors, however, have a reasonable chance of attaining a relatively advanced age[4] (Table 4-2).

One other interesting aspect of the variation in death rates and life expectancies relates to differences observed among the races. It is probable that differences are related more to social and economic factors than to racial characteristics. In general, they appear to be more circumstantial than inherent. This is exemplified by the fact that blacks in Europe and North America, although subject to a somewhat lower life expectancy and higher death rate than whites, nevertheless are in a decidedly more advantageous situation than members of the black race who still live in Africa. Furthermore, the discrepancy between the rates for whites and blacks in the Western Hemisphere has consistently become less. That the problem is not simple, however, is indicated by the situation in Hawaii, where the life expectancy of native Hawaiians is signifi-

cantly less than that for other races at every specified age except under 1 year. Caucasian-Hawaiians also have a shorter life expectancy than whites, Japanese, and Chinese who live on the islands. The explanation for this and similar phenomena remains to be determined.

EXTENT OF WORLD HEALTH PROBLEMS

Any attempt to understand world health problems must conclude that the sciences of biology and climatology are prerequisites. The cultural development, physical development, eating habits, clothing, housing, and at least to some degree, methods of political organization of humans are determined largely by biologic and climatic factors. This applies especially to our reaction to the environment. By like token, most of the preventable illnesses to which we are subject involve other biologic beings: bacteria, viruses, protozoa, helminths, insects, and the like.

Some examples may serve to illustrate these points. Since we are satisfactory hosts for the plasmodium of malaria and since we share this unfortunate role with the mosquito, it is obvious that, in the absence of scientific interference, human beings affected by malaria are most frequently found in areas where the climate is most conducive to the propagation of the mosquito. Such conditions are found especially in the warm, moist tropical and subtropical zones of the world. In contrast, as expected, the serious pulmonary infections occur most often in less temperate climates with wider and more frequent variations in temperature. These climatic conditions are conducive to frequent upper respiratory tract illnesses that often are precursors of more serious pulmonic diseases. Between these two situations one might point to typhus fever, which requires environmental and climatic conditions that are not so cold as to discourage the propagation of the louse vector yet are cold enough to cause the human host to wear considerable clothing, sometimes in a continuous and unwashed manner. If conditions are such as to combine a cold climate with continued inaqequacy of water, thereby precluding bathing and the washing of clothing, so much the better for lice and some other body-contact insects that may cause disease.

In view of the foregoing, one would rightly expect

TABLE 4-2. Infant and early childhood mortality rates, 1970-1975

	Infant mortality (per 1000 live births)	Early childhood mortality 1-4 years) (per 1000 population at risk)
More developed regions		
Country range	8.3-40.3	0.4-2.0
Less developed regions		
Northern Africa	c. 130	c. 30
Sub-Saharan Africa	c. 200	>30
Asia	c. 120-130	>10
Latin America	<100 (probably c. 85-90)	c. 6.0

From World Health Forum 2(2):264, 1981.

to find the greatest amount of preventable disease in the warmer areas of the earth. If the factors of biology and climatology are correlated with the degree of economic development and applied scientific knowledge (and, indeed, the latter would appear to be a function of the former), one observes a broad zone on the world globe, with necessarily indefinite borders and certain exceptions, that in general overlaps the equator about 20 to 25 degrees both north and south. This zone includes the areas in which the bulk of preventable infectious diseases and premature deaths now occur.

To most of those who reside permanently outside the zone, the extent of preventable disease seems incomprehensible. Nevertheless, as Russell[5] has said, "Nothing on earth is more international than disease." A few examples may illustrate.

The most widespread diseases result from infection by human feces. Included are infectious diarrheas, intestinal parasites, typhoid and paratyphoid, bacillary and amebic dysentery, infectious hepatitis, and cholera. Infectious diarrheas kill several million infants and young children (one third of deaths in this age group) each year in Africa, Asia, and Latin America.[6] The numbers of intestinal parasites are enormous. The World Health Organization estimated that worldwide in 1971 there were 650 million people with the roundworm *Ascaris,* 450 million with the hookworm *Ancylostoma,* 350 million people with amebiasis, and 350 million people with trichuriasis.[7] Some idea of the damage inflicted by such parasites may be gained by extrapolating from the earlier notable analysis by Stoll.[8] The 650 million people with roundworms would probably contain a total of 18 billion adult ascarids, which would equal the combined weight of almost 1 million adult men. The amount of food they rob annually from the intestinal tracts of those afflicted could feed the entire populations of Cambodia or Ecuador. This many adult worms broadcast from 30 to 40 thousand tons of microscopic eggs over the landscape to infect still other victims. Beyond these effects, the tremendous amount of malnutrition and anemia, with concomitant increased susceptibility to various acute communicable diseases, that results from the burden of helminthic infestations constitutes an ongoing disaster. A somewhat bizarre parasitic infestation, dracontiasis, is worthy of mention for its unusual nature and its handicapping effect.

The organism is a nematode *Dracunculus medinensis,* or the guinea worm, acquired by drinking water containing the minute crustacean *Cyclops,* which has ingested the larvae that the adult worm has discharged into the water. Eventually the adult worm, which is sometimes as long as a meter and develops in the tissues from the swallowed larva, surfaces, usually on the human foot, and completes the cycle by discharging more larvae into the water. In the process general symptoms as well as severe crippling may result. An estimated 50 million persons are affected by it.

Speaking of parasitic infestations as a whole, Stoll[8] dramatically described their significance by saying, "Helminthiases do not have the journalistic value of great pandemics like flu or plague . . . but to make up for their lack of drama, they are unremittingly corrosive."

It is impossible even to estimate the numbers of cases and deaths from typhoid and paratyphoid fevers, salmonellosis, shigellosis, the complex of so-called food poisonings, or infectious hepatitis. It is certain, however, that their incidence is tremendous. Cholera has been reported in more than 80 countries in Asia, Africa, and Europe since 1961. The disease waxes and wanes but can move with great rapidity, and at present it is spreading.[9] In 1979 there were 54,817 cases reported to the World Health Organization from 42 countries. The Director General of the World Health Organization once said that one fifth of all deaths in the world were attributable to faulty environmental conditions. He pointed out that probably three fourths of the world's people drink unsafe water, dispose of human excreta recklessly, prepare milk and food dangerously, and live in a primitive state of insanitation. Such conditions, hence such disease consequences, exist predominantly in the rural agricultural nations. As evidenced by data from developing countries, in 1975 only 22% of the rural populations had access to community water supplies in contrast to 77% of urban dwellers. With regard to adequate excreta disposal facilities, the figures were 15% for rural populations and 75% for urban populations.[10]

The large group of vector-borne diseases must next command attention. Only a few of the most important can be mentioned. Malaria occupies the predominant position. It is still probably the leading cause death in the world despite the strenuous national and international efforts to control if not eradicate it. The success of the 1950s and 1960s has been thwarted by a combination of mosquito resistance to insecticides, escalating costs, population movements, and in some areas national and international strife. In just the 4 years from 1972 to 1976, the number of new cases of malaria increased about 230% in Indonesia, Sri Lanka, and the Indian subcontinent. About 1.7 billion people live in areas where the disease continues to be transmitted despite control efforts, and an additional 352 million live in infected areas with no antimalarial efforts.[11] There are now a record 400 million cases in the world.

Trypanosomiasis, or sleeping sickness, spread by the bite of the tsetse fly, is of particular importance in a broad band across sub-Saharan Africa. If not treated early it is usually fatal. During the colonial era of the early twentieth century it became widespread. Epidemics, especially in Uganda and the Congo, were estimated to have caused the deaths of half of the population. In company with malaria, it bars effective use of tremendous areas that many consider to contain some of the world's best agricultural and grazing land. The total area involved is about 4.5 million square miles, half again as large as the continental United States.[12] Chagas' disease is a form of trypanosomiasis that exists in rural Mexico, Central America, and parts of South America. About 7 million people are estimated to be affected in South America. It is spread by the bloodsucking Reduviidae, or kissing bugs. Although Chagas' disease is not nearly as serious as its African counterpart, cardiac complications are common.

Bilharziasis, or schistosomiasis, spread by snails, affects the populations of large irrigated parts of northern Africa, northeastern South America, Japan, and southeastern China. It has been estimated that in the Middle East about 30 million people, or 90% of the rural population, suffer from this debilitating disease, which generally reduces productivity by at least one third. In Egypt about three fourths of the population is affected. Lower Egypt is affected more than upper Egypt as a result of large new areas irrigated in relation to the high Aswan dam. Worldwide it is estimated that 180 million people are infected.[7]

Filarial infestations are another cause of physical incapacitation and economic loss. *Wuchereria bancrofti,* spread by several species of mosquitoes, is found in most tropical countries, especially in Indonesia, northern Australia, parts of South Asia, Japan, Africa, the West Indies, the northern coast of South America, and the eastern coast of Brazil.

In addition *W. malayi* occurs in the Malay peninsula, Sumatra, Borneo, New Guinea, India, Indochina, Sri Lanka, and southern China. Onchocerciasis, a type of filarial infestation, spread by the black fly *Simulium,* is endemic to parts of Mexico, Guatemala and Venezuela, parts of Central Africa, and especially West Africa where "river blindness' from the disease has led to depopulation of fertile river valleys. The total number of people affected by onchocerciasis has been estimated at 20 million.[13] With reference to blindness as a whole, there are estimated to be about 24 million blind people in the world, over 30 million of them in the lesser developed countries.[6] Among the major causes, in addition to onchocerciasis, are trachoma, xerophthalmia from vitamin A deficiency, gonorrhea and syphilis, measles, cataracts, and glaucoma. Prevalence rates in some areas are very high, for example, upper Ghana, 6.5%; Egypt, 2.6%, Chad, 3% to 5%; rural northern Sudan, 4.5%; India, 1.5%; Pakistan, 4.3%; Yemen, 4%; and Uganda, 1.8%.[14]

Three other diseases, plague, leprosy, and tuberculosis, merit comment. Historically so important, human plague is by no means eradicated. Its incidence varies considerably from year to year. Between 1958 and 1977 it was reported in 45,296 people in 29 countries, nine of them (Bolivia, Brazil, Burma, Ecuador, Madagascar, Peru, United States, Viet Nam, and Zaire) reporting cases practically every year. From 1973 to 1974 there was a 400% increase in cases and deaths, 678 cases reported in 1973 and 2,755 cases in 1974. By 1978 cases had dropped to 766 and deaths to 31.[15] Meanwhile it remains a smouldering threat to mankind.

Leprosy, another historically ancient disease, claims about 15 million victims worldwide. Only about one fourth receive any treatment. Southern India has the largest concentration, about 3% of the population of 300 million. Other areas severely affected are the People's Republic of China, many parts of Africa and southeast Asia, and many nations in Latin America. The recent development of drugs such as rifampicin and clofazimine combined with dapsone, as well as efforts to develop an effective vaccine, may spell some hope in future attacks on this disease.

Tuberculosis, which may rightly be regarded as a disease of poverty, still claims at least 3.5 million new patients each year, more than half of whom

die from it. Its incidence and prevalence closely parallel the degrees of economic disadvantage
among the nations. The World Health Organization
and other international agencies have been gradually breaking the chain of infection by means of
early case finding followed by chemotherapy as
well as extensive BCG vaccination programs. The
ultimate weapon, of course, is economic improvement.[6]

HEALTH PERSONNEL

One of the most serious problems is the shortage
of health personnel of all types throughout most of
the world. Indeed, the insufficiency not only of physicians but also of nurses, trained midwives, environmental health workers, and all other types of
health personnel has been referred to by the Director-General of the World Health Organization as
the main reason why health levels throughout the
world are not improving.[16] The supply of physicians
provides a good example, not only of the general
inadequacies in numbers but also of the greatly
skewed maldistribution (Table 4-1). In 1973 the
physician-to-population ratio in Israel was 1 to 400,
the most favorable in the world. For the USSR it
was 1 to 455; for New Zealand, 1 to 680; for the
United States, 1 to 720; and for Canada, 1 to 890
inhabitants. By contrast Niger had 1 to 63,000; Indonesia, 1 to 41,000; and Sudan and Vietnam, 1
physician to 29,000 inhabitants each. World regional figures reflected these variations. For Europe
the ratio was 1 to 1,000, but of the 22 nations reporting, 10 nations averaged 1 physician per 500
to 750 inhabitants. For the western Pacific the ratio was 1 to 2,500, varying from Australia's 1 to
680 to Laos' 1 to 39,000 inhabitants. For Latin
America the ratio was 1 to 3,500, varying from Cu-
ba's 1 to 1,220 to Belize's 1 to 5,700 inhabitants.
In the eastern Mediterranean region the ratio was
1 to 4,500 inhabitants. Of the 11 nations reporting
many had significant shortages, yet the area included Kuwait with 1 to 800 and Egypt with 1 to
2,500 inhabitants. The Southeast Asia region,
which includes Sri Lanka, India, Thailand, Burma,
and Indonesia, averaged 1 to 5,000, despite a highly
unfavorable ratio of 1 to 41,000 inhabitants for Indonesia, which has a large population. In Africa
south of the Sahara, with all but two countries reporting, the ratio was 1 to 18,000 inhabitants.

In addition to the many quantitative inadequacies, differences in extent and quality of education
of physicians must also be kept in mind. On the
brighter side, it should be mentioned that training
in public health has been increased significantly in
both quantity and scope. There are now about 150
recognized schools of public health in 50 or more
countries. Furthermore, postgraduate education in
such schools is broadening to include not only the
biomedical but also the behavioral and managerial
aspects of public health and its administration.

Recently some important steps have been taken
to improve the health personnel problem and the
distribution of health services. For many years the
World Health Organization and other international
health assistance agencies placed great emphasis
on the training of health care personnel of high
quality to work in upgraded treatment facilities
preferably related to professional schools. Experience demonstrated that this resulted in small proportions of the public receiving excellent care, and
very little of the benefit filtered down to the populations as a whole. Added to this shortcoming was
the tendency of many of the well-trained personnel
to succumb to the recruitment efforts of international agencies, corporations, and less needy, more
affluent nations.[17] Recognition of these and related
problems has resulted in significant changes in national and international policies during the past decade.[18] Attention has shifted from expansion of facilities and personnel for high-grade, hospital-based
therapeutic care largely in urban centers to improvement and extension of relatively rudimentary
health care services by primary health workers.
Preferably such personnel are locally recruited and
often supported by their communities. Their basic
training is typically specialized, and in preferred
situations they are supported by supervision or consultation from more highly trained professionals.[19]
Included are many types with many names: medical or health assistants, sanitarians, nursing auxiliaries, midwives or birth attendants, feldshers,
barefoot doctors, and many others. Another change
that has occurred is the legitimization in many
places of so-called traditional healers and some of
their procedures. In many instances traditional
healers have received training in certain aspects of
scientific medicine and public health, and in return
certain traditional medications and methods have
been adopted by practitioners of scientific medicine
and public health.[20] The goal of course is better
distribution of more and better health care.

ECONOMIC, SOCIAL, AND POLITICAL RELATIONSHIPS OF WORLD HEALTH PROBLEMS

From what has been presented, it is clear that most of the mass of preventable disease in the world is concentrated in what is commonly referred to as *developing* areas or countries. It should be recognized that the term is unsatisfactory and that citizens of countries so described often object to it. Perhaps such understandable objection based on commendable national pride may be somewhat assuaged by pointing out that the term implies that there is something worth developing—a situation not without its desirable aspect. It would seem equally obvious that one cannot speak, think, or act about the health problems of these countries or areas within an isolated substantive framework. Large proportions of the human beings who live in these areas, and they constitute most of the population of the earth, eke out a miserable existence under circumstances that are undesirable from many different standpoints, of which ill health is only one. Their housing is inadequate, their economy unbalanced, their food supply precarious, their methods of performing daily tasks primitive, their educational horizons limited, and their daily work relatively inefficient and unproductive.

What is cause and what is effect? Widespread preventable disease unquestionably serves as a barrier to progress in any direction, be it economic, social, or political. A population that is chronically ill understandably has a decreased productivity. Millions of man-days of work are lost annually because of typhoid, paratyphoid, the dysenteries, and enteritis. The loss of manpower in countries where malaria is widespread has been reported to be from 5% to 10% of the total labor force, with the greatest incidence of the disease occurring at the peak period of agricultural production. It was estimated by Russell[5] that any nation importing products of a highly malarious country pays the equivalent of a 5% malaria tax. For what the United States imports from such areas, this would amount to a hidden cost of hundreds of millions of dollars per year.

Widespread disease also serves as an effective barrier to the development of agricultural lands and natural resources. The effective settlement of such areas as Sumatra, Borneo, central Africa, large parts of South America, and until recently, the Terai of India, Pakistan, Nepal, and large parts of Sardinia, to mention only a few examples, has been prevented by disease, primarily malaria and other insect-borne diseases. The accomplishments in the last two locations give some indication of the potential elsewhere. The control of malaria in Sardinia during the 1950s paved the way for the resettlement of about 1 million Italians from the overcrowded mainland. Similar measures in the Terai have made it possible to open this great fertile area to agricultural development. For the world as a whole, the malaria eradication program begun by the World Health Organization in 1955 has accomplished much, although, as has been mentioned, there have been recent setbacks in some areas.[11] Even greater success has been achieved in the fight against smallpox, which appears to have been completely eliminated as a threat to mankind.

For the individual, educational and intellectual development is difficult if at all possible when the body is chronically drained of its energy by illness and parasites. This was illustrated in the Philippines some years ago when it was found that malaria control reduced school absenteeism from about 50% daily to 3%. At the same time industrial absenteeism was reduced from 35% to under 4%. Uncontrolled disease in the environment and the continuance of conditions that breed unproductivity and illiteracy also effectively discourage investment from within or without as well as industrial development. Finally, a low economy and standard of living attributable directly or indirectly to widespread ill health are a constant encouragement to political instability. Under such circumstances, people have many reasons for discontent and have little to lose in resorting to violence.

This situation, of course, is a vicious circle. Disease breeds poverty, and poverty in turn breeds more disease. A similar relationship exists between disease and illiteracy, political instability, and many other factors. It is difficult or impossible to state which factor is primary, which is cause, and which is effect. Once the cycle is established, however, it is clear that each factor contributes to the continuance of all other undesirable factors. This has been referred to as a cumulative causation.

The World Health Organization has emphasized this in its listing of some of the characteristics of underdeveloped rural areas.[21]

Economic stagnation
Cultural patterns unfavorable to development

Roots of public
health

Agricultural underemployment and lack of alternative
employment opportunities

Poor quality of life due to scarcity of essential goods,
facilities, and money

Isolation caused by distance and poor communications

An unfavorable environment predisposing to communicable diseases and malnutrition

Inadequate health facilities and lack of sanitation

Poor educational opportunities

Social injustice including inequitable land tenure systems and a rigid hierarchy and class structure

Inadequate representation and influence in national
decision making

To these should be added:

Suppression of women

Inequities based on race, ethnic background, or religious affiliation

Some of these relationships are illustrated by data
of Sagen and Afifi[22] presented in Table 4-3. It will
be observed that many more people live in the less
developed countries than in those that are more
developed. Beyond this, it will be noted that in the
case of every index (measuring health, agricultural
development, industrial development, education,
trade, food consumption, and so on), the less developed countries are significantly disadvantaged
as compared with those that are more developed.

The solution to the problem is not easy. Certainly
it cannot be accomplished by an attack on health
problems alone. In fact, such an approach would
carry with it certain real dangers, if indeed it really
were to succeed at all. Advancement must be made
in many fields simultaneously. In this regard the
statement of Myrdal[23] at the Fifth World Health
Assembly is worthy of note in summarizing the
complexity of the situation and outlining a guide
for effective, lasting action:

TABLE 4-3. Comparison of economic, health, and educational conditions in countries grouped by phases of economic development, 1975

Variables	Stage of economic development					
	I	II	III	IV	V	Total
Total population (millions)	365	1,113	1,337	396	798	3,954
Death rate	23.0	15.8	10.5	8.5	9.4	12.76
Birth rate	47.4	41.5	30.9	20.0	16.5	31.7
Fertility	222	202	176	85	77	148
Infant mortality	158.6	128.6	67.0	21.0	20.8	80.0
Longevity at birth	41.3	50.6	60.9	71.0	71.0	59.0
Gross national product	120	160	459	2,615	3,967	1,219
Energy consumption*	51.0	201	700	3,277	7,290	2,022
Percent labor force, agricultural	72.3	68.2	63.7	28.3	21.0	52.6
Percent urban population	6.7	13.3	30.3	41.5	45.3	26.4
Percent literacy	21.2	36.0	68.2	93.7	98.4	62.9
Total daily calories	2,092	1,979	2,201	2,673	3,131	2,254
Daily calories, carbohydrates	1,686	1,545	1,665	1,691	1,668	1,636
Daily calories, fats	295	257	350	619	1,043	480
Daily calories, protein	220	200	243	314	364	259
Daily calories, animal protein	36	31	77	123	202	93
Population per M.D.	28,234	9,355	2,812	745	564	7,067
Population per hospital bed	2,838	1,496	540	121	106	1,004

From Sagen, L.A., and Afifi, A.A.: Health and economic development, IIASA Research Memorandum 78-41, Laxenburg, Austria, 1978, International Institute for Applied Systems Analysis.
*Per capita annual commercial energy consumption in kg coal equivalent.

The task of social engineering is to proportion and direct the induced changes in the whole social field so as to maximize the beneficial effects of a given initial financial sacrifice. One important corollary to theory of cumulative causation is that a rational policy should never work by inducing change in only one factor; least of all should such a change of only one factor be attempted suddenly and with great force. This would in most cases prove to be a wasteful expenditure of efforts which could reach much further by being spread strategically over the various factors in the social system and over a period of time. What we are facing is a whole set of interrelated adverse living conditions for a population. An effort to reach permanent improvement of health standards aimed to have a maximum beneficial effect on the well-being of the people will, in other words, have to be integrated in a broad economic and social reform policy. Such a policy will have to be founded upon studies of how in the concrete situation of a particular country the different factors in the plane of living are interrelated and how we can move them all upwards in such a fashion that the changes will support each other to the highest possible degree.

More recently Newell,[24] discussing health care development as an agent of social change, has observed that health development is one part of community development efforts and that "the health of individuals and communities will improve if a continuing self-sustaining process of community development can be started." These and similar increasingly frequent views have resulted in both the World Health Organization[25] and the United Nations[26] taking firm stands that emphasize that improved health is fundamental and necessary to economic development.

HEALTH PROGRAMMING FOR DEVELOPING AREAS

Areas of the world in which socioeconomic development has been delayed are always confronted by many frustrating dilemmas. One of the most obvious is what to do first. It is understandable that many individuals and groups who have had to wait for the opportunity to move forward clamor for many different, divergent, uncoordinated, and sometimes impractical things. Among the many examples that could be described is a nation with a mammoth backlog of preventable illness and widespread malnutrition that, when offered public health technical assistance, vigorously requested an electron microscope and the services of a cardiorespiratory physiologist. Another country with similar problems held for a 1,000-bed general hospital, a 500-bed pediatric hospital, and a 500-bed

tuberculosis hospital, despite the fact that there were not enough trained personnel in the entire region, much less in the particular nation, to staff such institutions.

Such tendencies force the necessity of determining some reasonably satisfactory guidelines or priorities for the most logical and effective health activities. In doing so it is critical that the total needs, problems, resources, and aspirations of the nation or area be carefully considered.

Decisions relating to program choices should be based on two fundamental considerations or criteria:
1. The extent to which they strengthen the economies of nations by health benefits that release effective human energy, improve citizen morale, improve environment for local and foreign investment, and open new land and project areas
2. The extent to which they contribute to desirable political objectives by aiding the stability of governments, by reaching large populations with highly welcomed personal service programs, and by demonstrating deep human interest in the dignity of mankind

In recent years we have witnessed several very encouraging trends. Increasing numbers of developing countries have established planning units within their ministries of health. These have been strengthened, not only by the assignment of personnel from other parts of the government such as finance, but also by the provision of advanced training in planning and administrative management to promising individuals already within the ministries of health. These individuals have been assisted in this effort by the several international sources of fellowships. Equally important has been the concurrent establishment at the highest level of broad-based planning or development units, with health representation included, reporting directly to the head of government. These are fundamental steps not only for the avoidance of duplication or conflicts of interest but also for the assurance that critically important views and actions are not overlooked.

INTERNATIONAL HEALTH ORGANIZATIONS

It must always be borne in mind that effective lasting action can occur only on the local level where the people, their problems, their communities, and their governmental structures are found. Therefore international health work cannot be thought of as a field unto itself. It has meaning only in its relation to the many national and local components of the total world health picture. It is with this reservation that certain aspects of the development and present status of international health activities are presented.

World Health Organization

Movement toward international cooperation in health goes back several generations, based initially on concerns about epidemic disease.[27] The first crystallization was the First International Sanitary Conference in Paris in 1851. It is significant that each of the 12 participating countries was represented by a physician and a diplomat. This was followed by a series of similar conferences, and in 1903 plans began to be formulated for the establishment of a permanent international health agency. This became a reality in 1907, when 12 nations signed an agreement for the creation of the Office Internationale d'Hygiène Publique.[28] Meanwhile, for the same reason (i.e., concerns about epidemic disease), representatives of 21 American Republics met at their first International Sanitary Conference in Mexico City early in 1902. On December 2, 1902, the International Sanitary Bureau was established. This organization has functioned continuously with several name changes and, as the present Pan American Health Organization, is the oldest functioning international health organization. It also serves as the western hemispheric regional office of the subsequently established World Health Organization.[29]

The end of World War I led to the establishment of the League of Nations, which in 1921 formed a Health Organization. Because of obvious conflict and duplication as well as the desirability of broad international connections, the Office International d'Hygiène Publique merged with the Health Organization of the League of Nations, which continued to function, as did the Pan-American Sanitary Bureau, through the period of World War II.[30,31]

In 1944, while the war was still in progress and Paris was occupied by the Nazis, an international conference was held in Montreal to discuss the fate of the Health Organization of the League of Nations. Stemming from this and culminating at a

further conference in New York, in 1946,[32] a constitution for a World Health Organization was signed by 61 nations on April 7, 1948, and the organization came into official existence. The duties and powers of the Health Organization of the League of Nations and the health functions of the temporary United Nations Relief and Rehabilitation Administration were transferred to the new agency. Subsequently the Pan-American Sanitary Bureau (now the Pan American Health Organization), although retaining a separate identity, became the World Health Organization's regional office for the Americas.

On June 24, 1948, the first World Health Assembly convened in Geneva with delegates from 52 member states plus observers from 11 nonmember states, and 10 international governmental organizations.[33] By 1982 the World Health Organization had a membership of 158 nations, which makes it the largest of the specialized agencies of the United Nations. In addition, about 120 nongovernmental organizations maintain official relations with it. The United States has been an active member since the World Health Organization's formation in 1948.

The constitution of the World Health Organization, particularly in view of its definition of health as "a state of complete physical, mental, and social well-being and not merely the absence of disease or infirmity," has been aptly referred to as the Magna Charta of health because of its affirmation that health is "one of the fundamental rights of every human being, without distinction of race, religion, political belief, economic or social condition" and its recognition that "the health of all peoples is fundamental to the attainment of peace and security.[34]

With regard to its structure and management,[35] the headquarters of the World Health Organization is in Geneva, Switzerland. Regional offices are located at Brazzaville, for Africa; Washington, D.C. for the Americas (Pan American Health Organization); New Delhi, for Southeast Asia; Copenhagen, for Europe; Alexandria, for the eastern Mediterranean; and Manila, for the western Pacific. It is financed by prorated and special contributions from active member nations and from the United Nations Technical Assistance Board. Its budget for 1982 to 1983 was U.S. $484.3 million. An annual World Health Assembly, usually held in Geneva in May, determine international health policy and program and serves as the agency's legislative body. Each member nation is allowed three delegates but only one vote at the Assemblies.

An executive board has the responsibility of implementing the decisions and policies of the Assembly and deals with emergency situations in the name of the Assembly. Normally this technical nonpolitical group of 30 health experts, who are elected at the Assembly, meets twice a year. A secretariat, headed by a Director-General, includes a technical and an administrative staff located at the Geneva headquarters and in the regional offices. It is responsible for the day-to-day work of the organization. The World Health Organization avoids one of the basic errors of the health office of the former League of Nations, that of overcentralization, in that is provides for regional committees comprised of representatives of member states in each region. These regional committees formulate regional policies and supervise the activities of the regional offices. In addition, panels and committees on various pertinent subjects involve more than 12,000 experts in various fields to advise the World Health Organization of its activities and keep it up to date on current scientific research.

The mission or purpose of the World Health Organization has been summarized as follows[36]:

1. It is the one directing and coordinating authority on international health work. It is not a supranational ministry of health; rather, it is a worldwide cooperative through which the nations help each other to help themselves in raising health standards.

2. It provides to member countries various central technical services, that is, epidemiology, statistics, standardization of drugs and procedures, a wide range of technical publications, etc.

3. Its most important function is to help countries to strengthen and improve their own health service. On request it provides advisory and consulting services through public health experts, demonstration teams for disease control, visiting specialists, etc.

Periodically, the World Health Assembly establishes priorities. For the period from 1978 to 1983 it has specified six major areas of concern.[37]

1. Development of comprehensive health services
2. Disease prevention and control
3. Promotion of environmental health
4. Health manpower development
5. Promotion of biomedical and health services research
6. Program development and support

There are two important distinctions between the health office of the League of Nations and the World Health Organization, which replaced it. First, the functions and activities of the latter are extremely broad. For the first time in international affairs emphasis has been placed not on quarantine, checking epidemics, and other defensive measures but on positive, aggressive action toward health in its broadest sense. Second, whereas the former organization was an integral part of a political body, the World Health Organization, although related to the United Nations, is nevertheless a separate, independent agency with its own constitution, membership, and sources of funds. As yet, it is too early to determine with assurance what the future holds for this organization. Much depends on the ability of the nations of the world to live with one another in peace and cooperation. It has been commonly said that despite its political affiliation, the old health office was the most successful part of the League of Nations. In view of this, the World Health Organization can expect much greater success, effectiveness, and permanency.

Pan American Health Organization

The turn of the century saw the establishment in 1902 at the Second American International Conference in Mexico City of the International Sanitary Bureau, subsequently renamed the Pan American Health Organization.[38] Its headquarters is in Washington, D.C. As has been mentioned, this was the first permanent international health agency and the longest lived up to the present. It was organized to be governed by an elected directing council and a Director-General. It is supported by annual financial quotas contributed by each of the American Republics, augmented from other sources. In 1977 its budget was $70 million, of which about two thirds came from assessments of member nations and the remainder from the World Health Organization, other United Nations sources, and miscellaneous inter-American, national, and private contributions. Under the provisions of the Pan-American Sanitary Code, which was ratified by all 21 of the American Republics in 1924, the Pan American Health Organization became the center of coordination of international action and information in the field of public health in the Western Hemisphere. It holds an annual conference of high quality, which is attended by delegates from all member nations. Through its development it has been given the responsibility and authority to receive and disseminate epidemiologic information, to furnish technical assistance on request to member countries, to finance fellowships, and to promote cooperation in medical research. It has done much to promote professional education in Latin America.[38] It also serves as the regional office and agent in the Americas of the World Health Organization.

United Nations Children's Fund

The United Nations Children's Fund is an agency whose history and activities have been intimately related to those of the World Health Organization. At the demise of the United Nations Relief and Rehabilitation Administration in 1946, certain of its funds were transferred to a newly formed agency organized to assist especially the children of war-torn countries. The program gradually expanded to include other activities and other areas, particularly underdeveloped countries.

This agency has spent large sums of money, especially on food and supplies, for the promotion of child and maternal health and welfare activities throughout the world. Beyond this, however, and usually through partnership with the World Health Organization, it has been carrying out large and significant programs of BCG vaccination, yaws control, and malaria control demonstrations. The promotion of family planning in developing countries has been one of its major activities in recent years. Organized originally as a temporary emergency agency, it has filled such a need and attracted such support that in 1953 it was given permanent status and named the United Nations Children's Fund. One of its most interesting and valuable enterprises has been the International Children's Center, established in the late 1940s.[39] The center brings together and coordinates the efforts of many disciplines: pediatricians, social workers, psychologists, educators, and health and social administrators. It is concerned with all three aspects of child development: physical, mental, and social. Its international activities are fourfold: teaching of child welfare problems and methods, medical-social research work, documentation and publications, and cooperation in matters of child welfare.

Bilateral health assistance

So far, consideration has been given to the development of what have been commonly referred to as the multilateral organizations in public health, that is, organizations whose financing, staffing, policy making, and operations are entered into and shared by more than two, and usually many, nations. In addition, there exists another type of international health cooperation that is carried out by what are referred to as bilateral agreements and organizations. This comes about when two nations, for reasons of mutual interest, agree to work together on certain matters dealing with public health.

The U.S. Government became significantly involved in bilateral international public health activities as a result of World War II. In January 1942 the Foreign Ministers of the American Republics, concerned about world events, considered areas where cooperation among the republics of the Western hemisphere was necessary for the common good. Health needs were placed high on the list. They recommended that through bilateral and other agreements steps be taken to solve the environmental sanitation and health problems of the Americas and that to this end, according to capacity, each country contribute raw material, services, and funds. The United States was asked to accept the responsibility of leadership, and an Office of the Coordinator of Inter-American Affairs was established. Originally it was attached to the Office of the President of the United States, but later it assumed a governmental corporate structure with the name Institute of Inter-American Affairs. It was given the responsibility of initiating and conducting bilateral technical assistance programs in health, agriculture, education, and eventually other fields.

In intimate relationship with each of the other republics involved, cooperative health programs promptly were established with 18 nations of Central and South America. The activities of each were financed by contributions from both the United States and the other governments concerned, and the programs were determined jointly by an official of the host government, usually the Minister or Director-General of Health, and the chief of the group of professionals assigned by the United States to the host country.

From the beginning the program had four areas of emphasis: (1) the development of local health services through health centers; (2) the sanitation of the environment, with particular emphasis on water supply, sewage disposal, and insect control; (3) the training and full-time employment of professional public health workers; and (4) the education of the public in health matters. It stressed complete community health development under full-time trained direction with active community participation.

With the end of World War II and stimulated by the tremendous needs for rehabilitation throughout the world, by requests for assistance from newly formed nations, and by the proved value of the approach of the Institute of Inter-American Affairs, the United States organized a succession of agencies. These underwent a series of reorganizations and eventually in 1961 constituted the Agency for International Development (AID) within the U.S. Department of State.

AID coordinates its health planning and programs with the Office of International Health of the U.S. Public Health Service and with the World Health Organization and assists other nations by providing, among other things, technical and material assistance in a wide range of public health programs. At present, public health personnel financed by AID are engaged in numerous types of health programs in various countries throughout the world, in cooperation with the various assistance programs of the World Health Organization and other United Nations–related agencies, other nations, and private foundations. Many public health and related workers from the United States, representing a wide spectrum of professional disciplines, are involved in its programs. One of the most significant contributions of AID and of its predecessors has been in the field of training. Fellowships for advanced training in the United States and elsewhere have been granted to several thousand professional health workers of other countries, and many thousands more have been given in-service training in connection with ongoing cooperative health programs.

Although AID is one of the most significant channels for international health participation and assistance, United States activity goes considerably beyond it. By 1978, 23 different federal agencies were involved with total expenditures of $528 million. This does not include health care provided by the Department of Defense to eligible beneficiaries overseas, which costs about $625 million, or the $49 million contributed through international financial institutions. All these together in 1978 constituted a total expenditure for international health assistance and foreign health care of $1,202 million annually by the United States.[40]

In addition to the United States, several other nations provide technical and material assistance in health and other fields on a bilateral basis. Among these are Sweden, the United Kingdom, the Federal Republic of Germany, France, the USSR, and People's Republic of China.

Nongovernmental agencies

No summary of international health cooperation would be complete without mention of the great contribution that has been made by nongovernmental agencies. As far as "shirt-sleeve" technical assistance is concerned, undoubtedly the earliest endeavors were those of the various church missions and medical missionaries. In addition, there have been certain philanthropic foundations with interest in international health based on the highest altruistic motives. Among the many that might be mentioned are the Unitarian Service Committee; the American Friends Service Committee; the various Catholic Mission groups; the American Bureau for Medical Aid to China; the Foreign Mission Agencies of the Baptist, Methodist, and Seventh Day Adventist churches; and the Near East Relief agency. Representatives of all these have performed yeoman service, working hand in hand with the people of villages and farms in many lands on a basis of true friendship and equality.

Among the foundations, the Rockefeller Foundation is the best known in the field of international assistance in health. It has operated in almost all countries of the world in the 7 decades of its existence. Its significant contributions are many and include such activities as the control of malaria and yellow fever, the development of recognized centers of learning in medicine and public health, the provision of postgraduate fellowships to many individuals, and the demonstration of sound methods of organization and operation of health programs.[41] The Rockefeller foundation has been joined by several other foundations, notably the Kellogg Foundation, which has been especially interested in improving professional education in the Latin American countries.

Conclusion

To some, it may appear as if the programs of international health are too many, too varied, too dispersed, and too confusing. Although this may be true to some degree, it has been by no means unexpected or undesirable. The field of international cooperation for social and economic development is still rather new. Indeed, there are still many individuals in the world who do not comprehend the mutual cause-effect and supportive relationships that exist between the efforts to improve health and the achievement of socioeconomic development. This in itself represents one of the greatest challenges to health workers on both the domestic and the international levels. It has been necessary and logical to approach international health with a combination of caution and courage and often on the basis of trial and error, rather than to attempt to establish prematurely a fixed pattern that might have misled future growth and thought. In recent years a process of pulling the pieces together has begun in both the multilateral and the bilateral areas. It is to be expected that the future will see an ever more logical and fruitful organizational approach to the tremendous problems that still exist in public health throughout the world. In the process, the names of some organizations may change. If so, it should be borne in mind that only results count and that titles are incidental.

Finally, it must be realized that there will always be an important place for all three types of international health work: multilateral, bilateral, and nongovernmental. Each in its way augments the efforts of the others. Sound, effective, and cooperative correlation of all of their activities may result in the ultimate achievement of the universally desired goal of world health and through it, indirectly, world peace.[42]

REFERENCES

1. World health epidemiological report and world health statistics (annual), Geneva, World Health Organization.
2. The least developed countries, WHO Chron. **35:**223, June 1981.
3. World development report, Washington, D.C., 1979, World Bank.
4. The world's main health problems, World Health Forum **2**(2):264, 1981.
5. Russell, P.: A lively corpse, Trop. Med. News **5:**25, June 1948.
6. Zahra, A.: WHO's communicable disease programme, World Health, Nov. 1980, p. 3.
7. Health, Sector policy paper, Washington, D.C., 1980, World Bank.
8. Stoll, N.R.: This wormy world, J. Parasitol. **33:**1, Feb. 1947.
9. News item: Cholera in 1979, WHO Chron. **34:**315, July-Aug. 1980.
10. World Health Organization: World Health Stat. Rep. **29:**570, 1976.
11. The malaria situation in 1976, WHO Chron. **32:**9, Jan. 1978.
12. McKelvey, J.J.: Man against tsetse, Ithaca, 1973, Cornell University Press.
13. Onchocerciasis, WHO Chron. **30:**18, Jan. 1976.
14. Data on blindness throughout the world, WHO Chron. **33:**275, May-June 1979.
15. Plague surveillance and control, WHO Chron. **34:** 139, Mar-April 1980.
16. Mahler, H.: WHO at the crossroads, WHO Chron. **31:**226, June 1977.
17. Mejia, A.: International migration of professional health personnel, WHO Chron. **34:**346, Sept. 1980.
18. Hall, T., and Majia, A.: Health manpower planning: principles, methods, issues, Geneva, 1978, World Health Organization.
19. Training and utilization of auxiliary personnel for rural health teams in developing countires, WHO Tech. Rep. Ser. No. 633, 1979.
20. Morinis, E.A.: Two pathways in understanding disease: traditional and scientific, WHO Chron. **32:**57, Feb. 1978.
21. Djukanovic, V., and Mach, E.P.: Alternative approaches to meeting basic health needs in developing countries, Geneva, 1975, World Health Organization.
22. Sagen, L.A., and Afifi, A.A.: Health and economic development, HASA Research Memorandum 78-41, Laxenburg, Austria, 1978, International Institute for Applied Systems Analysis.
23. Myrdal, G.: Economic aspects of health, WHO Chron. **6:**207, Aug. 1952.
24. Newell, K.W.: Health care development as an agent of change, WHO Chron. **30:**181, May 1976.
25. Contribution of health to the new international economic order, WHO Chron. **34:**274, July-Aug. 1980.
26. Health as an integral part of development, Resolution 34/58, U.N. General Assembly, Nov. 29, 1979.
27. Goodman, N.M.: International health organizations and their work, New York, 1952, Blakiston Division, McGraw-Hill Book Co.
28. The evolution of international cooperation in public health, WHO Chron. **12:**263, July-Aug. 1958.
29. Acuna, H.R.: The Pan American Health Organization—75 years of international cooperation in public health, Public Health Rep. **92:**537, Nov., Dec. 1977.

30. Jones, N.H.: International public health: the organizational problems between the two World Wars, WHO Chron. **31**:391, 449, 1977.

31. Jones, N.H.: International public health: the organizational problems between the two World Wars, WHO Chron. **32**:26, 63, 114, 156, 1978.

32. U.S. Department of State: International Health Conference, New York, June 19 to July 22, 1946, Pub. No. 2703, Washington, D.C., 1947, U.S. Government Printing Office.

33. Doull, J.A.: The first world health assembly, Public Health Rep. **63**:1379, Oct. 22, 1948.

34. World Health Organization: Basic documents, ed. 22, Geneva, 1971, The Organization.

35. Introducing WHO, Geneva, 1976, World Health Organization.

36. Division of Information, World Health Organization: The World Health Organization, Geneva, 1967, The Organization.

37. The work of WHO, 1976-77, biennial report of the Director-General to the World Health Assembly, Geneva, 1978, World Health Organization.

38. Pan American Health Organization: The Pan American Health Organization: The Pan American Health Organization: what it is, what it does, how it works, Washington, D.C., 1972, The Organization.

39. Berthet, E.: Activities of the International Children's Center, Am. J. Public Health **48**:458, April 1958.

40. Bourne, P.G.: A partnership for international health, Public Health Rep. **93**:114, Mar.-April 1978.

41. Shaplen, R.: Toward the well-being of mankind, Garden City, N.Y., 1964, Doubleday & Co., Inc.

42. Mahler, H.: Blueprint for health for all, WHO Chron. **31**:491, Dec. 1977.

CHAPTER 5

Population and public health

Every wise gardener knows better than to crowd his luck by crowding his plants too closely. Even the most aggressive organisms, such as weeds, rodents, and noxious insects, do not increase and spread indefinitely.

Paul B. Sears

STORM WARNINGS

No discussion of the health of the people of the world can be viewed in perspective without consideration of the single most significant phenomenon in our history—the population explosion. The potential consequences of this biologic surge are so great and far reaching in terms of local and world politics, economics, ethics, and even ultimate existence as to justify great concern. Increasingly, public health workers are criticized for compounding the problems of the world by causing widespread overpopulation through their dramatic saving and extension of lives. Public health workers, sociologists, political scientists, and others have long been aware of a relationship between public health activities and increases in the populations of nations and of the world. Awareness has been sharpened by recent world events, especially the sustained postwar rise in birthrates in many areas and the growth and success of international assistance programs in health and sanitation. This awareness has reached the point of acute concern, which increasingly is voiced in part by questioning (indeed, even condemnation) of the activities of the "dangerous doctor," the "heedless hygienist," and the "cynical sanitarian." On the other hand, there are those who are optimistic about the ability of this planet to sustain life. In view of these divergent opinions, it is pertinent to consider some of the facts, problems, and interrelationships of this important question.

THE BIOLOGIC SURGE

Recent anthropologic research indicates that our species has existed for more than 2 million years.

One may assume that throughout this long period, multiplication occurred to the extent that our way of life and environment allowed. The best available evidence indicates that during most of our species' existence, increase was gradual and often precarious. It is estimated that by 6000 BC the total world population was probably only about 5 million, an amount that is now added to the present world population every month. At the time of Christ the population had reached about 250 million. Over 16 centuries were to pass before it doubled to about 500 million in 1650. Then an acceleration began; the population doubled during the next two and a half centuries and then doubled again in less than another century. It took all of our long history to reach the current figure of about 4.5 billion people, but it will require only about 40 more years to double that figure. If the current rate of increase—1.9% compounded annually—continues, by the year 2050 the world's population will reach an almost incomprehensible 15 billion, and this is only about 65 years in the future! Usually accepted estimates are that the earth can support a maximum of 15 billion people if all land cultivation is brought up to that of the Netherlands. It should be pointed out, however, that calculations such as this are subject to disagreement.

Overall, the world's population is currently increasing at the rate of over 200,000 per day, or about 75 million per year. This is equivalent to adding a city the size of Jersey City, St. Paul, or St. Petersburg each day or more than the total combined populations of the United Kingdom and the Scandanavian countries each year. The annual increase is also equivalent to about one-tenth the population

TABLE 5-1. Rate of population increase
by region, 1975

Region	Population (millions)	Annual increase (%)	Doubles (in years)
Europe	473	0.6	116
North America	237	0.9	77
USSR	255	1.0	69
Asia	2,255	2.1	33
Oceania	21	2.0	35
Africa	401	2.6	27
Latin America	324	2.7	26
World	3,967	1.9	36

of China. Indeed, the increase of the past decade is equal to the population of all Europe, exclusive of the USSR. The rate of increase is not the same, however, in all parts of the world. In the more developed nations it varies from only 0.2% to 1.8 % per year. This is in contrast with rates of 1.5% to 3.5% per year in the lesser developed nations[1] (Table 5-1).

DYNAMICS OF POPULATION GROWTH

When population growth data are studied, it becomes apparent that many forces in addition to public health are involved.[2] Thus the onset of the upswing in world population actually antedates the modern public health movement. A significant quickening in the rate of population increase began about 1650. It is difficult to determine the relative importance of the various factors that must have been involved in the reduction of mortality and in the resultant increase in population. However, the increases during the first part of this period could not have been caused by public health measures because few if any existed. Rather, the determining factors appear to have been changing social organization, a rising standard of living, gradually improved nutrition and work conditions, and the appearance of certain social reforms.

In Europe a significant excess of births over deaths was already well established by the eighteenth century. This produced a steady population increase despite fluctuations caused by frequent epidemics and occasional famine. Then in the mid-nineteenth century a great decrease in mortality began, with a consequent upsurge in the rate of population increase. A peak was reached in the early twentieth century, despite much emigration. This upsurge may be attributed to the development

of improved transportation, which facilitated a wider distribution of goods and people; to the technologic progress of the Industrial Revolution, which provided more goods and improved living conditions for greater numbers of people; and more recently, to the acquisition and wide application of a new knowledge concerning the cause and prevention of disease. Subsequently, despite a continued decline in death rates, population growth in Europe decelerated as a result of a rapid fall in birthrates.

Population growth in the United States differed from that of Europe in three respects. First, during the early nineteenth century the rate of natural increase was much higher than in Europe, probably because of the young average age of those who came to America. Second, throughout the rest of the century the rate of natural increase declined because of rapidly dropping birthrates. Thus in the United States, births per 1,000 women 15 to 44 years of age dropped from 276 at the beginning of the nineteenth century to 208 at the midpoint and to 130 at the end. Finally, despite this considerable slowing in natural increase, the flood of immigrants prevented a drop in the rate of total population growth.

The relationship between population changes and economic and social conditions was analyzed in *The Determinants and Consequences of Population Trends*,[3] issued in 1953 and updated in 1973 by the Population Division of the United Nations Department of Economic and Social Affairs. This extensive presentation indicates not only that many basic aspects of the problem have been scarcely considered but also that there is much disagreement about interpretation of much of what has been studied. One thing appears obvious: in relation to population change, no single factor (such as public health) can be considered alone as if in a social and historic vacuum. Indeed, a complex set of factors is involved in the dynamics of population growth, stability, or retrogression. A partial list includes areal limitations; climate; present size, spatial distribution, and age structure of the population; present and potential resources for food; availability and use of efficient agricultural implements, machinery, and techniques; availability and quality of housing; policies and practices with regard to public health and education; existence, availability, and use of natural resources and sources of energy;

methods of verbal and physical communication, with special emphasis on farm-to-market roads; trends toward urbanization and industrialization; tax and financial structure, especially the availability of short-term and long-term loans at reasonable rates of interest; policies relating to the composition, full employment, and adequate compensation of the labor force; and a multitude of cultural factors.

Space does not permit adequate consideration of these factors. A few examples, however, may serve to illustrate the manner and extent to which some of them may affect a population. It is well known that the addition of new sources or types of nutrients will result in increased bacterial growth or increased size of a herd. It is not surprising that this applies also to human beings. Thus in the eighteenth century the sweet potato was introduced in China as an inexpensive, easily grown and stored, and rich source of carbohydrate in place of or to supplement grain. As far is known, no other significant factor was changed. Within 50 years the population increased from an estimated 60 million to 160 million. It is also interesting to note that the inception of the population spurt in Europe dates from about the time of the introduction of the white potato from the Andean region of South America.

The larger the area effectively available to a species, the more the species tends to move and also increase. Thus an inoculum multiplies and spreads throughout a container of nutrient broth. This has also been the experience of humans, most noticeably when new lands were discovered or developed. It was obviously more than chance that the beginning population upswing in the world coincided with the great period of discovery, colonization, and exploitation, and with more dependable and rapid means of transportation.

In the final analysis, life depends on energy. The determinant school of sociology has analyzed the history of the human race from this viewpoint and had noted that each time a new source of power or energy was discovered, a period of unrest and strife occurred, resulting in a smaller number of units of people—clans, tribes, nations, or alliances. Then an increase in production and a great upsurge in population has followed.

However, as Sears[4] has observed, "No form of life can continue to multiply indefinitely without eventually coming to terms with the limitations of its environment. . . . Every wise gardener knows better than to crowd his luck by crowding his plants too closely. Even the most aggressive organisms, such as weeds, rodents, and noxious insects, do not increase and spread indefinitely."

Without doubt, public health measures have contributed to the increase in population during the past century. They have done so in four ways: (1) by improving the chances of fruitful conception, (2) by greatly increasing the chances of survival among infants and young children, (3) by preventing the premature deaths of many young adults who comprise the most fertile component of a population and the group with the longest period of future fecundity, and (4) by greatly reducing the number of marriages dissolved by the death of one partner. This too has allowed a longer period of effective conjugal life.

Among the social and economic factors related to the dynamics of population, consideration must be given to the extent of urbanization and industrialization. These are two of the most notable phenomena of our time and are closely related. They have an interesting two-phased effect on population growth—initial encouragement followed by secondary retardation. The sequence is complex but basically appears to be about as follows. Industry, concentrated in centers of population and offering a means to obtain cash income, tends to attract especially the more mobile, vigorous, and adventurous young adults. At first they tend to follow the old established, essentially rural customs of their kind—marry young and aspire to large families. Sexual union among them is more fruitful because of their youth and because of the long average remaining period of fecundity. To this extent, industrialization and urbanization result in a substantial initial increase in the rate of population growth.

However, with improved education, growing sophistication, stabilization of the labor force, the wish for an improved standard of living, social rivalries, and competition for time, energy, and income, there develops an emphasis on rationality and independence from tradition, with a breaking away from the traditional conservative cultural ties. Marriages are delayed, and families are kept small for the sake of more education, increased income, or improved social position. Children come to be considered less an economic asset and more an economic burden. Family life becomes less cohesive because individuals have many contacts outside the home. Since life becomes increasingly complex, sexual intercourse becomes less frequent or more vicarious, and chances of fertilization decrease. Added to this is the greater availability of methods of contraception and the knowledge and funds to obtain and use them. Hence industrialization and urbanization result eventually in a decreased rate of reproduction and population growth. This has been found to hold true in Eastern as well as in Western civilizations.[5]

Reference has been made to the lesser developed areas of the world. Understandably there is concern over the rapidly declining death rates occurring in these areas in the face of sustained high birthrates and resulting high rates of natural increase [6] (Table 5-2).

Certain considerations should be borne in mind, however. In such circumstances there are several reasons for rapid decreases in mortality at this time. These areas are suddenly benefiting from technical knowledge that required long periods of investigation and experimentation by the presently advanced areas. The practical and immediate application of this life-saving knowledge in the lesser developed areas is now possible at low per capita cost because of the development of relatively simple and inexpensive techniques and the provision of international cooperation and assistance. It is unfortunate that during the early and critical phase of these assistance programs, technical knowledge and the inclination and political courage to plan for and maintain a proper balance between life-saving measures and birthrates were lacking. Belatedly, family planning activities are now encouraged and included in technical assistance programs to developing countries. One hopes that the ecologic balance has not been already so upset as to make these efforts too little and too late.

Another important reason for the rapid decline in mortality is the great striving for independence and national identity throughout the world. In the lesser developed but recently independent nations, great emphasis is understandably placed on catching up as quickly as possible in education, in health, and in technical, industrial, and economic progress. Because so much is needed, achievements have been rapid and dramatic. It would be unrealistic, however, to expect improvements in health or other fields to continue indefinitely at the present rate. In the field of health, preventable communicable diseases have accounted for a large part of the illness and death, and it is in this area that almost all the gains have occurred. Other gains will take longer and will be more difficult to achieve. The situation was well stated by Woytinsky and Woytinsky[7]:

The growth of world population in the past three hundred years obviously does not express the secular trend and cannot be projected indefinitely into the future. Rather, it has been a unique, unprecedented and unrepeatable phenomenon of limited duration. It had a beginning in the not too distant past, and it will have an end, perhaps, in the not too remote future. The slowing down and levelling off of growth in world population seems unavoidable. The question is only when will growth stop and at what level.

The possibility of a reversal must always be kept in mind. Overwhelming uncontrolled population increase itself would eventually produce a stifling effect. Furthermore, despite the great improvements that have occurred in the mortality picture, if concurrent progress in fields other than health

TABLE 5-2. Estimated population, birthrates, death rates, and rates of natural increase, world regions by state of development, 1975

Region and Country	Estimated population mid-year 1975 (in thousands)	Births per 1,000 population 1975	Deaths per 1,000 population 1975	Rate of natural increase 1975 (percent)
World	3,994,275	26.6	11.2	1.54
Less developed regions (Exc. China)	1,987,281	38.2	14.6	2.36
Less developed regions (Inc. China)	2,863,281	30.8	12.0	1.88
More developed regions	1,130,994	16.1	9.4	0.67

From World fertility patterns, Supplement to Population Reports, Series J, Washington, D.C., 1977, George Washington University Medical Center.

does not occur, a slump in the curve of health progress may be anticipated. Thus Stolnitz,[8] has viewed social and economic factors more as permissive than precipitating, stating: "It is obvious that the impact of medical skills on today's underdeveloped areas can be enormous. Whether the permissive elements will also be adequate is perhaps the foremost problem confronting half the world's population." Already, a Zero Population Growth movement is underway,[9-11] and its goal appears to be approaching achievement in several nations, including the United States.[12]

It should not be overlooked that some of the same social and economic factors that affect mortality also affect fertility. The relationship of these factors to mortality is not necessarily the same as their relationship to other factors that contribute to population change. Thus factors that contribute to mortality decline may not necessarily raise the rate of population growth, since they may also contribute to a decline in the birthrate. In this regard, public health activities can contribute to improved school attendance and intelligence, to industrial development and urbanization, to higher general income levels and improvement in the standard of living, and to an understanding of physiologic and reproductive functioning. Of all pertinent factors, two merit special mention—the extension of education and the enhancement of the social position of women. In all instances where improvement of these has occurred, the birth rate has declined.

Of necessity, much has been left unsaid. No mention has been made of the potentials of more efficient land use, development of new agricultural techniques, improvement of plant and animal strains, application of nuclear energy to power development, irrigation, water desalinization, food preservation, more adequate use of solar energy, reduction of food wastage by insects and vermin, chemical soil treatment, and hydroponics; and there has been no mention of the release of land for food use as a result of inexpensive artificial fibers and plastics, the food value of algae, the possibilities of sea farming and sea breeding, the possibility of more artificially manufactured foods, and the need for less energy as a result of increasing mechanization of farms and industry. The technologic possibilities of the future seem vast indeed and give some reasonable cause for optimism and hope.

POPULATION AND ECONOMIC PROGRESS

One of the most fundamental facets of a culture or society is productivity of the individual and the group—the degree of success to which people can feed, clothe, and house themselves, and those dependent on them. In the simplest sense this constitutes the economy of the individual or the group. The concept of both society and its economy implies people, and the plurality of the word *people* implies relationships, one type of which is interdependence and mutual support. But there is always the potential reverse relationship of competition and mutual destruction. Either relationship appears to be the result of the degree of balance or imbalance between the two dependent variables mentioned—the nature of a population, on the one hand, and of its economy, on the other.[13]

A population necessarily depends on its economy, whereas economic development in turn requires a population and is pursued to serve that population's purposes. Theoretically at least, the greater the population, the more will be its productivity. On the other hand, the greater the population, the more it must produce. Furthermore, the more a population grows, the broader and deeper must be its economic base. The breadth and depth of the economic base are dependent in turn on the resources that nature has made immediately and potentially available. These have tangible limits, and the avoidance of their depletion depends on careful husbandry and conservation to allow for whatever natural regeneration and replenishment may be possible.[14]

To this point, the word *population* has been used in a loose and general sense. It is important to consider certain of its components. Each population contains a proportion of socially dependent nonproducers—the young, the elderly, the infirm, and the unemployed. It must be recognized also that these groups are constant consumers. Indeed, at least two of the groups, the young and the infirm, in many societies such as that in the United States tend to consume proportionately more of the products and services of society than does the rest. Obviously, therefore, the more dependents there are in a society the greater the need for a large corps of producers. Any circumstance that alters the number and proportion of the various types of dependents and producers affects the economy. Similarly, any change in the extent or nature of the economy tends to affect the number and proportion of dependent nonproducers. The most obvious effect is an increase in unemployed persons. Usually close on the heels of unemployment, however, comes a decrease in the number of conceptions and births. Excellent examples of this sequence were provided by the economic recession and a major steel strike that occurred in the United States in the late 1950s[15], as well as similar more recent economic events. If a lowered economy persists in a society, financial inability to obtain adequate nutrition and preventive and therapeutic medical care as well as other necessities and amenities results inevitably in an increase in the number and proportion of individuals who become acutely and chronically ill. Finally, because of the interplay between these last two effects, there eventually occurs at least a temporary increase in the proportion of dependent adults and elderly persons.

Much of the problem with which we are confronted results from the different rates and timings of these and other changes. To consider this in another dimension, certain highly and rapidly effective disease preventive measures have made it possible within a relatively brief period of history for large numbers of otherwise doomed infants and children not only to survive but also eventually to become parents, resulting in a subsequent "baby boom" that can exacerbate population and economic problems. Not so prompt has been the effect on the number and proportion of persons of advanced age. Not so prompt also have been changes in cultural attitudes with respect to family size, the roles of women and children in society, attitudes toward fertility, and the control of conception to compensate in time for the population changes noted. As Sears[4] has pointed out, this delay, uncertainty, and confusion are understandable in view of the overwhelming force of the reproductive urge, "whose consequences are far less immediate and far more complex than those that may result from mixing a solution or throwing a switch." The individual beset by this natural urge is equally beset by inertia, custom, tradition, and the voices of his or her time.

Chisholm[16] the first Director-General of the World Health Organization, expressed a similar opinion in relation to underdeveloped areas. He considered it impossible under current circumstances for foreign development assistance to be increased sufficiently to make possible the necessary rapid economic development in the face of high birth and survival rates. He stated:

There are limits to the amounts of capital that can be absorbed usefully in an underdeveloped country at a given time. There are limits to the speed with which the people can be educated or trained. There are limits to the rate at which public administration can be improved, and to the rate at which public service can be expanded. And clearly, all these limits are narrowed by rapid population growth.

Many insist, however, that public health workers should be seriously concerned and pessimistic about the distribution of the world's food products and especially about the possibility of significant improvement of the standard of living of the average person during the remainder of this century.[17,18] Chisholm[16] illustrated this by pointing out that whereas a per capita income of $100 annually in a situation with a 1% population growth per year would increase to $135 annually over a 10-year period, it would increase to $106 annually in the face of a 3.5% population growth per year. As he indicated, several places in the world had already approached or reached the latter high rate of population increase.

It has become commonplace to compare the economically more advanced countries with those that are economically less advanced. One can compile a long list of variables, such as in Table 4-2, that measure different aspects of social and economic development as well as political stability and sophistication and find, as one would expect, a remarkable consistency of relationship. Then one can examine the densities of population and their respective rates of increase and income. Here the relationships are less clear cut and evident. The populations of Japan and the Netherlands are as dense as those of Egypt and Sri Lanka; those of Great Britain and the eastern United States are as dense as the populations of the Balkans and Indonesia. To pursue this further into another dimension, one might compare the natural resources of the eastern United States with those of Indonesia and still be left with some unanswered questions.

It would appear, therefore, that no simple direct relationship exists between socioeconomic status and population. One is forced to conclude that the relationship is affected by or dependent on a third set of variables, and evidence appears to be mounting to point to the importance of the degree to which the combination of mobility, urbanization, mechanization, and industrialization has become a fundamental part of the way of life. This even appears to hold true in areas devoted essentially to mineral extraction and agriculture. Thus the populations of areas that pursue such ends in a large-scale, mechanized, or industrialized manner fare better, at least temporarily, than do those that retain the more simple, primitive, and individualized way of life. This was illustrated some years ago by Gordon and coworkers[19] in a comparison of three groups of nations (Table 5-3). They indicated that the greater the degree of industrialization, hence presumably urbanization, mechanization, and mobility, the greater will be the degree of balance between birthrates and death rates. (It should be noted that in the interval since the study, several nations, notably the USSR and Japan, have clearly shifted into the industrialized group.) The same observations have been emphasized more recently by Robert McNamara, President of the World Bank.[5]

The fact that there is a worldwide trend toward urbanization and industrial development, as well as toward more efficient agriculture, would seem to provide some basis for optimism. These twin changes not only result in more food and goods for more people at less unit cost, and indirectly force facilities for greater mobility, but also tend to increase the ratio of those who recognize a smaller family as an advantage. This is related to a departure from outdated traditional beliefs, practices, and customs regarding family size, the purpose of the individual, interpersonal relationships in general, and the roles of children and women in particular.

Meanwhile it is worth emphasizing the conviction that some social scientists have done a disservice to the concept of economic development and to the recipients of its benefits by totally decrying its effect on existing mores and social organization as if they should be regarded as completely inviolate. To the contrary, one should frankly recognize that it is sometimes critically necessary to change family and group attitudes and practices to reduce birthrates as well as illness and death rates and to improve individual, group, and national living standards. To do otherwise is most unrealistic. Indeed, that in essence is what health education is all about. Some, for example, have advocated almost total emphasis on agricultural programs to the exclusion of efforts in other areas of economic development. This would be disadvantageous in the long run because the life of the typical farmer is highly traditional, and merely to make it tolerable would remove the necessity or incentive for him to alter or adapt his attitudes and behavior toward many things, especially his family's size and purpose.

To carry this line of reasoning into the area of health programs in relation to economic development and population control, it might be considered

TABLE 5-3. Vital balance in three world areas by degree of industrialization

Nature of group	World population (%)	Death rate	Birthrate
Industrialized	20	10	15
Relatively balanced and stationary populations with relatively low birth and death rates and incipient population decline (USA, United Kingdom, Scandinavia, France)			
Transitional	20	15 to 20	25
Somewhat imbalanced and expanding populations with significant control of deaths and beginning control of births (eastern and southeastern Europe, USSR, Japan, Brazil, Argentina)			
Preindustrial	60	30+	35+
Relatively balanced populations with high birth and death rates but with high population expansion potential (Asia except USSR and Japan, Africa except South Africa)			

Modified from Gordon, J.E., Wyon, J.E., and Ingalls, T.H.: Public Health as a demographic influence, Am. J. Med. Sci. **227:**326, March 1954.

best under ideal circumstances, especially during a transitional period, to emphasize activities in certain selective areas such as:

1. Activities that tend to emphasize urban industrial areas more than rural agricultural areas
2. Activities that tend to favor presently productive components of the population more than dependants
3. Activities that tend to aid potential producers more than postproducers
4. Maternal and child health activities that convince women of the advantages of having fewer but healthier children
5. Activities that tend to improve the social and political position of women
6. Activities that tend to develop new sources of security for the individual in place of institutions that tend to encourage large families

In considering the foregoing, however, it must be realized that the circumstances that led to industrial and economic development in the West were different in certain important respects from those confronting much of the remainder of the world, including Asia, Africa, and much of Latin America.[20] In the West, as has already been indicated, urbanization and the introduction of successful attacks on the resulting rising mortality have accompanied industrialization. In fact, for a significant period economic and industrial development in western Europe and the United States has depended on a lowered mortality in company with a sustained high birthrate and immigration rate for its continuance. During that period, industry could be considered to have consumed human life at a rate faster than it could be produced locally. By contrast, the present situation elsewhere in the world is quite different. By virtue of the sudden importation and application of certain products and techniques of the industrial culture, death rates are declining rapidly in the face of sustained or even increased birthrates. As a result, populations are soaring. The significant point is that these changes are deterrents rather than necessary concomitants of the hoped-for economic, social, and industrial development. Many authors have commented on the dangerous time lag between lowered death rates and lowered birthrates. Another dangerous time lag to which perhaps not enough attention has been given is summarized by Van den Haag[21] in the following way:

The endogenous industrialization of the West was prepared for by a cumulative historical development starting at least in the Renaissance, and including the rise of individualism, rationalism, empiricism and science, the fall of feudalism, and numerous other changes which led to the attitudes associated with successful industrialization. The sudden introduction of an alien economic system without historical preparation is a far more difficult and dangerous operation. It is unavoidable by now, but we must be prepared for undesirable side effects.

The phenomenon is further compounded by the agglutination of large numbers of persons in urban centers, not because growing industries can absorb them but because of the magnetism of the hoped-for amenities for a life-style that is not yet there to enjoy.

The foregoing comments apply to only a few of the many complex aspects of the relationship of population to socioeconomic development. Although concern over these problems is rapidly increasing, it is by no means new. The lack of reference to Malthus may have been noted. In its place, attention is called to a statement made in 1908 by Carver[22] of the Harvard School of Theology.

Fundamentally there are only two practical problems imposed upon us. The one is industrial and the other moral; the one has to do with the improvement of the relations between man and nature, and the other with the improvement of the relations between man and man. But these two primary problems are so inextricably intermingled, and they deal with such infinitely ranging factors, that the secondary and tertiary problems are more than we can count.

But whence arises that phase of the conflict with nature out of which grows the conflict between man and man? Is man in any way responsible for it, or is it due wholly to the harshness or the niggardliness of nature? The fruitfulness of nature varies, of course, in different environments. But in any environment there are two conditions, for both of which man is in a measure responsible, and either of which will result in economic scarcity. One is the indefinite expansion of human wants, and the other is the multiplication of his numbers.

The difficulty therefore is that all the intimate, interlinked phenomena discussed do not proceed apace, and some of them eventually end up counterproductive. It sounds satisfying to speak of the potentials of increased production of food and goods by the application of new methods and technology so that the needs and wishes of more people can be met. But this assumes that there is no limit or end point to development and production on a finite planet. Such a view is obviously illogical and folly. It also ignores the fact that although production of food and manufactured goods is shifting from first into second gear, the production of more people or consumers has been and still is racing ahead in ultrahigh gear.

The concerns and warning of Reverend Carver two generations ago have been updated, documented, and dramatically voiced by the so-called "Club of Rome,"[23,24] a loosely organized group of leaders in a variety of disciplines, professions, and occupations. Beginning in 1968, the group arranged for extensive and continuing amounts of data to be sent for computer analysis to a research group at the Massachusetts Institute of Technology. The data relate to six factors: (1) rate of population increase, (2) rate of food production, (3) rate of urbanization, (4) rate of industrialization, (5) rate of natural resource consumption, and (6) rate of environmental pollution. Their initial conclusions were that no matter what combinations were put into the computer model, only one appeared to offer hope for the continuation of the human species. This was an immediate and significant cutback on all six factors together. To make an exception of or to underemphasize even one of them would invite failure and ultimate disaster. On the basis of past and present human behavior, it is unrealistic to expect the kind of total worldwide coordinated effort indicated.

Human beings, especially those responsible for education, industry, politics, theology, medicine, and public health, who play such determinant roles in the life and future of society, have now reached a point when a critical and prompt decision must be made, a decision that no degree of euphoria or optimism can allow to be delayed any longer. Something has to give. We must either face reality and take rapid and forthright steps toward the deceleration of the increase in our numbers and of the misuse of our self-limited environment or accept the inevitable widespread political unrest, pestilence, and famine. Thus all the hard-won gains of our species would be lost.

What may be concluded so far? First, public health effort has saved lives but thereby has contributed to population increase; second, public health is only one of many factors involved in both social improvement and population increase; third, public health measures tend to be more rapidly successful than do activities in other fields; fourth, interrelationships among all the fields involved are still little understood in terms of cause and effect; fifth, assistance to underdeveloped communities or areas should be multidisciplinary and never limited exclusively to public health or any other single field of endeavor and should always be associated with family planning programs; sixth, in conducting public health programs anywhere, rather than attempt the impossible of bringing about public health changes entirely within existing cultural patterns, as if they were static, public health workers should encourage changes that are consistent with the realities of desirable dynamic, social, and public health improvement; seventh, there are valid reasons to believe that time may be running out more rapidly than previously realized and that prompt and coordinated worldwide efforts in several problem areas are critically indicated.

FAMILY PLANNING PROGRAMS

In view of the foregoing, it is obvious that efforts toward agricultural or industrial development or individual family or community self-sufficiency must be accompanied by population or fertility control. Furthermore, data exist to indicate that the incidence of infant mortality, maternal mortality, prematurity, mental retardation, congenital malformations, and brain damage is significantly higher than average among fourth and subsequent births, among births to older women, and among first births to girls in their early teens.[25] These undesirable phenomena are more likely to occur when pregnancies follow each other rapidly in economically underprivileged women whose health is below normal as a result of poor living conditions, undernutrition, and inadequate medical care. It has been estimated that in the United States about 2,200 infant deaths would be prevented annually among some 500,000 low-income patients if they were provided with voluntary family planning services.[26]

With reference to maternal risks, it has long been known that puerperal death rates increase significantly with increased age and multiparity of the woman. In addition, a study by the World Health Organization has noted that 10% of maternal deaths are caused by abortions, many of which are induced because of large families.[27] The removal of the mother by premature death or by invalidism especially in such instances is a family catastrophe. Practical availability of family planning services would go far to eliminate these needless causes of suffering and death. Parents with large families are most apt to be inextricably caught in the dependency vortex, and children born into it escape only with great difficulty. All aspects of living tend to be inadequately attainable—housing, food, recreation, education, and health. Such families also tend to be more frequently broken.

For these and many other reasons, fertility control or family planning has been promoted for many years in the United States as well as in some other parts of the world. Until recently, however, the promotion has been largely by some private physicians and several private or voluntary organizations. Without question, the greatest credit must go to the Planned Parenthood Federation, founded by the courageous and dauntless Margaret Sanger, who persisted over many difficult years for the fulfillment of an idea she considered humane, honorable, and important. Progress was discouragingly slow because of a variety of cultural blocks, political opposition, and technologic inadequacies. Gradually professional organizations also took a positive position. At present the list includes the American Public Health Association, the American Public Welfare Association, the American Medical Association, the National Academy of Science, and the United Nations and its various specialized agencies such as the World Health Organization, the United Nations Educational, Scientific, and Cultural Organization (UNESCO), and the United Nations Children's Fund (UNICEF). These actions have coincided with several significant scientific and technologic advances, particularly the development of relatively inexpensive, easily used, and increasingly effective methods of contraception.

At the same time and for a complex set of reasons, a remarkable change in public attitude toward the subject has occurred. Greatly improved and extended public education, the rigors of economic depression and wars, affluence, the emancipation of women, the development of mass communications—these and many other factors have led to a considerable liberalization of public, religious, and political attitude. Of great impact in the United States have been the forthright statements of recent Presidents, beginning with John F. Kennedy. Another significant milestone was the invalidation by the U.S. Supreme Court on June 7, 1965, of the 1879 Connecticut anti–birth control law. The Court ruled that such legislation violated the constitutional right of married couples to privacy.

Federal, state, and local health, welfare, and related agencies have adopted enlightened policies at an increasing rate. The first state-supported family planning services in local health departments were established in 1937 in North Carolina. Six other southern states soon followed (Alabama, Florida, Georgia, Mississippi, South Carolina, and Virginia). Services were incorporated into maternal health clinics and home nursing programs and served primarily rural rather than urban areas. Mention should also be made of the development and operation during the 1930s of a large number of birth control clinics in Puerto Rico, using funds from the Children's Bureau. In response to the need and to changing attitudes, the federal government through its pertinent agencies became actively involved in a wide variety of research, training, subsidy, and service programs in this field. By now all states are included. Unfortunately policies vary considerably, as does the effectiveness with which they are carried out. With reference to this, a study of 56 metropolitan counties with the largest number of infant deaths, accounting for 26% of the national need, indicated that only about one fourth of the women who needed subsidized family planning services were actually obtaining them from some source. Only about one half of the services obtained were provided by health departments. By the mid-1960s schools of medicine, nursing, and public health had begun to present special seminars and courses in family planning.

In July 1969 an important step was taken on the national level by the creation of a Commission on Population Growth and the American Future to study the various ramifications of the problem and to make recommendations relating to national research and action policy.[28] World-wide, although about 46 million women were using an IUD or the pill, by 1970 the need was far from met. Of 500 million women of childbearing age and facing the risk of an unwanted pregnancy, as estimated 70% were using no contraceptive method.

Methodology

The importance of the subject justifies a few words about methods of contraception. The origins of attempts to prevent conception are lost in primitive history. The Ebers Papyrus, 1550 BC, includes an interesting recipe for a medicated tampon to control fertility. The compound consisted of a mixture of acacia and honey, which was to be inserted into the vagina as a suppository. Interestingly, on fermentation acacia breaks down into lactic acid, a rather effective spermicidal agent.[29] Some indication of the wide variety of materials since used is presented in a study by deLaszlo and Henshaw.[30]

At the present time there exists a wide variety of behavioral, physiologic, chemical, and physical methods of contraception. They differ considerably as to effectiveness, acceptability, cost, and other factors. The use of many of them requires or indicates the assistance, advice, or supervision of a physician or other properly trained person. To a considerable extent, the ultimate choice depends on individual preference. The amount of research that is being carried out in this field is such as to anticipate further radical discoveries, hence changes in methodology.

Among the areas of active investigation are once-a-month oral contraceptives that combine a long-acting estrogen and a progesterone, a progesterone-impregnated Silastic vaginal ring implanted for a month at a time, a year-long capsule of progesterone for subcutaneous implantation, a long-lasting injectable preparation of medroxyprogesterone acetate, a postcoital, or "after-the-fact," pill based on a prostaglandin derivative, and the synthesis and possible use of the luteinizing hormone–releasing factor (LH-RH, or LRF) of the pituitary gland.[31,32] All the foregoing are for use by women, as of course are the various intrauterine devices. For men, in addition to condoms and to vasectomies, which are being done increasingly in the United States and several other countries, there have been unsuccessful attempts to develop a contraceptive pill based on pituitary gonadotropin suppressants; to inhibit sperm production by the administration of large doses of androgens, which unfortunately increases the risk of heart attacks; and to develop a number of nonsteroid sperm-suppressive compounds for oral use (unfortunately these have been either toxic or could cause genetic damage). Attempts to immunize men with testicular antigens and protein hormones have so far met with limited success, but research in this direction is very active.[33]

Special mention should be made of abortion, the oldest and still probably the most widely used method of birth control or family planning. Because of the severe physical and psychologic risks of self-induced, unsanitary, or unskilled abortion, induced abortion was condemned until recently by most societies. However, in the United States and many other nations, despite the considerable emotional, religious, and political conflicts that the subject has engendered, an increasing number of public and professional organizations as well as political jurisdictions have endorsed and approved medically induced abortions for a variety of reasons and justifications, including family planning. Recent reports in the United States indicate about 270 legal abortions per 1,000 live births, and in some other countries, such as Japan, the rate is much higher. The beneficial effects on maternal mortality have been notable. In Great Britain, out of 160,000 legal abortions performed in 1972, there were only 10 deaths, which gave a maternal abortion death rate of 6 per 100,000 compared with a former rate of 12 per 100,000. For simple abortions performed at less than 13 weeks gestation, the rate was only 3 per 100,000.[34] During the first year of legal abortion in South Australia, deaths attributable to abortion dropped to zero, and the total number of women dying in childbirth fell sharply.[35] In mid-1970, New York State liberalized its laws concerning abortion. During the 3 years from July 1970 to June 1973, almost 600,000 legal abortions were performed in New York City. Only 20 of the women involved died, giving a rate of only 2 deaths per 100,000 legal abortions. The comparison with the national maternal mortality rate of 24 per 100,000 live births in 1972 needs no comment. Beyond this, there was a beneficial effect on maternal mortality as a whole. During the 3 years preceding liberalization, the maternal mortality in New York City was 51 per 100,000 live births. During the first 3 years of liberalization it dropped to 38 per 100,000 live births.[34] Although most agree that abortion is a "second best" approach to family planning as compared with successful contraception, the evidence of the beneficial effects of properly performed abortion in place of self-induced, unsanitary, and unskilled abortion is incontrovertible. During the late 1960s and early 1970s efforts were begun by a number of groups, especially those involved in women's rights and maternal health, to obtain a national policy to legalize and make available medical abortion for those who wished it. Finally in 1973, the U.S. Supreme Court invalidated all restrictive abortion laws. However, this progressive step continues to be attacked by certain other groups despite majority support.

REFERENCES

1. World population data sheet, Washington, D.C., 1975, Population Reference Bureau, Inc.
2. Stanford, Q.H.: The world's population: problems of growth, New York, 1972, Oxford University Press, Inc.
3. The determinants and consequences of population trends, New York, 1973, United Nations.
4. Sears, P.B.: Pressures of population, an ecologist's point of view, What's New **212:**12, 1959.
5. McNamara, R.S.: Th world's population problem: possible interventions to reduce fertility, Public Health Rep. **93:**124, March-April 1978.
6. World fertility patterns, Supplement to Population Reports, Series J., Washington, D.C., 1977, George Washington University Medical Center.
7. Woytinsky, W.S., and Woytinsky, E.S.: World population and production; trends and outlook, New York, 1953, The Twentieth Century Fund.
8. Stolnitz, J.: Comparison between some recent mortality trends in underdeveloped areas and historical trends in the West. In Bourgeois-Pichat, J., and Pan, C., editors: Trends and differentials of mortality in underdeveloped areas, New York, 1956, Milbank Memorial Fund.
9. Ehrlich, P.R.: The population bomb, New York, 1968, Balantine Books, Inc.
10. Notestein, F.W.: Zero population growth: what is it, Family Planning Perspectives **2:**20, June 1970.
11. Olson, M.: The no-growth society, Daedalus, Fall 1973, p. 229.
12. U.S. population in 2000: Zero growth or not? Population bull. 30, No. 5, Washington, D.C., 1975, Population Reference Bureau.
13. Interrelationships between health programmes and socio-economic development, Public Health Papers No. 49, Geneva, 1973, World Health Organization.
14. Ogburn, C.: Population and resources: the coming collision, Population Bull. 26, No. 2, Washington, D.C., 1970, Population Reference Bureau.
15. Westoff, C.F., Potter, R.G., and Sagi, P.C.: Some selected findings of the Princeton fertility study, 1963, Demography **1:**1, 1964.
16. Chisholm, B. In Jones, J.M., editor: Does overpopulation mean poverty? Washington, D.C., 1962, Center for International Economic Growth.
17. Hauser, P.M.: Demographic dimensions of world politics, Science **131:**3414, June 3, 1960.
18. Mahler, H.: WHO at the crossroads, WHO Chron. **31:**226, June 1977.
19. Gordon, J.E., Wyon, J.E., and Ingalls, T.H.: Public health as a demographic influence, Am. J. Med. Sci. **227:**326, March 1954.
20. Coale, A.J., and Hoover, E.M.: Population growth and economic development in low-income countries, Princeton, 1958, Princeton University Press.
21. Van den Haag, E.: Population and economic development, What's New **214:**4, 1959.
22. Carver, T.N.: The economic basis of the problem of evil, Harvard Theol. Rev. **1:**1, Jan. 1908.
23. Meadows, D.L., and others: The limits to growth, New York, 1972, Universe Books, Inc.
24. Meadows, D.L., and Meadows, D.H., editors: Toward global equilibrium, Cambridge, Mass., 1975, Wright-Allen Press.
25. Bonham, G.S., and Placek, P.J.: The relationships of maternal health, infant health and sociodemographic factors to fertility, Public Health Rep. **93:**283, May-June 1978.
26. Family planning and infant mortality: an analysis of priorities (mimeographed report), New York, 1967, Planned Parenthood-World Population, p. 8 ff.
27. Beck, M.B., Newman, S.H., and Lewit, S.: Abortion: a national public and mental health problem, Am. J. Public Health **59:**2131, Dec. 1969.
28. An act to establish a commission on population growth and the American future, Public Law 91-213, 91st Cong. S. 2701, March 16, 1970.
29. The first prescription for control of fertility, MD **9:**58, July 1963.
30. deLaszlo, H., and Henshaw, P.S.: Plant materials used by primitive peoples to affect fertility, Science **119:**626, May 7, 1954.
31. Duncan, G.W.: Fertility control: contributions for the future. In Progress in drug research, Washington, D.C., 1969, Pharmaceutical Manufacturers Association.
32. Arehart-Treichel, J.: Birth control in The Brave New World, Science News **103:**93, Feb. 10, 1973.
33. Contraceptives for men, MD **16:**88, Oct. 1972.
34. Barnett, M.: Legalized abortion credited with some health advances, Hosp. Tribune, Feb. 11, 1974, p. 5.
35. Hosp. Tribune, March 26, 1973, p. 2.

PART TWO

The basis for public health

Public health work, by definition, is carried on mainly under governmental auspices. Despite this, as Kaufman,[1] a political scientist, says in an article that should be studied by all in the health field:

Experts whose careers will unfold in the public arena . . . pay little attention to politics in the training of their successors and in the conduct of their own research. Politics is treated as an intrusion to be ignored at best, condemned at worst.

He indicates three reasons why such an attitude is wrong. First, specialists such as those in public health all believe that everyone should know more about their field of interest, yet they keep their expertise among themselves. Second, neglect or denunciation of politics threatens the democratic process.

If every apprentice is trained to suspect and despise politics and to dedicate himself to remove his occupation from the political arena, an ever-increasing and more influential segment of the population may acquire a disrespect for the processes which are the core of a democratic policy. Moreover, if every specialty seeking exemption were in fact removed from the arena of partisan contention, the decision-making machinery of the society, deprived of an ultimate adjudicating authority mediating among the specialists, might grind to a stop.

Third, politics provides an essential sociologic input. As Kaufman strongly emphasizes:

neglect of political factors in the study of public health problems and programs omits a critical element in understanding, planning and executing public health services. For whether they like it or not, the practitioners of the public health disciplines are deeply immersed in a political environment. The ones who succeed are the ones who learn to understand it, adjust to it and turn it to their advantage. But few of them, in their formal training or in their professional research literature, receive any assistance in this vital aspect of their work.

The same is even more true of law. Usually the extent of exposure to the legislative process, even of those who reach other professions, is limited to a secondary school or college course in civics, which may include a few paragraphs about how laws are made. The following two chapters on government and on law, with emphasis on their relationship to public health, are presented with the intent to remedy partially these earlier educational gaps.

REFERENCE

1. Kaufman, H.: The political ingredient of public health services, a neglected area of research, Milbank Mem. Fund Q **44**:13, Oct. 1966.

CHAPTER 6

Government and public health

Government is a contrivance of human wisdom to provide for human wants.

Edmund Burke

FUNCTIONS OF GOVERNMENT

The particular political system that exists determines the role of government in relation to health. Public health programs are financed and the broad organizational patterns for their implementation are determined by governmental policy decisions. In general, a governmental system performs two functions. The first function is political. There must be a forum for debate on issues that exist or arise and an appropriate instrument for their solution. A structure must be provided to make possible the achievement of the aspirations and goals of society. The determination of the role of government in relation to health is an important part of the political function of government. The second general function is the provision of services and regulatory activities.

Public health workers need to be knowledgeable about the service and regulatory functions of government. Because the political functions of government cannot be separated from the service and regulatory functions, it is imperative that those who work in public health understand the political structure and functions of government as well. This is the major purpose of this chapter.

POLITICAL SYSTEM

Until recent years many regarded political science as a static description of formal organizational structures such as legislatures or political parties along with normative political theory. Political scientists now describe politics as a dynamic system. The political process is the system used by people to negotiate policy when differences exist, especially value differences regarding such things as welfare, the criminal justice system, education, and health. The institutions of government, especially the elected legislative bodies, serve as the forums in which the search for policy occurs. The administrative agencies of government often provide an opportunity for more in-depth, often narrower debate about the fine details of the policies as they have been developed by elected officials. The nature of these institutions and their relationships must be understood to gain an understanding of the political process and thus the role of government in health.

The basic outline of this system is contained in the Constitution. It is a federal system that is defined as "one where the governmental powers are divided by terms of a written constitution between a general government and the governments of territorial subdivisions, each government supreme within a sphere marked out in the Constitution."[1]

In this country the territorial subdivisions are states. Traditionally they tend to be apprehensive of the powers of the national or central unit of government. This may be understood in the light of history. Some states actually existed as distinct entities. For example, Vermont was independent between 1777 and 1791, as was the eastern part of Tennessee between 1784 and 1789. Texas was an independent republic from 1836 to 1845 and exchanged diplomats with the government of the United States. Hawaii, before becoming a territory of the United States in 1900 and eventually a state in 1959, also was an independent nation.

It is often overlooked that not until the American Revolution was almost won did the original 13 colonies think seriously about union. Many influential people insisted that each colony should be a distinct and separate nation. The Continental Congress ultimately solved the problem by devising a union of states. The decision was made by a narrow margin of votes.

The politically dominant state

In forming a union the colonies, which were now called states, did not surrender their individual rights and prerogatives. Instead they took the attitude that most governmental problems would continue to be met and solved best on a separate and independent basis. Relatively few matters of common interest and concern were to be referred to the overall federal government established by their union.

They recognized that they had common interests in matters of defense against aggression, and that therefore a single national army and navy should be established, consisting of men from all the states. Each state, however, organized and still maintains its own militia. The logic of a single agency to deal with matters of international diplomacy was similarly realized, and a federal Department of State was established. To finance these activities of common concern, a national treasury and taxing system were instituted. Subsequently, as additional common problems developed or were recognized, other federal agencies were established.

From the beginning, the states were explicit with regard to functions and authorities delegated to the federal government. These were specified in Article I, section 8 of the federal Constitution and subsequent amendments. The first 10 amendments were known as the Bill of Rights, and they specifically curtailed the power of government, both the national government and that of each of the member states. The tenth amendment stated that "the powers not delegated to the United States by the Constitution, nor prohibited by it to the States, are reserved to the States respectively, or to the people." This amendment has enormous significance for the understanding of public health, since health is not mentioned as a function of the national government in the Constitution. The authority of the national government is contained in three places: (1) the Preamble to the Constitution, which states, "We the people of the United States, in order to form a more perfect union, establish justice, insure domestic tranquility, provide for the common defense, promote the general *welfare,* and secure the blessings

of liberty to ourselves and our posterity, do ordain and establish this Constitution of the United States of America"; (2) section 8 of Article I where it states, "The Congress shall have the power to lay and collect taxes, duties, imposts and excises, to pay the debts and provide for the common defence and general *welfare* of the United States"; and (3) section 8 of Article I which states that Congress has the power "to regulate commerce with foreign nations, among the several States, and with the Indian tribes." These provisions, dealing with the common welfare and the regulation of interstate commerce, paved the way for the expansion of the national government in the health field since the 1930s, but its increased role has been implemented almost exclusively through the states, not directly by federal action. In contrast, most state constitutions explicitly recognize the police power of the state and the responsibility for the welfare of its citizens. The police power role authorized the control and abatement of nuisances, which can span the gamut from a weed-infested vacant lot to the licensure of nursing homes. The welfare role was specified by the adoption of the Elizabethan poor law (1601), which said that it was the responsibility of the most local government to aid and support those who were not otherwise provided for.

The power and authority of the states have been eroded in the last 50 years by the expansion of the national government's taxing and spending programs but, as previously noted, the federal interest has had to be carried out through the states and the local units of government: air pollution policy is developed at the national level but it is implemented through the state agencies; Medicaid has been implemented through the states as have programs to control lead poisoning, to cope with toxic wastes, and to treat venereal disease. Even the vital statistics reporting system, developed at the national level, depends on voluntary compliance by the states—a compliance that is virtually assured by the fiscal support and reporting power of the National Center for Health Statistics. It is the fiscal carrot, which often becomes a stick, that makes it possible for congressional or presidential interest to be implemented through the state governments.

CHANGING CONCEPTS OF FEDERALISM

Federalism has not remained static. The interpretation of the respective responsibilities of the state and national governments under the Constitution has changed considerably throughout United States history. Many people today regard the federal government as the ultimate source of power and money. Although they do so with increasing justification, this was not always the case. The original concept of state supremacy has been briefly discussed. Suffice it to say that in spite of recent trends, the principle is not dead.

For a considerable period of United States history the federal government seemed somewhat distant to the average citizen. This early relationship has been described by Brogan.[2]

It should be remembered that is was quite easy for the settler in the Middle West to have no dealings at all with the government of the United States. He paid no direct taxes; he very often wrote no letters and received none, for the good reason that he and his friends could not write. Yet the only ubiquitous federal officials and federal service were the Postmasters and the Post Office. There were no soldiers except in the Indian country; there were federal courts doing comparatively little business. True, the new union had built the National Road, down which creaked the Conestoga wagons with their cargo of immigrants' chattels. It fought the Indians from time to time and it had at its disposal vast areas of public lands to be sold on easy terms and finally given away to settlers. But no government that had any claim to be a government at all has had less direct power over the people it ruled. Politics was bound, in these conditions, to be rhetorical, moralizing, emotionally diverting, either a form of sport or a form of religion. The political barbecue, the joint debates between great political leaders were secular equivalents of the camp meeting and the hell-fire sermon.

Even the inhabitants of the older seaboard states shared this relationship. As Brogan continues:

Few things, on consideration, prove less surprising than the evaporation of federal authority over the South once secession was adopted. Almost the only federal institution that meant anything to the common man was the Post Office—and by a statesmanlike turning of the blind eye, the new Southern Confederacy continued to allow the federal government to deliver the mail even after the seceding states had formally broken with the Union.

As time passed, with increasing urbanization, education, mechanization, travel, industrialization, and interstate and international problems, the national government came more and more into focus in the citizens' eyes. At the same time there began to develop a blurring of the image of local and state government. Much of this had to do with increased needs and demands in relation to sources of revenue. There was a period when local governments were essentially self-sufficient, but as the demands made on them increased, they looked more frequently to the state governments for assistance. Up to a point these local appeals were within the financial ability of the states, but gradually they too became inadequate to meet many of the newer, more complex, and expensive problems. As White[3] described it in 1939:

The states as instruments of progress are definitely losing ground. Their leadership, with rare exceptions, is mediocre; their administrative organization, again with occasional exception, is inadequate. . . . It seems possible indeed that the future structure of the American administrative system will rest primarily on the national government and the cities, at least so far as the urban population (now approaching 60 percent) is concerned.

This had changed dramatically by the 1970s when many states began to be featured in the national news media as providing the leadership needed to solve complex problems. State governors were younger, better trained, and nontraditional in their political roots. A new breed of administrators was functioning at the state level too—a younger, more independent (independent of traditional political ties, that is), and better trained work force with business and public administration training.[4] For a period of time mayors of major cities seemed to hold the lead roles in public policy formation, particularly during the Johnson years (in the 1960s), as federal grants-in-aid were channeled directly from national agencies to the mayors rather than through the states. This began to change again with the Nixon administration and more strikingly with the Reagan administration, placing more emphasis on state-level officials.

Originally, federal powers were limited to affairs of interstate and international concern. Many aspects of social, scientific, industrial, and political development in the United States have made an increasing degree of centralization of power necessary. To allow for this change and still maintain the basic principles of federalism, national agencies have increasingly resorted to indirect but constitutionally permissible techniques that have resulted in increased centralization of power in state governments themselves and more significantly in federal agencies. This movement received great acceleration during the 1930s, when the widespread economic depression dealt a devastating blow to local and, to a considerable extent, state finances, rendering them incapable of meeting the demands placed on them. Local governments, having fruitlessly appealed to their state capitals for assistance, turned to Washington as the only source of relief. In light of the underlying social and economic causes, these trends continued and increased.

There are many methods short of total assumption of power and function that may be used to achieve a practical measure of centralization. Perhaps the simplest is the offering of advice and information by a federal agency to the states or by the states to the local governments. This is so common in the field of public health as to have become one of the prime activities of state and federal health agencies. It is only a short step from the transmission of printed advice and information to visits of state and federal consultants, followed by the loan of personnel as resident consultants, especially in the face of local shortages in personnel. Federal personnel, originally intended as consultants, may be assigned to direct state or local health programs. Field technical units, developed by state health departments to assist local units in many instances assume the authority to supervise and even determine local health programs. Thus activities designed for the purpose of rendering advice and information develop into programs of cooperative or outright centralized administration. A variation is a program of inspection and advice, often without authority, to bring about compliance with state or federal recommendations. The inspecting and advising officials, for example, may merely report their findings to the central authorities, who may then promote additional legislation that often gives them increased supervisory powers. This has occurred, for example, in matters of hospital construction and inspection of sanitary or environmental installations.

On the surface the requirement of periodic fiscal and service reports appears innocuous, and it is justifiable to obtain and share information concerning the problems and the programs. Theoretically a state or local health department has the right to organize its records and reports any way it sees fit to serve its purposes. However, after the right to require certain reports is obtained, the next step is to standardize them. In more than one instance this has resulted in a change in the local program itself, the local personnel following the path of least resistance, especially if financial grants are involved. This has occurred in varying degrees, for example, as a result of requirements for reports of births, deaths, and communicable disease and for standardized fiscal reports of state and local health departments to federal health agencies. An accelerating technique is to appoint a local official as the local representative of a state or federal agency. Thus many local health officers have appointments as collaborating epidemiologists of the Public Health Service or inspectors for the Food and Drug Administration and follow the national agency's procedures.

In some areas local activities are subject to direct supervision and review by the higher government. For example, local assessments often must be reviewed and approved by a state board of equalization or by state tax commissioners. Prior permission may be required and is especially effective when the higher level of government participates in financing as in major pollution control programs.

Of a similar nature are approval requirements for the appointment and removal of local officials. In many states it is the prerogative of a local government to select its own health officer, but in practice this is often not the case. Approval by the state health officer is often required. In some states local health officers are appointed and removed directly by the state board of health or the state health director. The local health officer serves as the state health officer's representative in carrying out state laws.

The extent to which the average county health officer is affected by these influences may be pictured somewhat as follows. In the first instance the local health officer may be recruited by and trained under the auspices of the state health department. Appointment, if not made directly by the state health officer, will probably require state approval. Monthly activity reports will have to be made to the state health department on standard forms and a record of all work kept in a form prescribed by the latter agency. By virtue of the local health officer's probable designation as registrar, births and deaths will be reported to the state health department on forms, this time developed and prescribed by the National Center for Health Statistics. If appointed a collaborating epidemiologist, it will be necessary for the health officer to send weekly reports to the Center for Disease Control of the Public Health

Service as well as to the state health department. The maternal and child health program may necessitate operation, inspection, and approval of clinics and hospital facilities, based on standards developed and required by the federal Maternal and Child Health Program or since 1981 by the state program director. Arrangement for the use of x-ray equipment and for hospitalization of persons with tuberculosis will in most instances be made with the state agency. Finally, it will probably be convenient if not necessary to obtain educational materials, biologics, and even office forms and supplies through the state health department.

All this may appear to virtually destroy any independence of action and thought by the local health officer, but the relationships also represent needed resources, even though they are sometimes overly encumbered with red tape. Considering the limited resources available in the majority of local health departments, the involvement of the state is necessary to adequately carry out state laws. This is not true in the larger, more fully developed local health agencies, and they have customarily resisted strong state guidance and control, often turning directly to federal sources of money and technical assistance. This pattern is changing once again as the Reagan administration channels block grant funds to the states, and the states begin to distribute both the funds and the controlling requirements to local agencies.

Details of contracts and the design of hospitals and health centers were specified as conditions for approval of plans by state and federal agencies when federal construction grants were available. Increasingly, many types of licenses are being placed within the jurisdiction of state health departments and through them the federal health and environmental agencies. The Emergency Maternity and Infant Care Program administered by the Children's Bureau through the state health departments during World War II and the many programs authorized by Social Security legislation (Medicare, Medicaid, Comprehensive Child Health Services, etc.) provide examples of the centralizing influence of the right to determine standards.

The federal government cannot dictate to the states the manner in which they should organize their governmental structure, establish their policies, or conduct their programs. However, actual dictation of these matters is not necessary for federal agencies to play a part in the direction of public health services throughout the nation. The signif-

icance of holding the purse sttings is well understood by all. Among many examples of federal influence on state government organizational structure are the rapid formation of state maternal and child health divisions after the passage of the Sheppard-Towner Act and, more recently, the establishment of separate environmental protection agencies by many states soon after such an agency was formed on the federal level.

Grants-in-aid may be made with rigid restrictions on their use, as in categoric or special project grants, or they may be made with only very broad outlines as to their use as in block grants for general preventive health services. Generally the government that contributes the most money to an effort has the greatest influence on how that money can be used. Occasionally, however, a federal grant may cover only a small proportion of the total effort, yet still require conformance of all related program activities with the federal requirements. Categoric and block grants differ primarily in the degree to which they centralize control of the program at the federal level. The contrasting arguments go as follows: the advocates of centralization insist that state and local officials will not generally respond to the needs of dependent people. Therefore along with federal money must go federal requirements, or the intended beneficiaries will not receive the intended benefits. The supporters of decentralization, on the other hand, insist that problems and the ability to respond to problems differ in each community and that money and other scarce resources can be more efficiently and effectively used when the local community has virtually unhindered control over the grants. Although it is difficult to obtain unequivocal evidence on the subject, it does appear that many states tend to withdraw from social programs or reduce their commitment when federal requirements are nonspecific or noncontrolling. Certainly this happened when the original Sheppard-Towner Act expired in 1929 (see chapter on Maternal and Child Health). It appears to be happening currently as Congress and the Department of Health and Human Services make it easier for the states to reduce their expenditures in the Medicaid program. If those reductions in effort are known to cause severe harm, then a case can be made for centralizing control of the programs, but in most instances no such clear-cut relationship can be established between the services rendered and the social benefit obtained.

Rudolf Klein,[5] in discussing the dilemma in a paper prepared for the Royal Commission on the National Health Service, shaped the argument as follows:

The Commission will have to decide whether the state of the art in health services planning is so well developed that it is sensible to endorse the kind of centralizing tendencies that have developed out of the desire to promote equity. If the Commission concludes—as it seems to me that they ought, on the basis of the available evidence—that the state of the art is still very primitive, that there are frequent fluctuations in fashions leading to the adoption of new policies on such issues as the best size for a hospital, then clearly they will also be led to endorse a policy of decentralization. If policy making is seen as a search process, of trial and error through experiment, then diversity becomes desirable in its own right—a value to be pursued, even if it means putting less weight on considerations of equity and uniformity. In turn this would suggest a more limited role for central government in assessing the outcome of local experiment and defining the outer limits of tolerance for diversity, rather than establishing uniform norms throughout the country.

Federal grants-in-aid usually require adherence to certain steps. First, the state must formally accept the terms of the grant, sometimes by means of legislation authorizing a state agency to provide the services. Preparation for use of the grant must be made by preparing and submitting specific plans and by establishing whatever organizations or agencies are indicated for their fulfillment. Plans are approved centrally by a national agency that administers the grant. Usually, but not always, federal grants must be matched in part by funds of the state or local government. The program or project itself is carried out by state or local agencies but is subject to federal as well as state and local inspection and audit. Often payment is made to the state only on satisfactory completion of the project or an agreed-on part of it. Sometimes partial payment is made in advance.

Several means of central influence and control are evident from the steps just outlined. The federal agency may refuse to approve a state or local plan or program or assist it financially because of unsatisfactory organization or procedure. Payments

may be withheld if conditions of agreement are not observed. Furthermore, the state or locality has little or no recourse beyond the federal agency administering the grant. The application of central influences such as these has occurred frequently in the field of public health. To benefit from grants-in-aid administered by many federal agencies, the states have found it necessary to establish or remodel their personnel standards and merit systems to the satisfaction of the federal agencies. Record systems, auditing procedures, clinic and hospital construction and maintenance standards, and many other factors have been similarly affected.

The tendency toward centralization has been most evident in the fields of highway construction, education, and social security. It is interesting to study the similarities in the patterns followed in these three areas of public administration. Of particular interest to those engaged in public health work may be a comparison of the history of federal interest in public roads and in maternal and child welfare. The national government first became concerned with highways in 1893, when it established the Office of Road Inquiry, later the Bureau of Public Roads. The original bill establishing this agency included the following statement:

It is not the province of this department to seek to control or influence said action [in building highways] except in so far as advice and wise suggestions shall contribute toward it. . . . The department is to furnish information, not to direct and formulate any system of organization, however efficient or desirable it may be.

From the date of its establishment until 1912, the Bureau of Public Roads restricted itself to experimentation, advice to state and local highway officials, dissemination of information, and construction of demonstration roads.

In 1912 an act was passed authorizing construction of post roads, followed in 1916 by a more potent Federal Highway Act that set up a system of grants to the states to assist them in meeting the increased demand for good roads and the increased cost of building better types of roads. Where originally the county governments had the chief responsibility for the construction and maintenance of highways, this responsibility and its accompanying authority passed first to the states and then to the federal government. States now receive a large part of their highway funds through federal grants-in-aid, and the Bureau of Public Roads of the Department of Transportation establishes the standards, approves plans, audits the accounts, and inspects the completed work. The effectiveness of these indirect forms of control is indicated by the fact that in 1916, when the Federal Highway Act was passed, 15 states had no highway departments. By the following year every state had a recognized highway department acceptable to the Bureau of Public Roads.

Compare with this the act of 1912 that established the Children's Bureau, directing it to investigate and report "... upon all matters pertaining to the welfare of children and child life, among all classes of people ..." It was designated as a clearinghouse for information on child health and was authorized to carry on research and field studies. During the first 7 years of its existence, the Children's Bureau adhered strictly to these specified functions. In 1921 with the passage of the Sheppard-Towner Act, the Children's Bureau was authorized to participate in the promotion of maternity and infancy programs throughout the nation by means of federal grants to the states. Thus the bureau received its first major administrative responsibilities. As in the case of highways, some states anticipated the passage of the Maternity and Infancy bill and created maternal and child health bureaus or divisions to administer the funds they would obtain if and when the bill became law. Accordingly, by the beginning of 1921, 33 such state agencies had been established, and during the following 2 years 14 more were created. By 1929 maternal and child hygiene bureaus or divisions had been formed and were functioning in the territory of Hawaii and in all the states except Vermont, where the work was carried on under the immediate supervision of the state health officer.[6] In administering the act, the Children's Bureau, as had the Bureau of Public Roads, set standards, approved projects, inspected work within states, and audited accounts.

When the Sheppard-Towner Act expired in 1929, 35 states decreased their appropriations for maternal and child health programs and 9 eliminated them altogether. The programs were reestablished beginning in 1935 with passage of the Social Security Act. This may serve to support the argument that the states are less inclined to aid dependent groups than the federal government, but it also typifies the argument against the grant-in-aid process, since it clearly encourages states and local governments to embark on new or expanded ventures that they might not otherwise consider and that may not even be particularly important in that jurisdiction—

or perhaps considerably less important than some other major problem. The overall record of federal grants-in-aid shows that they have stimulated growth and have not just replaced locally derived tax revenues with federal revenues. This stimulation can and has caused some units of government to extend their commitments beyond their abilities, and such governments, just like families with overextended credit obligations and rising interest rates, may have to terminate a program when grant support declines or is eliminated.

While it is often claimed that federal grants-in-aid support the whims of individuals in Congress or in the administering national agency, it seems more tenable to argue that the acts were passed and the programs developed to meet public demands and needs that could not be met or were not being met by state and local officials even though some unbalanced priorities were created in some areas. As noted earlier, the national government, although it has a substantial capacity to generate tax revenues and to borrow money, has only a limited ability to carry out human service programs or programs of environmental control directly. The reverse is the situation with state and local governments, which are often called on to carry out national initiatives not because of any deliberate usurpation of state and local autonomy but as a simple matter of administrative efficiency. Moreover, it would be difficult to avoid the conclusion that federal grants-in-aid have provided both the technology and the money to make substantial improvements in public health programs. The ideas and the creativity have often come from individual state or local health departments, but the ability to support diffusion of the concept and the practice has emanated from the federal structure.

The states today are performing many more functions than in the past and until recently have increased expenditures for domestic programs at a rate greater than that of the federal government. Today the United States is essentially an urban society with a population (in 1981) of about 230 million, over three fourths of whom reside in metropolitan areas. The process of urbanization demands that the relationships among the levels of government be redefined. A strict demarcation between the responsibilities of the state and national governments is no longer possible. Federalism is in the process of being redefined. Whether changes in federal structure can occur rapidly enough to allow the governmental system to perform its functions adequately in the future is one of the most crucial problems facing American government today.

ORGANIZATIONAL STRUCTURE

The organizational structures of the state and national governments are basically similar. Early in U.S. history a system of checks and balances was devised and applied to both. Each has three branches: the executive or administrative, the legislative or policy-making, and the judicial. On the national and, with one exception, on the state level, legislatures are divided into two houses.

All local governmental units are creations of the state. As a result, the character of the various local units varies from one section of the country to another. The state-local government relationship is defined as a unitary system; that is, powers are conferred on subdivisional governments by the legislature of the state government.

The primary units of local government are the city, village, township, county, and special purpose districts. In addition to these units, many special authorities, intergovernmental compacts, and cooperative service arrangements might be considered components of today's local governmental structure. There were nearly 80,000 local units of government in 1980: 18,862 municipalities, 16,822 townships, 3,042 counties, 25,962 special districts, and 15,174 school districts.[7]

Municipal government

Municipal units are incorporated, that is, they are granted separate legal existence by the state to perform functions other than those resulting from state policies. Cities are governed under special charters, general laws, optional laws, or home rule charters. Before incorporation the area is part of the sovereign state and shares in the benefits and legal exemptions of its sovereignty. On receiving a charter, the municipality becomes a corporation and as such can have a corporate name and seal; own and convey real and personal property; raise monies by taxation, borrowing, or issuing bonds; make and enforce its own local laws; and sue or be sued under its corporate name. It differs, however, from other corporations

in that it has two kinds of functions. There are, on the one hand, certain public functions in which the municipality acts for the sovereign state and concerning which it cannot be sued without its consent. In most states, fire and police protection and public health activities are considered public functions. There are, on the other hand, many activities in which a municipality is engaged primarily or exclusively for its own interests. Examples of these are the construction and maintenance of streets; municipally owned and operated transportation systems; water, gas, and electricity plants; and public hospitals. In most instances a municipality is considered subject to suit concerning these activities.

City governments may take one of several forms. The oldest type is what has been termed the weak mayor-council plan. In this plan the citizens elect by popular vote a mayor and usually a bicameral council of considerable size consisting of councilmen-at-large, plus a number of aldermen from each ward or district of the city. The mayor in such instances is often a member of the council and holds essentially an honorary social office, serving as the officiating representative of the community and as little else. Although this is the oldest type of municipal government in America, it is rapidly becoming outmoded because often it has been fraught with inefficiency and chicanery. The strong mayor form of local government is an adaptation of the older form. Here the legislative branch is reduced to a single council chamber, usually with far fewer members, all of whom are elected at large. The mayor is still elected for a limited term but is given greater executive powers and prerogatives, including increased power of appointment of department heads and other officials and greater control over the budget. In most instances the council may reduce budget items proposed by the mayor but may not add or increase items.

The early years of the twentieth century saw the development of two new forms of city government that have attempted to approach the management of civic affairs on a more business-like basis. The first of these, the commission plan, came about as a result of the devastating earthquake and flood of 1900 at Galveston, Tex. The corrupt and inefficient weak mayor-council government found itself incapable of coping with the emergency situation and literally collapsed. Through the efforts of prominent citizens, a substitute form of government was established. Under this plan a functional commissioner was elected by popular vote for each department. The commissioners ran the city somewhat like the board of directors of a business corporation. Although numerous communities adopted this form of government, experience indicated that it has practical disadvantages. In many instances agreement among the several commissioners has become impossible. In other instances the commissioners in charge of public finance or of the legal department have found themselves in a position to control the activities and plans of the other departments. As a result, the past three decades have seen a gradual rejection of the commission plan of government.

The city manager type of government also developed as an aftermath of a catastrophic flood, this time in Dayton, Ohio, in 1913. The experience of Galveston was duplicated, and in the place of the ineffective weak mayor-council system was substituted a plan whereby only a relatively small council was elected. This council of perhaps 20 to 25 laymen had no administrative duties; technical qualifications were therefore unnecessary. Their meetings usually required little time, their chief functions being the determination of general community policies and the employment of a salaried city manager whose tenure generally depended on satisfactory service. Again, this was an attempt to operate a city government as a business corporation, with the employed city manager acting in an administrative capacity similar to that of the general manager of a private corporation. The use of this plan has been confined almost entirely to small- and intermediate-sized cities. The extent of its adoption, however, has continued to increase, and some counties, particularly on the West Coast, have adopted it.

County government

The county is the one almost universal unit of American government. The boundaries of counties originally were determined essentially in terms of the distance a constituent could ride on horseback or in a buggy from home to the county seat and back again within one day. The entire land area of the United States is divided into counties, 3,042 of them, with spectacular variation in size and population. They vary in size from Kalawao, Hawaii, with a mere 14 square miles, to the 20,117 square miles of San Bernardino County, Calif., which is larger than the states of New Hampshire, Vermont, Massachusetts, Rhode Is-

land, and Connecticut combined. In terms of population, at one end of the scale is Loving County, Tex., with fewer than 100 people and at the other extreme is Los Angeles County, bulging with over 7 million people.

At times and in some places, county governments seem almost irrelevant. The five counties of New York City have virtually yielded their governmental authority to the city government. Some counties have no more than 200 residents, and others serve predominantly rural populations with no city of 10,000 population. Yet they serve a uniquely and currently increasingly important role. Certain legal differences exist between cities and counties. Cities have charters and exist as corporations. They generally may do anything they are not prohibited from doing by some superior law such as a state law or the state constitution. Counties are to an extent administrative creations of the state and may do only those things they are explicitly permitted to do or commanded to do by state law. Although counties may have some degree of independence, they are basically administrative units of state government, and their principal officers have their superior analogues in the state government: the state health officer, the state treasurer, the state attorney general. County administration has been handicapped by the legal relationships with the state. The flexibility that generally makes it possible for a city to frame a charter and determine its form of government and policies in line with its needs has not usually existed for counties. Instead they have had to accept whatever pattern of government the state legislature allowed, sometimes without regard for the limited financial resources or variability of the counties. As a result, larger counties often must operate through a governmental structure they have long since outgrown, whereas small counties are burdened by law with a system they do not need and cannot afford. County home rule is now provided for in some states. This allows counties to frame, adopt, and change their own charters. County home rule as a general principle has been concerned only with allowing the county to establish its governmental structure and has not increased its ability or freedom to enter fields of activities that have generally been forbidden for the county and retained by the state. Often freedom to determine structure has also been limited, since many states constitutionally or legislatively have required that certain county officials be elected even in a county home rule system.

The economic and social life of most counties is geared primarily to agriculture. A lesser density of population, with people living further apart, results in greater self-reliance and less social friction. Whereas city streets exist primarily for the inhabitants of the city, roads in rural areas are necessary for all travelers as well as for those residing locally. Beyond the problems of the individual household and farm, the county seat commands most of the attention of the rural population. To most it represents the prime social, recreational, educational, governmental, economic, and shopping center. The last is perhaps the most significant. Galpin,[8] in his classic studies of life in rural Wisconsin, summarizes:

> It is difficult, if not impossible, to avoid the conclusion that the trade zone about one of these agricultural civic centers forms the boundary of an actual, if not legal, community, within which the apparent entanglement of human life is resolved into a fairly unitary system of interrelatedness. The fundamental community is a composite of many expanding and contracting feature communities possessing the characteristic pulsating instability of all real life.

The results of these differences between rural and urban areas are reflected in the form of local government. Rural governmental machinery is simpler. Fewer officials, boards, and commissions are needed. The officals, boards, and commissions that do exist are usually subject to little or no supervision. Since counties for the most part need state functions on a smaller scale, much of the administrative work is either performed or supervised by state officials. The functions of the county are colored by the circumstances of its origin. In the political field it conducts elections to provide a basis for local representation in the state legislature. Its own legislative powers are almost nonexistent, except for a limited authority to enact certain local ordinances permitted or encouraged by the state. In the fields of administration and service, it serves as the basis for the state financial levy, assessment, and collection; directs many school affairs; con-

structs and maintains roads and bridges; provides public health services; engages in some licensing, in the letting of local contracts, and in the making of local appropriations; and determines salaries of local officials. Many of these functions are increasingly being assumed by the state governments themselves. Reasons include the increased cost of road construction and the increasing professionalization, expansion, and improvement in public health, public welfare, and public school services. In terms of judicial functions the county, through its court, probates wills and registers deeds. It presents a convenient unit of area for the local administration of the state law. The local justice of the peace is the lowest rung on the state judicial ladder. Counties also serve as the territorial units for the establishment of courthouses and penal institutions.

Perhaps the greatest of all deterrents to good county administration is the almost universal lack of centralized administration. In the great majority of instances there is no chief executive to correspond with a mayor or a governor. Some county governments consist of a small board of supervisors or commissioners with considerable administrative authority within the confines of state law. In other jurisdictions, there may be as many as 50 or even 130 commissioners. The voters are often faced with a long array of candidates for a wide variety of jobs. Talent is often in short supply, at least in terms of the technical skills needed to manage many of the functions, and responsibility and authority are widely diffused.

Often the elected supervisors must share authority with an elected sheriff, coroner, treasurer, tax collector, engineer, auditor, and superintendent of schools. The county sheriff is elected to protect life, liberty, and property and to carry out the judgments of the court. The office of county coroner involves the performance of autopsies and the holding of inquests concerning persons who have died suddenly or violently, without medical attention, or under suspicious circumstances. An important officer is the county clerk, whose function is to collect and safeguard public records (including in many instances vital statistics), to issue licenses, to open and adjourn court sessions, and to keep a record of court proceedings and the proceedings of meetings of various county boards. In some places a separate recorder of deeds is elected to keep a record of land titles.

A prosecuting attorney is usually elected to prepare evidence for the juries and to prosecute accused persons on behalf of the county. The county treasurer has the responsibility for receiving, recording, and disbursing all funds expended by the county, usually regardless of their source. An assessor is necessary to list taxable persons and property and to assess them at a fair evaluation. In a few states a special tax collector is elected, and in many states a county auditor is chosen to audit county funds and expenditures. In some states this function is carried out by the county board itself or by its financial committee. The invitation to fiscal folly involved in either case is obvious. School boards are generally elected either at large or by district representation separately from the rest of the county government. The superintendent of schools is generally elected by popular vote, although in some states the superintendent is appointed either by state authorities or by the county school board. In many instances this person is the highest paid and most influential official in the county. Other miscellaneous officers may be elected because of local need or tradition.

Last but not least among the county officials is the county health officer. In most instances the health officer is unique in not being locally elected. The tendency has been to consider this a professional position and one that can be entrusted only to a specially qualified person. Frequently, local governments experience difficulty in filling this position and turn of necessity to outside agencies such as state health departments, civil service commissions, or schools of public health for assistance. As a result of this and other factors, a tendency has developed for many local health officers to feel more responsible to the state than to the county government that they serve. In many jurisdictions, the position of local health officer is honorary but with little real honor. State laws often require that it be a physician, and because there is not any large staff or program to administer, the most prominent physician in the county or the physician who is closest to the leading elected official is asked to serve usually without remuneration. This accounts for the considerable difficulty in identifying official local health departments, since such individuals are often listed in directories of local governmental officials but have no real status or function. With a staff of three to five workers, they are called on once every 2 weeks or so to sign the payroll.

The picture of county government is distinctly different from the political portrait of cities. Since most county officials are representatives of a higher level state official and carry out state functions, they tend to develop a much closer relationship with the state government than do city officials who have more independence in establishing programs, raising money, and working with the national government. Until recently, mayors were more involved with and influential in national government transactions, while county officials were much more caught up in the political process of forming and running the state government. The counties after all run the elections, and they often run the candidates too. Partially as a result of some creative leadership provided to the National Association of Counties by means of a Ford Foundation grant in 1958, partially because public demand for better government has introduced a sense of reform, and partially because of the expansion of grants-in-aid, especially those that go through states to their administrative subdivisions (the counties), this pattern is changing. During the first half of the 1980s mayors are having a more difficult time making their needs heard, while the long-standing relationships between state and county officials are functioning relatively smoothly as they attempt to rework the flow of federal grants-in-aid.

Special districts

Special districts are the most varied of all local units of government. They usually are established to deal with a particular problem, such as water, sewage, air pollution, and the like. To finance the specific undertaking, special districts have recourse to taxation, assessment, or charging rates based on service costs.

Metropolitan government

It is evident that many reforms are indicated in local government. One of the most pressing is the need for consolidation. It seems inevitable that this will come about, and symptoms are already evident in many fields of public service and in certain parts of the country. The changes are difficult to accomplish, however. The provision of public health services in many areas on a multicounty basis is one example of this trend. The regional approach may be of considerable value in defining and locating public health problems, in revealing causal factors, in creating public consciousness concerning them, and in arriving at methods for their solution.

Attempts have been made to provide a governmental structure for metropolitan areas through a number of mechanisms. In one, intergovernmental agreements and contracts that allow for the provision of a single service on a regional basis are negotiated. Another that has not been used widely consolidates certain county and city services under the same administration. In another type of city-county consolidation, the limits of the city are extended to the county boundaries. This also results in the elimination of one unit of government.

Possibly the most effective structure for metropolitan government so far is the metropolitan federation. Municipalities in the metropolitan area continue their separate existence. Functions of regional interest, however, are transferred to a new central federated government. Examples of federated government include those of the Municipality of Metropolitan Toronto, Miami-Dade County, Nashville-Davidson County, and the Metropolitan Corporation of Greater Winnipeg. Since the formal legal mechanisms for metropolitan government in most areas have been lacking, informal voluntary bodies such as councils of governments have been formed. The membership on bodies such as these includes representatives who participate on a voluntary basis from the various governing units. The weakness of voluntary associations is that they have access to authority only through their member bodies.

Another approach to solving the problem of a multiplicity of political jurisdictions in relation to one service area is the nonprofit corporation. Nonprofit corporations, with their boards of directors selected on a regional basis, may assume in a variety of ways effective and efficient administration of publicly financed projects. The result of an increase in the number of such corporations, however, could be a loss of control, manageability, and public accountability.

It is evident that a type of local governmental structure that can adequately meet the needs and demands of an urban society still does not exist in the United States today. The incremental changes that have occurred facilitate the performance of the service functions of government but hinder the performance of political functions. They do not provide a structure in which regional issues can be debated and resolved. Progress along these lines is necessarily slow. Consolidation of local governmental units presents a most difficult political task with many factions ever alert to oppose it. County voters and county lines as they now exist are important to office holders, local merchants and bankers, political party workers, many property owners, and local newspapers; for patronage purposes they are important to local, state, and federal political factions. Today the inability of the governmental system to respond to demands made of it as a result of outmoded structure contributes in a large degree to the inability of the public health agency to solve health problems with the scientific expertise and knowledge that presently is available.

Despite the shortcomings discussed, it is increasingly apparent that counties, given expanded powers and efficient organization, could occupy a uniquely advantageous position because their territory is large enough to address realistically problems that are too great for other types of local governments to handle. Almost half of the nation's metropolitan areas are encompassed essentially by one county. Even in multicounty regions or metropolitan areas, two or several counties can more easily coordinate their activities and programs than can dozens or even hundreds of fragmented and sometimes gerrymandered municipalities and special districts. Such smaller cities, towns, and districts generally lack the revenues or qualified personnel to meet satisfactorily the growing demand for improved governmental service including the many social programs mandated by the state or federal governments.

GOVERNMENTAL REVENUES AND EXPENDITURES[7,9]

It is now incomprehensible that in 1913 the total expenditures of all levels of government in the United States were a mere $2.8 billion. Even on the eve of the nation's involvement in World War II in 1941, the figure had risen only to $25 billion. Since 1950, as illustrated in Table 6-1, dramatic increases have occurred in the amounts of revenues and expenditures on all levels of government. Thus between 1950 and 1980 overall revenues and expenditures increased 14-fold.

The fiscal requirements of the different levels of

TABLE 6-1. Revenues and expenditures (in billions of dollars) 1950-1980, United States

Year	Revenues				Expenditures			
	All	Federal	State	Local	All	Federal	State	Local
1950	67	44	11	12	70	42	11	17
1960	153	100	26	27	151	90	22	39
1970	335	206	69	60	333	185	56	92
1980	932	564	213	156	959	526	173	259

From Bureau of the census: Statistical abstracts of the United States: 1981, ed. 102, U.S. Government Printing Office, Dec., 1981.

government vary considerably relative to each other. In 1980, for example, the $959 billion of direct governmental expenditures was distributed as follows:

Expenditures (in billions of dollars)	Federal	States	Local	Total
Amount	$526	$173	$259	$959
%	55.0	18.0	27.0	100.0

Such figures indicate that the federal, or national, government is the big spender compared to state and local governments. However, it is difficult to estimate total governmental expenditures accurately because of the amount of intergovernmental transferring that occurs from the federal government to the state governments and from the states to local governments. In 1980 it was estimated that the state and local governments spent $432 billion, of which 18% came from federal sources, 66% from state and local taxes, and the rest from miscellaneous sources and charges. The states directly spent $173 billion plus $84.5 billion in intergovernmental transfers, mostly to local governments. If Defense Department expenditures and expenditures from the Social Security trust fund are removed from the direct federal expenditure estimate, it is clear that the delivery capacity, in terms of services and benefits, is at the state and local level.[9]

The magnitude of intergovernmental transfers can be appreciated from the figures in Table 6-1, since the figures reveal expenditures after intergovernmental transfers. Total federal outlays in 1980 were about $617 billion. The table shows that the federal government spent directly considerably

less than it received in revenues, but it transferred large sums to the states and to local governments. Local governments, for example, spent $259 billion in 1980 while receiving from their own revenue sources only $156 billion. Local governmental tax revenues were estimated at $83.5 billion while total local expenditures from own funds were estimated at $117 billion, suggesting that local units of government received $33.5 billion from nontax sources such as fees. During that same year, local governments spent approximately $215 billion, the difference ($215 billion minus $117 billion) coming largely from intergovernmental transfers.[9]

Intergovernmental transfers include not only federal transfers to states but also to local governments. Also included are substantial state-to-local transfers of both state and passed-through federal grants. Not all of the federal funds indicated as intergovernmental transfers are for the exclusive benefit of states and localities. Substantial proportions are earmarked for defense, highways, airports, railroads, natural resource development, and similar purposes. Of the remainder, major amounts are earmarked for specific programs. Thus in 1978 about $3 billion were for specific health activities and over $19 billion were for welfare, the largest part of that for Medicaid.

REVENUE SHARING

The preceding discussion has illustrated that state and local governments, in the face of increased population, urbanization, demands for public services, and greater citizen expression are hampered by an outmoded system of revenue resources. While the states have acknowledged the significant increases in federal subsidies and grants-in-aid, they have been tied to the categoric wishes of the federal government that may not conform to state or local ideas about problems, needs, and priorities. Although they have the right to apply for federal assistance, state and local decision-making authority is limited. Beyond this is the difficulty of balanced and long-range planning and financing. Democratic governments find it difficult to plan or budget for more than one year at a time. A partial response was the passage of the National Health Planning and Resources Development Act (P.L. 93-641). An additional complaint is the considerable amount of red tape, paper work, conferences, and reports required for each of the individual grants by each of the federal offices and agencies involved. An important step was finally taken by Congress in the passage of the State and Local Financial Assistance Act of 1972. This enabled and required the federal government to share revenue with the states and through them as specified in the law, with local jurisdictions. Such shared funds in the form of block grants replaced certain of the previously existing categoric grants-in-aid.

To meet increasing fiscal demands, units of government at all levels are engaged in a constant search and struggle for additional sources of revenue. Each unit of government, maintaining its own revenue and taxation system, finds itself increasingly in conflict with the others. In the early days of American history, the most lucrative, stable, and accessible form of taxation was on general property. Since originally most governmental functions took place at the local level, the general property tax was reserved largely for use by local governments. As a result, even today the general property tax represents the major source of income for local governments, accounting in 1979 for about 57% of city and 80% of county tax revenues.

Beyond the general property tax, cities and counties have access locally only to fees from licenses, permits, assessments, fines, and forfeitures, and institutional funds and earnings. In 1979 these accounted for 25% of city and 13% of county revenues. For some time the tendency has been for local governments, both city and county, to give way to the state and federal governments when new revenue sources are discovered or in cases of tax conflict.

This dilemma in which local governments now find themselves would not be so acute if the general property tax had remained as useful as it once was. Unfortunately, this tax has become increasingly difficult to administer, has been repeatedly subject to personal and political manipulation, and even if correctly applied may sometimes jeopardize individual property owners on whom it is levied. To assess the value of personal property honestly and accurately is in itself a difficult and costly procedure. Added to this is the fact that most tax assessors are local individuals who by virtue of their local election are subject to feelings of indebtedness and favoritism. It is not surprising that the administration of the general property tax not only has been lax and inefficient but often has been used as a political tool.

Another factor to be considered with regard to the general property tax is that much property is exempt from taxes. Typically, for example, the following are not subject to taxation: public property, places of religious worship and burial, charitable institutions, educational institutions, funds or property held or used as endowment by such institutions, real and personal estate of any public library and of any literary association connected with such a library, books, philosophic apparatus, paintings and statuary of any company or association kept in a public hall and not held as merchandise or for sale or gain, farm products grown in the state and remaining in the hands of the producer during the year after their production, and personal property and homesteads up to a certain amount.

Although the property tax remains the principal source of tax revenue for local government, it has adverse effects on inner city housing, perpetuates conflicts between business and home owners, has an inverse relationship to ability to pay, and retards the revitalization of major urban areas.[10] Because of these reasons, added to escalating housing costs, there is a growing feeling that home assessment for tax purposes can be raised beyond the homeowner's control or ability to pay. This had led to citizen reaction against all uncontrolled governmental spending and taxes, beginning in 1978 with an overwhelmingly supported referendum in California to limit property taxes severely, and has continued during the early 1980s.

GRANTS-IN-AID

Grants-in-aid represent one form of transfer of public funds for the purpose of equalizing revenue among the several levels of government and among the states and their contained local areas. No reasonable person would sanction the continuance, for want of adequate funds, of insanitary conditions, and of inadequate public health programs in some areas that might adversely affect others. This being the case, it becomes necessary to provide some method for assisting the smaller or less favored units of government to meet their obligations.

A second justification for the increasing use of grants-in-aid may be found in the situation previously discussed; that is, the local government units are more restricted as to types of revenue and are administratively in a disadvantageous position for levying and collecting some of the more lucrative sources of funds. Few would deny the right of local governments to share in the fiscal benefits of automobile excise taxes, since the local areas must share in the building and maintenance of the roads over which vehicles travel. It would be confusing, however, to say the least, should each locality attempt to apply and collect its own automobile excise tax. A revenue such as this is obviously collected more efficiently by a higher level of government.

A third purpose of grants-in-aid, as was indicated in the discussion of centralization, is to provide some measure of supervision or control over the activities of the lower units of government. Related to this, and arising as a result of it, is a fourth purpose of grants-in-aid: the enforcement of minimum standards on the recipient of the grant. Undoubtedly, few things have been as influential in promoting the employment of qualified local public health personnel, for example, as have been the conditions attached to grants by both state and federal health agencies.

The idea of grants-in-aid is by no means new, having been first applied in this country in New York State in 1795 for the improvement of schools in the poorer, particularly rural, areas of that state. Federal grants to states began as early as 1808, when Congress instituted an annual appropriation to assist the states in the development of their respective militia. No conditions were attached to these grants, and no federal supervision was exercised. Perhaps the next development of significance was the passage in 1862 of the Morrill Act, which entitled each state to a grant of public lands based on the total number of its members of Congress. The only condition was that not less than 90% of the gross proceeds was to be used for the establishment and maintenance of agricultural and mechanical colleges. Subsequent acts added to the

original provisions an annual grant of cash to each state. In 1887 the Hatch Act was passed, which provided $15,000 per year to each state for the establishment of agricultural experiment stations. With this act there was instituted the condition of submission of an annual financial report, followed 8 years later by provision for a federal audit. This established a pattern that has never since been altered.

The rising tide of federal influence in state and local affairs is well illustrated by another phase of social security, relief for dependents. Traditionally the care of such individuals in America has been a local and often a private affair. The economic depression of the 1930s changed all this when, because of lack of funds, first private charity, then local governments, and in turn state governments found themselves incapable of meeting the tremendously increased demands. Only one other source of assistance remained—the national government—largely because of its power to borrow money and adopt an out-of-balance budget. As a result, numerous federal agencies that provided for the first time a basis for a broad system of federal social security were established. These agencies concerned themselves with dependent children, the unemployed, the handicapped, and the aged.

The changes that have occurred in the relationship between the federal and state governments have also resulted in some change in the relationships between state and local governments and between local and federal governments. Theoretically the national government has no relations with cities. However, even antedating the depression there had appeared signs to indicate closer contacts between national and municipal authorities. Federal agencies had developed standards in weights and measures, traffic and safety, zoning and building, highway construction, and milk sanitation and had carried out studies and surveys on local education, finances, crime, vital statistics, and public health. In addition, federal agencies were actively engaged in a cooperative sense in food and drug control, municipal water supplies, sewage disposal, and other fields. The economic depression of the 1930s and subsequently World War II accelerated the intimacies of these relationships. Although the federal agencies operated for the most part through the state governments as an intermediary, they did in some instances deal directly with cities.

As has been noted previously, big-city mayors, the U.S. Conference of Mayors, the Urban League, and other organizations brought city and nationally elected and administrative officials into increasingly close contact. When the national government built and staffed regional offices, they were located in the nation's large cities: New York, Boston, Atlanta, Kansas City, Chicago, Dallas, Denver, San Francisco, and Philadelphia. This brought the federal program managers who often made grant decisions into much more intimate contact with the urban officials who wanted the money and had the organizations needed to implement the programs. The power of the states was not usurped, but the state legislatures, long dominated by more rural interests, were simply bypassed as city and federal officials found that they had more in common. The state scarcely noticed or cared. In 1965 Congress established the new federal Department of Housing and Urban Development, and federal involvement in the nation's cities became still more pervasive. With a well-trod path to Washington rather than to their state capitals, the cities were not prepared for the new federalism coupled with the severe budget cuts of the Reagan administration. From an administrative point of view, it makes sense for the federal government to deal directly and exclusively with the 50 states, especially with massive reductions in the personnel necessary to administer hundreds of grants. Similarly, it makes sense for the states to work with their administrative subdivisions, the counties. The new federalism of the 1980s promises not only major reductions in social programs at all levels, but major changes in the political relationships among the three levels of government.

Federal grants-in-aid for public health work began with the passage of the Chamberlain-Kahn Act of 1918. Stimulated by the increased threat of venereal diseases during World War I, Congress provided an appropriation of $1 million for each of 2 years to be distributed to the states on the basis of population. The program was administered not by the Public Health Service but by an interdepartmental social hygiene board. After the second year the appropriation was cut and then finally eliminated.

The next use of federal grants for public health purposes was in the field of maternal and child health. Again as a result of increased interest during the war, the Sheppard-Towner Act of 1921 was passed. It provided grants of $1.24 million a year to the states for 5 years "for the promotion of the welfare and hygiene of infancy."

The sound, effective, and equitable distribution of grants (or subventions) presents a difficult problem. Not infrequently plans have resulted in more aid being allotted to wealthier communities than to those most in need. By distributing grants on the basis of taxable capacity either directly or indirectly through matching requirements, by granting equal amounts to all communities, or even by granting on the basis of population alone, there is a tendency, if anything, to increase the inequities.

The great increase in the numbers and types of grant-in-aid programs in the health and health-related fields in the past 4 decades has created serious problems of mangeability. The Eighty-ninth Congress alone passed acts that created 21 new health programs, 17 new educational programs, 15 new economic development programs, 12 new programs for cities, 17 new resource development programs, and 4 new manpower programs. Until 1981 nearly 200 different federal aid programs existed, financed by over 500 separate appropriations, 21 federal departments, 150 Washington bureaus, and 400 regional offices. Funds for programs were channeled in different patterns under a variety of rules and regulations.

The last fairly complete resumé of the federal grant system was that developed by Zwick and Behney for 1975.[11] The amounts of money changed considerably by 1981, but the basic distribution of programs was more or less the same. The Reagan administration proposed converting these categoric programs and many others in nonhealth fields into 15 large block grants, which would provide the states with greater flexibility and fewer administrative controls. Two of these block grants were to encompass 26 categoric aid programs in public health. Congress adopted a bill calling for four block grants: a general preventive health services block grant; an alcohol, drug abuse, and mental health block grant; a maternal and child health block grant; and a primary care block grant to encompass federal programs in support of community health centers. The process was remarkable. Under the 1974 Budget Act, Congress found itself forced to vote on a total figure for major areas such as health and then to reconcile the statutes that authorized programs and expenditures with the budget ceiling. In 5 short weeks in the fall of 1981, Congress rewrote most of the public health laws developed over the prior 45 years (The Omnibus Budget Reconciliation Act, P.L. 97-35) and reduced the authorizations substantially. When it came time to appropriate money, the programs were cut even further. The states, through the National Governor's Association, supported the block grant concept even though it was apparent that there would be much less money available for local programs. Few of them realized just how severe the cuts would be. The administration compared the 1982 spending levels and their 1983 proposals with 1981 expenditures. That, however, failed to account for inflation. The appropriation in terms of services was more sharply curtailed than the appropriation of dollars.

An added feature would come back to haunt the states in their quest for less federal supervision. While the Reagan administration truly wanted to return control to the states, budget cutting was an even higher priority. Program and planning concepts were jettisoned in Congressional–White House negotiating sessions in favor of maintaining the targeted cuts. When the lobbyists for some of the categoric programs approached the budget committee staff members, they were asked to refrain from protesting the block grant move and the cuts since the cuts were sure to be made. In exchange they were often offered language that specified that "no less than the amount of money spent in the prior year shall be spent for disease X or program Y." When the hearings were held, the strongest advocacy groups were thus neutralized and only the weaker ones protested the new block grants with the smaller dollar amounts. When the states finally got the grants, they found the restrictions virtually intact and much less money with which to work. Not only that, but alternative sources had also dried up. In prior years if the appropriation of funds to support the community mental health centers was not up to the expectations of the center directors, the directors could learn to bill Medicaid more vigorously and bargain for a larger share of the state's Title XX money for social services. But this time all of the appropriations were cut, and virtually all public health programs in the United States were faced with sharp reductions at the very time when the people who needed their services the most were losing their jobs and other sources of support.

Block grants do offer the recipients the opportunity to become creative and to tailor their programs to their problems and the expectations of their communities. But two essential features of a successful block grant program were ignored: restrictions on how the money is to be used have to be minimized, and the funds must be adequate so that all of the grant managers, thrown together in the same box, can at least start out with the assurance that their rent is paid and their doors can stay open. This did not happen. Federalism in the United States has been dramatically altered, just as it was in 1935, and the outcome will not be clear for many years.

REFERENCES

1. Snider, C.: American state and local government, New York, 1965, Appleton-Century-Crofts.
2. Brogan, D.W.: The American character, New York, 1944, Alfred A. Knopf, Inc.
3. White, L.D.: Introduction to the study of public administration, New York, 1939, Macmillan, Inc.
4. Wright, D.S., and Dometrius, N.: State administrators: their changing characteristics, State Government **50,** Summer 1977.
5. Klein, R.: Evidence to the Royal Commission on the National Health Service, J. Health Polit. Policy Law **3**(1):11-19, Spring 1978.
6. U.S. Children's Bureau: The seven years of the maternity and infancy act, Washington, D.C., 1931, U.S. Government Printing Office.
7. Bureau of the Census: Statistical abstracts of the United States: 1981, ed. 102, Washington, D.C., 1981, U.S. Government Printing Office.
8. Galpin, C.J.: The social anatomy of an agricultural community, Res. Bull. 34, University of Wisconsin Agricultural Experiment Station, Madison, 1914, University of Wisconsin Press.
9. Significant features of fiscal federalism, ed. 1979-1980, Advisory Committee on Intergovernmental Relations, Washington, D.C., October 1980, The Committee.
10. Netzer, D. In Mitchell, W.E., and Walter, I.: State and local finance, New York, 1970, The Ronald Press Co.
11. Zwick, D.I., and Behney, C.J.: Federal health services grants, 1966-1975, Public Health Rep. **91:**493, Nov.-Dec. 1976.

CHAPTER 7

Law and public health

The law is the last result of human wisdom acting upon human experience for the benefit of the public.

Samuel Johnson

THE IMPORTANCE OF LAW

A conference in 1961 sponsored by the American Public Health Association and the U.S. Public Health Service concluded that public health workers were inadequately informed and trained in the legal aspects of public health and in the legal framework within which public health programs are designed and activated.[1] This is not surprising, since education about law for other than law students is one of the most neglected aspects of American education despite its impact on people.[2] In his discussion of the implications of this, Wing[3] notes that too often health personnel view the law as "merely a separate discipline or a system of institutions and activities . . . separate from the institutions and activities of concern to public health." However, as indicated by Clute,[4] the fault is not limited to the health and teaching professions:

As man finds himself beset today with problems that threaten his health and even bring into question his continued existence, it is vitally necessary that he use to the full every possible means of solving his problems. One such means is the law. Yet so far is the law from being used to the full, that it is little understood by health professionals, and, indeed, is hardly even in their thoughts. At the same time, lawyers have little understanding of health matters. In the interests of mankind, it is essential that this gulf be bridged, and without further delay. This will require, among other things, a much more fundamental understanding of the nature of law by health professionals; the establishment of much more solid and durable cooperation between the professionals in health and in law, at every level from education to the solving of problems in the field; and the serious examination of the undeveloped potentialities, as well as the shortcomings, of the law for solving the problems of human welfare.

Fortunately, one may point to the appearance during recent decades of not only an increasing number of specialists who have bridged the legal and public health fields but also a growing amount of literature concerning the relationships between law and public health.[5] Especially useful have been the series of articles that have appeared in the *American Journal of Public Health* under the by-lines first of Forgotson and currently of Curran.

It is impractical, indeed impossible, for health workers to attempt to function without at least a general familiarity with the legal system. To provide this is all that is attempted here. Beyond this readers are urged to acquire a familiarity with the legislation, legislative structures, and legislative procedures of their respective communities, states, and nations, especially as they relate to health matters.

The legislative process involves the interaction of the three basic branches of government that are usually interlocked by a system of checks and balances. Thus in the United States of America, on which much of the following is based. the *Executive* may veto legislation or sign it into law, the *Legislature* may introduce and enact a law and can override a veto by the Executive, and the *Judiciary* may discard a law if it considers it in violation of basic freedoms and rights. To these three may be added the operating or enforcement agencies that are held responsible for carrying out the intent of the legislation; these also may be a significant source of proposed legislative additions or changes. With this in mind, participation by public health workers in the legislative process was encouraged at a World Health Organization Conference of Directors of Schools of Public Health in 1966. The conference report[6] stated that "Legislation is an essential element of public health administration, not only for the control of various activities but increasingly as a means of facilitating or permitting the carrying out of certain activities that promote health." Indeed, as several writers[7,8] on the subject have pointed out, everything that is done in a health agency has a basis in law and is subject to legal sanctions of one type or another. As for official health agencies, in addition to their service functions, many activities involve the enforcement of law.

DEFINITION OF LAW[9,10]

Much has been written dealing exclusively with the nature and definition of law. It is interesting that although the average citizen probably considers law as an exact and strictly defined field, its mere definition presents the members of the legal profession with perhaps their most difficult problem. Law, at least in a democracy, depends in the last analysis on the collective wishes of the people; and the type and extent of their wishes vary through place and time. It should be realized that human behavior is subject to a never-ceasing process of evolution, as are also the social factors determining or influencing it. However, this has not always been the case. It is worthwhile to consider in considerable abbreviation the changes and evolution that have occurred in legal attitudes and definitions as they relate to the United States. Blackstone,[11] the great English jurist, considered law as a "rule of civil conduct prescribed by the supreme power in a state, commanding what is right and forbidding what is wrong." It should be noted that he refrained from including the criteria involved in determining "right" or "wrong" at any particular time. As has been noted elsewhere, those who developed the government of the United States subscribed to the concept of natural law, essentially fixed and immutable. This concept led to and supported a laissez-faire type of government that interfered with the individual to a minimal extent. It carried over into the late nineteenth century. Thus, C.C. Langdell,[12] the first Dean of Harvard University Law School, wrote in 1886 that ". . . the law is a science" and that ". . . all the available materials of the science are contained in printed books of judicial opinions." As the twentieth century was approached, several prominent jurists, notably Oliver W. Holmes[13] and James B. Thayer,[14] insisted that legal doctrine should be regarded basically as the historical product of social conflict and political compromise.

Early in the twentieth century, a group of progressive legal theorists and practitioners including Louis Brandeis, Felix Frankfurter, Ezra Pound, and James Landis urged consideration by the courts of nonlegal facts in relation to the interpretation and application of the law.[15] At the same time Woodrow Wilson[16] still considered law as "that portion of established thought and habit which has gained distinct and formal recognition in the shape of uniform rule backed by the authority and power of government." During the 1920s and 1930s, a group referred to as "legal realists" appeared. They were strongly critical of classical and professionally self-centered lawyers. They advocated the application of various sociologic disciplines including anthropology, Freudian psychology, political science, and statistics to the interpretation of law in relation to behavior. In stronger words they sought to deny "the autonomy of legal science" and sought to expose it as "a smoke screen disguising the realities of human motivation."[17] The great depression of the 1930s brought about a fundamental change in legal thought under the banner of the so-called "legal process" school. It considered the lawyer to have "a social role with definite social expectations" and therefore he should "coordinate his role with those of other role-players in the legal process." Further, it sought to demonstrate that "the courts were often not the institutions best equipped to make many judgments of social importance and that therefore judges should often defer to the policy resolutions made by legislatures, administrative agencies, other judicial systems, or by private parties themselves."[18]

The foregoing would appear to support the view of Wing[19] that law be seen as "other than a set of specific answers to specific questions; it is better thought of as a set of rather vague principles that may or may not be applied in a given situation depending on a number of factors and considerations."

CHARACTERISTICS OF LAW

A law implies an actual or potential command, and a command signifies nothing more or less than a wish or desire. However, the commands and desires of law differ from ordinary personal commands and desires in that they (1) represent community desires or commands, (2) are applicable to all in the community, (3) are backed by the full power of the government, and (4) provide for all people the administration of justice under these laws. Wilson's definition might be considered to be appropriate, since it either states or implies all of the characteristics mentioned.

PURPOSE OF LAW[20]

The primary purpose of law might be said to be the promotion of the general good by the regulation of human conduct to protect the individual from other individuals, groups, or the state, and vice versa. To effect such protection, it must be possible for the individual, the group, and the state to predict within reasonable limits the probable course of judgment in the event of an infringement of the law. Therefore another purpose of law is to assure, insofar as possible, uniformity of action to prevent errors of judgment or improper motives or actions on the part of judicial officers. It is often said that the wheels of justice turn slowly. The rate would be impossibly slow if the accumulative experience of earlier judges were not available to the people and to the courts. This also is a purpose of law.

The most fundamental means by which law endeavors to carry out its purposes is the definition of rights and duties existing between individuals or groups. Legal relationships form the essential subject matter of law, and rights and duties are the most important of legal relationships. A legal right is a power, privilege, or interest of an individual or group that is recognized and protected by law. Simultaneously the law imposes on all others the obligation to refrain from violation of the right. Thus the possession of a right by one person always implies a corresponding duty on the part of some other person or persons to respect that right. For example, A and B enter into a contract. The legal relationship may be expressed as either A has a right that B perform an act or B owes A a duty to perform an act.

Rights are of two kinds, primary and secondary. Primary rights are those that result merely from an individual's existence as a member of society. A citizen holds these primary rights against the entire community individually and collectively, and the community and each of its individuals own him a corresponding duty to refrain from violating them. Thus a citizen's person and property are held to be inviolate; that is his primary right, and all others owe a duty to respect it. Such rights exist not by virtue of any action taken or decision made but are the kind of rights that were termed "natural rights" by eighteenth century legal theorists. They are sometimes spoken of as "rights in rem" and "rights of ownership." Their violation is considered a civil wrong (a tort) or a crime, depending on their magnitude and on whatever statutory law declares them to be. Libel, slander, trespass, negligence, and the like are civil wrongs or torts. It is increasingly difficult, however, to determine just balances or limits for rights and duties and indeed to decide whether they result from rights or duties in rem or ownership. Examples of these dilemmas may be found in relation to tobacco smoking and to aspects of environmental pollution,[21] as well as to the privacy of personal health and medical records.[22,23]

Secondary rights are those superimposed on primary rights as a result of individual action and decision. They are not held against all other persons generally but only against a specified person or group. These rights arise as a result of contract. For example, A and B enter into a contractual agreement. Before the contract their legal relationship, consisting of rights and duties owed each other, was fixed and equal. Now, as a result of the contract, their legal relationships are different. A's previous primary rights are now increased by a secondary right that B carry out the action agreed on in the contract. This new right differs in kind from primary rights, first, because it is not simply caused by A's existence but results from a mutually agreed on contract and, second, because it is a right held against B alone and no others.

Remedial rights are sometimes referred to as a third form of rights. They come into existence on the violation of the legal primary and secondary rights just discussed. In other words, they are rights resulting from a personal injustice and are held against the individual committing the legal wrong. What they really amount to is a right of reparation, usually in the form of a money judgment. All that is meant by saying that a person has a remedial right is that if he appeals to the court, he will in all probability be rendered a favorable verdict. As Justice Holmes observed, a remedial right is in the nature of a prophecy.

SYSTEMS OF LAW
Development[24,25]

The concept of law has gone through many changes throughout the centuries of recorded history. With primitive man it apparently originated as a combination of gradually developing customs based on tradition and supposedly divine dictates. Perhaps the chief function of the patriarchs of a tribe was to define the practices evolved and followed by their predecessors, and these customs were gradually given the significance of established precedent and law. As to the meaning or reason for such laws, it was the theory of the Hindus and Chinese that laws were an essential necessity of human society, as a result of the innate depravity of man. As evidenced by human nature, laws were necessary to prevent violence and injustice. Therefore it became a primary duty first of the tribal leaders and ultimately of their successor, the state, to formulate and enforce rules of human behavior and conduct.

The Grecian theory of law was somewhat different and followed in general the basic philosophic pattern of their civilization. The Greeks argued that all necessary social laws really existed in nature and were merely waiting to be discovered, similar to the principles of physics. In fact, nature was thought of more or less as an expression of the total of all universal law. This concept that law exists perpetually, waiting to be discovered as natural truths, held sway for over 1,700 years, passing through Stoic philosophy, Roman law, the principles of the Christian Church, and on through the medieval civilizations and governments. It is significant that the men who founded the North American Republic and formulated the Declaration of Independence and the United States Constitution with its Bill of Rights had as their legal background the natural theory of law. It is noteworthy that the basic idea of the Declaration of Independence deals with the natural rights of men, which are to be *secured* rather than *granted* by government.

Since the establishment of the republic, the concept or theory of law in the United States has undergone considerable change, especially since the beginning of the twentieth century, so that legislation is now seen merely as a manmade device for the regulation and control of human conduct to assure the ultimate wishes of the greatest number or of the dominant groups in the community.

Statutory law

At the present time almost the entire western world is governed by a combination of two distinct systems of law: (1) statutory law, based essentially on Roman civil law, and (2) the common law of England. The earliest known recorded statutes were those of Hammurabi (2067-2025 BC) for the Babylonian empire. Roman law began its development very early in the Roman state. To these were added innumerable unwritten laws that ultimately, as a result of the Institutes of Justinian and others, were codified into a system of written law so perfect that even today it serves as the basic law of most European countries. Its geographic adoption was related, of course, to the paths of Roman conquest, which brought the Roman legal code into most parts of the continent. After the decline of the Roman Empire, the resulting daughter nations retained the Roman legal system, since they had little other pattern to follow. Subsequent states, such as the members of the American Republic, provided legislatures to make whatever laws were necessary for government, and the resulting collections of legislative acts constituted the statutory law. For a time an attempt was made to adhere rather strictly to statutory law, but as societies became more complicated, especially as a result of urbanization and industrialization, innumerable additions had to be made in the form of specific interpretations, court decisions, and rules and regulations. The result is that at the present time, for example in the United States, written or statutory law constitutes only a small part (about 2%) of all existing laws.

Common law[26]

It was recognized at an early date that statutory law was in many cases too general to be directly applied to particular cases. As a result, there followed the development of courts, the judges of which were expected to be guided in their specific decisions by the established customs of the community. England took particular strides in this direction. Essentially this recognition of the legal importance of custom represented a practical recognition of the rights of a people to take part in the making of the rules and laws governing their conduct and relationships. This was a great step toward liberty. A custom, to be entitled to consideration in law, must meet certain conditions. First, it must have existed for a long time or, as Blackstone put it, "have been used so long that the memory of man runneth not to the contrary." It must be followed continuously, that is, constantly observed and respected whenever an occasion for its observance or respect arises. Second, it must have a peaceful purpose and be reasonable and not inconsistent with the general spirit of the law. Third, it must be definite rather than vague and must be considered binding on all people. Fourth, it must be consistent with all other customs of society.

Stare decisis

With the gradual development and extension of use of the common law courts, another practical procedure soon became indicated. The administration of justice would have become impossibly slow were it necessary to judge every particular controversy directly against existing written law and custom. Therefore the doctrine of stare decisis (the decision stands) developed, whereby a rule of law, whether based on custom or on being recognized by the courts and thereby applied to the solution of a case, formed a precedent that should be followed in all similar cases thereafter unless subsequently deemed absurd or unjust or unless repealed by the legislature. As summarized by Kent[27]:

A solemn decision upon a point of law arising in any given case becomes an authority in a like case, because it is the highest evidence which we can have of the law applicable to the subject and the judges are bound to follow that decision unless it can be shown that the law was misunderstood or misapplied in that particular case. If a decision has been made on solemn argument and mature deliberation the presumption is in favor of its correctness; and the community has a right to regard it as a just declaration or exposition of the law, and to regulate their actions and contracts by it. It would, therefore, be extremely inconvenient to the public, if precedents were not duly regarded and implicitly followed.

The American colonies, having been settled primarily by people of Anglo-Saxon origin, had as their original legal basis the written law existing in England at the time of their migration plus the vast volume of common law that had evolved in England up to that time. It naturally followed that there was superimposed on this an additional and ever-increasing amount of common law based on the social customs that evolved on the new continent. For example, the law governing the state of Indiana consists of the following:

FIRST. The Constitution of the United States and of this state.

SECOND. All statutes of the general assembly of the state in force, and not inconsistent with such constitutions.

THIRD. All statutes of the United States in force, and relating to subjects over which congress has power to legislate for the states, and not inconsistent with the Constitution of the United States.

FOURTH. The common law of England, and statutes of the British Parliament made in aid thereof prior to the 4th year of the reign of James I (except the second section of sixth chapter of 43rd Elizabeth, the eighth chapter of 13th Elizabeth, and the ninth chapter of 37th Henry VIII) and which are of a general nature, not local to that kingdom and not inconsistent with the first, second and third specifications of this section.*

Added to this is all the common law evolved in Indiana since the inception of its statehood. Statements similar to this are to be found in the constitutions or statutes of each of the American states with the exception of Louisiana, for which the Napoleonic Code provides the legal base.

Equity or chancery

Up to the time of William the Conqueror (AD 1066) the administration of justice was limited to the application of existing laws. However, William the Conqueror assumed the doctrine that the sovereign was the ultimate source of all justice and that he himself was above the law. Hence the well-known saying, "The king can do no wrong," developed. Therefore he and the English rulers who followed him for a considerable period dispensed justice as they considered desirable or expeditious.

Thus if some wrong were committed for which the law offered no true remedy or if the plaintiff believed that the law had not given him complete justice, the king could be appealed to for assistance beyond the power of the courts. As common law courts came to depend more and more on precedents as guides in their dispensing of justice, they became more and more rigid. Accordingly the king was appealed to with increasing frequency, so much so that the king's chancellor, who was other-

*Section 1-101 (244) Burns Indiana Statutes Annotated 1933.

wise spoken of as the "keeper of the king's conscience," was made responsible. This was eventually followed by the establishment of separate courts of chancery or equity, the essential purpose of which was to render as complete justice and restitution as possible, going beyond the dictates of existing laws if necessary. As time went on, such courts became strictly limited to situations for which no adequate remedy or solution was offered by the regular law courts. Eventually, however, as chancellors and their courts rendered more and more decisions and judgments, they too, as a matter of course, became more or less bound by precedents, sometimes defeating the original purpose of their existence.

This system of equity as a supplement to the written and common law was also brought to America and established as a part of its legal structure. Separate chancery or equity courts still exist in a few states along the eastern seaboard and in the Southeast. Otherwise, for practical purposes the same court now sits as a court of law, dispensing strictly legal judgments, and again as a court of equity, administering relief in cases for which the law as it exists offers no remedy. Equity serves as the basis for the proper administration of justice in many cases of public health concern, reference to a few examples of which will be made.

Certain principles have been laid down to define the natural sphere of interest and applicability of equity. They may be summarized as follows:

Equity will not suffer a wrong without a remedy. This is very fundamental, considering the reason for the development of equity.

Equity delights to do justice and not by halves. Thus it is the intention of equity that all interested parties be present in court and that there be rendered a complete judgment adjusting all rights for the plaintiff and preventing future litigation. An example of this is presented by a case* questioning an amendment to a Wisconsin statute relating to the licensing of restaurants. A subsection had been added providing that no permit should be issued to operate or maintain any food-serving business where any other type of business was conducted unless the facilities dealing with the preparation and serving of food were separated from such other business by substantial partitions extending from the floor to the ceiling and with self-closing doors. The provisions of the sub-

section were applicable only to restaurants commencing business after the effective date of the subsection. In a mandamus proceeding in which it was sought to compel the state board of health to grant a permit to conduct a restaurant, the complainant contended that the added subsection was void under the federal and state constitutions in that it denied due process and equality before the law. The basis for licensing the business involved, said the court, was for the protection of the public health and safety. "If protection of the public health and safety requires partitions in case of a business subsequently to be commenced, then by the same token it requires them in case of existing businesses; and if one operating an existing restaurant is not required to maintain the partition, and one about to establish a restaurant is required to maintain one, then manifestly the latter is denied equal protection with the former." On this basis the supreme court sustained the contention of the complainant, declared the amending subsection void but allowed the existing statute to remain in force, and instructed the board of health to grant the requested permit, thereby adjusting all rights and preventing future litigation.

Equity acts in personam. A law court may merely render a judgment against a person's property rather than against the person himself. For example, the court may command a sheriff to seize and sell enough of the unsuccessful defendant's goods and turn over to the plaintiff sufficient proceeds to meet the money judgment of the court. Equity, on the other hand, commands an individual to perform or to refrain from performing whatever acts constitute the subject of the litigation. Such an action by a court of equity is known as injunction. Failure to obey the command of the court places the defendant in contempt of court and, thereby, subject to personal punishment. Thus if the sewage from the premises of one householder gives rise to an intolerable situation on the property of another, the ordinary court of law can merely render a judgment for money damages in favor of the offended property owner. This, however, does not solve the problem, since the original nuisance still exists. In equity, however, not only may there be rendered a judgment of cash restitution for damages already done but, in addition, the court may issue an injunction directing the person responsible to abate and prevent the nuisance from recurring in the future.

Equity regards the intention rather than form. This constitutes a weapon against legal decision. Law concerns itself with a strict interpretation of a form of a law transaction, or contract, but equity considers also the intent. This is illustrated by a case* involving the question of whether common-law marriages, which do not necessi-

*Wisconsin Supreme Court: State ex rel. F.W. Woolworth Co. v. Wisconsin State Board of Health et al., 298 N.W. 183 (1941).

*Superior Court of the State of Pennsylvania: Fisher v. Sweet and McClain et al., 35A 2nd 756 (1944).

tate a license, were included under a state law requiring premarital examinations as a prerequisite for marriage licenses. The superior court said that the act was clearly a public health measure designed to assist in the eradication of syphilis, to prevent transmission by a diseased spouse, and to prevent the birth of children with syphilitic weaknesses or deformities and should be construed so as to effectuate its purpose if at all possible. "Certainly," said the court, "the legislature never intended that such an important hygienic statute could be circumvented by the simple device of the parties entering into a common-law marriage without first obtaining a license."

Equity regards that as done which ought to be done. If a contract is broken, the court of law may render a money judgment for damages, whereas equity orders or commands (mandamus) that the contract be specifically performed. This is illustrated by the previously cited case of F.W. Woolworth Company v. Wisconsin State Board of Health et al.

Equity recognizes an intention to fulfill an obligation. If an individual promises or contracts to do a thing or if he has done anything that might be regarded as at least a partial fulfillment of the promise or contract, equity assumes that he intends to do it until the contrary is shown. This has sometimes served as a stumbling block to public health officials. For example, a person maintaining a public health nuisance may necessitate numerous fruitless visits and inspections on the part of public health workers. Finally, as a means of last resort the wrongdoer may be brought to court. If he can demonstrate to the satisfaction of the court that in some although inadequate manner he has followed the suggestions or commands of the public health official, the court may dismiss the case, saying in effect: "Why do you bring this man to court when he is taking steps to meet your requirements?"

Equity follows the law. In accordance with this maxim an equity court will observe existing laws and legal procedures, insofar as possible, without hindering its own function in the administration of justice.

Where there is equal equity, the law must prevail. If both parties to the litigation are judged to have equal rights, the case will be sent back to the law courts where the party with a right in law will have that right enforced.

The logic of this and the previous principle is obvious, considering the purpose for which equity was established. Equity is an adjunct to law, not a substitute for it.

He who comes into equity must do so with clean hands. If an individual claims a wrong, he himself must be free from a related wrong or the equity court will not listen to him. This was a factor in the well-known Chicago drainage canal case,* in which a court of equity refused a judgment against the city of Chicago for the city of St.

*Missouri v. Illinois, 180 U.S. 208, 2 S. Ct. 331, 45 L. Ed. 497 (1901).

Louis, partly on the basis that St. Louis itself contaminated its own public source of water.

He who seeks equity must do equity. This is similar to the previous principle in that not only must the plaintiff have clean hands but he must be and have been willing to do all that is right and fair as a part of a transaction or a judgment.

Equity aids the vigilant, not the indolent. This is known as the doctrine of laches and calls into effect the statue of limitations that fixes definite intervals within which legal action may be instituted after the cause for action has occurred or becomes complete. These time intervals are not the same for all actions and vary further among the states. If a person wishes to receive relief from an equity court, he must be prompt in applying to it. In other words he must not "sleep on his rights."

Administrative law

In the statutory legislation of an earlier day dealing with comparatively simple social and economic structures, the understandable attempt was usually made to include in the written statutes considerable detail with reference to the problem at hand. However, in more recent times, with the accelerating complexity of the social and economic systems and with ever increasing knowledge in all fields, it has become obviously impossible to include within the statutes sufficient detail to cover adequately all of the situations that might arise in the practical application of the true intent of the law. At the same time, United States governmental structure has become more and more complicated and has had more and more demands placed on it in the form of public services and regulatory functions previously unanticipated. The relative recency of the modern public health program provides a good example of this. To meet the situation, a considerable and increasing number of administrative agencies have been established by government, on a statutory basis, set up for the purpose of putting into effect the intent of legislation.

The procedure of passing enabling legislation written in more or less general terms was evolved. Such legislation includes clauses delegating administration and enforcement to a new or existing administrative agency, giving the agency the power and responsibility to formulate whatever rules, regulations, and standards where necessary for carrying out the purpose of the law. It naturally follows that such powers and responsibilities must be in conformity with all existing laws of the community, the state, and the nation. Thus although the legislative branch of government is the only body that may actually formulate and enact a law and although this power cannot itself be delegated, the legislature may delegate the power to make whatever rules and regulations are necessary to carry out the intent of the law. (In some states even administrative rules and regulations must be reviewed and approved by the state attorney general.) All such administrative rules and regulations, when properly formulated and when not in conflict with existing laws of the state and nation, have all the force and effect of law, even though they arise from an administrative agency and not from the legislature itself. However, their interpretation by the courts tends to be somewhat more rigid than the interpretation placed on the enactments of the legislature itself.

CLASSIFICATION OF LAW

For purposes of consolidation, a few words on the classification of law may be appropriate. Perhaps the simplest method of classifying laws is (1) by origin and (2) by application.

From the point of view of origin, law may be classified as follows:

Constitutional law—law developed by specially designated bodies or legislatures convened for the purpose of framing or amending a constitution

Statutory law—legislation that may arise from either representative assemblies or by the process of initiative and referendum

Decree or administrative law—rules, regulations, standards, orders, etc., issued by executive or administrative boards or officers within the sphere of their legal competence and responsibility to carry out the intent of statutory laws

Common law and equity—decisions made by courts in specific cases

Another approach classifies law into (1) *substantive law,* which provides the rules and requirements of conduct; (2) *procedural law,* which tells how to bring a lawsuit and how to prosecute; and (3) *remedial law,* or law of sanctions, which tells what remedies are available for breaches of the law.

From the point of view of application, law may be classified as follows:

Public law—law concerned with the establishment, maintenance, and operation of government; the definition, relationships, and regulation of its various branches; and the relationship of the individual or of groups to the state

1. *Constitutional law*—deals with the basic nature, structure, and function of the state in relation to the

powers of the various branches of government; sometimes includes a bill of rights
2. *Administrative law*—as discussed previously
3. *Criminal law*—concerned with offenses or acts against the public welfare and safety, such being considered as offenses against the state and varying from petty offenses and misdemeanors to felonies

Private law—law concerned with the rights and duties of individuals and groups in relation to each other; originally based largely on common law but increasingly becoming subject to statutes

COURTS

American government is based on the wise principle of the separation of powers. Accordingly, legislation can be formulated, considered, and ultimately enacted only by the legislative branch. After its enactment the legislature has no further concern with a law except for the possibility of subsequent amendment or repeal. On passage, a law is referred to the executive branch of government for its administration and enforcement. However, the constitutionality of the law and the manner of its enforcement are subject to review at any time on the initiative of the citizenry by the third or judicial branch of government, which is manifest by the actions of the courts. It is the duty of the courts to pass on the constitutionality of laws, to interpret them in the interest of justice and the public good, and to determine their validity whenever controversies related to them are brought before the court in the proper manner.

The jurisdiction of the court may be either original or appellate; that is, the courts may be a place where the merits of a controversy are originally passed on, or they may be a place to which an unsuccessful and dissatisfied litigant may appeal for a review of the action taken by a court of original jurisdiction. Using the judicial system of the states as a point of departure, their courts may be divided into three categories. At the top are the superior courts, including the state supreme court, the superior court, the court of appeal, or the court of civil appeals. Such courts usually have five to nine justices who hear appeal cases from the lower courts of the state and who have in some instances varying amounts of original jurisdiction. Appeals may be taken from here to the Supreme Court of the United States if the case involves the federal Constitution, federal laws, or treaties. Below the state superior courts are the intermediate courts, including the circuit courts, the district courts, the county courts, and the common pleas courts, the terminology differing in different states. These are courts of original jurisdiction and the first two hear appeals from lower courts in some states. In other states these functions are separated. It is to be noted that a county court, although locally elected and locally responsible for the administration of its verdicts, is actually part of the state judicial system. On the lowest or most local level are the locally elected justices of the peace, who in effect individually constitute the lowest rung on the state judicial ladder.

In addition, a state may set up certain special courts to deal with particular social problems such as juvenile delinquency, domestic relations, and industrial relations. On the municipal level of government, by virtue of a charter granted by the state government, an urban community may have the privilege of setting up certain courts of its own to administer justice in cases involving problems of concern limited to the municipality itself. Thus there are police courts with original jurisdiction in minor matters and municipal courts with original jurisdiction in more important cases; these municipal courts also serve as a place of appeal from the police court.

On the federal level is the Supreme Court of the United States, consisting of a chief justice and eight associates, to which cases may be appealed from the lower federal courts and state supreme courts in instances where the federal Constitution, laws, or treaties are considered to be involved. In addition, it has some original jurisdiction in interstate, maritime, and some other matters (see Article III, section 2, of the Constitution and the Eleventh Amendment). To expedite the federal judicial system, a number of intermediate courts have been established. Thus there are 10 federal circuit courts with appellate jurisdiction and below them over 90 federal district courts, which are the principal federal courts of original jursidiction. There are, in addition, federal courts for special purposes, such as the Customs Courts and the Federal Court of Claims. There might also be mentioned the increasing number of federal administrative boards, for example, the National Labor Relations Board, which have a certain amount of delegated original jurisdiction.

SOURCES OF PUBLIC HEALTH POWERS

Public health law may be defined as that body of statutes, regulations, and precedents that has for its purpose the protection and promotion of individual and community health. Although the term *public health* was not entirely unknown to contemporaries of the authors of the American Constitution, its present-day scope and significance were not conceived of. After all, there was no public health profession in existence, and science was not to enter the golden era of bacteriology until about 100 years later. Three quarters of a century were to pass before the need for establishment of the first state health department was to be felt. Still 40 years more were to pass before the formation of the first county health department. The founders of the United States cannot be censured, therefore, for not considering public health functions specifically in their organization of the new government. They were so remarkably astute and farsighted, however, as to provide for future developments in many fields by the use of certain broad and general phrases that in subsequent periods were to make possible broad interpretations of the Constitution, thereby allowing the introduction and inclusion of certain public health activities in the functions of the federal government.

By far the most important of these broad phrases is that occurring in the Preamble to the Constitution, which includes among the fundamental purposes of the government the intent to "promote the general welfare." This recurs in section 8 of Article I, which, dealing with the functions of Congress, gives it power "to lay and collect taxes . . . and provide for the common defense and general welfare. . . ." It is the generous interpretation of this by the Supreme Court that made possible the activity of the Children's Bureau in maternal and child health and the subsidization by means of federal grants-in-aid of state and local health programs by the Public Health Service. In fact, these and many other federal agencies owe their existence in large part to the intent that has been read into the "general welfare" phrase.

In addition, the varied and widespread activities of the federal government in fields relating to health have as their legal basis the manner in which numerous other clauses of the Constitution have been

interpreted. Thus the direction to Congress "to regulate commerce with foreign nations, and among
the several states, and with the Indian tribes" has
been construed to include such matters as international and interstate quarantine, sanitary supervision, vital statistics, and direct responsibility for
the health of the American Indians. The provision
for the establishment of "post offices and post
roads" has led to the right of the federal government
to bar from the mails material deleterious to the
public health. The power "to raise and support
armies" and to "provide and maintain a navy" logically placed responsibility for the health of the
armed forces (in recent years a not inconsiderable
fraction of the population) in the hands of federal
agencies. Complete and exclusive jurisdiction over
the inhabitants of the seat of the national government (the District of Columbia) is also specified.

The reader may be reminded at this point that
the United States, far from being one nation, is in
a true sense a federation of 50 separate nations,
called states, each with its own history, economic
and social problems, and still somewhat jealously
guarded intrastate interests. It will be recalled that
the members of the constitutional convention carefully guarded the rights of their respective states,
jointly turning over to the newly formed federal
government only such powers and activities as they
considered desirable and necessary for the common
welfare and survival of all. Matters that they could
adequately handle as individual states were retained by the states. Therefore the federal government truly was and is a creature of jointly concurred
action of the several states. Since the beginning it
has been inferred that all matters not specifically
mentioned in the Constitution and its subsequent
Amendments were questions to be dealt with primarily by the states. It is for this reason that the
more complete and coordinated organization of
public health activities is found on the state and
local levels. Each state has developed its own characteristic body of legislation and judicial interpretation as well as its own type of plan and organization for the implementation of its public health
laws.[28] Indeed, each state may do as much or as
little as it wishes within the limits imposed by national interest.

Although there are 50 differing sets of public
health laws and organizations, certain fundamental
legal principles are involved in all. A brief discussion of some of these fundamentals is necessary for

further consideration of sources of public health
powers.

Eminent domain

The first of the basic powers of a state is that of
eminent domain, sometimes referred to as the power of condemnation. This is the power or right of a
sovereign state to summarily appropriate an individual's property or to limit the individual's use of
it if the best interest of the community makes such
action desirable. In so doing, however, the state
must provide an equitable compensation. In effect
the state has the right to demand the sale or limitation of use of private property. The distinction
between the exercise of the power of eminent domain and actions on which legislatures may insist
without compensation is not clear-cut at any given
time and varies from time to time. The history of
zoning measures to control the height of buildings
has been cited as a good example of this. At first
the state attempted to control the height of buildings by purchasing from individuals their primary
right to build on their own property above the height
that was considered most desirable from the community standpoint. Since this action was upheld in
the courts, it was resorted to by more and more
people in more and more communities until it got
to the point where, as Ascher[29] aptly stated, it re-
sembled the economy of the mythical village of Bal-
lycannon, where everyone made his living by taking
in his next-door neighbor's washing. In other
words, when resorted to on a wide scale, use of the
power of eminent domain amounts to individuals'
(as taxpayers) purchasing the exercise of a right
from themselves as private citizens. Inevitably,
such a procedure becomes ineffective as a measure
of control. Recognizing this, the public through its
legislatures may finally say, "We shall forbid this
particular action or use by the individual," and the
courts more often than not will uphold the action.

In a certain sense, the procedure followed by
some health departments in the past of paying an
allotment to chronic carriers of typhoid bacilli to
make sure of their refraining from engaging in food-
handling occupations represented the purchase by
the state of an individual's primary right. The states
in most instances finally simply forbade such activity by these persons.

As pointed out by Ascher, it is interesting to note that those who attempted to bring about a form of building control that eliminated the necessity of compensation deliberately avoided a test case for about 10 years. Finally, when the Ambler Realty Company protested the restrictions of its use of land by the village of Euclid,* the U.S. Supreme Court upheld this arbitrary use of the police power in a sweeping opinion that had as one of its basic contentions that over 900 cities were already subject to zoning and about one half of the urban dwellers of the nation lived under the benefits of zoning procedures. This is perhaps another way of saying that within a relatively short period of time the social concept of zoning had become part of the custom of American communities and that its requirement could be considered as having become part of the common law.

Laws of nuisances (noscitur ad sociis)

Long before the United States and its government were conceived, the concept was developed by medieval legal theorists that whereas "a man's home is his castle," an individual's use of his private property could be detrimental to others. The use of private property is unrestricted only as long as it does not injure another's person or property. If this occurred, a nuisance was considered to exist, and the individual whose person or property was injured could seek assistance from the courts. Innumerable examples of this exist in the field of public health, especially with regard to the salubrity of the physical environment. For example, an individual property owner has the right to dispose of his sewage in any manner that he may see fit, provided that it cannot actually or potentially affect another. If he allows raw sewage to flow onto the land of another, a social injustice has obviously occurred, and the health and well-being of others have been placed in jeopardy. Legal relief against nuisances may be obtained in the courts by means of (1) a suit of law for damages resulting and/or (2) a suit in equity to forbid or abate the nuisance.

It is perhaps unfortunate that a large proportion of public health officials still consider the use of the law of nuisances as one of their most important if not their chief legal recourse. The pursuit of this point of view eventually leads to many difficulties and dissatisfactions, since the law of nuisances is subject to increasing limitations.

In the first place, there are many things or uses of things that do not intrinsically constitute a nuisance but are merely in the wrong place. An example of this is provided by the case of Benton et al. v. Pittard, Health Commissioner, et al.,* in which the plaintiff protested the establishment and operation by a health department of a venereal disease clinic in a residential district. The complaints were that the disease of the patients who would congregate in the neighborhood "were not only communicable but were offensive, obnoxious and disgusting; that the clinic operation would be offensive to the petitioners and that their sensibility would be injured; and that their dwelling would be rendered less valuable as a home and place of residence." The defending health officer and county commissioner filed an answer and a general demurrer, a form of pleading that although admitting all the facts, challenged their legal sufficiency to constitute a cause of action. The judge, after hearing both sides, denied the plaintiff's request for an injunction and sustained the demurrer. On being appealed, however, the Georgia Supreme Court stated that the fact that the clinic was to be operated as a public institution would not alone prevent it from becoming a nuisance if located in a residential section and that the statutory provision requiring the care of venereally infected persons did not imply the right to perform such care in any location. "In other words, a nuisance may consist merely of the right thing in the wrong place regardless of other circumstances." On this basis the judgment of the original trial court was reversed.

Another factor tending to limit the value of the law of nuisances is that a great many of the legal doctrines and decisions dealing with nuisances and their abatement were developed before the germ theory of disease became established scientific fact. During most of its development, no obvious factual or scientific data existed on which to base conclusions, and those appearing in court in such cases were merely pitting their opinions against the opinions of others. This left the court as its only final recourse the expression of its own opinion. As a result, a mass of unsound and unscientific deci-

*Village of Euclid v. Ambler Realty Co., 272 U.S. 365 (1926).

*Georgia Supreme Court: Benton et al. v. Pittard, Health Commissioner, et al. 31 S.E. 2nd 6.

sions has been built up, which because they are precedents, continue to influence the public health problems of present-day communities. This also partly explains why many supposedly modern health departments are required to expend much time, energy, and funds in activities that have little relationship to public health, for example, garbage and refuse control.

Still another difficulty is caused by the fact that recourse to the law of nuisances does not overcome one of the rules of law. Decision by a law court that a nuisance exists may result in damages being paid to the plaintiff but does not necessarily effect the solution or abatement of the noisome circumstances. There is, of course, the possibility of resorting to a court of equity with the hope of obtaining complete justice. However, here again it is found that a rule of equity may provide a way out for the defendant in that if he can demonstrate to the court's satisfaction his intention or, better yet, partial action to abate the nuisance, the case in all probability will be dismissed from court. The thought might arise that the situation could be improved by trying to bring about more up-to-date judicial interpretations and judgments regarding nuisances. Although theoretically possible, the task involved to accomplish this would be enormous. Furthermore, even if modern present-day standards could be made the basis of definition, these standards and definitions might become outmoded with the passage of time.

Police power[30]

There remains another means of legal recourse for the public health official to consider, that is, the police power that the sovereign state possesses. As a matter of fact, public health law owes its true origin and only real effectiveness to this inherent right of the state. Police power originated in the so-called law of overruling necessity, which claims that in times of stress such as fire and pestilence, the private property of an individual might be summarily appropriated, used, or even destroyed if the ultimate relief, protection, or safety of the group indicated such action as necessary. Through time this concept expanded to include even activities designed for the prevention of causes of social stress. The U.S. Supreme Court has on numerous occasions not only upheld the principle of the police power of the state but also has defined its scope in sweeping terms to include, as did Chief Justice Marshall, all types of public health laws and to ac-

knowledge the power of the states to provide for the health of their citizens.* It should be noted, however, as Justice Brown stated, that ". . . its [legislature's] determination as to what is a proper exercise of its police powers is not final or conclusive but is subject to the supervision of the court."†

One of the best definitions of the police power was given in the case of Miami County v. Dayton,‡ in which the court defined it as "that inherent sovereignty which the government exercises whenever regulations are demanded by public policy for the benefit of the society at large in order to guard its morals, safety, health, order and the like in accordance with the needs of civilization."

Although the possession of police power is fundamentally that of the sovereign state, the legislature of the state may for practical purposes delegate it to an administrative agency acting as its functional agent. The use of the police power is not a matter of choice when it has been delegated to a governmental agency. The agency has a definite and legal responsibility to use it, but *is accountable for the manner in which it is used*. When the means for action are made available, the public officer responsible may be compelled to exercise the police power delegated to him if the public interest indicates such action. Failure to do so makes the public official guilty of malfeasance of office. However, although application of the police power may be indicated and demanded, the manner in which it is employed is usually left to the discretion of the administrative officer; that is, the public officer may select methods of enforcement, formulating rules, regulations, and standards as he deems necessary unless the statutes that made him responsible specifically prescribe the method of procedure.

An important case§ in point was the decision of the U.S. Supreme Court in 1978 to uphold the decisions of a series of lower courts that the searches and inspections of business premises by inspectors of the Occupational Safety and Health Administration without warrants was a violation of the Fourth Amendment of the Bill of Rights. This is of signif-

---

*Perhaps the best known case is Gibbons v. Ogden, 9 Wheat. 1, 6 L. Ed. 23 (1824).
†Lawton v. Steele, 152 U.S. 133 (1893).
‡Miami County v. Dayton, 92 O. S. 215.
§Marshall v. Barlow's Inc.

icance to public health workers. As Curran[31] comments,

Most lawyers familiar with the case law of the Supreme Court in the past two decades would have thought that the type of warrantless inspections in OSHA were of doubtful constitutionality. However, legislative draftsmen do not always follow such guidelines when the overall objectives of the inspection program are believed to be right and proper and where such inspections are thought "necessary" to the regulatory scheme of the legislation. There is also a practical assumption that most people will allow the inspections anyway, either because they wish to cooperate with the program in the best interests of safety and health, or because they think the inspector "must have" a legal right to enter. All sorts of federal and state laws have granted inspection authority to firefighters, health inspectors, mine-safety officials, and many others, all essentially on these grounds.

The position of a public health officer as related to the summary abatement of a nuisance, was well stated by the Iowa Supreme Court in a case* involving such action by a health department in enforcing an ordinance dealing with the improper and indiscriminate dumping of garbage. In upholding the action of the board of health, the court stated that although nothing in the statute granted to the officers immunity from the consequences of unfair or oppressive acts, "the particular form of procedure prescribed may vary from the customary procedure, but essential rights are not violated by granting to the board the right, in an emergency, to proceed in the abatement of a nuisance detrimental to public health, and it is safe to say that most cases calling for action on the part of boards of health are matters requiring immediate action." Of perhaps greater significance, the court went on to say that even though the courts had not been uniform in their holdings, it believed that the weight of authority as well as reason and necessity prescribed that in cases involving the public health, in which prompt and efficient action was necessary, the state and its officers should not be subjected to the inevitable delays incident to a complete hearing before action could be taken.

The careful distinction between the power of inspection and the right of privacy has become in-creasingly important as a result of a ruling of the California District Court of Appeals.* The court held that the entry by a health inspector into a private residence for the purpose of a routine housing inspection at a reasonable time and on presentation of proper credentials was not a violation of the Fourth or Fourteenth Amendments of the United States Constitution. "The court reasoned that the ordinance in question was part of a general regulatory scheme which was civil in nature, limited in scope, and could not be exercised except under reasonable conditions." The court then defined the conditions in which privacy may be restrained. "In those areas of exercise of the police power where the chance of immediate tangible harm is present, such as in premises which might present fire or communicable disease hazards, the right of privacy most probably will be accorded only that constitutional protection that is given to property or economic rights. In intimate or personal activities not at all likely to cause immediate danger to life or limb, the right of privacy will approach the more protected constitutional position of freedom of expression."[32]

On appeal, however, the Supreme Court† held that administrative searches for housing violations are significant intrusions on the privacy and security of individuals—interests that are protected by the Fourth Amendment against arbitrary invasions by government officials and enforceable against the states under the Fourteenth Amendment. The court declared that such searches when authorized and conducted without a warrant procedure lack the traditional safeguards that the Fourth Amendment guarantees to the individual. This is true, the court added, whether the discovery of a violation on the initial inspection leads to a criminal conviction or results only in an administrative compliance order.

The court noted the following three significant reservations to its general holdings:

1. Nothing in the opinion is intended to foreclose prompt inspections, even without a warrant, that the law has traditionally upheld in emergency situations.

2. In the light of the Fourth Amendment's requirement that a warrant specify the property to be searched, "It seems likely that warrants should normally be sought only after entry is refused, unless

---

*Iowa Supreme Court: State v. Strayer, 299 N.W. 912 (1941).

*Camara vs. San Francisco, 277 A.C.A. 136 (1965).
†87 S. Ct. 1727 p. 1734 ff (1967).

there has been a citizen complaint or there is other satisfactory reason for securing immediate entry."

3. ". . . The requirement of a warrant procedure does not suggest any change in what seems to be the prevailing local policy in most situations, of authorizing entry, but not entry by force, to inspect."[33]

The right of a legislature to delegate rule-making power to an administrative agency has been questioned many times, but only in one instance has such power been denied to a state or local board of health. This occurred in Wisconsin,* where it was held that the State Board of Health was simply an administrative agency and that no rule-making powers could constitutionally be delegated to it. On the other hand, the Ohio Supreme Court stated that "the legislature in the exercise of its constitutional authority may lawfully confer on boards of health the power to enact sanitary ordinances having the force of law within the district over which their jurisdiction extends, is not an open question,"† The question was more or less settled by the United States Supreme Court, which held the following:

(1) That a State may, consistent with the Federal Constitution, delegate to a municipality authority to determine under what conditions health shall become operative.

(2) That the municipality may vest in its efficiency broad discretion in matters affecting the applicability and enforcement of a health law.

(3) That in the exercise of the police power reasonable classification may be freely applied and that regulation is not violative of the equal protection clause merely because it is not all-embracing.‡

It is obvious and logical that a municipality or an administrative agency in dealing with questions concerning the public health, for example, can act only when it has been given specific authority for such actions and that the ordinances adopted by the legislative body of the municipality must not only be limited to the subject matter of the power delegated but also must not conflict with or attempt to set aside any provision of the Constitution, of the state law, or of any other sanitary regulations of the state. The same conditions apply to regulations adopted by local boards of health. They can apply only where the subject matter has been placed by law under the jurisdiction of the local board of health.

*State v. Burdge, 95, Wis. 390, 70 N.W. 347 (1897).
†Exparte Co. 106 O.S. 50.
‡Zucht v. King, 260 U.S. 174, 43 S. Ct. (1922).

Police power, administrative law, and judicial presumption

The delegation to administrative agencies and officers of the right and power to formulate rules, regulations, and standards to implement the intent of legislation has given rise to a relatively new and increasingly important branch of law and source of enforcement powers. It is unfortunate that in the public health profession there are still many who do not adequately realize the great administrative possibilities presented by sound administrative law.[34] There are many communities that although sometimes possessing adequate enabling legislation for various public health activities, have only limited control because of the failure of their health officials to make the rules, regulations, and standards necessary for the proper and adequate implementation of the statutes. Failing to establish a solid legal background based as much as possible on sound scientific criteria and standards places the public health official, the department, and the community at an unnecessary and unwarranted disadvantage.

Even if existing legislation is adequate, something more is needed. The health official must "do his homework" thoroughly. As Grad[8] has indicated, "cases, particularly those to enforce environmental health regulations, are won or lost long before they get into court." Samples must be collected, labeled, analyzed, dated, and recorded properly, legally, and accurately. Photographs and depositions should be obtained if pertinent and helpful. Witnesses should be found, and *facts* must be arranged and presented in a clear and orderly manner. In the discussion of the law of nuisances, mention was made of the undesirable possibility of the public health official being in the position of pitting mere opinion against that of the defendant. The court's only alternative in such a situation would be to express its own opinion regarding the desirability of the action rather than its legality. Ideally it is only the latter with which the courts are essentially concerned, and as much as possible it is preferable that they not have to make decisions regarding the sense or desirability of an action.

When a scientist, a health officer, or another expert is in a position to provide the court with definite regulations and standards based on scientific criteria or group judgment, especially if they have been drawn up with the idea of administering legal advice, the judge of the court is no longer in the somewhat embarrassing position of having to balance what amounts to the personal opinion of the plaintiff against that of the defendant and then being forced to make a decision by expressing a personal opinion. The very existance of sound rules, regulations, and standards serves to pass the burden of proof from the administrative agent to the defendant in the case so that the judge can avoid conflict and save time and face by saying, for example, that the defendant has not presented evidence to show that the health officer did not fairly apply the rules, regulations, or standards that by virtue of their development are more or less accepted without question. Thus there has been established what is termed a *judicial presumption* in favor of the findings, conclusions, and recommendations of the enforcing administrative official.

To obtain the maximum amount of judicial presumption, certain conditions are desirable and should be borne in mind. First, laws and ordinances should contain only broad principles, delegating authority to the enforcing or administrative agency for the development of the necessary details. Second, such rules, regulations, and standards as may be indicated by the law or ordinance should be carefully formulated. Third, they should be based as much as possible on accepted scientific facts or authoritative group judgments. Fourth, it is desirable that they be written with the aid of an administrative lawyer. Fifth, advantage should be taken of the opportunity presented in the process of making the rules, regulations, and standards to lay the foundation for their ready acceptance by the public and the courts of the community. This is meant to imply that the process presents an important opportunity for education and persuasion as well as democratic participation. If those who are to be affected are consulted in the writing of a regulation, they will develop in the process an understanding that is a first step toward voluntary cooperation, acceptance, and self-enforcement. At the same time, the public health administrator is provided with an invaluable opportunity to determine in advance how far the community is willing to go.

Licensing

A related method of legal enforcement and control is found in the technique of licensing. The legality of the principle of licensing as a method of control and enforcement as well as a source of revenue to meet the cost of the administration of a law has been well established and accepted for a long while. However, intent and methods of licensing are constantly subject to questioning in the courts, as are all other methods of enforcement. Licenses may be granted or revoked under conditions imposed by public health authorities, provided that there is a statutory basis for the licensing and there is no oppressive, discriminatory, or arbitrary action involved in their application.

An example to illustrate the latter is that of a city board of health that voted that after a certain date no more milk distributor licenses would be granted to persons who were not residents of the city.* The plaintiff operated a well-qualified dairy 6 miles beyond the city limits and brought suit to compel the issuance of a license, charging that the regulation was discriminatory. The state law said, "Boards of health may grant licenses to sell milk to properly qualified persons." The court held that the word "may" in the state law should be construed as meaning "shall" so that a local board of health, existing by virtue of state law, had no alternative but to issue a license to any person who satisfied the sanitary requirements. More pertinent to the question at hand, it further held that the limitation on nonresidents was unreasonable and arbitrary and that if it had been included in a law instead of a resolution, it would have been ruled unconstitutional.

On several occasions, licensing has been found useful by health authorities in accomplishing a certain amount of indirect control and prevention of problems not obvious from the primary purpose of the licensing. Several communities, for instance, have found it necessary to institute the licensing of individuals engaged in certain personal service occupations, such as masseurs and beauty parlor operators, in an attempt to stop advertising by prostitutes operating under the guise of these occupations. This particular use has caused no difficulty, since the right of health departments to maintain sanitary control over individuals engaged in personal services to prevent the spread of communicable diseases has been well established.

However, when an ordinance requiring permits or licenses can be shown to have no public health basis, it will probably be considered an infringement of personal rights by the court and declared

*Whitney v. Watson, 85 N.H. 238, 157 A. 78 (1931).

invalid. This is illustrated by the case* of a city board of health that passed a regulation providing that no person should engage in the business of undertaking unless duly licensed as an embalmer by the board of health. The Massachusetts Supreme Court held the regulation unconstitutional and invalid, saying, "We can see no such connection between requiring all undertakers to be licensed embalmers and the promotion of the public health as to bring the making of this regulation by the board of registration in embalming or the refusal of a license by the board of health on account of the regulation within the exercise of the police power of the state."

NECESSITY OF BASIC PUBLIC HEALTH LAWS

In a DeLamar lecture given in 1920, Freeman,[35] who was at that time Commissioner of Health of Ohio, said: "Every thoughtful sanitarian has in his mind the picture of that ideal system of health administration which would be founded on scientific principles, organized on the basis of administrative efficiency, and manned by a staff of trained workers filled with the spirit of public service. This ideal organization would have behind it a volume of law which, while fully recognizing the principles of individual liberty, would permit no man to offend against the health of his neighbor." Freeman added with considerable justification, "However thoughtfully a proposed measure may be prepared by its framers, it has by the time it is enacted into law usually been so altered by ill-considered, hasty or prejudiced amendment as to have lost all semblance of its original form." It is advantageous to consider some of the fields of public health activity in which fundamental legislation is desirable or necessary. The first of these is concerned with the registration or reporting of births and deaths. It is conceded by all to be well-nigh impossible to carry out a public health program in the absence of basic information concerning the circumstances surrounding birth and death. In most parts of the United States, it is the public health agency that is charged with the responsibility for assuring the collection of this information. To achieve this, it is necessary that each state have the appropriate legislation and administrative machinery to deal with mandatory reporting of these biologic events by those in the best position to submit such reports, the attendants at births and death.

Related to this is the need for legislation requiring the reporting and control of cases of certain types of illnesses, especially those of a communicable nature. To accomplish this adequately requires careful and exact definition of certain terms such as *cases*, *communicable*, and *isolation* and the listing of the morbid conditions to be included. In accord with what has been said elsewhere, such defining and listing is best accomplished by inclusion in the rules and regulations drawn up by the administrative agency rather than in the body of the statute, which should limit its concern to broad principles, responsibilities, and penalties. The desirability of this is particularly evident in light of the spectacular changes that have occurred in recent years in the areas of diagnosis, treatment, and social management of many of the communicable diseases. If details of reporting and control appear in the law, further scientific advances are certain to result in the necessity of either changing the law or allowing it to become hopelessly out of date.

In the field of food and milk control an enormous, confusing, and frequently contradictory mass of legislation and regulation exists. Undesirable as this situation is, all will agree that certain types of legal control are necessary. It is obviously important for a community to exercise some control over those who produce and handle its food and milk supplies.[36,37] This has been repeatedly upheld in the courts. With reference to milk, the Connecticut Supreme Court explained in an opinion: "The State may determine the standard of quality, prohibit the production, sale, or distribution of milk not within the standard, divide it into classes, and regulate the manner of their use, so long as these standards, classes, and regulatory provisions be neither unreasonable nor oppressive. The many recorded instances in which the courts have sustained this power of regulation bear witness to the liberality of their viewpoint where the public health and safety are concerned."* Judicial prejudice in favor of rules, regulations, and standards dealing with the sanitary quality of food and milk supplies has been extended far beyond the actual product itself. It has long been accepted as proper for the responsible health authority to formulate rules, regulations, and standards dealing with the sources of food and milk, the health and sanitation practices of all who come

*Wyeth v. Cambridge Board of Health, 200 Mass. 474, 86 N.E. 295 (1909).

*Shelton v. City of Shelton, 111 Conn. 433 (1930).

in contact with them, the sanitary facilities provided such persons, and the sanitary nature of all machinery, instruments, or utensils involved in their transfer from the source to the ultimate consumer.

In the field of general sanitation, including the sanitary problems involved in housing and industry as well as the supervision of water supplies, sewage disposal, and the like, basic legislation is necessary to place responsibility in the hands of the public health agency and to give it such powers as are needed to activate the intent of the law. Licensing of certain trades and occupations has been mentioned briefly. It is obvious that before such a procedure can be put into effect, the necessary legal justification must be brought into existence.

Perhaps the most fundamental of all such legislation is that enabling the establishment and development of local public health programs. Obviously, a local area, being ultimately subject to the state, should be granted the legal right to establish official activity dealing with the public health. The rapid expansion in recent years of local health work, especially on the county level, has developed increasing interest in the proper formulation of such enabling acts. In the first national conference on local health units held in 1946, Mustard[38] summarized the essentials that should be included in enabling legislation for local health work. These essentials are included here for their conciseness and inclusiveness and because they remain valid:

1. That this volume of law should provide assurance that there is a proper balance between local autonomy and state supervision.
2. That this volume of law should provide insurance that where a local unit of government is too small for effective public health administration, combinations of local jurisdictions may be made.
3. Insurance that health work locally will not be scattered among different elements of the local government.
4. Insurance that budgets for local health units be sufficient to meet at least a minimum in terms of funds, and to meet standards as to personnel.
5. No local jurisdiction will remain in want of health service, merely because of unfavorable financial position locally.
6. Supplementary to this insurance that even the poor areas will be included, there should be insurance that there will be adequate state aid.

7. Insurance that the whole state system of local health units will not be jeopardized by local option.

WRITING AND PASSAGE OF LAWS AND REGULATIONS

In a discussion of court actions. Tobey[39] stated:

These cases also demonstrate that the actions of public health authorities must be conducted in a strictly legal manner, with due guarantee of the constitutional rights of individual citizens and the people as a whole. If regulations or procedures are defective, the courts have no choice but to uphold the law as it should be, and this they will do despite their willingness to support all reasonable public health measures. Public health officials must bear in mind that prevention applies to law as well as to sanitary science, and they should see to it that legislation and law enforcement comply with adjudicated standards and modern jurisprudence.

Curran[40] also has expressed concern about the inadequate attention given to the development of regulations by public health workers. He pinpointed three areas of weakness in most health departments: (1) the departments' ongoing programs tend to operate ahead of the regulations; that is, the regulations have not yet caught up with what the department is actually doing; (2) the current regulations are too broadly worded to be used effectively; and (3) regulations are often based on model codes or the regulations of some other health department without sufficient regard for local conditions.

Many people complain about the terminology and complexity of laws and regulations and repeatedly call for simplification. On the other hand, as Curran[41,42] well points out, interpretation of the meaning of both common and technical terms is the source of much legal controversy. Exactly what is mean by *promptly, insanitary, filth, reasonable access,* and *informed consent?* Attempts to simplify the terminology in laws and regulations have an unfortunate tendency to magnify and multiply administrative difficulties and overload the courts with unnecessary litigation.

It might be well to consider briefly a few practical considerations with regard to the proper formulation of laws and regulations. Before doing so, it is worthwhile to repeat at least two important legislative handicaps to effective administration.[43] The first is that legislatures often attempt to do too much by writing into the law itself excessive detail with regard to administrative responsibilities, organization, itemized appropriations, and procedure. For example, in one state for many years the salaries of the state health officer and others were specifically limited in the state constitution; economic changes, competition for good administrative personnel, and progress in general were ignored.

The second legislative handicap is the sacrificing of long-term considerations to immediate, local, or personal advantage. There have been many examples of this in the field of public health. The logical solution to these handicaps may be found in the passage of legislation that considers general policy and leaves the details of procedure and operation to whatever administrative agency the legislature may see fit to hold responsible. This, of course, requires that administrative agencies assume their full responsibility in carrying out the intent of the statutes by adequately and effectively formulating and enforcing whatever rules, regulations, and standards are indicated.

Because of the number and significance of federal legislative actions, it is important that health personnel be familiar with the complicated process involved. The actual procedure followed in the enactment of legislation is essentially the same on the national and state levels of government. Basically there are 15 steps involved, but they really boil down to the following: (1) after a first and second reading by title, the bill is referred to a committee (or subcommittee), which may or may not hold hearings; (2) the bill is placed on the calendar of the entire chamber for a third reading and debate; (3) if passed, it then goes through the same process in the other chamber, and if passed there, it goes to the chief of state for signature. If he vetoes it, a two-thirds majority overrides the veto.[44] More specifically, on the federal level, a bill is born when it is introduced in either house by its congressional sponsors. Bills are assigned numbers in order of their introduction. Occasionally, identical bills are introduced in the Senate and House of Representatives; more frequently, many different bills are filed on any major issue. In both houses the bill is assigned to the committee having appropriate jurisdiction. There are now 22 standing committees in the House of Representatives and 20 in the Senate. Often, the bill is then referred to a subcommittee for special detailed study. It is in this phase that hearings are often held, and the original bill is often changed during "markup" or drafting sessions.

When the subcommittee completes action on the bill, it is referred back to the full committee, which must approve all recommendations and amendments before the bill can be "reported out" to the full House or Senate. If the committee does not report out the bill, the legislation is "killed." It goes no further in the legislative process unless by special petition of the full membership. Legislation can also be "bottled up" by committee chairmen who do not report the bill out of committee. Once reported out, a bill is placed on the legislative calendar in the Senate or on one of several calendars in the House of Representatives. In the House the bill then goes to the Rules Committee, where it is decided whether amendments will be permitted from the floor and the length of debate time is allocated. "Open rule" permits amendments from the floor; "closed rule" does not. The first House floor action is debate and vote on acceptance of the "rule" recommended by the Rules Committee, then on amendments, if an open rule is adopted. At this point the bill may be recommitted to committee for further study or voted on for final action. In the Senate there is no restriction on amendments, and debate time is unlimited unless there is a three-fifths cloture vote to cut it off.

When either chamber passes a bill, it must then be sent to the other chamber for acceptance, rejection, or alteration. If it is altered, the bill is sent to a "conference" committee, made up of senior members of the committees from both houses that worked on the legislation. Differences between the legislation passed by each chamber are ironed out in this committee. Occasionally they are unable to work out a compromise, and the measure dies.

If an acceptable agreement is reached, the revised bill is then sent to both chambers for final approval. If approved by both chambers, the new bill is sent to the White House for signing within 10 days. If the President does not act on the bill within 10 days, it automatically becomes law. However, if Congress adjourns before the 10-day limit expires, the President can "pocket veto" the bill by not signing it. Congress can override a Presidential veto with a two-thirds majority vote. If Congress does not override a veto, the bill is dead and the process must begin again with the introduction of new legislation.

Essentially the same sequence of steps is involved in the introduction, consideration, and passage of legislation on the state level, with the governor fulfilling the role played by the President on the federal level.

On the state and local levels, it has been customary in the United States for responsibility for the public health to be vested in a board of health that is directed to employ as its agent a health officer and whatever other personnel are needed to carry out its policies. It is much better that rules, regulations, and standards be passed by someone other than the enforcement officer. The public then believes that it is being treated more fairly and that the enforcement officer is not grinding his own axe. In turn the health officer is relieved of the onus of enforcing his own regulations and the risk of repeated personal liability. This alone presents an important justification for the interposing of boards of health between the legislative body and the functioning agency. With these words of introduction, the following suggestions are made concerning the formulation of rules and regulations by public health agencies:

1. First is the necessity that they be promulgated by a board of health or whatever other administrative agency in which this authority and responsibility is vested. Furthermore, the agency must have been properly created and legally existing in the eyes of the legislature. If any of its members have been improperly chosen, elected, or appointed, the entire board does not legally exist and all of its actions are considered invalid.

2. The actions of the board must arise by virtue of power and responsibility that has been delegated by either expression of implication to it by the state legislature.

3. The pronouncements of the board must relate and be limited to its legal jurisdiction and not infringe on the jurisdiction of another agency or another governmental entity.

4. The rules and regulations must not conflict with the Constitution and laws of the United States or with the constitution and laws of the state of which the agency is a part.

5. The rules and regulations must be reasonable and no more drastic than is necessary.

6. All rules, regulations, and standards must be adopted by a legally constituted board of health legally convened in an official session. No individual member of a board has power to enact a regulation any more than an individual Congressman has power to enact a statute. Final enactment can result only by a vote at a properly called meeting of the board, notice of which has been given to each of the members of the board and at which a quorum is present. To attempt to act on a regulation by means of telephoning or visiting the office or home of each member individually does not constitute action by a legally convened meeting of the board since it precludes debate.

7. Since a board of health regulation is in effect a law, it follows that the same care should be exercised in its formation as is exercised in drawing up a state or federal statute. The first consideration in this regard is proper form (including a title and enacting clause), a series of consecutively numbered articles each related to one subject, a statement concerning the time when the regulation is to become effective, and a statement of penalties involved in instances of proved infraction.

8. The ordinance or regulation must be precise, consistent, definite, and certain in its expression and meaning. The present tense should be used. It should be written for the public and especially for those who will be affected by it. Complicated, high-sounding phrases should be avoided, punctuation used sparingly, and parenthesis almost never used. Foreign or technical terms should be avoided if possible. It has been said that there can be a lawsuit for each extraneous or ill-chosen word and for every ill-advised punctuation mark.

9. If the legislature prescribes the manner in which regulations and ordinances should be passed, such prescription must be exactly adhered to. If, for example, it is specified in the state law that a proposed ordinance be read and voted on favorably at three successive meetings of a legally constituted and convened board, this cannot be fulfilled as has been sometimes attempted by having the clerk stand and read the ordinance and call for a vote three times during the same meeting.

10. The ordinance or regulation must be enacted in good faith and in the public interest alone and designed to enable the board of health to carry out its legal responsibilities. It should therefore be impartial and nondiscriminatory, applying to all members of the community.

11. In some states it is necessary that actions of boards of health be approved by the attorney general of the state.

12. On legal passage the final step is proper and adequate publication of the rule or ordinance in order that those who are to be affected by it shall have ample opportunity to be informed concerning it. This is usually carried out by means of publishing in the local newspapers.

Concerning this last requisite, Gellhorn[34] has commented that "regarding publication of administrative legislation the situation, especially in the states, is confusing almost to the extreme and eventual reform is certain to be demanded as a result of this disregard of the public interest in knowing what rules and orders they are subject to. Such lack of adequate publication has undoubtedly led to judicial hostility toward delegated legislation and authority."

A final caution might be given concerning the frequent practice of adopting or incorporating rules and regulations by reference. This procedure has the enticement of being convenient and easy, but it may give rise to legal difficulties in that only existing things can be legally incorporated by reference. Therefore each time the original regulation or law is changed, it is necessary to reincorporate by reference. Furthermore, it is legally impossible, although it is sometimes attempted, to adopt or incorporate a subject by reference on a blanket basis through time because such action amounts to committing the public to regulations that are not yet in existence. It is comparable to asking the public to sign a blank check.

This is not meant to condemn the technique of reference entirely, since its convenience amply justifies its use. However, it should be used with full knowledge of its limitations and potential disadvantages, some of which are illustrated by the case* of a board of health that adopted a regulation dealing with the sale of milk and milk products in accordance with the unabridged form of the 1939 edition of the U.S. Public Health Service Milk Ordinance. The publication of the new regulation did not contain the ordinance but stated that a certified copy was on file in the office of the board of health. The Ohio Supreme Court, in ruling on the case of a defendant charged with violating the regulation, stated, "The effectiveness of legislation by reference has been so generally recognized . . . that no very specific declaration appears in the reported cases." The court added, however, that "no by-law or ordinance, or section thereof, shall be revived or amended unless the new by-law or ordinance contains the entire by-law or ordinance, or section revived or amended, and the by-law or ordinance, section or sections so amended shall be repealed." As long as there was no violation of this section, the court said that it saw no objection to the incorporation by reference in a regulation of a district board of health on a duly enacted statute, or on a duly enacted ordinance that has been theretofore properly published. However, the Ohio Supreme Court was of the view that the publication of a board of health regulation, which omitted the rules of conduct to be observed and merely referred those

who might be affected to a copy of the terms on file in the office of the board of health, did not constitute proper publication as meant by the law and that until proper publication had been made, any such regulation was not effective.

LIABILITY AND AGENCY

To accomplish a desired purpose such as the completion of a contract or the rendering of a public service, practicality usually makes it necessary that the one (the principal) who is legally responsible for fulfilling the contract or for rendering the public service obtain an agent or agents to carry out the details involved. This relationship between principal and agents gives rise to an additional series of legal complications, especially in terms of those things for which the principal is liable and those for which the agent is liable. In public health work the citizens of a community as represented by their legally designated board of health may be considered the principal, whereas the health officer acts as the agent of the people and is responsible to the board.

The view has been held repeatedly by the courts, as illustrated by two cases* in which the courts observed that the authority for the appointment of a city health commissioner was precisely the same as that for the appointment of nurses and other employees and that the health commissioner was not a public officer but an employee under the direction, supervision, and control of the board of health.

The fundamental rule governing the relationship of principal to agent is that the principal is liable for contractual agreements or other acts of an agent, provided that the agent has acted within the real or apparent scope of his authority. It should be noted from this that the principal is not vested with a blanket liability for all contracts or all acts that might be carried out in his name but is liable only for those acts for which the agent has been given power by him. The most important and difficult problem is to define or determine the meaning and extent of the agent's real and apparent authority and power.

*Ohio Supreme Court: State v. Waller, 55 N.E. 2nd 654 (1944).

*Ohio Supreme Court: Scofield v. Strain, Mayor, et al., State ex rel.; Reilly v. Hamrock, Mayor, et al., 51 N.E. 2nd 1012 (1943).

The powers of an agent have been divided into real and apparent. An agent's real power consists of the expressed or implied authority delegated to him by the principal. Expressed powers are given usually in the form of actual and explicit instructions. Thus a board of health may instruct a health officer to control the spread of a communicable disease through the community.

Added to this expressed authority, the agent also has certain implied powers to find it possible to do whatever is reasonably necessary to carry out the instructions given. The health officer, therefore, on being instructed to control the spread of communicable disease, may correctly assume the implied power and authority to include whatever administrative procedures are reasonably indicated, for example, quarantine or contact examination, to accomplish the responsibility given in relation to the expressed powers.

Over and above real authority, expressed or implied, the agent has certain so-called apparent powers. In the use of these the agent really exceeds actual power and would be considered liable in many instances were it not for the concept that other persons under certain circumstances are correct in believing that the agent has power to act. The use of apparent power is involved in major part in the solution of individual problems, each with its own peculiar circumstances, and the test of its correct use is the determination of whether or not a reasonably prudent person in similar circumstances would have been justified in acting as did the agent on the behalf of the principal. This may be illustrated by the case of a health officer* who in the face of a smallpox outbreak hospitalized an individual erroneously considered to have smallpox, with the result that the patient became infected with smallpox while in the isolation hospital. Because the erroneous diagnosis was made in good faith by the attending private physician and similarly confined by the health department diagnostician after exercising due and customary care and judgment, neither the private physician nor the community through its authorized public health agents were held liable. "To hold otherwise," the court stated, "would not only invite indifference at the expense of society, but the fear of liability would well-nigh destroy the efforts of officials to protect the public health."

This emphasizes that an agent owes to the principal the exercise of a degree of care and skill that a reasonably qualified and prudent person in terms of the community involved at the time would be expected to exercise under similar circumstances. Therefore the professional agent, in this case a health officer, owes to the principal (the community) the exercise of a reasonable degree of care and skill as judged by the time and place. It should be noted that except where a contract exists to the contrary, no guarantee is involved that a certain result will be effected. All that is required by the law is the exercise of that degree of skill, knowledge, and care usually displayed by similar members of the profession under similar circumstances.

In the absence of malice or corruption or a statutory provision imposing the liability, health officers generally are not liable for errors or mistakes in judgment in the performance of acts within the scope of their authority where they are empowered to exercise judgement and discretion. Personal liability therefore depends on proof of bad faith, which "may be shown by evidence that official action was so arbitrary and unreasonable that it could not have been taken in good faith,"* Although obviously difficult to ascertain, bad faith has been demonstrated to the satisfaction of the courts, as in the case† of a smallpox patient who was forcibly transferred from her home to a dirty, insanitary cabin, for which action a health officer was understandably held liable.

It logically follows, however, that if reasonable and legal instructions have been given to an agent by the principal, it is the agent's duty to obey them or think that he or she knows a better way in which to accomplish the purpose desired. In such an instance should the agent willfully disobey the principal's instructions or laws, and injury or any other undesirable result follow, the agent is liable for whatever damages have been sustained as a result of this disobedience.

With regard to liability of the principal if it is a government, it must first be reemphasized that the state is sovereign and, as such, cannot be sued or held liable by its individual citizens except where it grants permission. Since county governments are

---

*Dillon's Municipal Corporations 771, as quoted by Tobey.[45]

*Kirk v. Aiken Board of Health, 83 S.C. 372 (1909).
†Moody v. Wickersham, 111 Kan. 770 (1922).

essentially local administrative and political units of the sovereign state, the same rule tends to be applied to them. However, there is an increasing tendency on the part of states to allow counties to be sued and to hold them liable whenever there is question or doubt. Municipalities are somewhat different in that they are corporations carrying on various functions and services. Some of these functions, for example, the operation of a transportation system or a water works, are considered private, and the city may be sued concerning them. However, other functions and services such as the maintenance of police and fire departments are public functions, and concerning these the city cannot be readily sued. Public health activities fall into this category. Some states have been highly specific in this regard, as evidenced by a Michigan Supreme Court decision that said: "The matter of public health is not local; it concerns the State. In matters relating to public health the city acts as an arm of the State, and the property whose use is devoted to the public health is used in the discharge of a governmental function."*

EXTENT OF USE OF LAW IN PUBLIC HEALTH

Seen in its proper relationship, legal enforcement represents only one of several ways by which an administrator acting as an agent of the community may bring about desirable results and effect conformity to the socially desired standards of the community. In effect, the administrator has three main tools or methods of approach at his disposal—education, persuasion, and coercion—and the extent to which the administrator successfully blends and balances them is one of the best measures of true administrative ability. As Tobey[45] has warned, "A health officer who is constantly involved in court actions, either as plaintiff or prosecutor or as defendant, would hardly be classed as an efficient public officer since he should be able to administer the public health of his community or State and enforce the public health laws in the great majority of cases by means of persuasion and education and by suitable action before the board of health." The efficient and reasonable health officer must be ready to recognize sincere and honest attempts to meet the standards set up by society when such attempts are within the range of social tolerance,

*Michigan Supreme Court: Curry v. City of Highland Park et al., 219 N.W. 74 (1928).

and he or she must be able to explain the tolerance point to the average citizen, the legislature, and the courts. On the other hand:

Many of the most important achievements of public health have had the support of laws and ordinances requiring conformity to specified sanitary standards. Without this support movements for the extension of public health work would have evolved more slowly and would still be far from their present state of development. Informed public opinion would have brought about great improvement, but more slowly. The coercive power must, therefore, be considered a powerful factor in the development of effective public health work, but is has definite limitations.[46]

The early history of public health in America might be characterized by almost complete dependence on legislation and its enforcement:

During the past generation the student of public health has witnessed a rapid shift in emphasis away from the doctrine of direct control toward that of education. This change has been due in no sense to the failure of the regulatory theory but rather to the broadening scope of public health that now includes problems of personal hygiene. . . . Even the exercise of the regulatory authority must rest on education, for an uninformed legislative body will not enact proper laws or appropriate funds for their enforcement, and an uninformed public will not tolerate regulations it does not understand or appreciate.[46]

Addressing essentially the same point, Miller and co-workers[47] observe:

A restraining influence on implementation of statutory authorizations is lack of money. And yet tremendous amounts of money are spent for health services. If that money is not spent in constructive ways then the responsibility may well rest with public health leadership that fails to provide enlightenment and programmatic vigor that can compete successfully in the nation's economic and political markets.

In most instances, social legislation is framed by persons who are somewhat more advanced in their social thinking than is the average citizen. Only relatively recently has the realization come about that legislation dealing with social concepts that are too far ahead of the citizenry as a whole is almost inevitably doomed to failure. Many tragic examples of this nature may be found in the history of public health. One of the best known is the fate of the

General Board of Health of England, established in 1848, which failed as a result of overenthusiasm because of Edwin Chadwick's social thinking and planning, which was too far ahead of the people of England at the time. At least one local health officer in America was literally tarred and feathered because of his persistent attempts to institute complete pasteurization of milk when the strongly opinionated citizens of his area were not intellectually prepared or ready for it.

As a result of the relatively recent realization that social progress of all types must be based on understanding and acceptance by the majority of those involved, leaders in the field of public health administration have turned increasingly toward emphasis on educational and persuasive action, minimizing the legal and enforcement approach. Boyd[48] pointed out that permissive legislation for the establishment of local health units in Illinois existed for 25 years, but as a result of the legislation alone, only six county health departments came into being. As a result of subsequent public educational methods, however, the citizens in most parts of the state expressed their desire for local health departments with almost no opposition.

The place of legal enforcement in present-day public health activitiy has been well stated by Lade[49] in discussing the control of venereal disease:

Now compulsion is not the only recourse in these cases—not even the first recourse. A substantial number of contacts resistant to examination and patients delinquent from treatment will respond to information, reassurance, persuasion, or assistance when unable to pay for examination or treatment. Indeed, the extent to which these measures are successful is to a degree a measure of the efficiency of a health department, and a demonstration of the superiority of our democratic government over a dictatorship. But there will always be a residue of cases resistant to all of these measures who are the kernel of the venereal disease problem. Here a show of force is frequently all that is necessary. Nevertheless, behind the facade there must be a solid structure of duly constituted authority, lest we have government by the whim of officialdom. Hence, law is necessary as an expression of sound medicolegal thinking in a problem which concerns all the people.

The changing epidemiology of venereal disease provides a good example of the need to attend to changes in health legislation. For a number of years beginning in 1935 public health departments found mandated premarital tests for syphilis productive. Accordingly, the states enacted the necessary legislation. Recent social and epidemiologic changes, however, have resulted in a newer cost-benefit ratio, in comparison with other case-finding methods, which has prompted many states to repeal the earlier laws.[50,51]

A contrary situation is found in relation to the trend of widespread repeal of state laws that require the use of motorcycle helmets. This is despite the proven fact that the fatality rate per miles of travel for motorcyclists is seven times the corresponding rate for automobile occupants and has increased 50% between 1975 and 1979.[52] Furthermore, it has been clearly shown that repeal of such protective laws is followed by a 38% increase in motorcyclist fatalities. It is instructive that a long series of state legislatures have turned deaf ears to such incontrovertible facts in favor of the vigorous and skillful lobbying activities of a minority of motorcyclists.[53] This should give public health and safety personnel great cause for concern and introspection, a concern admirably stated by Yankauer,[54] editor of the *American Journal of Public Health:*

The movement against vehicle safety standards is only one of many similar recent regressions. Such actions against the public health can only be viewed as symptoms of a sick society. It is an upside down world in which a basic public health principle, preserving life, has become the catchword for a zealous minority intent on its own narrow goals to the exclusion of all other considerations— a society where consensus about the public good is fractured by single-issue fringe elements. Therefore, it is not surprising that deregulation has become the order of the day, mindlessly sweeping the good as well as the bad into the same dust bin.

Obviously a balance is necessary. No single approach meets all situations, and not infrequently firm action must be taken. Curran[55] has taken health professionals to task in words worth careful attention: "Professionals in the health field have traditionally downgraded the use of legal sanctions. They have preferred to achieve their goals of better health for the American people through education. . . . Many professional public health people have forgotten that their basic responsibility is to protect and to improve the health of the masses of people and to use all effective public means to achieve it." An example relates to community protection against certain communicable diseases. The judicious withholding of mandated school attendance until immunization is obtained has proved effective in many situations.[56-58]

In noting an increasing legal activist role of health workers in company with the poor and with consumer groups, Curran[55] suggests, "In the future, we may look for greater participation in this field by 'traditional' health professionals and their 'traditional' professional organizations. Otherwise," he warns, "this will be another in the growing number of health fields taken out of the hands of the old-line health groups."

COURT PROCEDURE

Since despite all wishes to the contrary, every active health officer will sooner or later appear in court, it may be well to include a few words concerning court procedure. When court action appears to be necessary, all other efforts for the conformance to social standards and for the enforcement of a law or ordinance relating to them having failed, the first step is to bring charges against the offender. The party who initiates the action is called in law the plaintiff and in equity the complainant. The individual against whom action is brought is known as the defendant in both law and equity. In bringing charges against the defendant, one must first determine which court has jurisdiction. The same action may be interpreted as constituting any one of several different criminal acts, depending on the intent, the circumstances, the existing laws, and the consequences. Thus to give dangerous, contaminated material to an individual is considered an assault; to make it available to the public at large results in a criminal nuisance; and if sent through the mails, it is a breach of the postal regulations. The first two offenses are crimes under the common law or statutes of a state; the third offense is a crime under the acts of the Congress of the United States. As pointed out previously, violations of public health laws or regulations usually are considered misdemeanors. In any case infractions of these laws constitute a criminal act, so that the case is within the jurisdiction of a criminal court such as a police court.

The plaintiff then files with the court a complaint (sometimes referred to as declaration, information, petition, bill, or statement of claim) that has been drawn up by the plaintiff or, preferably, with the aid or a municipal, county, or state attorney. This should consist of a detailed statement by, for example, the health officer of the facts and circumstances leading up to the controversy and including the terms of any regulation or ordinance violated. The plaintiff should expect to prove the facts and circumstances beyond reasonable doubt in court with the aid of creditable witnesses to obtain a favorable judgment. The magistrate of the court then issues a summons ordering the defendant to appear in the particular court on a certain stated day and hour, and the summons is served in person to the defendant by an officer of the court. The purpose of the summons is to give actual written notice to the defendant that legal action has been instituted against him. Its personal service is essential, since a court is powerless to render a judgment against a defendant who has not been so notified. Each individual is entitled to his day in court to have the opportunity to bring out whatever defense he may find possible. The defendant now has a choice of six procedures:

1. He may ignore the proceedings, placing himself in default and inviting judgment against himself.

2. He may confess to the accusation of the plaintiff and again invite a judgment against himself.

3. He may enter a plea in abatement, questioning whether the court has power or jurisdiction to act against him and whether proper procedure has been followed.

4. He may file a demurrer, stating in effect that although he admits the truth of what the plaintiff states as a matter of law, the facts do not entitle him to recover.

5. He may file an answer or a plea consisting of a denial of the facts stated in the plaintiff's declaration.

6. Again, the defendant may admit the facts brought out by the plaintiff but bring out still other facts in avoidance or in excuse of those alleged by the plaintiff. Pleading continues until one side denies the facts claimed by the other, thereby raising an issue calling for a decision, and the case is then ready to go to trial.

Most public health legal controversies do not take place before a jury, although either side is entitled to a trial by jury if it so wishes. The first step in such instances is the impaneling of a jury, consisting of the calling of prospective jurors from an approved list and questioning them individually concerning prejudices for or against either litigant. The function of the jury is to decide questions of fact, in contrast to the judge's function of deciding questions of law. When the court proceeding gets under way, counsel for each side may make an opening statement that explains briefly what the counsel expects to prove. After this each side introduces its evidence.

All offenses consist of two factors, that is, the criminal act and the criminal intent, and both must be proved beyond reasonable doubt to demonstrate the commission of a crime. A criminal act is an action or omission that the law forbids. To be considered criminal, the act must be defined by a law or regulation forbidding its commission. The rule of law is strictly interpreted in favor of the accused, so that the act is not considered criminal unless it corresponds exactly with the definition contained in the law. The criminal intent is the state of mind of the accused at the time when the criminal act was committed. It involves a conscious recognition of the unlawful nature of the act, followed by a determination to perform the act. The courts presume the existence of criminal intent on the basis of the actual commission of the act, and it is usually unnecessary to produce evidence of criminal intent unless the accused attempts to prove that at the time the criminal act was committed he was incapable of determining or understanding its nature and unlawfulness or that the act was involuntary. Such proof must be based on (1) youth, (2) insanity, (3) mistake of fact, (4) accident, (5) necessity, or (6) compulsion. If the accused is able to do so to the satisfaction of the court, although the commission of a criminal act is recognized, the proved lack of criminal intent causes the court to consider that he did not perpetrate a crime, and the defendant will be declared innocent.

When all evidence has been brought forth, the judge instructs the jury concerning the law involved in the issues raised, and the jury then retires to decide on a verdict. When the jury renders its verdict but before the court pronounces judgment, the losing party may make a motion for a new trial. This may be granted if the court believes that an erroneous ruling has been made concerning the admission or rejection of evidence, if an erroneous instruction has been given to the jury, or if the verdict is obviously contrary to the weight of the eivdence given. If the motion for a new trial is refused, the court tenders its judgment. If the losing party still believes that there was a substantial error in the conduct of the trial, he may thereupon take the case on appeal to a superior court of appeal, in which case he is termed the *appellant* and the other side the *appellee*. The court of review or appeal is exactly what its name implies, since it does not conduct a new trial. It simply considers the record of the proceeding that took place before the inferior trial court and the exceptions taken to ruling of the trial judge with regard to procedure, pleading, admission of evidence, instructions, etc. If the court of review or appeals decides that a substantial error prejudicial to the losing side was made by the lower trial court, the judgment of the lower court is reversed and the case is remanded for a new trial.

EXPERT WITNESS[59]

Occasionally the public health worker takes part in a court proceeding not as a plaintiff or defendant but as an expert witness for either side or for the court itself. Whereas ordinary witnesses are restricted in their testimony to exact statements of facts, expert witnesses are called on to give opinion testimony. Before being considered an expert witness, evidence of competency must be presented to the satisfaction of both sides. In general, any licensed physician is considered to qualify as an expert witness in controversies dealing with medical questions. Specialization is not necessary, and the expert witness may give an opinion even if he never before saw either litigant and even if he never before observed a similar case. Expert witnesses are customarily compensated for their services, but compensation can never be contingent on the winning of the suit by the side for whom the individual appears as a witness.

Courts in general tend to be suspicious of any opinion or expert testimony, and its acceptance by the court depends largely on the manner in which it is given.[60] With this in mind, the expert witness should be well prepared for whatever questions he might anticipate will be presented. The witness should be serious and unassuming and present an attitude of wanting to assist an intelligent jury in their rendering of a verdict by offering whatever special knowledge he may possess. The expert witness should be free of partiality and bias, frankly and honestly admitting a fact even if it injures the side that employed him as a witness and honestly admitting lack of knowledge on a particular item if he does not have it. He should listen carefully to all questions and answer clearly, directly, and concisely in language understandable to the jury (with a simple yes or no whenever possible). The wise witness never volunteers information when on the stand, assuming that, if significant, counsel will bring it out. Perhaps the most fatal mistake that might be made by an expert witness, or any witness for that matter, is to allow himself to be successfully prodded into losing his temper.

Finally, health workers would do well to heed the dictum of a famous French expert in forensic medicine: "If the law has made you a witness, remain a man of science; you have no victim to avenge, no guilty or innocent person to save."

REFERENCES

1. Grad, F.P.: Public health law manual, ed. 3, Washington, D.C., 1973, American Public Health Association.
2. Freund, P.A.: The legal profession. In Lynn, K.S.: The professions in America, Boston, 1965, Houghton Mifflin Co.
3. Wing, K.R.: The law and the public's health, St. Louis, 1976, The C.V. Mosby Co.
4. Clute, K.E.: Law and health, some current challenges, Milbank Mem. Fund Q. **50:**7, Jan. 1972.
5. Curran, W.J.: Public health lawyers, Am. J. Public Health **59:**854, May 1969.
6. Report of Conference of Directors of Schools of Public Health, WHO Tech. Rep. Ser. No. 351, Geneva, 1967, World Health Organization.
7. Hamlin, R.H.: Public health law, or the interrelationship of law and public health administration, Am. J. Public Health **51:**1733, Nov. 1961.
8. Grad, F.P.: An effective legal enforcement program, Am. J. Public Health **59:**947, June 1969.
9. Gray, J.C.: The nature and sources of law, New York, 1909, Columbia University Press.
10. Cardoza, B.N.: The nature of the judicial process, New Haven, 1921, Yale University Press.
11. Blackstone, W.: In Lewis, W.D., editor: Commentaries, Philadelphia, 1897, Rees, Welsh & Co.
12. Sutherland, A.E.: The law at Harvard, Cambridge, Mass., 1967, Belknap Press.
13. Holmes, O.W.: The common law, Boston, 1881, Little, Brown & Co.
14. Thayer, J.B.: The origin and scope of the American doctrine of constitutional law, Harvard Law Review **7**(3):129, Oct. 1893.
15. Akerman, B.A.: Law and the public mind: by Jerome Frank, Daedalus **103:**119, Winter 1973.
16. Wilson, W.: The state: elements of historical and practical politics, Boston, 1918, D.C. Heath & Co.
17. Akerman, p. 119.
18. Akerman, p. 123.
19. Wing, p. 163.
20. Gurvitch, G.: Sociology of law, New York, 1942, Alliance Book Corp.
21. Curran, W.J.: A constitutional right to a healthy environment, Am. J. Public Health **67:**262, March 1977.
22. Curran, W.J.: The privacy protection report and epidemiological research, Am. J. Public Health **68:**173, Feb. 1978.
23. Lappé, M., and Myers, B.: California's new birth certificate law: some lessons to be learned, Am. J. Public Health **69:**706, July 1979.
24. Cardoza, B.N.: The growth of law, New Haven, 1942, Yale University Press.
25. Seagle, W.: The quest for law, New York, 1941, Alfred A. Knopf, Inc.
26. Holmes, O.W.: The common law, Boston, 1881, Little, Brown & Co.
27. Kent's Commentaries, Lecture 21.
28. Miller, C.A., and others: Statutory authorizations for the work of local health departments, Am. J. Public Health **67:**940, Oct. 1977.
29. Ascher, C.S.: The regulation of housing, Am. J. Public Health **37:**507, May 1947.
30. Freund, E.: The police power, Chicago, 1904, Callahan.
31. Curran, W.J.: Administrative warrants for health and safety inspections, Am. J. Public Health **68:**1029, Oct. 1978.
32. Forgotson, E.H.: 1965: the turning point in health law—1966 reflections, Am. J. Public Health **57:**934, June 1967.
33. Edelman, S.: Search warrants and sanitation inspections—the new look in enforcement, Am. J. Public Health **58:**930, May 1968.
34. Gellhorn, W.: Administrative law: cases and comments, Chicago, 1940, Foundation Press, Inc.
35. Freeman, A.W.: Public health administration in Ohio, DeLamar Lectures, Johns Hopkins University School of Hygiene and Public Health, Baltimore, 1921, The Williams & Wilkins Co.
36. Tobey, J.A.: Legal aspects of milk control, Washington, D.C., 1924, Reprint 939, U.S. Public Health Service.
37. The legal phases of milk control, Washington, D.C., 1929, Reprint 1343, U.S. Public Health Service.
38. Mustard, H.S.: Legal aspects of planning for local health units, Am. J. Public Health **37**(suppl.):20, Jan. 1947.
39. Tobey, J.A.: Recent court decisions on milk control, Washington, D.C., 1933, Reprint 1555, U.S. Public Health Service.
40. Curran, W.J.: The preparation of state and local health regulations, Am. J. Public Health **49:**314, March 1959.

41. Curran, W.J.: Problems in drafting and interpreting health regulations, Am. J. Public Health **67:**768, Aug. 1977.

42. Curran, W.J.: Common sense in enforcement of inspections and regulations in occupational health and safety, Am. J. Public Health **68:**73, Jan. 1978.

43. White, L.D.: New horizons in public administration, Tuscaloosa, 1945, University of Alabama Press.

44. Fischer, J.: How our laws are made, Washington, D.C., 1971, U.S. Government Printing Office.

45. Tobey, J.A.: Public health law, New York, 1947, Commonwealth Fund.

46. Anderson, G.W.: In Graham, G.A., and Reining, H., editors: Regulatory administration, New York, 1943, John Wiley & Sons, Inc.

47. Miller and others, p. 945.

48. Boyd, R.F.: Legal aspects (of local health units) from viewpoint of a state health department, Am. J. Public Health **37**(suppl.):31, Jan. 1947.

49. Lade, J.H.: The legal basis for venereal disease control, Am. J. Public Health **35:**1041, Oct. 1945.

50. Kingon, R.J., and Wiesner, P.J.: Premarital syphilis screening: weighing the benefits, Am. J. Public Health **71:**160, Feb. 1981.

51. Felman, Y.M.: Repeal of mandated premarital tests for syphilis: a survey of state health officers, Am. J. Public Health **71:**155, Feb. 1981.

52. Watson, G.S., Zador, P.L., and Wilks, A.: Helmet use, helmet use laws, and motorcyclist fatalities, Am. J. Public Health **71:**297, March 1981.

53. Baker, S.P.: On lobbies, liberty, and the public good, Am. J. Public Health **70:**573, June 1980.

54. Yankauer, A.: Deregulation and the right to life, Am. J. Public Health **71:**797, Aug. 1981.

55. Curran, W.J.: Making new health law: "Sue the bastards," Am. J. Public Health **60:**2016, Oct. 1970.

56. Anthony, N., and others: Immunization: public health programming through law enforcement, Am. J. Public Health **67:**763, Aug. 1977.

57. Yokan, C., and D'Onofrio, C.: Application of health education methods to achieve higher immunization rates, Public Health Rep. **93:**221, May-June 1978.

58. Robbins, K.B., Brandling-Bennett, A.D., and Hinman, A.R.: Low measles incidence: association with enforcement of school immunization laws, Am. J. Public Health **71:**270, March 1981.

59. Curran, W.J.: The doctor as a witness, Philadelphia, 1965, W.B. Saunders Co.

60. Association of the Bar of the City of New York: Impartial medical testimony, New York, 1956, Macmillan, Inc.

CHAPTER 8

Organization of public health in the United States

We trained hard . . . but it seems that every time we were beginning to form up teams, we would be reorganized . . . what a wonderful method it can be for creating the illusion of progress.

Petronius
Satyricon

INTERGOVERNMENTAL RELATIONS

For many years public health programs in the United States were organized and operated along relatively simple lines (see Chapter 2). Relationships among the official health agencies of the three levels of government were usually quite clear. They might be summarized as follows:

1. In accord with the federal Constitution, each sovereign state determined the form and function of its official health agency.
2. The local health agencies, as they were developed with the approval of and some support from the state, served in effect as agents of the State Health Department.
3. The national health agency dealt essentially with interstate and international matters and on request assisted the states in various types of emergencies.

As time passed, a number of forces led to significant and lasting changes in these relatively comfortable arrangements. Prominent among these forces were (1) economic fluctuations; (2) changes in revenue potentials; (3) societal needs and demands; (4) population changes in numbers, concentration, and mobility; and (5) scientific and technologic developments. The great economic depression of the 1930s and the responses of the Roosevelt administration appear to represent the overall watershed between the established roles of the past and the rapidly emerging roles of the future. Certainly of the five forces mentioned, the first—economic fluc-

tuations—accelerated, if not indeed triggered, the other four. It is interesting to observe how essentially the same process appears to be recurring at the present time, although the direction of change seems to be somewhat reversed.

Public health organization on all three levels of government understandably paralleled the socioeconomic development of the nation. Thus for a long time the concept of governmental involvement in any type of health activity either was not even considered a possibility or, if attempted, was viewed as an unwarranted intrusion into personal and private affairs. This was especially so on the local level. Governmental operation of a postal system was understandable and welcomed, roads were accepted with the reservation that they be constructed and maintained locally, but health matters were essentially one's own business. As the nation grew in size and complexity, it became increasingly evident that such restrictive views could no longer serve the best interests of the people. Not only were areas of governmental action expanded but the respective roles and relationships of the federal-state-local partnership were more definitively determined. As things now stand, a 1980 symposium[1] on the subject outlined these roles and responsibilities as follows:

Federal government

1. To develop broad national goals and standards for personal health for the country as a whole.
2. To help equalize the ability of the states to achieve these national goals and standards.

The basis for public
health

3. To monitor the performance of the states and to facilitate improved achievements.
4. To take direct steps in those areas in which national action is essential for the protection and enhancement of personal health.

State governments
1. To prepare detailed plans in the light of national goals and standards.
2. To develop and acquire necessary resources for the implementation of these plans.
3. To assign responsibility for the delivery of personal health services and to facilitate effective and efficient delivery of these services in innovative ways.
4. To monitor performance to ensure that state plan objectives, standards, and targets are met.

Local governments
1. To serve as the grass roots voice of citizens in the development of national goals and standards, as well as in the development of the plan of their respective states. This includes identifying needs, highlighting the underserved and unserved, and providing feedback on the effectiveness and efficiency of current services.
2. To be an active partner with the state government in the financing, organizing, and delivery of personal health services for its own citizens in the light of their unique needs and circumstances but in full conformity with the state plans and with national goals and standards.

Jain[1] suggests that his summary of the symposium while

seemingly utopian . . . attempts to balance the tension among the three dominant societal values of our time, viz., liberty, equality and resource-reality (federal government ensuring equality of opportunity, state and local governments ensuring availability of needed services in the light of their unique circumstances, and grass roots accountability of decision-makers resulting in increasingly effective and efficient use of finite resources).

In this sense, he believes, it may serve the future well.

LOCAL PUBLIC HEALTH ORGANIZATION

In a system in which three interacting levels of government are involved in health affairs, it is somewhat difficult to decide the most logical point at which to begin discussion. The choice has been made in favor of local public health organization, because it is on the local level that the most direct and intimate contact with the client public occurs. There are 3,135 local health departments in 47 states and the territory of Puerto Rico. They play an important role in providing most of the direct community health services including epidemiology, immunizations, perinatal care, public health nursing, environmental health protection, and various other services depending on need and resources. In 3 states (Delaware, Rhode Island, Vermont) and 6 territories (the District of Columbia, Guam, the Northern Mariana Islands, American Samoa, the Trust Territory, and the Virgin Islands) there are no local health departments. In these, the state health agency or another public agency provides the community health services. In fiscal year 1980 expenditures of local health departments totaled $2.4 billion of which $1 billion were intergovernmental grants (Table 8-1).[2]

It has been pointed out earlier that for a long time personal health needs were regarded as an individual responsibility. The exception was in the event of an epidemic. It is understandable therefore that the earliest local public health organizations had their genesis in relation to disease emergencies of various types. This sense of local determinism has by no means disappeared, as evidenced by emphasis on revenue sharing and the recent trend away from categoric grants in favor of block grants. It is also evidenced by even the most cursory comparison of the organizations and programs of the local (and state) public health agencies. Considerable variation is observed despite professional models

TABLE 8-1. Local health department (LHD) expenditures, in millions of dollars, by source of funds, fiscal year 1980

Source of funds	Intergovernmental grants to LHDs	Additional funds to LHDs
State funds	$ 576	$ 78
Federal grants and contracts	321	88
Local funds	73	1,046
Fees, reimbursements, other	48	180
TOTAL public health—local	1,018	1,392

Modified from National public health program reporting system: Public health programs 1980, Washington, D.C., 1980, Association of State and Territorial Health Officials.

and standards and despite grant carrots and sometimes even mandate. Tilson[3] notes that "the reluctance of local governments to assume responsibility
for funding of public health services is reflected by
a broad spectrum of unreadiness—even inability—
to undertake the sort of rigorous administration of
public health services needed to make the 'model'
work."

Considerable light has been shed on the types of
and reasons for the variations in local public health
programs by an extensive study of state-local relationships conducted by DeFriese, Miller, and their
coworkers.[4,5] They surveyed 68% of local health officers throughout the United States inquiring about
jurisdiction, organization, finance, functions, staffing, training, salaries, and other characteristics.
The information obtained indicated four patterns
of organizational structure based on the operative
administrative relationships between local health
departments and state and local government: (1)
centralized, (2) decentralized, (3) shared control,
and (4) mixed centralized-decentralized. It was
noted that the funding of the centralized departments differs from the other three types in that
they receive significantly higher proportions of their
budgets (nearly 50%) from federal and state
sources. "Shared" and "mixed" structures rely on
federal and state funds for about 30% of their budgets, and for organizations with decentralized
structures the figure is only slightly more than 20%.
This prompted the comment that program directors
of "centralized" departments were more apt to be
influenced by forces external to the local community.

Of particular interest are the differences that
were found in program emphasis among the four
types of organizational structure[5]:

(1) "shared" structured departments are more involved
in environmental surveillance activity; (2) "mixed" forms
of organization are more involved in health education; and
(3) "centralized" organizations are more involved in direct
patient care delivery while giving less emphasis to local
health code enforcement. Health departments with stronger local control and influence (i.e., decentralized) appear
to have placed more emphasis on local code enforcement.

It is evident that sources of funds do indeed influence programs hence organizations significantly,
and that the greater the support from state and
federal sources, the greater the involvement in direct medical service delivery possibly at the expense
of so-called traditional public health programs.

To carry out its mandate, the official public health

agency in rural or small urban situations requires
only a relatively simple type of organizational structure. Legal responsibility for the public's health is
commonly given to a local board of health, the
members of which are usually appointed by the
locally elected officials—in cities by mayors and in
counties by boards of supervisors or their equivalent. The board of health usually appoints and employs a county health officer, frequently subject to
approval by the state health department. Increasingly state health departments have established
standards and qualifications that must be met by
those appointed to local public health positions.
This type of state supervision has met with relatively little local resistance, since in most instances
local units of government have found it necessary
to turn to the state health department for assistance
in finding capable candidates.

The employment of all other personnel is customarily a prerogative of the local health officer but
is subject to merit system and equal opportunity
regulations if they exist. Depending on the size and
nature of the jurisdiction, the health officer's staff
usually consists of one or more workers in environmental health, public health nursing, health education, and office management. Nutritionists, public health dentists, and representatives of other
professions may be employed even in small local
agencies, again depending on local needs, wishes,
and resources. The workers in environmental
health may consist of combinations of engineers,
professionally trained sanitarians, or sanitary inspectors trained on the job.

Usually, approximately one half of the funds and
one half of the positions of the local health department are devoted to public health nursing. Even
the smallest local health unit will or should have
several nurses on its staff. One of the nurses, selected on the basis of training, experience, and personality, should be appointed as supervising nurse.
Where several office workers are employed, one
should be designated to serve as office manager and
to supervise the work of the others. All members
of the staff should be ultimately responsible to the
county health officer, who in turn in responsible to
the board.

When funds and candidates are not available to
make possible the employment of the necessary
personnel or when employment of full-time employees is not practical, as is often the case in staff-

ing clinics, the gap may be filled by the part-time employment of private practitioners or by the use of services of district or state agencies. Wherever possible, however, the employment of full-time personnel is recommended. Obviously it is desirable that at least the health officer and the supervisory staff have specialized training in public health.

In the larger local units of government, particularly municipalities or combinations of them with their surrounding county areas, more extensive personnel and organization are obviously required. In general, the distribution of types of personnel per unit of population is similar to that followed in the smaller areas; various numbers of different types of specialists are added to meet the needs of the particular situation. The larger and more complex programs necessitate a more formalized organizational structure with the bringing together of similar and related functions into divisions and bureaus. Although there is no standard organizational structure, certain functional divisions are nevertheless almost universally encountered. Thus there usually exist units responsible for health statistics and records; sanitation, sanitary engineering, or environmental health; maternal and child health; public health nursing, either as an entity or integrated with the activities of several of the other divisions; laboratory service; epidemiologic service, or communicable disease control; mental health; and health education. Increasingly one also finds units for adult health, chronic disease, and medical care. Each category large enough to make up a unit should have its own director and possibly subdirectors. The direct professional service activities of those in the top administrative positions become greatly reduced, giving way to functions of a managerial and supervisory nature.

With the increased trend toward core city-suburbia complexes as well as metropolitanization, a growing movement is underway toward merger of even large city and county health departments. About 20% of all local health departments involved a city with one or more counties.[5] The establishment of public health organizations on the basis of these larger units of local government or combinations thereof has been necessitated by a consideration of the number of people and the size of an area required to raise enough public tax funds to support at least a minimum of staff of qualified

public health workers. The trend, although fraught with difficulties of a political and fiscal nature, to the extent that it succeeds, can only bring about greater efficiency and improved public service.

Periodically, The American Public Health Association has issued official policy statements regarding the responsibilities and services of local health departments.[6] The Association emphasizes that the fundamental responsibilities are (1) to determine the health status and needs of the people in its jurisdiction, (2) to determine the extent that these needs are being met by effective measures currently available, and (3) to take steps to see that unmet needs are satisfied. It also emphasizes the role of the local health department in social planning, especially in the areas of medical care, regional planning of health services, effective use of existing resources, and efficient delivery of traditional services. It notes that "changes in demand for both health services and delivery techniques are requiring health agencies to modify their programs. . . . These changes will have a great impact on program organization and financing. . . . Thus, it is likely that existing programs, and existing ways of doing business within many health agencies, will be put in new organizational, institutional, and personnel settings." It then predicts that "how health agencies adjust to these changes and how aggressive they become in terms of moving ahead with comprehensive health services for their constituent populations within this context, will to a large degree determine the future of public support for health programs." This was essentially the theme of the National Commission on Community Health Services[7,8] in the late 1960's, that in the years ahead each community would have to make maximum collaborative use of all of its health-related resources regardless of formal organizational or other distinctions.

The Association's policy statement lists the following functional areas "to indicate the scope of the obligation of local government to see that these services are provided either by its own official health agencies, or by direct arrangement with other agencies, institutions, or providers":

A. Community Health Services
   1. Communicable Disease Control
   2. Chronic Disease Control and Medical Rehabilitation
   3. Family Health, including prenatal, well child, crippled children, school health and family planning programs

4. Dental Health
5. Substance Abuse
6. Accident Prevention
7. Nutrition Services and Education
B. Environmental Health Services
1. Food Protection
2. Hazardous Substances and Product Safety
3. Water Supply Sanitation
4. Liquid Waste Control
5. Water Pollution Control
6. Swimming Pool Sanitation and Safety
7. Occupational Health and Safety
8. Radiation Control
9. Air Quality Management
10. Noise Pollution Control
11. Vector Control
12. Solid Waste Management
13. Institutional Sanitation
14. Recreational Sanitation
15. Housing Conservation and Rehabilitation
16. Environmental Injury Prevention
C. Mental Health Services
1. Primary Prevention of Mental Disorders
2. Consultation to Community Resources
3. Diagnostic and Treatment Services
a. Outpatient
b. Emergency
c. Short term hospitalization
d. Day care and night care services
e. Aftercare services
f. Diagnostic and evaluation services for the mentally retarded
D. Personal Health Services
1. Personal Health Services, per se
2. Health Facilities Operations
3. Emergency Medical Services
4. Home Health Services
5. Employee Health Programs

6. Medical Care for Inmates of Prisons and Institutions
E. Processes Common to all Services
1. Health Data Acquisition and Processing
2. Agency Program Planning
3. Interagency Planning
4. Comprehensive State and Regional Health Planning Participation
5. Disaster Planning
6. Health Education of the Public
7. Health Advocacy
8. Continuing Education of Health Personnel
9. Involvement of Non-Agency Health Personnel
10. Research and Development
11. Community Involvement
12. Organization of Health Agency
13. Policy Direction of Health Agency
14. Staffing
15. Financing
16. Relationships with State and Federal Health Authorities

The list represents more than an ideal—it is a professional goal that has been approximated by a number of local health agencies. Overall, however, the reality leaves many gaps. A general indication of this may be obtained from Table 8-2, which presents the broad program areas to which local health agencies devote funds available to them from the several sources. The inclusion of state health expenditures is to clarify several points that might otherwise raise questions.

It will be noted that local health departments obtain almost one half of their monetary support from the

TABLE 8-2. State (SHA) and local (LHD) health agency expenditures, in millions of dollars, by program areas, fiscal years 1980

Program areas	Direct SHA expenditures		SHA intergovernmental grants of LHAs		Additional LHD expenditures		Total LHD expenditures	
	$	%	$	%	$	%	$	%
Personal health	2,512	73	833	82	1,000	72	1,833	76
Environmental health	225	7	92	9	228	16	320	13
Health resources	328	10	37	4	33	2	70	3
Laboratory	147	4	18	2	44	3	62	3
General administration	223	6	38	4	87	6	125	5
TOTAL	3,435	100	1,018	101	1,392	99	2,410	100

Modified from National public health program reporting system: Public health programs 1980, Washington, D.C., 1980, Association of State and Territorial Health Officials.

state health agencies. This includes most federal grants, which are channeled through the state. It will be noted further that intergovernmental grants to local health agencies vary in relation to program purpose. Almost one half of local expenditures for personal health services derives from intergovernmental grants, and even then the state health departments themselves spend significantly more for this purpose than do the local health departments. In contrast, the proportions are reversed in relation to environmental health activities, with local health agencies spending one third again as much in dollars and twice the proportion of their total available funds as do the state health agencies. But again the picture is reversed with reference to expenditures for health resources (such as personnel development) and laboratory services. These are areas in which the state health agencies are in a much better position to act effectively and efficiently both for their own and for local health department needs. The data in the table illustrate very well the extent and nature of the interdependence of the health agencies on the two levels of government. To significant degrees, the local health agencies depend on the state agencies for fiscal support and certain types of services, and the state health agencies depend on the local agencies for much of the program implementation. Not only is a workable state-local partnership necessary but there often are times when it is difficult to know where one stops and the other begins.

STATE PUBLIC HEALTH ORGANIZATION

A recent discussion by Clarke[9] of the role of states in health services delivery was introduced with a statement relevant to the subject to be considered.

The role of states in the delivery of health services is a difficult one to assess. The states are involved in such a wide variety of health activities, have such different administrative structures as well as varying competence and sophistication, that it is almost impossible to characterize "the states" in anything but abstract terms.

In addition, states by their very nature are subject to certain conflicts and limitations. It is true that they are sovereign and subject to the federal constitution only up to a point. As sovereign governments they have comprehensive authority that includes the protection of the health, safety, and general welfare of their citizens. Yet they lack the considerably greater federal fiscal power and the public intimacy that local governments may have. Nevertheless, they are sufficiently large and conveniently accessible to attract the diligent attentions of a wide variety of special interest groups for undesirable as well as desirable purposes. These and related factors have led to a common criticism especially by academics and federal officials of state governments as inept, corrupt, inefficient, and lacking in social leadership. Such defamations necessarily tend to affect attitudes toward the state health agencies. History, however, does not provide clear validation of these views. State health departments developed on their own initiatives, many of them when federal activities were limited. They played a major role in the development of public health laboratories, sanitary engineering, and the formation of networks of county health organizations. Despite accusations of program limitations to the contrary, the scope of their health activities is, in the words of Clarke, "truly awesome, and capable of reaching into almost every facet of health care delivery."

Each state and territory has vested some one agency with primary legal responsibility for overseeing the public's health. Typically, this is a state department of public health (or some similar title). As on the local level, the state health department should provide the leadership and oversight on its governmental level in public health matters with other agencies acting in this field as collaborating or auxiliary agencies. In general terms, the American Public Health Association has listed the following as responsibilities of state health departments.[10]

1. To develop effective relationships with the elected officials and bodies of the state government in order to represent public health interests and goals to them and to obtain both the necessary legal basis and funds for meeting its responsibilities
2. To provide leadership in a multiagency framework of health services that can offer guidance to colleague agencies in the fulfillment of their services and goals
3. To support a division of responsibilities between state and local health agencies under which the state agency sets statewide health policy and standards, while most actual health services are provided locally
4. To provide leadership and assistance to local communities and their health agencies by the allocation of state and federal grants for health programs

5. To maintain surveillance of the state of health and illness and of environmental conditions throughout the state and its components in order to respond promptly and effectively both to emergencies and to emerging problems
6. To promote and develop statewide plans, objectives and programs that will provide maximum health benefit at both the state and local levels
7. To work with federal health agencies in the development of national health policies, and to make most efficient use of transferred federal funds for the maintenance of necessary existing programs and the stimulation and development of new activities
8. To develop and maintain effective cooperative relationships with voluntary health and human welfare agencies and with pertinent professional organizations
9. To encourage public or consumer representatives and groups to participate in the study of health problems and in the shaping of health programs and policies
10. To conduct a vigorous and effective health information and education program throughout the state
11. To assure the adequacy and standards of personal health services to all the citizens throughout the state
12. To promote quality professional education and practice as well as in-service training, in partnership with the organizations and institutions representing the several health professions

From this one can classify state health department functions into the several categories of statewide planning, intergovernmental relations, intrastate agency relations, and certain statewide policy determination, standard setting, and regulatory functions.

In fulfilling their many responsibilities, all of the 50 states have developed their own unique pattern. Some have strongly centralized organizations, whereas others have decentralized to varying degrees. The subdivisions or functional units within the structure of state health departments vary greatly, both in number and in manner of emphasis and arrangement.[2] No two state patterns are identical, but some similarities are to be noted. Thus the Association of Management in Public Health found that in two thirds of the states the director of public health had a span of control encompassing seven divisions or bureaus. This conforms essentially with the findings of The Association of State and Territorial Health Officials reporting system,[2] which are presented in Fig. 8-1. Shown is the struc-

ture of a hypothetical state health agency with the programs most frequently found within each of the organization's components.

As presented in Table 8-2, direct expenditures of state health agencies in 1980 totaled $3,435 million. In addition, the state health agencies made grants of $1,018 million to local health agencies. Of this total of $4,453 million, 57% represented state funds, 35% came from federal grants and contracts, and 8% from local sources in the form of various fees and reimbursements. Of the federal funds, 52% were grants and contracts from the Department of Health and Human Services, 42% from the Department of Agriculture, 3% from the Environmental Protection Agency, and 2% from the Departments of Labor, Education, and Transportation and certain regional commissions. Almost all of the Department of Agriculture funds came from the Special Supplemental Food Program for Women, Infants, and Children. With reference to the $798 million of the Department of Health and Human Services grants and contracts, more than one half was from the Health Services Administration for Maternal and Child Health, Crippled Childrens' Services, and Family Planning. The next largest proportions were from the Centers for Disease Control (14%); Medicare and Medicaid (11%); and the Alcohol, Drug Abuse, and Mental Health Administration (7.5%).

Actually, the organization of state health policy and service is much more complex than even the foregoing would seem to indicate. Over the years, an ever-increasing number of official state agencies have become involved in one or another aspect of health. Among the hundred or more that might be listed are departments, boards, or commissions concerned with health, mental illness, crippled children, cancer, tuberculosis, social service, welfare, Social Security, medical care or institutions, education, recreation, food and dairy products, agriculture, natural resources, conservation, migrant labor, immigration, industrial relations, mines, public safety, and many others. Estimates of the number of different agencies that perform clearly health functions in a single state vary from 10 to 30 or 40. Furthermore, many agencies may share responsibility for specific health activities, such as accident prevention, health education, and health planning. Some states have attempted coordination by the

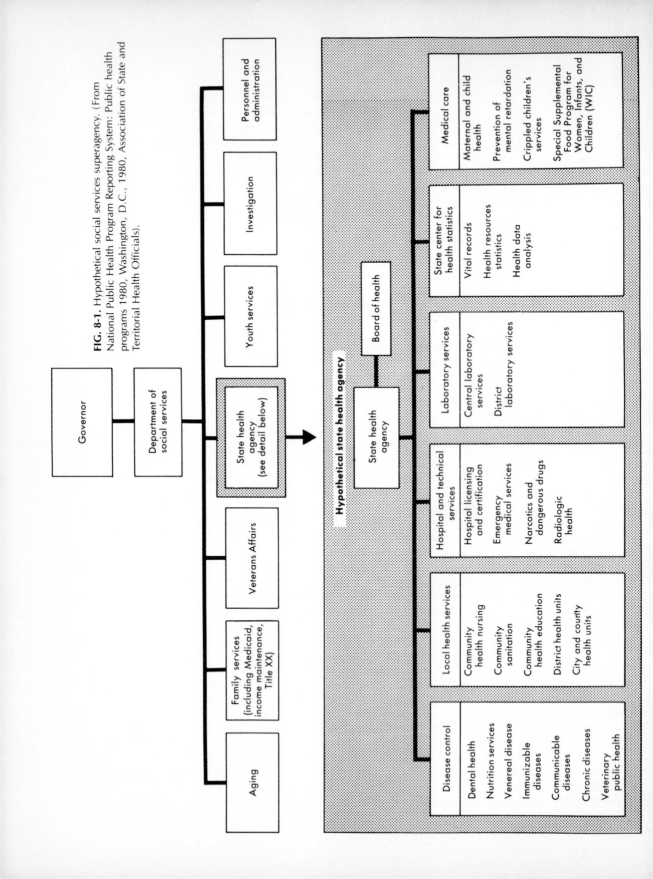

FIG. 8-1. Hypothetical social services superagency. (From National Public Health Program Reporting System: Public health programs 1980, Washington, D.C., 1980, Association of State and Territorial Health Officials).

Governor

Department of social services

State health agency (see detail below)

Aging

Family services (including Medicaid, income maintenance, Title XX)

Veterans Affairs

Youth services

Investigation

Personnel and administration

Hypothetical state health agency

Board of health

State health agency

Disease control

Dental health
Nutrition services
Venereal disease
Immunizable diseases
Communicable diseases
Chronic diseases
Veterinary public health

Local health services

Community health nursing
Community sanitation
Community health education
District health units
City and county health units

Hospital and technical services

Hospital licensing and certification
Emergency medical services
Narcotics and dangerous drugs
Radiologic health

Laboratory services

Central laboratory services
District laboratory services

State center for health statistics

Vital records
Health resources statistics
Health data analysis

Medical care

Maternal and child health
Prevention of mental retardation
Crippled children's services
Special Supplemental Food Program for Women, Infants, and Children (WIC)

establishment of organizational units of human or social services, environmental protection, or comprehensive health planning (Fig. 8-1). Unfortunately, however, many such "superior umbrella agencies" have accomplished relatively little other than the bringing together in one large organizational unit a number of supposedly related but sometimes diverse programs or agencies. The extent to which this has resulted in genuinely greater coordination or improved operational relationships seems somewhat debatable. Often little has resulted beyond making it more complicated and difficult for those outside the agency to locate and relate to the programs with which they hope to have dealings. As a result, complaints are often voiced of another bureaucratic layer and an additional source of directives and report requirements.

FEDERAL PUBLIC HEALTH ORGANIZATION

The many federal agencies that have responsibility for one or more aspects of public health fall into four categories. The first is concerned with broad health interests. The only example is the Public Health Service. The second is concerned with special groups in the population. Examples are the Administration on Aging, the Agricultural Extension Service, the Bureau of Indian Affairs, the medical divisions of the army and the navy, and the Veterans Administration. The third category includes agencies concerned with special problems or programs, such as the Office of Education, the Federal Trade Commission, the Bureau of Labor Standards, the Bureau of Labor Statistics, many bureaus within the Department of Agriculture (animal industry, entomology and plant quarantine, dairy industry, production and marketing, human nutrition, and home economics, etc.), the Bureau of Mines, the Maritime Commission, the Social Security Administration, and the Bureau of Employees' Compensation. The fourth category is concerned with the international health interests of the United States. In addition to the Office of International Health of the Public Health Service, there are the Agency for International Development of the Department of State and the international health activities of several other departments such as Defense and Agriculture. Their functions range from direct personal or technical service to regulation, research, education, and grants-in-aid.

The Public Health Service. The Public Health Service is recognized as the focal point of health concerns of the United States. At the time of this writ-

ing (1982), the Public Health Service is directed by the Assistant Secretary for Health, who serves also as Surgeon General. It is organized into five functional units: (1) the Centers for Disease Control, (2) the Food and Drug Administration, (3) the Health Resources and Services Administration, (4) the National Institutes of Health, and (5) the Alcohol, Drug Abuse, and Mental Health Administration. In addition, the Office of the Assistant Secretary has several staff offices directly related to it. These are concerned with management; with health policy, research, and statistics; planning and evaluation; intergovernmental affairs; and health promotion. There are also offices for legislation, international health, population affairs, and other special concerns (Fig. 8-2). For decentralization of services and more effective assistance to states, 10 regional offices are maintained in Boston, New York, Philadelphia, Atlanta, Chicago, Kansas City, Dallas, Denver, San Francisco, and Seattle. In addition to a National Advisory Health Council, a number of special advisory councils and committees composed of nongovernmental experts are available to many of the institutes and programs. Each year the Assistant Secretary for Health meets at an annual conference with the state and territorial health officers and with certain other special groups.

The five components of the Public Health Service function in a variety of ways. To a considerable extent, the responsibilities of the Health Resources and Services Administration and the Alcohol, Drug Abuse, and Mental Health Administration are met by means of grants and contracts with other governmental agencies, private institutions, and individuals. One exception is the Indian Health Service in the Health Resources and Services Administration, which provides hospital, clinical, and other health services for Native Americans on reservations and for Eskimos. The National Institutes of Health and the Centers for Disease Control carry out extensive intramural and extramural research both on their own and by means of grants and contracts in the United States and other parts of the world. In addition, the Centers for Disease Control serve directly as the epidemiologic surveillance and emergency unit for the nation, and the National Institutes of Health have the added responsibility of the National Library of Medicine, the Fogar-

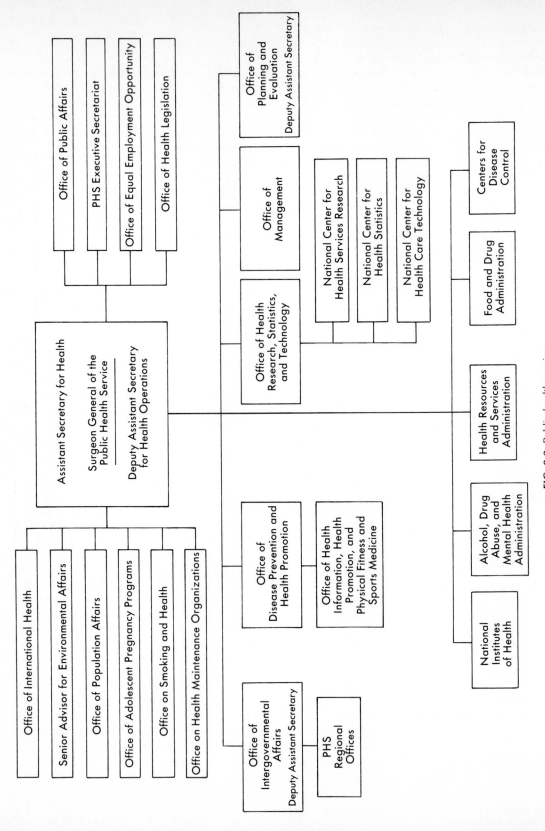

FIG. 8-2. Public health service.

ty International Center for Advanced Studies in Health Sciences, the National Center for Biomedical Communications, and the National Clinical Center. The Food and Drug Administration, by means of its field and laboratory staff, maintains surveillance over the safety and efficacy of foods, food additives, pharmaceuticals and other drugs, cosmetics, and a wide variety of consumer goods including toys and flammable fabrics. It also is responsible for the control of nostrums and medical charlatans.

In view of the foregoing, it is clear that the administration of grants and contracts constitutes a very important aspect of the function of the Public Health Service. The number of grants in the health field grew spectacularly since the mid-1950s and by 1979 numbered many thousands in relation to 69 programs. This accumulation necessitated the development of "an administrative machinery that became," as Assistant Secretary Brandt[11] described it, "for all intents and purposes, a program in itself." Furthermore, Brandt indicated the program was expensive, unwieldy, and often unfair and unresponsive and caused state and local governments as well as the private sector to forfeit a significant amount of their jurisdictional liberty. Because of this, the Reagan Administration in 1981 proposed two block grants in health. One would consolidate 11 health service grants and the other 15 preventive health programs. This would allow state health authorities, within certain general guidelines, to make their own decisions regarding program emphases so that they would be more responsive to the needs of their citizens. While the Ninety-seventh Congress agreed in principle, its bill consolidated 21 grant programs (rather than 26) into four block grants as follows:

1. Alcohol, drug abuse, and mental health
2. Maternal and child health services
3. Primary care (Community Health Centers Program)
4. Preventive health

In addition, a number of other categoric aid programs were authorized.

The Department of Health and Human Services. In the years that followed the establishment of the Federal Security Agency in 1946, various federal health programs in addition to the Public Health Service were transferred to it. Most significant among these were the Children's Bureau and the Social and Rehabilitation Service from the Department of Labor, the Food and Drug Administration

from the Department of Agriculture, the National Office of Vital Statistics from the Department of Commerce, the health and medical functions of the Bureau of Indian Affairs from the Department of the Interior, and the Administration on Aging. Eventually, on April 11, 1953, Congress established a Department of Health, Education, and Welfare as part of President Eisenhower's reorganization of the Executive Branch of the government. The purpose was to bring into closer functional relationship and to improve the administration of the important health, education, welfare, and Social Security functions then being carried on by the federal government. Up to the present this plan has succeeded only partially; the functions, relations, and organization of the basic components have not yet meshed substantially toward a clearly defined and understood purpose or mission. This had led some to refer to the department as an enormous social welfare "holding company," a "bureaucratic maze" for which no effective guide exists or perhaps is even possible.

The Department of Health, Education, and Welfare therefore was not truly an administrative or functional unity. It consisted of units of different organization, expertise, and interests. Most units have strong traditions and histories that antedate the department considerably. Many have separate, strong, and effective congressional ties and public or professional constituencies and do not hesitate to use them unilaterally. Yet, there is a clear need for a more effective operational relationship among those working in the components of human services. Awareness of this, and the consequent chronic administrative frustration, is evidenced by the many reorganizations that have occurred during the past 2 decades.[12] In 1967 a cabinet-level post of Assistant Secretary for Health was established to coordinate and direct the health-related activities of the Department. Then, in 1977, the positions of Assistant Secretary for Health and the Surgeon General were brought together in one person, obviating finally the confusion that resulted from the existence of the two separate positions in two different individuals. More recently, in 1979, Education was removed and established as a separate Cabinet-level department. The remainder was retitled the Department of Health and Human Services (Fig. 8-3).

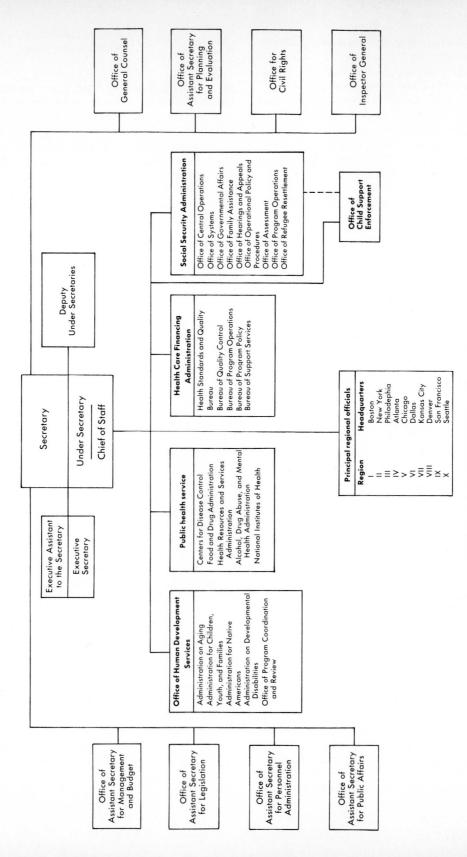

FIG. 8-3. Department of Health and Human Services.

Other federal agencies. The Department of Education is engaged in several activities related to health. It promotes programs of health education and school health and safety, engages in investigations relating to medical examination of school children and their teachers, promotes school lunch programs, and administers a grant-in-aid program for vocational education in health.

Several units of the Department of Agriculture engage in programs concerned with health. The Bureau of Animal Industry inquires into the cause, prevention, and treatment of diseases of domestic animals, which naturally have an influence on many phases of human health. Federal meat inspection services are administered by the Production and Marketing Administration, which also administers the Insecticide Act. The labor branch of this office finances medical care and health services for migrant farm workers. The Bureau of Dairy Industry is active in investigations and education relating to the sanitary production and handling of milk. The Bureau of Entomology and Plant Quarantine, although primarily concerned with the protection of crops from parasitic insects, necessarily contributes much knowledge and service to the control of insects affecting man. Active in research and service relating to foods, nutrition, and dietary habits is the Bureau of Human Nutrition and Home Economics, which with the agricultural extension service in cooperation with state land grant colleges has accomplished much in the improvement of rural health and nutrition.

In the Department of the Interior are several agencies with specialized interests in public health problems. The Bureau of Mines conducts an important health, sanitation, and safety program in relation to the mining and quarrying industries. In company with the Fish and Wildlife Service it is concerned with certain phases of the problem of stream pollution. The latter agency also contributes to health protection by promoting rodent control programs.

With the establishment of the Environmental Protection Agency at the end of 1970, most of the environmental health activities and responsibilities of the Public Health Service were transferred to it.

Federal agencies in international health affairs. Originally the interests of the U.S. Government in international health affairs were limited to measures designed to prevent the introduction of certain diseases. Developments in world history, economics, and methods of transportation, however, have made it necessary to adopt a broader viewpoint and to assume responsibilities of great significance to international public health. These newer responsibilities are of two types: first, participation in development of public health programs in other specific nations and, second, participation as one of a number of partners in the promotion of worldwide health. The most important federal agencies involved in these activities are the Office of International Health of the Public Health Service and the Agency for International Development of the Department of State.

The Office of International Health of the Public Health Service was established to coordinate and give general direction to all service activities in the international health field; to maintain liaison with agencies in this field; to represent the service in international health conferences; to direct a program of international exchange of health personnel and educational material; to draft sanitary conventions and regulations and reports required by international agreements; to collect and distribute data relating to foreign medical and health institutions; to supervise special health missions for foreign countries; to advise the Department of State regarding development of plans, programs, and policies for consideration by the World Health Organization and the Pan American Health Organization; and to advise the offices of the Secretary of Health and Human Services, and Surgeon General on international health matters. In relation to the foregoing, the United States government has representation in the World Health Organization, the Pan American Health Organization, and the Anglo-American Caribbean Commission.

The bilateral international health activities of the United States government are centered in the Agency for International Development of the Department of State. In the planning, staffing, and conduct of its health programs it relates not only to the Office of International Health of the Public Health Service but also to other significant parts of the United States government, to bilateral health assistance programs of other nations, and to any other official or nonofficial organizations concerned with health assistance to developing nations. Much of its work is carried out by means of contracts and other cooperative arrangements with state health departments, universities, schools of public health, and schools of medicine and professional associations or organizations.

REFERENCE

1. Jain, S.C.: Introduction and summary: role of state and local governments in relation to personal health services, Am. J. Public Health **71**(suppl.):5, Jan. 1981.
2. National Public Health Program Reporting System: Public health programs 1980, Washington, D.C., 1980, Association of State and Territorial Health Officials.
3. Tilson, H.H.: Intergovernmental relationships: more different, or more the same? Am. J. Public Health **71**:1103, Oct. 1981.
4. DeFriese, G.H., and others: The program implications of administrative relationships between local health departments and state and local government, Am. J. Public Health **71**:1109, Oct. 1981.
5. Miller, C.A., and others: A survey of local health departments and their directors, Am. J. Public Health **67**:931, Oct. 1977.
6. American Public Health Association: The role of official local health agencies, Am. J. Public Health **65**:189, Feb. 1975.
7. National Commission on Community Health Services: Health is a community affair, Cambridge, Mass., 1966, Harvard University Press.
8. National Commission on Community Health Services: Health administration and organization in the decade ahead, Cambridge, Mass., 1967, Harvard University Press.
9. Clarke, G.J.: The role of the states in the delivery of health services, Am. J. Public Health, **71**(suppl.):59, Jan. 1981.
10. The state health department: an official policy statement of the American Public Health Association, Am. J. Public Health **59**:160, Jan. 1969.
11. Brandt, E.N.: Block grants and the resurgence of federalism, Public Health Rep. **96**:495, Nov.-Dec. 1981.
12. Sims, L.B.: Organizational history of HSMHA, Health Serv. Rep. **88**:117, Feb. 1973.

CHAPTER 9

Voluntarism in public health

Defer not charities till death; for certainly, if a man weigh it rightly, he that doth so is rather liberal of another man's than of his own.

Francis Bacon

DEVELOPMENT OF THE MOVEMENT

While the official, governmental, or public health agencies were still in the process of development, a complementary and supplementary force appeared in the form of voluntary or nonofficial health agencies. These are supported by private funds or donations and are directed by individuals with varied educational and experiential backgrounds. They have no legal powers. Although not unique to the United States, they are especially numerous here, but that was not always the case. Until the late 1800s, organized charities were unpopular. According to Carter,[1] the New York *World* denounced the Red Cross in 1889 for helping the victims of the Johnstown, Pennsylvania flood, saying that the Red Cross had "introduced pauperism by giving out provisions and clothing to the more shiftless class," who desired only "to eat the bread of charity."

Early settlers in the United States were mostly white Protestants from England or western European nations, business-oriented people with no tradition of organized charity. Able-bodied people created wealth by farming, manufacturing, or trade, and if one thing failed, one could always migrate farther west and try again. Those who followed were either slaves, or later, people from eastern European traditions or other racial backgrounds. They were scarcely wanted, few in number, and of no great concern to the original residents and their descendents. Toward the end of the nineteenth century, however, spurred by rapid industrialization, immigrants began to play an increasingly important role. Their different traditions, often with backgrounds in socialism and late nineteenth century social protest, coupled with the spread of in-

vestigative reporting, reformism, and muckraking, changed the approach to welfarism dramatically. John D. Rockefeller, to change his image of imperial stinginess, established the Rockefeller Foundation with $100 million in 1913, making philanthropy more acceptable. The practice was repeated by Carnegie and Mellon and, by the time of the Great Depression, the private, voluntary health and welfare movement was well developed. By 1980, charitable giving for all purposes amounted to $47.8 billion.

The voluntary health movement began with the Anti-Tuberculosis Society of Philadelphia in 1892. Its development epitomizes the voluntary health movement as a whole. Encouraged by the formation of the local Philadelphia society, a group of unusually intelligent and enthusiastic private citizens banded together in 1904 to organize the National Association for the Study and Prevention of Tuberculosis. The membership of the group is worthy of special mention. It included Trudeau as president, William Osler, Bowditch, Bates, Janeway, Welch, Billings, Victor Vaughan, and other outstanding individuals. Among the six lay members of the board were Homer Folks, Samuel Gompers, and Edward T. Devine, who were most prominent in the development of social welfare in the United States. At that time tuberculosis caused 10% of all deaths and was the leading cause of destitution and orphanhood. From the beginning it was agreed that the control of tuberculosis should be a function of government, since voluntary funds could never hope to meet the total bill. It was recognized, however, that government action in a democracy does not necessarily precede or preclude public opinion and that both the public and the government needed to be educated. This the association believed it could do, and it proceeded with the eventual organization of 50 state associations and approximately 3,000 local affiliates.

At first the financing of the National Association for the Study and Prevention of Tuberculosis posed a difficult problem. It was temporarily solved by the Russell Sage Foundation, which assumed the responsibility for the 10 years from 1907 to 1917. Meanwhile, the Tuberculosis Christmas Seal idea had been developed in Denmark. This was considered an especially desirable fund-raising technique, since it gave individual citizens a personal interest in the fight against tuberculosis. The idea was quickly adopted in the United States, and by 1914 it provided the bulk of the funds, not only of the national but also of the state and local associations. The pattern of distribution of the proceeds was set from the beginning by the national association, which decided to assign most of the funds raised (95%) to the state and local associations while the national agency retained only 5%.

The National Society to Prevent Blindness was established in 1908, the Mental Health Association in 1909, the American Social Health Association in 1912, the American Cancer Society in 1913, the Maternity Center Association in 1918, and then, in rapid succession, the American Foundation for the Blind, The National Easter Seal Society for Crippled Children and Adults, and the Planned Parenthood Federation of America all in 1921. Current directories of national voluntary health organizations of all types include 1,200 to 1,500 references.[2,3]

NUMBER AND TYPE

Since the establishment of the Anti-Tuberculosis Society of Philadelphia in 1892, a confusing number of separate categoric voluntary health or disease-related agencies have been formed. They draw their support from literally millions of persons and serve millions of others in various ways. Not infrequently the development of these agencies has been related to certain strong and appealing personalities, such as Beers, Trudeau, Wald, and Franklin Roosevelt. One interesting aspect of their development is that although some agencies—such as the antituberculosis associations—began locally and spread upward to state and national levels, others—such as the National Foundation (origi-

nally the National Foundation for Infantile Paralysis)—began on the national level and spread downward. Still others, notably the mental hygiene associations, began on the state level and spread both upward and downward.

These agencies have been both effective and ineffective, efficient and inefficient, blessed and belittled, well and ill managed, intelligent and unreasonable, cooperative and uncooperative. These are only a few of the possible and inevitable outcomes of rapid development of a large number of independent undertakings. They have, however, one characteristic in common—they seldom die. Hochbaum[4] has summarized the all too typical sequence:

In a young organization, almost all its activities are geared to deal with the very objectives and purposes for which it was created—nothing matters as much as its self-avowed mission. Later, however, increasingly strong concerns develop to maintain and strengthen the organization for its own sake, to expand its activities, to stake out a scope of goals and activities, and to protect this domain against intrusion by other agencies.

In addition to paid employees, voluntary health agencies involve the time and often the money of at least 500,000 men and women who serve on boards or committees, as well as the time and effort of millions of other voluntary workers. According to the American Association of Fund-Raising Counsel, Inc., private philanthropy accounted for $4.4 billion in health expenditures for the year 1976. These figures exclude the American Red Cross, the large philanthropic foundations, industrial health services, and a large number of agencies that only incidentally furnish health services. The American Red Cross is in a class by itself; it had a peacetime membership of about 5 million people, which increased during World War II to 36 million people. There are about 4,000 chapters and 6,000 branches. During the 3½ years from the Pearl Harbor bombing to May 1945, contributions amounting to $654 million were raised. The American Red Cross is the only voluntary agency with quasi-official status; the President of the United States serves as its president, and the organization is regarded in effect as the official disaster relief agency of the nation.

As early as the close of World War I concern had developed about the growing number of fund-raising agencies. In 1918 the National Information Bureau that had been established laid down the following eight precepts to guide philanthropic agencies that might wish approval by that agency. So well were they stated that they have remained unchanged and useful ever since[5]:

1. Board—An active and responsible governing body (must maintain direction of the agency), serving without compensation, holding regular meetings, and with effective administrative control.
2. Purpose—A legitimate purpose with no avoidable duplication of the work of other sound organizations.
3. Program—Reasonable efficiency in program management, and reasonable adequacy of resources, both material and personnel.
4. Cooperation—Evidence of consultation and cooperation with established agencies in the same or related fields.
5. Ethical promotion—Ethical methods of publicity, promotion and solicitation of funds.
6. Fund-raising practice—In fund-raising:
   a. No payment of commissions for fund-raising.
   b. No mailing of unordered tickets or merchandise with a request for money in return.
   c. No general telephone solicitation of the public.
7. Audit—Annual audit, prepared by an independent certified public accountant or trust company, showing all income and disbursements, in reasonable detail. New organizations should provide a certified public accountant's statement that a proper financial system has been installed.
8. Budget—Detailed annual budget, translating program plans into financial terms.

Voluntary agencies concerned with health fall into several categories. Most important is a large group of agencies supported by citizen contributions and donations. These are divisible into the following four types, which demonstrate a remarkable degree of specialization:

1. Agencies that are concerned with specific diseases, for example, the American Cancer Society, the Cystic Fibrosis Foundation, the Epilepsy Foundation, The National Foundation, the American Social Hygiene Association (venereal diseases, narcotics, and alcoholism), the American Diabetes Association, and many more
2. Agencies that are concerned with certain organs or structures of the body, for example, the Eye-Bank Association of America, the National Kidney Foundation, the American Lung Association, the Association of Blood Banks, and the American Heart Association
3. Agencies that are concerned with the health and welfare of special groups in society, such as the National Council on Aging, the National Society for Autistic Children, the National Society for Crippled Children and Adults, and the National (black) Health Association
4. Agencies that are concerned with particular phases of health and welfare, for example, the National Safety Council and the Planned Parenthood Federation of America

The second large group of voluntary agencies engaged in health work is composed of foundations established and financed by private philanthropy. Prominent among these are the Rockefeller Foundation, the W.K. Kellogg Foundation, the Carnegie Foundation, the Commonwealth Fund, the Johnson Foundation, the Milbank Memorial Fund, the Mott Foundation, the Rosenwald Fund, and the Markle Foundation. Organizations of this type have functioned in a variety of ways, particularly by promoting and subsidizing local health departments, especially in rural areas, by supporting basic research and professional education, and by assisting in international health development.

The third main group of voluntary health agencies is made up of professional associations such as the American Public Health Association, the American Medical Association, the National League for Nursing, and their state and local affiliates. In addition to providing a meeting ground for professional workers in their respective fields, these associations do much to establish and improve standards and qualifications, encourage research, further health education, and promote programs.

Integrating or coordinating agencies such as community health councils and United Fund agencies constitute what may be considered a fourth group. Their purpose is the efficient funding and planning of the activities of the many specialized voluntary agencies.

A fifth group of nonofficial agencies that may be considered to have some interest in public health consists of an increasing number of commercial organizations that have found it worthwhile for one reason or another to participate in the health promotion programs. Notable among these are several large insurance companies that have carried out extensive and effective educational programs and demonstrations.

FUNCTIONS AND ACTIVITIES

The Gunn and Platt study and analysis[6] of voluntary health agencies listed eight basic functions of voluntary health agencies. These may be described briefly as follows.

Pioneering. Pioneering involves exploring or surveying for needs not being served and for new methods of dealing with needs already recognized.

Demonstration. Voluntary health agencies have rendered particularly significant service by carrying out or subsidizing experimental projects designed to demonstrate practical methods for improvement of public health and for the wider application of proved methods by official and other agencies. Projects have ranged from demonstration of the value of full-time local health departments, to home health care and delivery service, nutrition programs, and various planning and administrative procedures.

Education. Education is probably the single most important function of voluntary health agencies. In fact, it might be said that all other functions have education as their goal. Although activities in this field have been designed primarily for the public, many of the agencies have made provision for or have engaged in all types of professional training by means of fellowships, in-service training courses, and the maintenance or subsidization of field training areas.

Supplementation of official activities. With no legislative restrictions to encumber them, voluntary health agencies have frequently been able to assist official health agencies, which often have been unable to institute new programs because of political restrictions or public reservation. In such instances the voluntary agencies have played an important role by bridging the gap between currently accepted practice and more advanced scientific knowledge. Usually when this is done, the custom has been to provide assistance for a limited period of time, at the end of which the government is expected to carry on.

Guarding citizen interest in health. Voluntary health agencies, because of their nature, representation, and support, have often been in a position to guard the public interest, not only by promoting the official health program but also by defending it against political and other interference. By like token, they have sometimes found it necessary to subject official health agencies, programs, and officials to study and criticism. This can cause ill feeling, and some health officials have looked on voluntary agencies as presumptuous and interfering. Health departments, however, being official, tax-supported agencies, should expect to be subject to criticism by the citizenry and the various groups that represent them.

Promotion of health legislation. On every level of government there is a constant stream of proposed health legislation of concern to the public. A great source of strength in this regard can be the voluntary health agencies that are active and influential in the community. With a prime interest in health matters and representing large numbers of voting citizens, the opinions of these agencies carry much weight.

Planning and coordination. Group planning and coordination have been particular concerns of community health federations and councils and of health divisions of councils of social agencies. With the development of many voluntary agencies and the potential for overlapping and conflict, there is a need for coordination and collaboration among them. Beyond this is the need for coordination between the programs of the voluntary agencies and those of the official agencies in the community.

Development of well-balanced community health programs. The development of well-balanced community health programs is really the overall goal or result of the several foregoing purposes and functions. By protecting and promoting the official health department, by increasing the health consciousness of the community, and by providing funds and facilities where gaps exist, the voluntary health agency may make the difference between a mediocre community health program and one that is truly effective.

FINANCING

Important to the understanding and evaluation of voluntary health agencies is the manner in which they are financed. The professional associations are supported by membership dues, whereas the health activities of commercial agencies are usually financed by budgetary items designated for education or public relations. The philanthropic foundations, of course, owe their existence to large bequests from wealthy individuals. The large voluntary health agencies are supported by relatively small contributions or donations from large numbers of individuals. Several techniques have been developed by these organizations, each guarded jealously by whatever agency first devised and used them. Some of these techniques have been spectacularly successful, depending in many instances on emotional rather than intellectual appeal, carefully developed and conducted by promotional agencies that specialize in the business of fund raising.

The first and still one of the most successful methods is the Christmas Seal, previously referred to. As promoted for years, their cost of only a penny each appeared to be insignificant to most economic or social groups, most sales are in the form of several sheets of 100 each, and by now many millions of dollars are raised each year by the participation of millions of people. The fact that it is done represents at least a certain amount of educational impact on all groups in society, thereby making the fight against tuberculosis and other lung diseases truly a people's fight. An important additional incentive has been the identification of the Christmas Seal with Christmas greeting cards. This campaign has been so successful that several other agencies have adopted the technique, for example, the Easter Seal, inaugurated in 1934 by the National Society for Crippled Children and Adults.

Another effective technique was developed by the National Foundation for Infantile Paralysis. Associated with the name of Franklin Delano Roosevelt who was a polio victim, this foundation developed a custom of annual drives involving careful planning, organization, and promotional activities. For a number of years a gala ball to raise funds was held in the nation's capital, attended by many dignitaries. Similar events were held in cities, towns, and even small villages throughout the nation. Concurrently the public was deluged on the streets, in their homes, and in places of amusement such as theaters with requests for contributions to the March of Dimes. These techniques were amazingly fruitful and brought in large sums of money, most of which has been devoted to research, training, and education. The most spectacular contribution of the National Foundation for Infantile Paralysis was the sponsorship of the development of the Salk vaccine against poliomyelitis. In 1958 this organization changed its name to the National Foundation and expanded its scope of interest to include arthritis, birth defects, and disorders of the central nervous system.

Other methods used by various voluntary health agencies to raise funds include dues for nominal membership, the sale of educational literature, fees for services, personal solicitations, and direct mail appeal. Another innovation has been the use of radio or telethon programs, which has greatly benefited several voluntary health agencies. Certain of the techniques have caused considerable public resentment, particularly when pressure or embarrassment potentially enters into the appeal. Examples are the passage of contribution boxes in a lighted theater and the use of neighbors for personal door-to-door solicitation.

Recent years have seen an increasing trend toward consolidated fund-raising efforts. This is epitomized by the United Fund approach, begun in 1918, which, by major community effort, once each year raises funds for a large number of member organizations. At present there are several thousand United Fund agencies and Community Chests. The latter, unlike the United Fund agencies, primarily collect money only for local agencies. United Fund agencies allocate a certain proportion of the funds they raise to the United Health Foundations, Inc., which in turn supports a broad range of research and demonstration projects in universities, health departments, and other agencies. Some agencies refuse to affiliate with the United Fund, and inevitably new voluntary agencies appear; these add their special interest and separate appeals to that of the Community Chest or United Fund and allegedly create confusion. Recognition must be given to the natural wish of many people to contribute to one or a few causes in which they are personally interested rather than to what may appear as a large, vague, and indefinite fund.

United Fund drives are by no means universally endorsed. Their net effect has been to spread the base of giving among many low-paid employees, while corporate giving has declined as a percent of total charitable giving, amounting to only 5.3% of the total in 1980. Lower paid workers tend to give a greater percentage of their salary than do higher paid workers, and coercion of blue collar and clerical workers by fund drive organizers, supervisors, and personnel officers is common, frequently causing resentment. Many businesses find it useful to support the United Fund approach vigorously since, in addition to enabling a shift from corporate sources to employee giving, an active role may enhance the ability of the business to obtain favorable tax rulings, zoning changes, and traffic patterns from city councils. United campaigns set a target for fund raising for the area that is often derived politically, based on prior experience, rather than any real assessment of the community's needs. Since independent fund drives are vigorously discouraged by corporate leaders, the participating voluntary agencies may have little opportunity to acquaint the public with the real dimensions of specific problems.

An important consideration in connection with the fund-raising activities of voluntary health agencies is the cost of the fund raising and administration in contrast to actual public service. Attention was severely focused on this problem some years ago by the New York State Department of Social Welfare,[7] which reviewed the approximately 3,200 organizations that solicited public contributions for health, welfare, and educational purposes in that state.

They received a total of $324 million, of which about 13% was devoted to fund-raising costs. "Patriotic" and fraternal organizations raised $9 million, of which more than $5 million, or 57%, went for fund raising! When salaries, overhead, and other operating costs are added, sometimes there is little left for "charity." Fund raising *can* be profitable. Examples of extremes, however, should not be construed as condemning the many good organizations.

There does not appear to have been much improvement since then, but it is difficult to know what the figures actually mean. United Fund has fund raising as its principal business and necessarily has a different percent allocated to fund raising than might be the case for a service delivery agency. Some fund-raising campaigns, similar to political campaigns, may receive substantial support from participating businesses that can donate service rather than money yet obtain the same tax benefits. However, these "donations" do not show up as a fund-raising cost.

Hamlin,[8] as well as others, has called for the establishment of a uniform accounting system and a standard chart of accounts. Hamlin also emphasized that "it does not take over 100,000 voluntary agencies . . . to provide health and welfare services in the United States. A better job could be done by a smaller number and a greater joint effort. Fur-

thermore, it would then be simpler to provide for the new agencies which will be needed from time to time." Hamlin found the situation so confused and discouraging that he even urged the President of the United States to establish a permanent national commission on voluntary health and welfare agencies. However, there has been little evidence over the years to indicate any great interest in this on the part of the individual voluntary health agencies.

PHILANTHROPIC FOUNDATIONS

Philanthropic foundations have certain advantages over the voluntary agencies that depend on public donations. They can be more flexible and adaptive in their interests and activities, they are not directly accountable to the public, and they do not depend on repetitive fund-raising activities. There are about 26,000 private foundations in the United States with assets of more than $31 billion. Thirty-nine have assets of $100 million or more, and 133 have assets of $25 million to $100 million. These 172 foundations account for about one half of the total grant funds dispensed. In the past many foundations spent merely what their investments earned each year without regard to capital gains. The Tax Reform Act of 1969 changed this, and since 1975 the foundations must spend the equivalent of 6% of their total assets each year. About a third of the foundation grants are devoted to various aspects of health and welfare, usually for innovative purposes. Most of the large foundations now tend to emphasize studies and demonstrations of broad social consequence rather than large, expensive laboratory research projects. It should be noted that some of the smaller foundations have little if any active programs, and some obviously have been established for personal or familial tax-benefit purposes.

By contrast, some large foundations (and many not so large) have enviable records of efficient philanthropic management. Their essential purpose, which is to stimulate orderly human progress, requires intelligent management of their resources, and such organizations as the Robert Wood Johnson Foundation, the Rockefeller Foundation, and others have developed tough-minded approaches to the planning of social experiments and their evaluation. "Philanthropy is a complex process that is both an art and a science, and it must by necessity be creative."[9] Pointing to their wide involvement in all parts of the nation and throughout the world on matters of great social concern and urgency, Cunninggim[10] indicated that on balance, "tangibly and intangibly, foundations have done much of which they have cause to be proud." He concluded that at worst, some foundations may have been indiscreet or naive, but not wicked.

DESIRABLE AND UNDESIRABLE CHARACTERISTICS

It is apparent that voluntary health agencies have both desirable and undesirable features. On the favorable side is the fact that these agencies have developed as a result of spontaneous reaction by groups of citizens. Their leadership usually consists of devoted, intelligent, nonpartisan individuals. Generally, they have been established to meet a genuine and commonly felt need. Without question, public health in America could never have reached its present high level in the absence of the voluntary health agencies. They are unrestricted by statutory or program limitations or by partisan politics. Because they are so relatively unhampered, they can adapt their programs rather readily to changing needs and conditions, thereby often shortening the lag between the acquisition of new scientific knowledge and its application. They can be credited with much that has been accomplished in improved professional education, standardization of techniques and procedures, and research.

On the other hand, voluntary health agencies have certain undesirable features or disadvantages. Occasionally official health departments have had to conduct poorly balanced programs because of pressure from voluntary agencies. This may come about in two ways: A voluntary agency may exert pressure on the health department to overemphasize its particular interest or, contrariwise, some voluntary agencies have caused health departments to underemphasize certain programs because the voluntary agencies have wanted to monopolize activities in those fields. Such tactics may jeopardize appropriations for official health agencies. Similarly, despite the avowed purpose of leading the way until an activity is officially adopted, many voluntary agencies are reluctant to relinquish any parts of their programs. In fact, it is rare to find a voluntary agency closing up shop, as did the American Child Health Association when it had fulfilled its mission.

With the multiplicity of agencies, overlapping of function, high administrative costs, and growing confusion of the public are certain to result. This

is not surprising considering the frequent duplication of purpose and the multiplicity of appeals. Thus one still finds many communities in which several groups of nurses operate out of an equal number of agencies, visiting homes and working in clinics. Certain of the voluntary agencies do not accede to the policy of affiliating or even coordinating their activities with each other, much less with those of local official health organizations.

Finally, one of the most serious objections is that the public tends to contribute to the organization that makes the most emotional and persistent appeal and then believes that it has done its part toward the support of the entire public health program.

VOLUNTEERS IN SERVICE PROGRAMS

Volunteers are frequently used in public service programs. Some employed workers consider them to be a nuisance, whereas others think of them as an inexpensive way to expand services. Volunteers can add a great deal to virtually any public program, but their effective use requires skillful management by trained supervisors.

What makes people volunteer for work that others may see as a vocation? Such groups as the Association of Voluntary Action Scientists study voluntary action under a variety of circumstances. Sometimes called the study of altruism, experiments may involve stationing a car with a flat tire along the highway with a female participant standing by and looking helpless. Researchers conceal themselves and monitor the reactions of passing motorists. While the variables are numerous and difficult to control, Kemper[11] has reviewed the literature and concluded that about 20% of people will respond in a basic situation that requires their help but does not demand too much or expose them to danger. If manipulation is used, such as a direct verbal appeal for help, 40% of people exposed will respond with an altruistic voluntary action. When the elements of an emergency are present, the response rate increases to 60%.

People place themselves into volunteer service roles for a variety of reasons: sometimes out of commitment to the purpose of the organization such as the relatives of a suicide victim, sometimes as a way of receiving the experience and exposure needed to reenter the work force after a long hiatus in another role, sometimes for business purposes to establish a helpful image in a community for the new assistant vice president of a bank, sometimes as a way out of loneliness after being widowed or divorced, and sometimes simply as a way of filling a culturally acquired obligation to perform a community service. Occasionally the reasons are based in a personality disorder or a pattern of mental illness. Depending on the nature of the task, it may be extremely important for the organization to screen out certain kinds of motivations, such as the voyeur who wants to work for a suicide prevention organization where he or she will come into contact with disturbed people over the telephone. The best volunteer organizations are so successful in their recruitment and screening efforts that they are more difficult to get into than a regular employment situation.

Volunteers can be involved in virtually any task from sweeping floors to providing psychotherapy to psychotic children, depending on the abilities of the volunteers, the effort and skill of the organization, and the manager of the volunteer program. There are journals and organizations devoted to the subject. One thing is clear: volunteers can contribute many needed ingredients to the successful work of an organization often at a bargain price, but they are not inexpensive. It takes a real investment on the part of the organization to develop the roles, recruit people with a matching need to serve, and provide them with the work environment that can make their task effective and efficient. The purpose of the volunteer program may be to provide services without a large paid work force, to involve more people in the cause of the organization, to develop a stronger base for community advocacy, or to maintain flexibility in job descriptions and hours that may not be possible in a unionized or civil service job setting. Whatever the purpose, it should be made explicit to both the volunteers and the paid staff. Paid staff are often suspicious of the volunteer worker. They may fear job displacement or the motives of the volunteer. Some workers think that volunteers will only handle the glamorous jobs of the agency and will leave the staff worker with tedious tasks. Their stability over time is questioned as well as their motives. None of these fears need be true, nor need they hinder the effective incorporation of volunteers into the program. The program

or agency director should be clear about the reasons for wanting volunteer workers and should assign the volunteer program to someone who is committed to the purpose, knowledgable about volunteer work, or willing to learn.

Volunteers require both rewards for their efforts—genuine rewards of respect and support, not just symbolic awards—and the same discipline expected of others. They should and can be held accountable for the work they have agreed to do when they have agreed to do it, and they can and should be suspended or fired for the same reasons as a paid worker. They also should have the same appeal and grievance structure to protect them from supervisorial or agency abuse.

Volunteers may be demanding, but they offer many advantages in a variety of roles and for many purposes. However, the roles, purposes, and advantages should be explicit and clear and the program managers need to be genuine supporters of the effort, or it would be better not to get involved in the effort at all.

CURRENT TRENDS AND THE FUTURE

Nearly half a century ago, Marquette[12] called attention to three major developments that he considered were certain to have an important effect on the future of voluntary health agencies. First was the trend toward the allotment of federal funds under the Social Security Act to the Public Health Service and other governmental agencies for categoric attacks on important health problems such as venereal disease, tuberculosis, cancer, mental health, heart disease, and dental health. These allotments of federal funds intended for state and local as well as for national use were already making it possible for official health agencies to enter into territory previously occupied almost exclusively by the private health agency. The second development, which grew largely out of the National Health Conferences, was the increased appropriation of tax monies for hospital and medical services. Related to this was support for more governmental participation in public health, health education, mental health, the care of the mentally ill, the support of tuberculosis hospitals, facilities for convalescent care and rehabilitation, group hospitalization, and cash indemnity against sickness. A third development of great impact was the economic depression of the 1930s, followed by a trend toward higher taxes. Working together, these latter factors served to eliminate some large fortunes and to reduce somewhat the inclination of many people to contribute to what they increasingly considered to be governmental responsibilities.

In light of what has occurred since, Marquette's observations appear to have been generally accurate. Previously the respective traditional roles of governmental and voluntary health agencies were more clearly defined. Education, experimentation, demonstration, and the provision of direct personal services were regarded as the strengths and proper domain of voluntary agencies. The great expansion of governmental planning and financing of health programs of all types has brought about a shift in the traditional roles. Whereas the fundamental distinction between the freedom of the voluntary agency and the statutory requirements imposed on governmental agencies remains, that distinction is becoming increasingly hazy. Community sanctions tend increasingly to limit the freedom of action of voluntary agencies, while a plethora of special grants now provide governmental agencies with greater program flexibility. As a result, today there are many areas in which both types of agencies are in a position to render essentially the same types of services for the same kinds of individuals.

Related to such factors as the nation's economic growth, the population increase, changes in age distribution, and the remarkable mobility and urbanization of American society, several other developments have contributed to the shift from voluntarism to official agency action. Among these are (1) the spectacular advances in medical science, (2) a growing demand by the public for health services now possible as a result of these advances, (3) an affluent society that can and is increasingly willing to support these services through taxes, (4) a considerable improvement in the educational level of most citizens, and (5) the development of a national social philosophy that regards health as a fundamental human right to be guaranteed by the government. Added to this was the impact of mandated citizen participation in health planning, financing, and surveillance beginning in 1966 with health planning legislation.

The voluntary health agencies are now faced with the problem of reacting to these trends. Some have already accepted the policy that when a tax-supported agency develops to the point where it can take over the work, the private agency should vacate the field. To decide logically on a sound future course, these agencies would do well to subject themselves and their communities to careful scru-

tiny to reevaluate problems that do or may exist and their relationship to them in comparison with other, essentially governmental, sources of solution. Reevaluation is further indicated for bringing up to date the position occupied by the voluntary agency in the community and its relation to all other official and nonofficial organizations. Accordingly, many voluntary health agencies have established appraisal or evaluation committees. The United Fund agencies have played an important role in the encouragement of this procedure. In speaking of agency appraisal, the National Health Council has encouraged each voluntary health agency to establish[6]:

. . . machinery for the periodical appraisal of the agency, at intervals of perhaps five years, by qualified experts with wide knowledge of the field of activity as well as of agency and community organization. This is particularly needed in the swiftly changing trends that are ahead. Valuable as is self-analysis, the outside and objective approach reduces the likelihood that smugness or self-satisfaction will establish itself. Such an appraisal should consider (a) adequacy and effectiveness of program; (b) financial status and future; (c) cooperative relationships; (d) adequacy of staff and executive direction; and (e) future opportunities and functions. Properly planned and carried out with the full cooperation of board and staff, such an appraisal will be worth more than it costs. Funds should be set aside and gradually accumulated for such an accounting and future planning. No agency would think of omitting its yearly financial audit merely to save the cost. It is even more important to have an audit of the organization itself made at intervals in order to determine how wisely it expends its money.

In addition to the evaluations sponsored by voluntary agencies themselves, the past 20 years have seen the development of community-wide surveys performed by outside experts. Many of these have been sponsored by the combined fund-raising organizations with financial support coming from any one of several sources: the local community fund, the council of social agencies, private subsidies, or the local government itself.

The National Health Council has attempted to provide leadership to the voluntary health agencies in adapting to changing times. At the time of its organization in 1920 it was hailed as one of the most important steps taken in the field of public health up to that time. Its avowed goals included consolidation of funds and facilities; increased efficiency of action through joint planning, housing, and programming; and the provision of services and conferences conducive to evaluation. Its program has not been as successful as originally hoped—among other reasons, because of resistance by many agencies to the idea of unification for fear of loss of agency identification.

Several other steps worthy of mention have been taken to keep voluntary health agencies up to date and to increase their community value. For many years many agencies were directed by interested lay persons. At first they served without pay, but that policy was soon recognized as being administratively unsound. Increased employment of full-time agency directors led to a recognition of the need for some type of training. As a result, in-service training courses and other types of programs designed to fill the need have been established and conducted. In addition, many executives of these agencies now hold graduate degrees from accredited schools of public health or from other pertinent educational institutions. Increasingly such degrees have become requisites for employment.

That voluntary health agencies should find themselves in the position of having to give way here and tighten up there is neither surprising nor undesirable, nor do these trends necessarily indicate their approaching demise. As aptly stated by Marquette[12]:

There is really no occasion for leaders outside the tax supported health field to have any concern as to the continued importance of their work. It is rather a matter of elasticity and adjustment. Everybody in the public health field knows that so much remains to be done and that we fall so far short of using effectively the instruments that medical science has placed at our disposal for combating disease, that the combined public and volunteer health forces will be needed for years to come. It must all be properly integrated and the private agency must see the changing picture and be ready to modify its role.

However, as stated in the Hamlin report[8] "If the unstinting philanthropic spirit of the American people is to be translated into the greatest public good and their confidence in the agencies maintained, the structure and objectives of voluntary agencies should be reviewed and modernized." The study committee believed that five major steps were available to voluntary agencies:

1. Stronger voluntary agency leadership
2. Higher standards for local affiliates
3. Increased participation in organized planning
4. Better reporting of programs and accomplishments
5. Greater emphasis on research and the application of new knowledge

In the interest of objectivity, it must be observed that the need for increased attention to each of these five items applies equally to official health agencies. Furthermore, if voluntary and official health agencies not only both did these things but did them in concert, the health of the public would be the better for it. Both are needed. As far as the voluntary and philanthropic health agencies are concerned, many have commented that the importance to the imaginative and perhaps unorthodox investigator of another door to knock on for necessary assistance besides that of the government should not be underestimated. Viewing this from another vantage point, Mackintosh[13] has noted that "in the United Kingdom, as people stand and watch the vast changes in health and social work that have characterized the middle of the twentieth century, especially toward the 'Welfare State,' they sometimes wonder whether there is still a place for voluntary action. Excess of officialdom carries its own hazards, notably in the suppression of the individual and his independence."

With massive cutbacks in national support for human service programs during the early 1980s, President Reagan called on the private and voluntary sectors to take up the slack, to replace governmental bureaucracies with caring community organizations. It does seem that voluntary organizations have been squeezed into tighter boxes in recent years by official programs and official funding source requirements. They have shifted to a highly bureaucratic, grant-seeking stance. There are signs of a reinvigoration of a more pragmatic and practical voluntarism with self-help groups, insurance company–sponsored efforts to encourage economic development in slum areas, and coalitions of business and political leaders to regulate the health industry by economic pressure rather than governmental processes, but the entire effort cannot replace the huge amounts of federal money that have been withdrawn from social programs. With budget cuts of $35 billion in 1981 and more in subsequent years and an entire private charity budget of $47.8 billion in 1980, the capacity is just not there, but that should not detract anyone's attention from the need to reincorporate voluntarism into the fabric of public health.

REFERENCES

1. Carter, R.: The gentle legions, Garden City, N.Y., 1961, Doubleday & Co., Inc.
2. Wasserman, P., editor: Health organizations of the United States, Canada, and the world: a directory of voluntary associations, professional societies, and other groups concerned with health and related fields, ed. 5, Detroit, Mich., 1981, Gale Research Co.
3. Farley, L., and Farley, B., editors: 1980-81 National directory of health/medicine organizations, Bethesda, Md., 1980, Science and Health Publications, Inc.
4. Hochbaum, G.M.: Health agencies and the Tower of Babel, Public Health Rep. **80:**331, April 1965.
5. Lear, J.: The business of giving, Sat. Rev. **63,** Dec. 2, 1961.
6. Gunn, S.M., and Platt, P.S.: Voluntary health agencies: an interpretative study, New York, 1945, The Ronald Press Co.
7. Report of the charities registration bureau, Albany, 1958, New York State Department of Social Welfare.
8. Hamlin, R.H.: Voluntary health and welfare agencies in the United States, New York, 1961, Schoolmaster's Press.
9. Shaplen, R.: Toward the well-being of mankind: fifty years of the Rockefeller Foundation, Garden City, N.Y., 1964, Doubleday & Co., Inc.
10. Cunninggim, M.: Private money and public service, New York, 1972, McGraw-Hill Book Co.
11. Kemper, T.D.: Altruism and voluntary action. In Smith, D.H., and associates: Participation in social and political activities, San Francisco, 1980, Jossey-Bass, Inc.
12. Marquette, B.: Is the private health agency on the way out? Am. J. Public Health **29:**46, Jan. 1939.
13. Mackintosh, J.M.: Voluntary action in the British health services. In Galdstom, I., editor: Voluntary action and the state, New York, 1961, International Universities Press.

PART THREE

Management of public health programs

Management and *administration* are among the most misunderstood words in the lexicon of public service. To many citizens, they are synonymous with bureaucracy. To many elected officials, they mean the expenditure of money for something other than direct service to people. To the staff in a public agency, they often mean "those" people who are thought to be in a position to move obstacles either into the path of a good idea or out of the way. But no organization can get its work done effectively without skilled administrators, people who understand civil service systems and their purpose, collective bargaining, budget building, fiscal control, the politics and process of planning, and the necessity for good public relations.

A department of health is a public agency created to perform several types of public tasks. Its functions may be categorized as (1) provision of health leadership in the community; (2) service in clinics, labs, and even hospitals; (3) control of certain human activities such as the regulation of food service establishments, nursing homes, and people with tuberculosis; (4) education of the public about positive health behavior practices; and (5) protection of people, records, and the environment. To perform these tasks well requires more than skilled clinicians and technicians; it requires people who know how to organize the work of different parts into a whole, who know how to plan for the future, who know how to work with the most valuable resource in public health through effective personnel management and career development, who know how to properly safeguard the public trust in the monies appropriated and creatively use them to meet genuine community needs, and who know how to help the public understand the work and value of public health through education and thoughtful public relations efforts.

The administration of public health programs has changed greatly in recent years with the advent of more purposeful planning efforts, affirmative action programs, collective bargaining in many communities, increased attention paid to the involvement of citizens in the design of their own programs, more elaborate approaches to budgeting (such as zero-based budgeting and planning systems), and the general realization that all resources, including tax dollars, are scarce and becoming scarcer and have to be used judiciously.

The internal organization of many agencies has undergone constant experimental change; and administrative analysts, functioning first as consultants and then as employees of health agencies, have accelerated the development and acceptance of greatly improved procedures. These changes have also brought about better coordination of staff activities within organizations and, in addition, have resulted in greatly expanded interagency coordination. This, incidentally, has been one of the many factors involved in the expansion of national administrative power and influence at the expense of the states, and of the states at the expense of the local governmental units. During this same period, there has come about a more practical attitude toward the establishment of better management practices. Administrative and service responsibilities of health departments have expanded greatly. In this category are included responsibility for standards, construction, supervision, and sometimes operation of various health facilities. There has been a steady shift away from law enforcement by court action to administrative regulation, with a further, concurrent shift away from the use of laws and regulations for health promotion to the educational approach wherever possible. In the past decade there has been a countertrend toward aggressive court action in certain spheres as the natural adversity of relationships has become more ap-

parent, particularly in the area of pollution control
and health rights. Each of these changes has
placed additional emphasis on effective administration and has forced public health administrators
to accept a broader view of their responsibilities.
These changes and practices are discussed in the
following chapters.

CHAPTER 10

Managing organizations

In good administration, every decision should be made at the lowest possible level of command. Otherwise, there is little or no use for the creation of a pyramid of organization.

Lent D. Upson

PURPOSES OF ORGANIZATION

A popular cartoon shows two people slouched in easy chairs, feet up, with the legend "Next week, we've got to get organized." Whenever two or more people set out in pursuit of something, the effort has to be organized if it is to be successful and efficient. To administer such an effort involves organization of the parts, management of resources, and constant evolution of the policy and purpose that brought about the effort in the first place. The definition of an organization is the same as the definition of a system: a body of two or more people (or parts) engaged in the pursuit of common goals.[1] Management (some prefer *direction* or *administration*) consists of all "organizational activities that involve goal formation and accomplishment, performance appraisal, and the development of an operating philosophy that ensures the organization's survival within the social system."[2] An organization is an "open" system in that it interacts with its environment (other organizations and systems), is subject to disease and injury, and can benefit from skillful diagnosis and treatment. An organization is very much a human system, and the parts must be so related that appropriate consideration is paid to the needs and proclivities of humans.

GENERAL PRINCIPLES OF MANAGEMENT

Certain basic principles of management have been understood for a very long time. Without intending to intertwine religion and the state, it is worth reflecting on Moses' father-in-law's advice:

... the people stood about Moses from the morning unto the evening. And when Moses' father-in-law saw all that he did ... he said: "... why sittest thou thyself alone, and all the people stand about thee from morning unto even?" And Moses said unto his father-in-law: "... when they have a matter, it cometh unto me; and I judge between a man and his neighbor ..." And Moses' father-in-law said unto him: "The thing that thou doest is not good. Thou wilt surely wear away, both thou, and this people that is with thee; for the thing is too heavy for thee; thou art not able to perform it thyself alone. Hearken now unto my voice, I will give thee counsel: ... thou shalt teach them the statutes and the laws, and thou shalt show them the way wherein they must walk, and the work that they must do. Moreover thou shalt provide out of all the people able men ... men of truth, hating unjust gain; and place such over them, to be rulers of thousands, rulers of hundreds, rulers of fifties and rulers of tens. And let them judge the people at all seasons; and it shall be that every great matter they shall bring unto thee, but every small matter they shall judge themselves; so shall they make it easier for thee and bear the burden with thee. (Exodus 18:13-22)

An organization can be as small as two or three people or as large and complex as the U.S. Department of Health and Human Services, but the basic principles remain the same: there has to be a purpose, an ability to carry out that purpose, some means of knowing if that is being done, and some means of deciding what action to take. This process is similar for any living organism. Mintzberg,[3] in one of the best current books on organization, states "The structure of an organization can be defined simply as the total of the ways in which it divides its labor into distinct tasks and then achieves coordination among them." Mintzberg's diagram (Fig. 10-1) has five parts: a strategic apex, a middle line, the operating core, and the

171

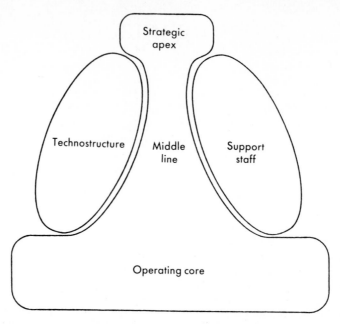

FIG. 10-1. Mintzberg's diagram of an organization. (From Mintzberg, H.: The structuring of organizations: a synthesis of research, 1979. Reprinted by permission of Prentice-Hall, Inc., Englewood Cliffs, New Jersey.)

technostructure and support staff, which sit on either side of the middle line. The strategic apex includes the top policy makers of an organization as well as the chief executive. These functions may be separated into a board of directors and a chief executive officer or merged into one person, depending on the size of the organization, the environment in which the organization operates, and the idiosyncrasies of the people who designed the organization. The operating core includes the people who perform the real work of the organization, such as nurses, practicing physicians, engineers, and sanitarians. The middle line includes the managers and line supervisors who supervise the work of the major divisions of the organization, often with considerable latitude. Mintzberg makes an important distinction between the support staff, which may include clerical workers, data processing personnel, cafeteria staff, and maintenance personnel, and the technostructure, which consists of analysts and planners who seek ways to organize and standardize the work of the organization. The technostructure is growing in size and significance in public health organizations. The five-part structure developed by Mintzberg is fluid and serves well to illustrate the malleability of what were once described as rigid principles of organization. It is a "scalar" structure (see Fig. 10-2) with an apex, a line of command or supervision, and a work force, with each box on the chart (or each bureau) responsible to one person above in the chain of command.

Mintzberg has also identified five coordinating mechanisms within the organization:

1. The process of mutual adjustment by and between people
2. The direct supervision of one or more people by a designated supervisor
3. The standardization of work processes, such as typing
4. The standardization of work outputs, such as the management of patients who have been discharged from a state mental hospital
5. The standardization of worker skills, such as the employment of licensed personnel.

The three standardizing mechanisms require and allow varying degrees of control by the analysts in the technostructure.

Max Weber is usually held accountable for the invention of the term *bureaucracy*.[4] His influence on the organization of governmental agencies has been strong, but in the last 2 decades, the inflexibility of the bureaucracy has increasingly yielded to the heterogeneous pressures of environment, purpose, and personality. Mintzberg[3] has described five forms: the simple structure, the machine bureaucracy, the professional bureaucracy, divisionalization, and adhocracy.

Simple structures are usually small, centralized in control, and young. They are rarely found in government since they are characteristically entrepreneurial and lack the complex patterns of accountability to elected officials, boards, and legislative bodies, which are a ubiquitous part of the governmental process.

Machine bureaucracies depend on standardization of process for coordination and are characteristic of large, old organizations with a fairly well-understood product. Many regulatory bodies are typical machine bureaucracies, and the style is characteristic of some environmental health agencies, which depend on inspections and rules to carry out their purpose.

The *professional bureaucracy* is a common concept in health agencies. The professional is in essence a standardized worker who has acquired skills, indoctrination, and socialization from the tradition and practice of professional organizations and academic training centers external to the bureaucracy. As such the professional worker, who cannot take the time to develop individualized treatment programs for each situation, usually tries to define a problem by placing it into a familiar diagnostic category so that a regimen of treatment can be used. For example, there are certain approved procedures for the diagnosis and treatment of tuberculosis and, although the worker has substantial independence to make judgments about which diagnosis and treatment to select, both are well categorized and the exercise of judgment is usually limited to the selection process. Health organizations have a difficult time organizing and coordinating the work of professionals, who wish to work independently, and the analysts, who try to standardize and coordinate the work of the organization, either for the presumed efficiencies that come with standardization or to satisfy some requirement for accounting for the work of the organization. The two often engage in a struggle for control that can result in oppressive burdens of paper work and activity reporting. In a sense, the professional bureaucracy decentralizes control to the individual worker, but the need for managers and analysts to standardize work, either to establish control or to respond to real or perceived requirements for upward accountability, confronts the organization with a constant conflict.

Divisionalized organizations are not common in the public sector. Although public health organizations are commonly compartmentalized into operating divisions, these are not autonomous organizations and cannot be dissolved or devolved by the agency director or the governing body without legislative approval.

Adhocracies have become the most popular concept in organizational theory in recent years. Originating in the fast-changing world of the National Aeronautics and Space Administration, adhocracies avoid standardization because of their need to diverge from established ways of doing things to solve new problems. Experts have a home base in units of similar experts and are extracted from the home unit and grouped together in interdisciplinary teams to work on specific problems or projects. These are known as matrix organizations, since workers may be part of two organizations at the same time, defying one of the classic principles of organizational theory. For example, the nurse may be a member of the nursing unit but may be placed on a committee with specialists from nutrition, social work, data processing, and health education to develop a nutrition strategy for pregnant teenagers. The style of the adhocracy may appear more stimulating and less contentious than the professional bureaucracy, but matrix organizations purchase their creativity at high cost. They practically double the number of managers needed to get the work done and they must not only tolerate diversity but protect it. It is difficult to nurture diversity in the public sector.

Most public health organizations have a variety of structural styles operating at any one time. The vital statistics office may function effectively as a simple structure. Its basic purpose is not the analysis of data, but the ministerial function of collecting it, cataloging it, safeguarding it, and providing people with necessary documents. The laboratory may work well as a machine bureaucracy with each technician following a carefully prescribed set of procedures. The pediatric clinic can function fairly efficiently as a professional bureaucracy and gets into real trouble only when managers attempt to erode the scope of professional judgment by task analysis and rigid job specifications. When it becomes necessary to look at the possibility of a genetic screening program for Tay-Sachs disease, staff from the vital statistics office, the laboratory, and the pediatrics clinic as well as others may be drawn together into an ad hoc task group to assess the size of the problem and consider intervention strategies.

Important to any organizational structure are the liaison devices described by Galbraith.[5] Liaison, an essential activity in coordinating the work of an organization, is accomplished by (1) direct contact between managers, (2) appointed liaison workers who have a communication function but no explicit authority to force coordination, (3) task forces, teams, or committees that involve the necessary managers but lack the authority to do more than recommend, (4) appointed managers who have some control over resources but still must rely heavily on negotiation to coordinate work, and (5) matrix organizations that adopt adhocracy as a work process. There is an apparent increase in the complexity and the cost of the liaison process moving from the first process to the fifth, but the cost and complexity may be a necessary price to pay for the work that has to be done.

It is apparent that many variables enter into the design of any organization: its size, its age, its mission, its enabling legislation, the nature of its work, the training and indoctrination of its workers, the nature of the problem with which it is working, and very importantly, the external environment. No one style, process, or structure can be prescribed as best for any organization, purpose, or environment. What does seem to be important is consistency in the design. A centralized chain of command would be inconsistent in a professional bureaucracy with coordination functions served through personal contact between managers, as would a matrix structure in a stable external environment with a consistent demand for an established service. Both would court disaster. The principle to be derived from this is that the design and management of an organization have to evolve from a continuing attempt to define its purpose, its environment, and

the nature of its human resources. Unlike a private sector enterprise, which can change its purpose, its structure, or even its resources to fit its need to increase or preserve profits, the public health agency must make many adaptive adjustments to achieve consistency in design. In fact, structural consistency is virtually impossible in most public agencies, given the diversity of expectations and requirements that make up their environments. This emphasizes that top managers need to be able to use adhocracy in their own environment even though it may be an inappropriate structure and style for the operating core of the agency.

Authority in an organization derives from the position of the office or job in the organization chart. Power, which is the ability to exercise that authority, derives from the personal influence the incumbent has over the work of others. In large organizations the gap between authority (the right to make a decision) and power (the ability to execute it) appears to be growing. Balance is important. It is easy for a strong leader to draw power away from the second-level managers, and an ineffectual leader may allow imbalance to occur by letting too much power drift into second- or even third-level management circles. If the health director establishes a strong office with powerful assistants and overdirects the program managers, the latter will either fight against such intrusions, leave the organization because they cannot achieve the professional satisfaction they need, or become passive and fail to provide the kind of technical and goal-oriented leadership needed. On the other hand, a director can allow authority to devolve too casually to second- or third-level managers who may not have the experience or the resources to handle it. If the missions and policies of the organization have not been debated and clarified, a spin-off of authority can lead to a power imbalance, resulting in poorly articulated programs and a confusing portrayal of policy to the public and to the personnel of the agency.

Participatory management has become very popular in recent years, with a number of industry success stories involving such diverse products as cars and dog food. In some cases, a small production team is formed, elects its own leader, and even manages its own employment. The team may determine its own work schedule and will prosper or flounder depending on the quantity and quality of its output. The design has interested workers in public health agencies, where concepts of professionalism and autonomy are characteristic of many of the personnel. However, although proprietary and private nonprofit health agencies may be able to function in less traditional modes, public agencies have accountability requirements that may make democratic management impossible. Usually the director of a public health agency is responsible directly or indirectly to elected officials who are accountable to the public in a very direct way. Program managers or staff who feel that they are accountable to their clients and who resist reasonable direction are in danger of becoming unaccountable. The public does not elect public health nurses or social workers and cannot effectively express dissatisfaction with a particular worker or manager by not patronizing the program or the agency. The public can insist, however, that the elected representatives see to it that civil servants carry out public policy in an acceptable manner. It is ironic that a line of direct accountability to the public and the lack of a profit motive may mean that public agencies cannot embrace participatory management styles as fully as can private sector enterprises.

The chief executive officer of a large private company must satisfy several constituencies: the board of directors, the employees, and the customers. As the organization matures and attains stability, the director becomes a satisficer rather than a maximizer in an effort to keep each group sufficiently satisfied that the organization can survive. The risk taking that went with maximization of one purpose in the creation of the enterprise is often muted, and the achievement of stability becomes a preeminent objective of the director. Public health directors have the same problem with the addition of an entailed clientele (private physicians, hospital boards, and other groups who often have in mind a specific role for the organization) that may exercise considerable control over the work of the agency either through political influence or through service on a board that sets policy for the health agency. Most organizations, just like organisms, react to challenge or the threat of injury defensively. The instinct is to preserve and stabilize by the elaboration of policy. Over time, the organization becomes encumbered by policies and reflexes, just as a living organism develops a plethora of immune response mechanisms and defensive reflexes. The isolated incident or criticism is seen as a sign that something may be wrong not with the organization but with its clients or its governing body, and the reaction is systemic. In a long-term care institution, if a patient becomes disturbed in the middle of the night and rips the sinks from the wall of the bathroom, the staff and managers are likely to pronounce a new policy: "Bathrooms will be locked after 9 PM; patients who need to use the bathroom after this hour should go to the nursing station." The incident should provoke some thoughtful inquiry into how people react to long-term institutionalization and the anomie that often sets in, but policy formation is easier and places the blame on the patient, not the system. After years of reaction, most bureaucracies become so encumbered with such an armor plating of policies that they cannot move. The final drama is public attack, a new administrator, and reorganization, followed by repetition of the process of bureaucratization. Shonick and Price[6] have described reorganization as one of the public agency's responses to stress. It is often wasteful and enervating. It might be possible to examine the process more carefully and design institutional barriers to bureaucratization. Advisory boards and consumer-controlled governing boards have been used in this manner, but the results have not been completely satisfactory. More research is needed to make public institutions more accountable and responsive without making them less efficient.

LEVELS OF ORGANIZATION

The legislative branch of government determines the areas in which a public agency must act and the boundaries limiting that action. The details of policy are usually delegated to a board or to a chief executive officer who is charged with the development of necessary rules to carry out the broad purpose of the law. The actions of the legislature, the board, and the chief executive officer are, of course, subject to adjudication by the courts.

Boards

Most agencies of state and local government are directly responsible to the chief executive. Schools and health departments are common exceptions. Boards of health were created for one or two reasons: the employed workers lacked expertise and needed the direction of competent citizens, and public health programs were thought to be too important to be vulnerable to the vicissitudes of electoral politics and the board was inserted between directly elected officials and the health department to protect the latter from the former. Although the continued existence of such boards is rarely questioned, circumstances and concepts have changed. Most well-organized health agencies have little need for volunteer advisors in professional and technical matters, and when they do need such assistance it usually can be obtained from another agency of government. As to political interference with public health, the contrary criticism has been heard more often since the 1960s. Health departments and boards of health have been attacked for their alleged unresponsiveness to community wishes and needs, and elected officials have expressed frustration with the independence of such boards and officials who do not have the same degree of direct accountability to the public.

In the early 1970s, Gossert and Miller[7] found that 40 states had policy-making health boards (4 states were without boards entirely and 6 had advisory boards) and that consumers occupied 12.5% of the 433 positions on the boards. By 1980, Gilbert, Moos, and Miller[8] found only 27 states with a policy-making board. Since 1900, all 50 state health agencies have been reorganized by statute at least once. Ten were the subject of new statutes between 1961 and 1970, and 23 were reorganized between 1971 and 1980. In those 23 reorganizations, 13 resulted in the disestablishment of a policy-making board of health. Of those that remained, 80% of the members were men and 90% were white. Consumers held 29% of the positions, and physicians and dentists held 40%. Overall, state health agencies were placed more closely under the control of the governors. The continued dominance of physicians raises questions about conflicts of interest, since most state health departments have some regulatory or licensure functions relating to the practice of medicine. Most boards do not reflect the population of the community.

The average size of the state boards of health found in the study by Gossert and Miller was nine members. These are usually appointed by the board of supervisors, the mayor, or the governor for overlapping terms. In several states the appointment must be made from a list of nominees submitted to the governor by the state medical association, and in Alabama the board is the state medical association. No recent surveys of local boards of health have been reported, but their structure is generally the same as that of the state boards.

At the local level concerned citizens have begun to question the continued dominance of the medical profession and other providers on boards of health. Before boards are restructured, their role needs to be defined. In some attempts to do this, board members have listed as many as 17 different functions, including provision of technical expertise, the watchdog function, provision of consumer feedback, education of the community, fund raising, program and agency protection from real or imagined threats of elected leaders, a hearing panel for complaints, development and analysis of health-related legislation, promulgation of regulations, and a forum for public debate and deliberation. Members selected for one of these purposes may be ineffective for another, and it would be impossible for any one member to be useful for all of the suggested purposes. If the board members and those who appoint them are unclear about the purpose of the board's role, confusion will ensue, resulting in either constant fighting or lethargy and inattention. The purpose of the board has to be thoughtfully defined, and the number of different purposes should be limited so that a small number of members can accomplish them with a reasonable degree of success.

Perhaps the most important role for boards of health, exclusive of their responsibility for developing necessary regulations, is to expand the deliberative capacity of local government. Unlike the federal government and most state governments, local governments have little if any capacity to conduct a full deliberation of public policy issues. They usually combine legislative and executive functions as well as some judicial functions in a board that serves more as a board of directors than a legislative body. Moreover, they must consider issues relating to public welfare, transportation, highways, hospitals, garbage, taxes, zoning, health, recreation, and law enforcement without a committee structure or enough staff to assist them in studying the issues. They often have to rely on brief interactions with agency directors and interested citizens and then arrive at a decision or postpone it until some external event forces a decision. A board of health specifically organized and composed for this purpose could provide the community with the opportunity for expanded deliberation of public issues; after analysis of the debate and distillation of the points raised, such a board could provide the elected officials with a better sense of the community's needs and expectations. In addition, the process could take much of the heat of debate out of the council chambers and into the community, where full and sometimes angry expression of opinions may do more good.

Conflict between the board members and the executive officer may develop in several ways. The executive officer, either because of dogmatic personal forcefulness or preoccupation with daily work, may ignore the board. If the board and its traditions are weak, the health director may get away with it. On the other hand, there may be one or more particularly active and forceful board members who, because of enthusiasm or a wish to express power and influence, may step beyond their prerogatives and attempt to enter the field of operations. In addition to these situations, there is the type of executive who because of personal weakness or of particular confidence in the board may try to pass responsibilities to it. The ideal relationship between an executive officer and a board is a delicate one wherein both parties must be constantly alert to their own responsibilities and prerogatives and those of the other party. The field of operation belongs to the administrative or executive officer, who in turn must respect the functions and responsibilities of the board by keeping them informed, asking their advice, and including them in planning.

Most communities also have one or more community mental health center boards and may have a state-mandated board for mental health services as well as alcoholism programs, drug abuse programs, services for the developmentally disabled, and other groups. There may also be a health planning council. Federal and state governments have required such a proliferation of advisory and governing boards in recent years that the communities to be served have become confused and tired. Membership requirements are usually different enough to preclude combining or merging boards, even if the various constituencies would tolerate such a move. Unless a local board of health can be thoughtfully designed and appointed, it may isolate the health agency director from other more aggressive and even more important boards. State and federal laws that stand in the way of developing constructive linkages and networks of citizen boards should be amended, and health agency ad-

ministrators and their boards should exert considerable effort to integrate and coordinate the work of the various boards.

Advisory committees

Advisory committees are formed for one or more of three reasons: (1) because the board of health or the health director needs technical advice in certain areas, (2) because not enough interested groups can be accommodated through appointment to the board of health, or (3) because the principal legislative or executive body of the jurisdiction does not want a board of health between itself and the health department but cannot afford to deny citizen input and oversight altogether. Often these committees are required by federal or state legislation, although the trend in recent years has been to insist that such groups have some real governing authority over the program. They may be advisory to the board, the chief executive officer, or a program manager.

Advisory committess are of two general types— constituent and technical. Members of constituent advisory committees may be chosen for their personal qualifications or because they represent social, professional, client, or other groups in the community. The chief advantage and use of constituent advisory committees is as a channel through which the community, on the one hand, and the health department, on the other, are kept aware of each other's thoughts, plans, and actions. Members of technical advisory committees assist the administrative officers of the public health agency in the formulation of plans and in the development and application of various techniques of value in the public health program.

Advisory committees have no direct power but can exert considerable influence, either through the quality of their advice or their political pressure, or both. When they are seen as an irrelevant nuisance by the health director and treated as such, they become useless at best and dangerous at worst. Kept from participation, an energetic advisory board will forcefully intrude on the operational domain. Although these groups have sometimes been created capriciously by federal or state law or regulation, they should always by taken seriously. Membership should be carefully developed, not to assure homogeneity but to assure that responsible and thoughtful members become involved. Providing effective staff support and liaison to the advisory group are not skills that can be assumed casually. They require thought and training. The relationship is an important one because the advisory committee may have considerable influence over what can and cannot be done. When a health director asks for advice from a group of citizens, willingness and ability to accept that advice are important attributes.

Administration

Most organizations are hierarchical in nature and structure with the chief executive officer at the apex. In public health agencies the chief executive officer is the health officer or director of health. The director is responsible for carrying out the mission of the organization, usually expressed in statutory language, and has three functions: political leadership, management of the agency's resources, and ceremonial representation. The inherent politics of the role are often denigrated, yet any position that involves the development of a pattern of action emanating from an ideologic base in an often vaguely worded statute is a political position. The director has the opportunity to emphasize, to obscure, to create, and to resist—in short, to direct.

The importance of the ceremonial mission is often overlooked. Those who seek power as a goal may be disappointed with the perquisites of position, but those who acquire it by pursuing the goals of public health may be surprised at the status accorded the position. To most people in the jurisdiction served, the position is an important one and is treated with respect and trust. The presence of the health director at community functions may occasionally expose him or her to real anger and frustration, but even that is an indication of the expectations of the community.

The director's position differs in other ways from that of the staff of the agency. Although most workers are employed by the civil service system, the director often is appointed either by the elected executive or by a board and may be fired just as easily. The director of a public health agency occupies a position whose functions are often specified in statute, whereas the staff works with job specifications developed by the civil service system. In the private sector, a chief executive officer can usually do anything that is not prohibited by law or forbidden by policies of the board. The public sector manager can do only those things permitted or required in the governing statute.

Whether continuing in office or starting out in a new position, the director should do three things: (1) read and know the law because it describes what is supposed to be done and to some extent how it is to be done, (2) study the needs of the community because they may not be the same as what the law allows and requires, and (3) evaluate the resources available because they indicate what can actually be done. Review of the statutes may take the director into several different code books and reveal a number of functions that are not being served. Some laws were passed without real legislative intent to implement them and without any appropriation to make implementation possible. Sometimes the agency and its director have decided to ignore or postpone implementation of the law. It is important for the director to find out what happened and why and to ascertain just what legislative leaders know about the situation and what they may want to have done. Some activities of the agency may not be identified in the law and a similar search for reasons is important. If the activity is important but subject to contest, such as a regulatory action, it would be well for the director to explore the possibility of obtaining specific legislation to support the need.

Examining a community's needs has become so fashionable as to have its own jargon: *needs assessment*. This is sometimes a code phrase for unfocused data that are collected while people try to figure out what to do. Important data sources should be identified and studied. This includes data from the census on housing, living conditions, and socioeconomic status; vital statistics data, which can reveal differences between the jurisdiction and the nation; welfare data, which can pinpoint the areas with a high concentration of frail elderly people, women with dependent children, and disabled individuals; and health services data, which have been assembled since 1966 in most communities by health planning bodies. The review of such data by people trained in public health and epidemiology can do much to define the real needs of the community. The results should be compared with the statutory specifications of purpose, and the gaps will identify the major areas of work and planning in the years ahead.

Finally, having identified what is allowed, required, and needed, the director has to measure the resources available both in the agency and elsewhere in the community. They will rarely be sufficient to meet either the needs or the requirements, and that realization forces the process of setting priorities—one of the most important tasks for any public health agency director. (Some of the techniques for doing this are described in the chapter on planning and evaluation.)

Before considering the organization of resources, it would be useful to reflect on the nature of the administrator. Historically the public health officer or director has been a physician de jure, if not de facto, (in law, if not in fact). Since it was usually impossible for economic reasons to employ a physician full time for such purposes in most local health departments, the law allowed part-time appointments or the appointment of a state health department physician as the local health officer of several counties. In the early 1970s the Health Officer's Section of the American Public Health Association changed its name to the Health Administration Section. This reflected the growing number of graduates from programs in health administration and the trend toward allowing nonphysician health officers to be appointed at both the state and the local level. By 1978, only 21 states required that local health officers be physicians, and nonphysicians filled about one third of all local health department director positions.[9] Miller and associates[10] found that two thirds of the local health directors were physicians but only 23% had both a physician's degree and a master's degree in public health.

The consolidation of health agencies with other human resources agencies at the state level, such as welfare, probation, and social services, has resulted in new, cabinet-level secretaries being appointed with more ecumenical and more overtly political backgrounds, although there is usually a physician somewhere in the agency who heads the frankly public health part of the organization. Wright and Dometrius[11] concluded that although state-level health directors were still generally white male physicians, the trend toward women and nonwhites was measurable. They also noted a younger group of leaders who saw themselves as more independent of traditional professional ties as well as electoral politics and who had had more business and public administration training.

Before 1935, physicians with training in public health were the exception as health officers. This is still true, but in most of the large urban health departments as well as state agencies, the directors are more often physicians with postgraduate training in public health. Not many of them set out to be health officers. Most physicians have found themselves in the situation by happenstance and have acquired the training on the job and through later enrollment in a school of public health. Many began in public health clinics or in tuberculosis, venereal diseases, epidemiology, or maternal and child health programs, functioning as clinicians. The traditional pattern of making the physician the head of the "team" meant the gradual assumption of administrative duties, often followed by more formal assignment of such tasks. Since there are usually few physicians to fill such roles, when vacancies occur the board of health or the mayor or governor often assumes that a physician is required, and the transition from part-time employed clinician to public health director is made. The transition is one of position, not capabilities, however. Medical school is a poor place to learn how to be an effective administrator: the orientation is toward individual autonomy and decision making. The work of such professionals is standardized, and efficiency depends on the ability to classify problems and apply standard solutions; the urge to solve problems by diverging from accepted norms is necessary in administration but not a characteristic of the clinical professions. When teamwork is involved, the physician is usually in a fairly autocratic position. These are not the circumstances that characterize the job of public health administration. Some physicians have made the transition well, but that has been a function of their personal characteristics, not of their training as physicians.

In the last 20 years, many local legislative bodies have become aware of the complexities of public health administration and the cost of medical care, particularly if they are responsible for a public hospital. It is difficult to disagree with a physician or any other professional, particularly in a public setting, which has made it doubly difficult for such general purpose legislative bodies at the local level

Management of public
health programs

to treat the public health programs and more especially the budget with the same scrutiny and inquiry they accord to the sheriff, the engineer, the librarian, or the welfare worker. Faced with rising costs and demands and the professional mystique of the physician, local elected officials have turned to more business-oriented directors. The professional public health administrator is a relatively recent but gradually more common leader in city and county health agencies.

Leadership is a popular but poorly understood concept. How does someone lead? Partly by position, which conveys authority, but the power to use that authority constructively comes from less objective assets. It is clear that an effective leader has to have a good grasp of the purpose and the methods of the organization being led. Beyond that, training in administration is a major asset. Both in the private and in the public sector, boards are looking for people who are comfortable with accounting terminology, are at ease with computers, understand (without being overly fascinated by) cost-effectiveness studies, and know enough about personnel administration to keep the agency and the elected leaders out of court. Most important of all, given the basic knowledge to use the agency's resources intelligently, is the leader's use of power. Power is the ability to get things done. The ability to get things done has much to do with productivity. Workers are more productive when they can exert more control over their environment, when they can, as individuals or as a group, bring enough of the tasks together to be able to carry out a whole task, not just an isolated piece of it. A supervisor or agency director becomes more powerful by devolving rather than accreting power, since productivity is increased. In short, a leader can only acquire the power needed to lead by learning how to devolve it to others. This is not simply the process of delegation—the location of the decision-making authority at the lowest level in the organization at which a decision can be made—but the development of strong program leaders who can enter into contest with the agency director and each other for the expression of ideas and their implementation. It requires an individual who is secure in knowing what is being done rather than doing it all personally. It requires much hard work, but basically it depends on training, personality, and experience.

THE SCALAR PRINCIPLE

The term *scalar principle,* referred to in the preceding discussion of the general principles of management, consists of the administrative arrangement of the functional groups or units in steps as in a scale (Fig. 10-2). Each of the steps, usually referred to as divisions or sections, is determined usually on the basis of purpose, discipline, or function, such as water control, family planning, or nursing. The confusion from different terminologies is somewhat unfortunate; *department, division, bureau, service,* and *office* often are used interchangeably if not haphazardly in the structural plans of many organizations. Actually it matters relatively little how the terms are used as long as they are used in a consistent manner and are understood by those involved.

The fundamental concept of the scalar principle is unity of command, with lines of authority and responsibility in which every individual in the organization is directly responsible to only one superior and through that person ultimately answerable to the head of the organization. As mentioned earlier, the rigidity of this concept is weakening. In theory, all intra-agency communications and actions are supposed to follow these lines and should never cross them. Each superior block in the organizational chart can serve as a filter for information passing in both directions. As a filter, the person in that box may inadvertently or intentionally block a signal that should pass through or may allow too much noise to get through, obscuring signals. The process of filtering noise and signals inevitably results in a reduction and distortion of the information that does get through. In designing an organizational chart, administrators need to be sure that they maximize information flow without overloading the circuits or adding to the noise and confusion.

Some administrators believe that the charts make little difference and that the effectiveness of the organization depends on the personnel, not the design of the chart. Others go to the extreme of mechanizing their management by believing that complex charts will make things happen properly regardless of the individuals in the boxes. Neither approach is realistic. The organizational chart has two purposes: (1) it reveals the emphasis that the administrator places on different activities and programs, and (2) it outlines a facilitative approach to communications. The fact that the organizational chart conveys impressions about how the designer

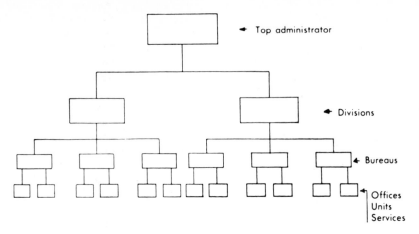

FIG. 10-2. The scalar process.

feels about certain activities or persons is often missed by administrators. Both the staff of the agency and groups within the community will interpret the chart with great care to see how they or their interests are valued. The perceptions they develop, whether or not they are accurate, will have a great deal to do with how they react to the administrator/designer. The chart should not be drawn in such a way as to force relationships or communications to flow in an unnatural or unpopular manner. Properly designed, it can help clarify for both staff and community how signals are meant to move through the organization. It should also facilitate the best proclivities of both groups while attempting to minimize counterproductive tendencies.

Although the organization should not be designed to fit the personalities of the workers, it cannot ignore them. The design should be seen as a dynamic blueprint: one that can and will change to facilitate needed improvements but that was, after all, thoughtfully planned in the first place; it will not be redrafted every time there is a personnel change or a new idea. The units to be headed by subleaders should be established or differentiated on the basis of functional definition. The trend has been to provide a small number of relatively large major divisions, each with a major purpose and each further subdivided into smaller units, if necessary, on the basis of subfunctions.

Although sound in theory, this is more easily said than accomplished, since many instances arise in which two or even more departments or

other organizational units are involved and appear to have valid claims. Should the industrial hygiene program be placed in a state health department or in a state labor and industry department? If the former is decided on, should responsibility for the program be delegated to the division of environmental health or the division of medical services; or should it be set up as an entity in itself? Should the school health program be in the department of health or in the department of education? Whether assigned to one or the other, the school health program involves safety, sanitation, medical services, and education, each of which extends into other fields.

Although it is best for the individual division or bureau to be concerned with a particular function, each should contribute to an overall major purpose of the department and not be allocated to the department as a result of a search for a roosting place. Occasionally it is found expedient and practical to form administrative units on bases other than functional. They may be determined by geographic area, such as the Tennessee Valley Authority, or by type of clientele, such as the Department of Public Welfare or the Veterans Administration.

Should an organization conform geographically to already existing governmental boundaries, or should new boundaries be established based on the nature of the problem to be met or the distribution of the public to be served—a catchment area? The size and boundaries of a problem-oriented/resource-oriented catchment area, being divorced if necessary from political boundaries, may be determined on the basis of population, trading or economic areas, topographic considerations, or convenience of officials and citizens. These are relatively easy to readjust with little or no friction, in contrast to service areas whose boundaries conform to those of established political units. The effect of the latter is commonly seen when attempts are made to expand the jurisdictions of local health departments either by combining a city with its surrounding county or by combining two or more counties. Vested political interests are disturbed. The National Commission on Community Health Services[12] recommended that "the planning, organization, and delivery of community health services . . . be based on the concept of a 'community of solution'—that is, environmental health problem–sheds and health marketing areas, rather than primarily on political jurisdictions."

Nevertheless, the administrative district based on problem or service needs has limited governmental status, no independent existence, and usually no power to raise revenue in its own right and by its own action. It can easily find itself standing alone and helpless. Hence, public health units in the United States are based on politically defined units of government: municipalities, counties, combinations of counties or combinations of counties and municipalities, and states.

Span of control is a time-worn phrase in organizational theory. It has been common practice to organize spans of control in sixes since some early theorists believed that administrators could not deal effectively with more than six different personalities, programs, or divisions. No single rule can be applied. In some tasks, it may be better to develop a tall, narrow organization with a single leader, two or three boxes on the chart reporting to the strategic apex, and no more than a few program directors reporting to each of those managers. A flat organization is one in which the span of control is broad and shallow with many program directors reporting directly to the chief executive. The latter is useful when it is desirable to reduce administrative control and forestall attempts to stultify the individuality of program leaders. The taller, narrow organization is more effective when there are many legalistic functions to be carried out and tight supervision is necessary to assure precision in the output. The same

purpose can be served by more rigid standardization of process.

The best plan is one that groups functions in such a way as to enable responsiveness to the jurisdiction served rather than to the administrative controls placed on the agency. The contrary pattern has, unfortunately, prevailed in the United States. National agencies are established with their own mandates but with little understanding of how such activities are carried out on the local level. The state agencies that receive the national funds to carry out the program are encouraged to organize so that they can respond to the national initiatives. This is often incongruent with the way the services must be delivered locally, yet the administrative requirements of the sponsoring national agency may override the service delivery requirements at the other end and dictate an administrative form that does not follow function. This has been especially evident in the development of environmental protection programs at the national level where water pollution has been seen as a wastewater treatment problem, whereas in some states water pollution is clearly a matter of acid mine drainage that is not amenable to control through the construction of sewage treatment plants. Ideally each layer of government should be so designed as to conform to the needs of its receiving constituency rather than its sponsoring constituency. It should absorb the administrative problems of confusion rather than pass them along to the local level where the ultimate purpose is served.

Organizational units may be formed around purpose, place, function, process, or discipline. Public health agencies have had a difficult time with organizational theory because some programs are organized around their client group or their purpose, such as venereal disease control or maternal and child health programs, while others are organized to fit the place, such as a district office that attempts to provide comprehensive services. Other groupings are formed around a discipline such as nutrition, which has a specific purpose, while other discipline groupings such as nursing have at best a very broad purpose. The nursing division in most health departments does not have a nursing program but provides trained professionals to serve a variety of programmatic needs. This is not necessarily a significant problem until the jurisdiction becomes enamored of program planning processes and directs each operating unit to write a program plan following a specified format. This is easier to do in a functional unit such as tuberculosis control, where objectives can be stated numerically, than in nursing, where function ranges from prenatal care to hospice care for the terminally ill.

It is not difficult to accommodate this conflict when all of the boxes on the same level of an organization chart have the same grouping rationale, such as the support service units that may be grouped on a line below the director's office. It does become confusing when different grouping concepts occur on the same line, since those programs or functions are often treated the same administratively. It is not necessary to reshape valid program decisions to fit an organizational chart design, but such problems usually point to a conceptual issue that has more important ramifications than design aesthetics.

STAFF SERVICES

For a considerable period, all divisions of public agencies were more or less self-contained units performing all of the activities and functions necessary for their operation and maintenance. Beginning about 1900, with the expansion of public service and its increased specialization, various functional units of a staff nature were separated from the operational unit. Activities of this type were brought together to form what are referred to as staff agencies, which are usually aligned structurally in close relationship with the chief executive officer of the organization. Still more recent has been the tendency to develop these staff agencies into a combination of service and control units.

Staff agencies do more than study, plan, and advise. Their purpose is to facilitate the work of administration. They assist the line or functional units by working with them but without infringing on their authority or responsibility. Lines of authority, command, and responsibility should not pass through them. Instead, these agencies are situated in an "off line" position as adjuncts to the office of the chief executive. Because of this rather special status, their purpose and value tend to be misunderstood. Staff assistants do carry implied authority in that they serve as personal representatives of the chief executive. As such, their opinions are not viewed as their own but as reflections of what the chief executive wants done. To be effective, staff assistants have to have a full understanding of the policy and even the style of the chief executive so that these can be conveyed accurately and consistently. Moreover, program administrators

have to be guaranteed access to the chief executive whenever they believe that the staff guidance offered is at variance with the facts or with program policy. The chief executive and staff assistants have to be very cautious about developing lines of communication that bypass the responsible administrator of a division or program. There may be times when this is necessary because of an emergency or the incompetence of the bypassed administrator, but such occasions are usually indicative of a management problem that needs attention.

In categorizing staff agencies, Mintzberg[3] distinguishes between the technostructure and other support services. The difference in the public sector is more apparent when looking at local or state government as a whole than when looking at the health agency by itself. Support service staff groups may provide clerical support, housekeeping support, fiscal reporting services, and some personnel services. The technostructure is involved more in analysis, evaluation, and planning, and the personnel are not always under the control of the managers of the health agency at the state or local level. In the public sector they are more likely to be placed in separate organizations formed to exercise budgetary control and financial accountability. While such staff units usually lack a statutory assignment for programmatic review, the function is often assumed since the financial officer is appointed by the elected chief executive and the role may offer some additional opportunity to gain political control over the professional bureaucracy. When a vacant position is to be filled, the health agency director theoretically needs to requisition an eligible candidate from the civil service system. In practice, the request often has to be approved by the director of finance who may question the wisdom of the program as well as the authority of the health director and the expenditure of funds, which if unspent might be available for some other purpose in the next fiscal period. The advent of the technostructure has presented new problems for governmental agencies where program directors guard their statutory prerogatives and traditions from elected officials who need to gain control of the bureaucracy. The best way to avoid the confrontation is for the director of the health agency to become a more effective manager and to gain better control of the bureaucracy so that the mayor or the governor will have less need to do so.

One of the auxiliary services that sometimes gives rise to controversy is that of central purchasing. Although this office is intended to assist the functional units, there is a division of authority between the unit that uses and the one that purchases. Theoretically the functional unit decides on the articles or material needed and describes them on a standard form, specifying the quantity required, the desired time and place of delivery, and any special considerations of the purchase in question. This requisition may include the names of preferred manufacturers when one commerical product is considered superior to those of other companies. The requisition is sent to the central purchasing office, usually after it has been examined by the comptroller or fiscal officer to be certain that sufficient funds are available. Actual purchase may then be made by the central purchasing officer, usually on the basis of open competitive bids. The authority to purchase is vested solely in the purchasing agent. On delivery, inspection and even laboratory tests may be carried out to ascertain the quality of the materials supplied.

The controversy revolves around whether the purchasing officer should have the right to modify a requisition either quantitatively or qualitatively. The extent of this authority depends on the policy of the particular organization and occasionally on legal requirements. Another objection concerns the delay encountered in obtaining the materials. Functional units complain that by the time delivery is made, the need has passed. Many organizations have attempted to solve this problem by allowing direct purchase of emergency material and specialized equipment under specified circumstances, as well as the use of "open" contracts for some supply items.

Technical staff personnel are specialists. Whenever such technical specialists are loaned to line units, they should be answerable to the director of those line units rather than to some technical headquarters or to the agency's chief executive. The relationship of the technical field staff to the functional line unit poses several problems. The objective is to provide a smooth effective channel along which the knowledge and resources of the central organization can flow to local units without destroying the initiative of the local personnel or impairing the authority of the director of the local unit.

Complete autonomy of the local units tends to inhibit the flow of technical service and advice from specialists in the central office to their counterparts on the local level. On the other hand, for central office specialists to have direct authority over corresponding specialists on the local level interferes with the coordination of the activities of the local organization. When this occurs, the director of the local unit may be reduced to little more than an administrative clerk.

As in the case of the administrative staff, care must be taken to assure understanding, both on the state and on the local level, of the purpose and function of the technical field staff. In turn, the members of the field staff must gain the trust and confidence of the local personnel. The most important step toward this goal is for the chief executive of the state or central agency to choose the members of the field staff as much for their skill as consultants as for their technical knowledge and ability. Coordination of the policies and methods of approach is extremely difficult. A program director on the local level is likely to have several consultants from the state agency in the office during the same period. One approach to the problem is to have all technical field consultants who go into the local units originate from a single coordinating division in the central agency. All requests for field consultation are channeled through the director of the local unit, on the one hand, and the director of the division of local health service, on the other; the latter is usually designated as deputy state health officer.

Organizational change

Organizations may have either a functional structure or a product-oriented structure. The product-oriented structure is more characteristic of private sector entities, especially profit-making ones, while functional structures are a characteristic result of the governmental process and of the civil service system of personnel management (see chapter on personnel). Functional structures are not well thought of in business schools or schools of public administration, and many health agency directors have attempted to reorganize public health functions into a product-oriented array of activities. As previously noted, many states have reorganized their health agencies in recent years, and the same thing has occurred at the local level. Some of the more complete reorganizations have occurred in Florida (1975), Minnesota (1976), West Virginia (1977), and Michigan (1978). All of the efforts have emphasized the reorganization or the development of local or community health services. Michigan's effort was a recodification of all state laws affecting public health, but its full implementation at the local level has not yet been realized. The changes in Minnesota and Florida have been well documented.[13,14] Both efforts are described as decentralizations, but they are very different.

The Florida reorganization stemmed from the Health and Rehabilitation Services Act of 1975, which required the state agency to "establish measurable program objectives and performance criteria for each program it [sic] operates" and conduct studies of "relative cost and effectiveness."[13] The Minnesota law, by contrast, has as its purpose "to develop and maintain an integrated system of community health services under local administration with a system of state guidelines and standards."* The Florida effort emphasized the role of the technostructure at the state level, whereas the emphasis in Minnesota is on community capacity building under a variety of arrangements to be selected by the community, not the state. The impressive effort in Florida used almost every acronymic device popularized in the management literature of the 1960s and 1970s. Organizational development (OD) was used when professional resistance was detected, and a host of reports and computerized management information system documents have been generated. The base of the system rests on the Program Activity Report (PAR) to be filled out by each employee at the local level for each activity performed. These are keypunched and filed and then manipulated to produce an impressive array of tables. The planners have tried to standardize activities so that they can be categorized and given a number. From examining the reports it is easy to see how professionals at the service delivery end of the system, who do not like to think of their work as "standardized," manage to satisfy the needs of the analysts without really changing their activities very much. The statewide system is impressive, and the work that was done to develop and implement it is worthy of study by those with a similar job to do, but the impression that is gained is one of process overcoming purpose. The organization (the state health agency) has taken the ultimate step of

devolving the entire operating core of public health, and the technostructure has become the new operating core with standardization and analysis as it objective. The results of the effort in terms of services, costs, or the availability and use of resources have not been reported.

The Minnesota change emphasized community development from the outset, and control by a technostructure was minimized. Considerable latitude was left to local communities, which could choose a single-purpose department and board or various consolidated or integrated models. The reports indicate that virtually the entire state is covered by the community-based system after 5 years and that local per capita support for the community health agencies has increased from a statewide average of $4.49 in 1973 to $14.60 in 1979. This is not to suggest that a strong management information system is undesirable—quite the contrary, but the impetus in Florida appears to have been managerial control ("more bang for the buck") while the emphasis in Minnesota, in the law and in the state health agency's effort, has been on service development under the auspices of community agencies.

Reorganizations can be sponsored for a variety of reasons. The change in West Virginia was partly because of an effort by the governor to gain some control over the state health agency, which was run by a board and a director resistant to gubernatorial exhortations. Reorganizations can occur because of external dissatisfaction with the costs of management or the lack of attention to a favored program or constituency. They may be generated by community groups who do not feel the agency has been effective in meeting perceived health needs in contrast to the agency's tradition of enforcing the health laws. They may be necessary because of a change in federal laws that make it necessary for a state to change to conform to the structure of the national agency and receive its share of the money. They may come about because a new health agency director does not think that the agency is well positioned or designed for the role it is to assume. The reasons for a reorganization effort will have a strong influence on the nature of the new structure. Dr. Harry Seidman, who had many years of experience in what formerly was known as the Bureau of the Budget, has said that "reorganization has become almost a religion in Washington. Reorganization is

*Minnesota Statutes section 145.911.

deemed synonymous with reform and reform with progress. For the true believer, reorganization can produce miracles."[15] Many people feel that noticeable changes in personnel and in organization structure are necessary to establish a new director's position, but dramatic cosmetics such as that may result in more losses than gains. Exhaustive attention to the nature of the organization, its resources, and its leading personnel is the first task to be undertaken by any new agency director, and dramatic changes should be avoided until the evaluation has been completed. This should be done within the first 3 months, or the momentum necessary to make dramatic changes, if they are necessary, may be diminished by increasing familiarity with the present structure.

Reorganizations have emphasized consolidations, with the number of new consolidations formed being slightly greater than the number of old ones dissolved. About 17% of the local agencies studied by Shonick and Price were in some combined form, sometimes with a public hospital, sometimes with other human service agencies. These combined agencies covered areas with about 29% of the total population of the country, which indirectly confirms the hypothesis that such consolidations are more likely to be formed in metropolitan areas. The movement is not rapid but is steady even though some consolidated agencies have been subsequently disaggregated.[6] Geographic combinations have progressed no more rapidly. In 1945 Haven Emerson proposed that nearly 70% of local health agencies should be in combined form with two or more counties. By 1977 only 8.7% of reporting jurisdictions had such a form.[17] The theoretic logic of consolidation ignored political reality.

Decentralization is a popular term in organizational formation or reformation efforts, but the term is poorly understood. It is not the relocation of service centers so that transit time is reduced and access is made easier. Relocating staff relocates people. Decentralization involves the relocation of power and can occur with or without a geographic relocation of people. It is important to realize that an agency director can decentralize responsibility without the requisite power to meet that responsibility. If both responsibility and authority are decentralized to a community program or a division director, the recipient program director may hold

that authority tightly, and the process of decentralization will stop abruptly. Decentralization involves the devolution of both authority and responsibility onto the lowest units in the organization that have the ability and resources necessary to make the decisions involved in carrying out the purpose of the unit. In a professional bureaucracy, decentralization is actually accomplished down to the individual worker, since management is relying on the standardization of professional skills to obtain the coordination necessary to accomplish the organization's mission. Yet many forces exist that try to extract some of the power: civil service systems with job descriptions, employee unions with an interest in confining work, fiscal officers and controllers who need to make standardized reports, and funding agencies that require performance audits and activity accounts to justify continued funding. The effort to standardize is strongly resisted by the workers and is sometimes distorted by managers when it is necessary to protect what they are doing from the changes the funding agency wants to make. When federal and state requirements in California reduced support for social services but left intact the funding for eligibility workers, activity reports dutifully reflected a decrease in activity by social workers and an increase in work by eligibility workers. The actual work done changed very little and the local welfare agencies were able to continue as they had. (It should be noted that they continued because they felt that what they were doing was more important than what the state wanted them to do.) Decentralization of authority and responsibility in a human services agency is one of the most effective ways to move toward the agency's goals, but only when top management and unit supervisors have a reasonable degree of agreement about those goals and a willingness to absorb the additional work of diversity and dissent.

Service integration is another common term that has become less precise with repeated use. Integration may mean a series of administrative steps taken to obtain greater control over a diffuse array of human services, or it may mean an attempt to bring service providers into a closer working relationship at the community level so that more efficient and effective services can be delivered. Once the term became popular, there were federal Service Integration Programs and state Directors of Integration Programs. One could anticipate the formation of a National Association of Service Integration Program Directors (NASIPD). Integration is a process, not a program. It is only of value if it achieves some higher goal than integration itself: more effective services, more efficient services, better access, less reduction when budgets are cut, or less waste. The National Academy of Science's Institute of Medicine began a study of service integration in 1981 that proposed to "focus on relationships between 'integration as a set of administrative techniques or structural arrangements on the one hand, and integration as a characteristic of services or their manner of delivery, on the other,' not just on presence or absence of integrative devices drawn from a typological laundry list which may or may not form a coherent program or make a difference."[18] Perhaps a better word is *coalition*. As resources available for public health work and other human service programs decline, it is essential that providers, especially at the local level with commitment to the effort at the state and national level, acquire the resources needed to do a job by negotiation and coalition building with other provider organizations rather than through acquisition. Public health agencies, community health centers, community mental health centers, social service agencies, and other organizations all have service obligations that are increasingly difficult to fulfill because of repeated budget cuts. Whatever shape the integrative effort takes, it is necessary for the organizations to look to each other for shared resources. The Institute of Medicine study will describe several cases thoroughly in an effort to see what works and why.

CONCLUSION

This review of the principles of organization is necessarily incomplete. Laws, expectations, and concepts are changing so rapidly that a description of how things function and are organized today will be out of date tomorrow. State legislatures, the Secretary of the U.S. Department of Health and Human Services, and local governments are all reacting to economic stresses and the demands of their constituents for more accessible and acceptable health programs by reorganizing and regrouping existing services. But organization and reorganization are not effective substitutes for careful deliberation about where we are going and how we plan to get there. Only then can form follow function and function follow purpose.

REFERENCES

1. Levy, S., and Loomba, N.P.: Health care administration: a managerial perspective, Philadelphia, 1973, J.B. Lippincott Co.
2. Duncan, W.J.: Essentials of management, ed. 2, Hinsdale, Ill., 1978, Dryden Press.
3. Mintzberg, H.: The structuring of organizations, Englewood Cliffs, N.J., 1979, Prentice-Hall, Inc.
4. Gerth, H., and Mills, C.W.: Max Weber: essays in sociology, New York, 1946, Oxford University Press, Inc.
5. Galbraith, J.R.: Designing complex organizations, Reading, Mass., 1973, Addison-Wesley, Publishing Co., Inc.
6. Shonick, W., and Price, W.: Reorganizations of health agencies by local government in American urban centers: what do they portend for public health? Milbank Mem. Fund Q. **55**:233, Spring 1977.
7. Gossert, D.J., and Miller, C.A.: State boards of health: their members and commitments, Am. J. Public Health **66**:486, June 1973.
8. Gilbert, B., Moos, M.-K., and Miller, C.A.: State level decision making for public health—the status of boards of health, J. Public Health Policy **3**:51, Mar. 1982.
9. Cameron, C., and Kobylarz, A.: Nonphysician directors of local health departments: results of a national survey, Pub. Health Rep. **95**(4):386, July-Aug. 1980.
10. Miller, C.A., and others: A survey of local public health departments and their directors, Am. J. Public Health **67**:931, Oct. 1977.
11. Wright, D.S., and Dometrius, N.: State administrators: their changing characteristics, State Government **50,** Summer 1977.
12. National Commission on Community Health Services: Health is a community affair, Cambridge, Mass., 1966, Harvard University Press.
13. Bigler, W.J., Mittan, J.B., and Wisthuff, R.: Florida's new local health unit management system, Tallahassee, Fla., July 1981, Department of Health and Rehabilitation Services.
14. Hossler, J.L.: Community health services: Minnesota's experiment with decentralized health services, Minneapolis, Oct. 1981, Minnesota Department of Health.
15. Sims, L.: Organizational history of HSMHA, Health Serv. Rep. **88**:117, 1973.
16. Shonick, W., and Price, W.: Organizational milieus of local public health units: analysis of response to a questionnaire, Public Health Rep. **63**(6):648, Nov.-Dec. 1978.
17. Pickett, G.E.: The future of health departments: the governmental presence, Ann. Reviews of Public Health **1**:297, 1980.
18. McGeary, M., Darling, H., and Evans, C.: A study of the integration of health services at community and state levels, Background paper No. 1, Washington, D.C., revised, Aug. 12, 1981, Institute of Medicine's Committee on Services Integration.

CHAPTER 11

Planning

Is it that some high Plan betides,
As yet not understood,
Of Evil stormed by Good,
We, the Forlorn Hope over which
Achievement strides?

Thomas Hardy

EVOLUTION OF PLANNING

Few topics in health administration are as controversial as health planning. It seems as if no two people mean the same thing when talking about it. At the core of the confusion is a reluctance to accept the political nature of planning. Many planners insist that planning is an objective way to make decisions and that politics and planning are antithetic to one another. That belief is delusional. Even at the microlevel, where, for example, two hospitals are considering a shared laundry service, the final choice is political, since one hospital usually gives up something to get something. At the state level, the linkage becomes more apparent and more important. Planning is the process of determining how to achieve an objective once the objective has been defined. The effect of planning is to clarify the differences between alternatives, and in most important decisions, clarification narrows the superficial differences and exposes the value differences as the principal issues. Whenever two or more people have to make a choice involving values, the process of decision making is political. The reluctance of planners to understand and accept that allows the mythology rather than the reality of planning to dominate discussions about the subject and reduces the usefulness of planning in public health.

It is widely believed that planning and collecting more and better information make decision making easier. The opposite is probably true. Simple problems are simple because the issues are clear and there is little value conflict. Elaborate planning is rarely needed. Important problems are hard to solve because issues are not clear and because value judgments are involved. In such cases, more and better information only serves to strip away the rationalizations of those with different values, finally exposing the basic conflicts and making the choice very difficult. For example, is prison meant to be punitive or rehabilitative? Most societies do neither well and both badly because they cannot decide. Although elected officials may ask for better data so that they can make a decision, they are probably better off not making a clear choice because it could not be accepted for long. Is a welfare worker supposed to get public assistance for those who need it or reduce the size of the dole? The answer is to help those in need and to keep those who would cheat from doing so, but that answer masks a deep-seated and shifting belief as to just who are the "truly needy." More and better information will not make the choice any easier, but it does help to keep people from deluding themselves.

Planning as a formal process was not common in public health until the work of the American Public Health Association's Committee on Administrative Practice and Evaluation in the 1920s. As funds for public health programs increased, as the perimeters of the field were extended by legislation, as public demands and expectations increased, and as government and management in general became more sophisticated, health agencies became more visible and more accountable. Planning became more important. In the mid-1960s concern for efficiency in government coupled with apprehension over the rising cost of medical care and the persistent evidence that many people still did not get the care they needed prompted President Johnson and the Eighty-ninth Congress to begin a series of initiatives with far-reaching effects. The President required his cabinet officers to incorporate sophisticated planning techniques into their budget-making procedures. An Office of Health Planning was established in the Department of Health, Education, and Welfare, but it remained in an "off-line" position (out of the mainstream of decision making) and had little impact on budget and program strategies.

The Comprehensive Health Planning Act

Congress attempted to develop health planning systems throughout the country by passing the Comprehensive Health Planning and Public Health Services Amendments in 1966 (P.L. 89-749). The new law attempted to move the responsibility for health planning to the states and to subareas within the states. The local or "area-wide" organizations were known as "B" agencies, and the state agencies that were to assimilate the area-wide plans into a single statewide plan were known as "A" agencies. The designations came from the pertinent sections of the law, 314(b) and 314(a), respectively.

The comprehensive health planning legislation did not include authority over the federally funded (Hill-Burton) hospital construction program or the new Regional Medical Programs, which were to extend medical training and services from the major medical centers to the communities of each state. The "B" agencies had to rely heavily on local support for their budgets and had no real authority over federal grants to community agencies. The law contained an unfortunate restriction in its statement of purpose, which was "to support the marshalling of all health resources . . . to assure comprehensive services of high quality for every person, but without interference with existing patterns of private professional practice of medicine, dentistry and related healing arts." This paradox was repeated in other health legislation in the 1960s and reflected a major problem of Congress in the latter part of the twentieth century. In earlier days national legislation had been more local in scope, and compromises occurred between a dam in one jurisdiction and a post office in another. Neither may have been needed, but when completed the dam held water and the post office held mail. With the increasing involvement of the federal government in the broad issues of health and welfare,

which had been traditionally reserved to the states, compromises began to occur within the context of the bill itself in an effort to get enough votes for passage. Thus we got an increasing number of creations that combined a dam and a post office, the result of which could hold neither water nor mail. Health statutes that might have been landmarks in the history of public health were internally compromised with conflicting values and the inevitable problem of interpretation by administering agencies, interest groups, and the courts.

All of the states formed comprehensive health planning "A" and "B" agencies, but if their purpose was to rationalize the distribution of health resources and to contain cost increases, they failed. If their purpose was to involve citizens in making decisions about health affairs, an arena heretofore reserved for the providers, and to broaden community awareness of the workings of the health system, they partially succeeded. They were required to have a majority of consumers and to reflect the broad ethnic, racial, and socioeconomic groupings in the communities. Congressional expectations and those of the interested public health groups were not met and were not realistic. The comprehensive health planning agencies did involve a lot of people in thinking about health services in an orderly way and subjected many provider plans to public scrutiny and debate. However, the provider groups were better organized, had more knowledge about the systems, and easily dominated the debates.

Congress moved to strengthen the process with the National Health Planning and Resources Development Act of 1974 (P.L. 93-641). The new law required the governors to designate health service areas to include between 250,000 and 3 million people. Once the area designations were approved by the Secretary of the Department of Health, Education, and Welfare, groups within the areas could apply for designation as the Health Systems Agency (HSA) for the area. The law required a consumer majority and went further in specifying limits on provider representation. Two other provisions were remarkable: (1) although the areas were designated by the governor, the HSAs made their application to the Secretary of Health, Education, and Welfare and became accountable to the Secretary rather than to the governor or to the community served, and (2) although it was possible for a council of governments or a general-purpose government to apply for status as an HSA, the law made that difficult with the result that most of the planning agencies (180 of the 203 formed) were private, not-for-profit organizations accountable to the Secretary of Health, Education, and Welfare in Washington.

Congress's national priorities were specified in section 1502 of the act: improved access to primary care for medically underserved groups and communities, consolidation and better use of hospitals, the development of medical group practices and health maintenance organizations, improved quality, better management and cost controls, and health promotion and disease prevention. Each HSA was to develop a health systems plan and an annual implementation plan. The Statewide Health Coordinating Council, which was partly made up of representatives from the HSAs, was to meld the health systems plan into one state health plan. The staff work was to be done by the State Health Planning and Development Agency. In 13 states the health service area was the entire state, which meant that the statewide HSA and Statewide Health Coordinating Council, together with the State Health Planning and Development Agency, were all writing health plans for the same area.

The new agencies had more authority than the predecessor comprehensive health planning agencies. The Hill-Burton hospital construction program and the Regional Medical Programs were abolished, and some of their functions were assigned to the HSAs. As the new agencies grew in experience, they were to get increasing grants of authority from the Secretary of Health, Education, and Welfare, which finally encompassed approval authority over most applications for the use of federal health funds except those used to purchase medical care (such as Medicaid and Medicare), federal subsidies to educational institutions for the training of health workers, and research grants from the National Institutes of Health. The latter two exclusions reflected the power of the medical schools, which could scarcely condone community control over such enterprises. The law also established a National Council on Health Planning and Development, which was to advise the Secretary and adopt national standards for health services.

One of the more complex and controversial sub-jects encompassed in the health planning legislation was the certificate of need. During the early years of the formation of hospital planning councils and the Hill-Burton program, need, at least operationally, meant the need of the hospital—its physicians, its administrator, and its board. So long as they could substantiate their need for equipment or additional beds, the need was accepted as real. By 1966 and in the spirit of that time, need meant what the community needed. Since it was really the community that paid for the program or the construction through health insurance, foregone property taxes, or direct, tax-supported subsidies, the added investment required some assessment of whether the community really needed it. The 1974 health planning legislation required each state to pass a certificate of need law to qualify for designation of the State Health Planning and Development Agency and the rest of the health planning apparatus. A proposal to build or initiate a program or acquire equipment that would cost more than $100,000 had to be reviewed by the HSA. The tests were whether or not the new effort was congruent with the needs described in the health systems plan, whether the plan was feasible and affordable, and whether it was the least costly of all the alternative ways of meeting that need. The recommendation of the HSA went to the State Health Planning and Development Agency, which had a specified period of time to either approve or disapprove the proposal and state its reasons. Lacking approval, the program could not be implemented, or if it was implemented, it would not be eligible for reimbursement by any of the federal medical care payment schemes such as Medicare and Medicaid. In some states, denial of a certificate of need meant that the facility could not be licensed.

The National Health Planning and Resources Development Act represented a conviction by some in Congress that the concept of community health planning was sound but needed more authority over community programs and better financial support. It incorporated fiscal information into the planning data base for the first time. Earlier health planning efforts had ignored fiscal realities, assuming that if the plan was all right, the money would be available. The 1974 law included a requirement to review from time to time the appropriateness of existing facilities and to make plans for their discontinuation or other changes that might be desirable. Amendments to the law in 1979 were extensive but largely procedural.

Ultimately 203 HSAs were designated by the

Secretary, although three subsequently lost their designations for failure to meet the requirements of the law (Los Angeles County, Clark County, Nevada, and Topeka, Kansas). Puerto Rico was placed in a special category.[1] One hundred and eighty of the agencies were private, not-for-profit organizations, and 23 were a function of regional planning bodies or a local general purpose government. There were 13 statewide HSAs and 16 interstate agencies, which required complex efforts on the part of two states. The National Council on Health Planning and Development found that 50,000 volunteer participants were contributing 1½ million hours of time to the effort: 9,000 on HSA governing bodies, 2,000 on statewide Health Coordinating Councils, 16,000 on subarea advisory councils, and the rest on committees and task forces.[2] The National Council and the American Health Planning Association (an association largely representing HSA directors) claimed impressive reductions in capital expenditures and other improvements as a result of the health planning effort. Others have claimed that it has been an expensive failure. Once again the truth lies somewhere between expectations and reality.

PROBLEMS WITH HEALTH PLANNING

To plan effectively there must be some understood and broadly accepted sense of purpose—a direction. Some believed that the purpose of the health planning process was cost containment, others thought it to have been improved access especially for the "have nots" of society, and some thought the sole purpose was to turn over health planning to consumers at the community level. There were some who believed that key congressional aides were acting on an agenda set in the 1930s to centralize planning and resource allocation and that the health planning laws were an elaborate attempt to create failures leading to a centralization, first at the state level, then at the national level. The former Surgeon General, Dr. Julius Richmond, stated that we did indeed have a national health policy: to extend and improve health services to all Americans, to conduct an elaborate program of research, and to promote health and prevent disease.[3] This policy or purpose, if it does exist, meets the test of general acceptability but tends to be reflective more of interest groups than of any real consensus. The National Council on Health Planning did not promulgate national standards until March 1978,[4] and they were so highly specific in some areas, such as computerized axial

tomography, and so general in others, such as the supply of hospital beds (4 per 1,000 people), as to require a series of special conditions and qualifications and to provoke inquiry as to the comprehensive nature of the few standards developed. Many believed that if the purpose of the law was to develop a pattern of community health planning, national numerical standards encumbered with a series of qualifications would be an inappropriate way to fulfill that purpose. Still others thought that there should be even more rigid standards at the national level.

The certificate of need process was seized on by HSAs and state agencies as their most important task and reform tool. Yet it was a very complex and flawed concept. It amounted to a form of licensure, but standards were lacking. It meant that volunteers who often had very little concept of such matters would review complicated financing and service delivery plans that were worth millions of dollars to boards, physicians, construction companies, and equipment manufacturers. Denials of any significant nature often ended in court, and the proceedings were tortuous at best. Well-monied corporations with multimillion dollar investments at stake were pitted against small, understaffed, and underpaid state health planning agencies. The concept also had some aspects of an anticompetitive nature, since the practice involved review of a proposal against the suppositions of an approved plan. If a second proposal to do the same thing was received a few days later, it followed the same mandatory process with a specified number of days in review. If the first proposal in the pipeline of review was approved, the second proposal, even though it might have been a better one, would be disqualified since by the time its due date arrived, the need had been filled by the first proposal. Some agencies attempted to solve this by batching competing proposals. The process became entangled in antitrust laws since it sometimes involved extending franchises to existing providers at the expense of would-be competitors. An important experiment in regulation was moved to nationwide implementation before sufficient experience had been accumulated to give it a reasonable chance to work, and state health planning agencies became hopelessly entangled in the review and approval process without an adequate base of guidelines, precedent, and practice.

Management of public
health programs

TABLE 11-1. Consumer representation of HSA
governing councils

Category	Number	Percent
Sex		
Male	2041	43
Female	2664	57
Age		
18-34	797	17
35-64	3179	68
65+	729	15
Income		
Less than $10,000	692	15
10,000-24,999	2121	45
25,000 or more	1599	34
Race		
Black	695	15
White	3743	80
Other	267	5

From the National Council on Health Planning and Development: Report on consumer participation in the health planning program, Feb. 6, 1981, U. S. Department of Health and Human Services.

Many states found themselves faced with the task of having to complete a host of separate plan documents for the Department of Health, Education, and Welfare (a title V plan, an alcohol plan, a mental health plan, a 314[d] plan, a plan for the developmentally disabled, an aging plan, a title XX social services plan, a title IV-B plan for child welfare services, to name just a few) with little support for their efforts to bring the planning processes together at the state agency level. The national program planning requirements were all separate and different, and there was virtually no interest on the part of program managers at the national level in having their plans merged with those of any other program. As a result, a new initiative, the Planning Reform Demonstration Project, placed in the office of the Assistant Secretary for Intergovernmental Affairs in 1978, funded efforts in 10 states to attempt to develop a consolidated plan. The effort was commendable, but the Assistant Secretary and his regional counterparts had an uphill battle with the central program managers, since the consolidators had little authority over the separators.

Citizen participation, although impressive when looked at from one angle, was weak when seen from another. The National Council on Health Planning saw the benefits of involving 50,000 people in health planning, but this participation in community decision making concerning a $200 billion plus industry represented 0.03% of the adult population of the country. In Los Angeles, 9,058 people (0.2% of the population) voted for the 150 seats available in the health planning system, and those who remained involved were those with the greatest need or interest to stay involved—scarcely a representative group.[5] The National Council concluded that the consumers on the HSAs suffered from a relative lack of knowledge and that they lacked an organizational base that could have made them more effective vis-a-vis the providers. The Council report[2] urged dedicated staff support for the consumers and less paperwork and jargon, recommendations that were not at all likely to end either the flow of paper and jargon or the influence of staffs with their own biases. The Council did find a surprisingly good distribution of consumer members, in contrast with the predecessor comprehensive health planning (b) agencies (Table 11-1). Although scarcely reflective of the composition of the groups targeted in the purpose of the act, the makeup of the governing bodies is fairly reflective of the voting public.

The General Accounting Office conducted two major reviews of the health planning process and found it to be inadequate to the purposes stated in the enabling legislation. In particular, the General Accounting Office concluded that the objectives adopted by HSAs lacked the essential ingredient of measurability (discussed later), that there were far too many objectives (a hundred or more in some cases) to allow any hope of implementation, that objectives were frequently unrealistic and did not take into account either available resources or the feasibility of acquiring the needed ones, and that they lacked a realistic set of implementing recommendations.[6] The report recommended that the Department of Health and Human Services (the successor agency to the Department of Health, Education, and Welfare) play a stronger role in HSA and state plan development (contrary to those who felt the purpose was to encourage diversity in problem solving at the local level), that single HSA states be allowed to combine the Health Systems Plan and the State Health Plan into one document, and that the HSAs be required to pursue implementation of a more realistic set of objectives.

The National Academy of Science's Institute of Medicine also studied the health planning program and found that it had substantial potential.[7] The Institute encouraged the diversity and decentralization other critics had decried. It found that the process had been an important experiment in forming relationships between government and the private sector and between consumers and providers. The Institute identified three functions for the planning program: to provide an open and participatory structure, to contribute to a redirection of the health system, and to contribute to cost containment. These are a more modest set of expectations, and they were within the grasp of most HSAs, although some may claim that the cost of attaining such a modest set of objectives would be too high.

If diversity of problem solving is seen as an important objective, the Institute of Medicine's study seems to reflect fairly on the experience. The problems have stemmed from the lack of understanding and acceptance of these functions and from the belief by most HSA governing bodies that they were apolitical planning groups rather than voting bodies of citizens, all of whom had an interest in what was going on and whose personal interests were often in conflict with the interests of some other people or groups in the community. Some national strategists expected entirely too much, and some HSA staff and board members shared those unrealistically high expectations. The accountability of the HSAs to the Secretary of Health, Education, and Welfare (now Health and Human Services) rather than to the community served, the flawed effort to wrestle with national standards, and the intense legal battles over project reviews and certificate of need reviews embroiled the HSAs in a governmental experiment too far reaching to be achieved in so short a time.

Most public health officials at the local level stayed apart from the community health planning process, missing its importance and assuming that they had the health planning responsibility in their community anyway. They not only failed to become involved, they tended to ignore the new planning bodies when they developed proposals for new services or changes in old ones and were subsequently puzzled and even angered when the councils sought to interfere in those plans. That mistake became more serious in 1974 when the new and stronger law was under consideration. During the debates about accountability and the role of local general-purpose government in forming HSAs, congressional leaders indicated their dissatisfaction with the participation of local government in health planning. While the legislative liaison worker (lobbyist) for the National Association of County Health Officers was able to force a floor colloquy that opened the door slightly for local government, the law clearly favored the better organized comprehensive health planning agencies, which had everything to gain and nothing to lose by dedicating themselves to the shaping of the new legislation. If they could not gain designation as the successor agencies, they would suffer bureaucratic death.

The reduction of health planning

Local health officers and their state-level counterparts may have been realistic about the immediate impact of community planning on public health programming. Gorham, who had had much to do with the development of sophisticated planning procedures in the U.S. Department of Health, Education, and Welfare, said that "anyone in government knows that most decisions on spending emerge from a political process and are most heavily influenced by value judgments and the pressures brought to bear by a wide range of interested parties."[8] He knew that government leaders, both elected and appointed, had program preferences often unrelated to costs, benefits, or efficiency. They may be related to an influential constituent or to a personal experience with alcoholism, cancer, or heart disease. Nonetheless, the community health planning experiment offered a new chance to develop a larger constituency of public involvement in health.

Given more time the process might have matured and achieved some of the effectiveness experienced in counterpart agencies in England. However, President Reagan was intent on eliminating the process partly in response to intense pressure from vested interest groups such as the American Medical Association and the American Hospital Association and partly because of his own commitment to a society regulated by a "free market." In his 1982 budget he proposed no funds for the HSAs. Congress provided $64 million dollars by means of a continuing resolution (in contrast to the inadequate $127 million that had been available in the prior year) and allowed any governor to certify by October 1, 1981, that the state agency could perform the work of the HSAs, with the result that the Secretary would dedesignate the HSAs in that state. Five governors did just that (Ohio, Alabama, Nebraska, Louisiana, and Missouri), and the HSAs lost their designations and their federal funds. The remaining agencies did not have sufficient funds to continue and made plans to cut back, shut down, solicit private donations from the community (an unlikely prospect for a quasiregulatory agency), or form private consulting agencies in an already cluttered competitive market. State agencies showed no signs of support for the community planning bodies. In 1982 the President returned to his elimination agenda and proposed $2 million to close the remaining HSAs.

While some HSAs will continue to function in a limited capacity for awhile, the experiment begun in 1966 is for the time being dead. Those who believe that the whole strategy had been part of a long-term effort to demonstrate that neither community nor state health planning could work and that only centralized control over health resource allocation efforts in Washington could lead to achievement of a national agenda of equity may look with satisfaction on the events of the last few years. Those who believe that the ability to carry out such planning is still so very primitive that only a policy of diversity and scanning for useful approaches to complex problems makes sense must now try to resurrect the idea of local health planning. It may be that the nation's most conservative president since the 1920s will foster the development of a more creative experiment at the community and state level than would otherwise have been possible.

THE PLANNING PROCESS

The comprehensive health planning ferment during the last 2 decades has obscured attention to planning as an administrative process. The framers of P.L. 89-749 and P.L. 93-641 had the establishment of community and nonprovider control over the allocation of health service resources as much on their minds as planning. The intense community struggle for control of the new health planning agencies tended to distract attention from the day-to-day realities of health planning, both in legislative bodies and in operating agencies.

Structure

Just where does planning fit in the operating agency? The answers illustrate some of the previous discussion about the political nature of the planning process. Levin[9] thought that the comprehensive health planning process failed because it was grafted onto administration when it should have subsumed it. However, that would intertwine decision making (a political process) with planning. If the planners or planning bodies subsume decision making, the planners become the new administrators and the purpose of planning turns out to be the substitution of a new leadership for the old one. Others think of planning as a scientific process separated from the more subjective realm of day-to-day management—an "off-line" location. Levy and Loomba[10] see planning as an "on-line" process with the planners very much involved in programming and implementation. In practice, planning is a process, not a product, and it is a process that should permeate all management and political systems. Planning is to administration as epidemiology is to disease prevention. Some agencies may establish a staff unit organizationally close to the director's office with analysis and planning as its function. This fits into what Mintzberg has called the technostructure[11] (see Chapter 10) and has a number of unfortunate implications for the HSA with a professional staff. A separate staff unit may be able to avoid the pressure to become involved in immediate problem-solving tasks and concentrate on long-range planning, but it has a penchant for attempting to analyze and standardize the work of others so that the work of the organization can be more systematically studied and planned. Such efforts are resented and resisted by the workers in a professional bureaucracy.

The breadth of the planning process will influence its organizational placement. Some have argued for a very broad scope that would include the environment in an ecologic approach to health planning. The broader the boundaries of the planning effort, the more likely it will come into conflict with other spheres of interest such as education and welfare. If health planners realize that employment has a major impact on community as well as family health and take a broad approach to their mission, they might try to incorporate vocational training and employment opportunity programs into the health plan, leading to wasteful battles with other agencies of government. The scope of planning should fit the agreed on mission of the agency. When it exceeds those boundaries, the planners and the agency director need to begin discussions with the planners and directors of other community agencies.

Health planning does impinge on other spheres

of interest and should be seen as one facet of social and economic planning. Many states developed large hospitals for the mentally ill and for tuberculosis patients in the nineteenth century and the first half of the twentieth century. These were usually located in isolated, rural communities. With modern treatment techniques, the number of people confined to such institutions has declined dramatically, especially since the 1950s. It is essential that those responsible for the management of such institutions consider alternatives for the future, including the possibility of converting them to more generalized use or closing them. The last alternative is often the most practical one because of the location and age of the facilities, but it is a difficult choice because the surrounding area is often dependent on such institutions for its economic stability. The mental health of a community is jeopardized by undercutting its economic stability, and health agency administrators should become involved in studies of the economic development of the area as part of the closure alternative. It can be argued that it would be better to continue less than optimal care for the patients in the institution if moving them to a better system would imperil employment opportunities for a large sector of the community. Such considerations raise the question of boundaries: how global does a health plan have to be to be comprehensive? Although health planners have to consider such issues as employment and economic development, they need to work with rather than try to usurp the work of those who have a responsibility for and skill in such efforts.

Some large state agencies and the national Department of Health and Human Services maintain separate planning units that often are involved in the study of technology or policy. In most state and local health agencies, planning is carried out at the program level and as part of the budget process (see Chapter 13).

Terminology in planning

A variety of terms have been invented and applied to the analytic processes of planning[12-13]: program planning, program analysis, decision trees, program cost accounting, cost-benefit analysis, cost-effectiveness analysis, planning-programming-budgeting systems, operations research, systems analysis, program evaluation and review technique, and automatic scheduling with time integrated resource allocation. Many of these names and methods are more or less synonymous, some represent parts of others, and many overlap. The more encompassing programs are planning-programming-budgeting systems, operations research, systems analysis, and program evaluation and review techniques. These techniques are concerned with the complete spectrum from fact finding, problem definition, goal setting, programming, controls, and evaluation with proper feedins and feedbacks of information, resources, and results to subsidiary or final outputs or solutions.

Planning-programming-budgeting-systems is a procedure intended to make possible the better allocation of resources among alternate ways of attaining a desired objective.

According to Hatry and Cotton,[15]

Its essence is the development and presentation of information as to the full implications, the costs and benefits of the major alternative courses of action relevant to major resources allocation decisions . . . Such problems as budget and implementation, manpower selection, the assessment of the work efficiency of operating units and cost control of current operations are generally considered to be outside the purview of PPBS [planning-programming-budgeting systems]. Cost accounting and non-fiscal performance reporting systems are very important in providing basic data required for PPBS analyses (as well as for fiscal accounting and management control purposes.) However, such systems are usually considered complementary to PPBS rather than directly part of it . . . The main contribution of PPBS lies in the planning process, i.e., the process of making program policy decisions that lead to a specific budget and specific multi-year plans.

Operations research originated from the efforts of scientists of many disciplines to solve military operations problems during World War II.[16] It is a term applied to "research into some or all aspects of conducting or operating a system, a business, or a service, while treating the system as a living organism in its proper environment. . . ." Operations research usually involves the development of a model, manipulation of the known variables, and forecasting of the results of the system under different conditions.

Systems analysis focuses on the first phases of planning-programming-budgeting systems or operations research. The process involves the definition of the problem, the projection of determinants of the problem, the generation of alternative approaches to solving the problem, the evaluation of the cost effectiveness of the alternatives, and the interpretation of the quantitative and qualitative results.

Program evaluation and review technique is adapted from the work-flow studies used in industrial management. It provides a graphic detailed representation of the components of a program during the planning of its implementation. It involves a breakdown of the project into subprojects with their objectives and the development of a network of activities necessary to move from one event to another. Time estimates are developed for each activity and then for the whole process, including the critical path, which is the longest path in terms of time from the beginning to the end. The network is a diagram of the events necessary to reach the project's objective, and it is under constant analysis to identify problem areas and to indicate whether predicted progress is being made.[17]

The iterative process

Planning is an iterative process with the results constantly feeding back into the cycle. The steps can be described in various ways, but the following are generally used in some form or another: (1) statement of a goal, (2) listing of problems in attaining that goal, (3) definition of objectives, and (4) exploration of various methods for moving toward the objectives. Then (5) someone has to choose which method will be used, and this has to be coupled with (6) priority setting. Finally, (7) the program has to be implemented and (8) evaluated. At this point, and all along the way, the process of iteration begins, with the results feeding back into the cycle and forcing a reappraisal of the goal, the problems, the objectives, the methods, and the priorities. Information about social and health status indicators, the law, the availability and cost of resources, political and social constraints and sanctions, and the effectiveness of different intervention techniques is essential to the process.

Goals. Goals are broad statements incorporating social values and policy into a statement of a desirable future status. Goal statements need not be immediately attainable nor involve numerical targets; but it is important that they reflect a social consensus and not contain an inherent conflict with the aspirations of the community. *Assuring all persons an opportunity to develop their capabilities so that they can live as independently as possible*

is a useful statement of a goal. To reduce dependency by guaranteeing every person an adequate income may be acceptable as a statement of personal principle, but it fails as a goal because it specifies the method to be used (a guaranteed annual income), one that is not generally accepted in the United States.

Problem definition. What are the obstacles that stand in the way of goal attainment? *Many children have a hearing problem that interferes with the development of language skills, psychologic growth and development, and learning skills.* This problem can be due to a number of causes and its prevalence is measurable. This statement has all of the ingredients of a useful and explicit statement of a problem: clarity, measurement, and an understanding of causality.

Objective. A statement of an objective must include (1) a realistic target, (2) a measurable target, and (3) the advantage of clarity. It should not make reference to a preferred method of reaching the objective, and it should not include a mixture of objectives that would necessarily involve the development of several different strategies. *The reduction of the prevalence of hypertension through better public education aimed at obesity* would be a poor statement of an objective. It says "reduce" without indicating from what to what; it selects public education as the method of choice when there are many other strategies that could be used for the reduction of hypertension; and it confuses obesity with hypertension without defining either.

To curtail the number of acute care hospital beds from a ratio of 4.3 per 1,000 persons to 3.8 by 1986 would be a useful statement of an objective. Presumably a goal of reducing the cost of health care has been accepted, and one of the problems has been found to be an oversupply of hospital beds (although the nature of these relationships is by no means clear). The objective is to reduce that supply by a measurable amount over a defined period. An objective that does not allow measurement should be avoided if possible.

Objective statements should be aimed at results or outputs, not inputs or activities, although this is not always possible. For example, most communities cannot reduce the incidence of polio since the incidence is usually zero. Since the relationship of immunization to the prevention of polio is well known and adequately measured, *the maintenance of a 95% level of immunization among schoolchildren* would be an acceptable objective. Stating objectives and measuring results in prevention programs are difficult. If an input or an activity is to be measured, its efficacy in attaining the real purpose of the program must be known. The relationship of restaurant inspections to the prevention of outbreaks of food-borne disease is a good example. The objective may be to reduce the frequency of outbreaks, but measurement is difficult. A "proxy" target of some number of restaurants inspected each year with correction of 75% of the deficiencies within 30 days could be used, but the staff should review what they know about the relationship of such enforcement activities to the possible spread of disease before adopting the indices.

Methods. Most program managers when asked to reach an objective will describe the existing method, but it is important that alternatives be explored and their costs compared. If an acceptable objective is to reduce the number of decayed, missing, and filled teeth in school-aged children from 2.9 to 2.5 over a 10-year period, all available technology should be explored to develop an array of methods. This might include the expansion of water system fluoridation, the use of topical fluorides, a program of preschool dental health education coupled with training and incremental dental care, and the possible use in the future of immunizing agents or other chemicals. The cost, the effectiveness, and the acceptability of each technique and the availability of necessary resources must be considered in the review.

Priorities. The choice of a method is intimately related to the process of establishing priorities. Program managers have to choose or recommend a method to accomplish an objective. This has to be done within the political framework for reviewing community priorities. Sometimes the elected community, state, or national leaders will have established priorities, as was true with the passage of the National Health Planning and Resources Development Act of 1974. More often it is a program or agency administrator who takes the analysis of problems and priorities to a decision-making body, such as a county commission or a governor and the legislature, with a recommendation. There are a number of ways to analyze priorities: the simplex method, the nominal group process, criteria weighting, decision alternative rational evaluation, or the priority rating process.[13]

The priority rating process has some of the advantages of several of the other techniques and serves as an effective learning process for the participants. As is true of the other procedures, it yields relative results that are useful for comparing different and competing programs or alternative methods for achieving the same objective. It cannot be applied to a single program as a method of evaluation. The members of the group have to work together throughout the process rather than separately, since definitions of the component parts of the process tend to be unique to each working group. Consistency across the scope of programs reviewed is necessary to get a useful relative ranking.

The first step is for the participants to list every activity or program under consideration. The list may easily number into the hundreds. The group then proceeds to analyze each program using a dynamic formula consisting of four components:

Component A: size of problem
Component B: seriousness of problem
Component C: effectiveness of the intervention
Component D: propriety, economics, acceptability, resources, and legality (PEARL)

The basic priority rating formula is:

$$\text{Basic priority rating (BPR)} = \frac{(A + B)C}{3} \times D$$

The range of scores for each of the four components is:

A: 0 to 10
B: 0 to 20
C: 0 to 10
D: 0 or 1

The maximum obtainable product of the four components (A, B, C, and D) is 300. By an arbitrary division of this maximum product by 3, the maximum score becomes 100. Every rating will then be in the range of 0 to 100. Component D, or PEARL, becomes 0 or 1, as shown later.

As in the case of many evaluative procedures, a large subjective element enters into this exercise. The choice and definition of the components in the formula and the relative weights assigned to them are based on group consensus. Some control may be achieved by the use of a precise definition of terms, the delineating of exact rating procedures, and the use of statistical data to guide ratings when feasible.

Component A: size of the problem. For purposes of assigning priorities, the size of the problem may be scored by the use of rates or the percent of the total population at risk for the problem under consideration. Many problems will be defined for very small population groups, making an incidence or prevalence rate per 100,000 people at risk a useful approach as in the following scale:

Incidence or prevalence per 100,000 population	Score
50,000 or more	10
5,000 to 49,999	8
500 to 4,999	6
50 to 499	4
5 to 49	2
0.5 to 4.9	0

The use of incidence or prevalence depends on whether the program is designed to prevent the occurrence or to reduce the prevalence of the problem through secondary or even tertiary prevention techniques (see Chapter 16).

Component B: seriousness of the problem. The seriousness of a problem is defined in terms of four factors: urgency, severity, economic loss, and involvement of other people. "Seriousness" is assigned a range of 0 to 20 in the formula, and each of the four factors is assigned a range of 0 to 10. It is possible to attain a mathematic score of 40, which exceeds the range, but it is rare that the combination of the factors accumulates to that extent. The most urgent or severe problems are usually individual problems that do not involve significant community disruption. The terms are all subjective, and several iterations of the process will be necessary before the group can begin to agree on its terms. *Urgency* can be used to define the emergent nature of the problem, such as emergency response to a car wreck, or the sense of community urgency if an unknown chemical is spilled by a tank truck. *Severity* may encompass estimates of the case fatality rate or the seriousness of the disability if the problem is rarely fatal. *Economic loss* is related to severity and may reflect both community costs or losses as well as family costs. The involvement of other people is related to the other factors as well and is most frequently an issue in rapidly contagious diseases such as measles in an unimmunized population. If the total score exceeds 20, it is arbitrarily truncated by the participants.

Component C: effectiveness. Effectiveness is of-

ten difficult to measure. The efficacy of most vaccines has been measured fairly carefully, but other interventions, such as the hospitalization of psychiatric patients or the use of supplemental nutrition for high-risk, low-income pregnant women, are less well evaluated. Most groups can make reasonably useful estimates, especially if the members have programs in competition, since they will contest unrealistic claims of effectiveness by each other. If the program reaches only 20% of those with the problem and is only 70% effective, then the effectiveness is $0.20 \times 0.70 = .14$, or 14%, and the rating would be quite low. Effectiveness is a multiplier in the basic priority rating formula, so its impact is powerful.

Component D: propriety, economics, acceptability, resources, and legality (PEARL). PEARL consists of a group of factors not directly related to the actual need or the effectiveness of the proposed intervention, but which determine whether a particular program can be carried out at all.

Propriety and acceptability are virtually synonymous. If economic resources are not available, if other resources such as physicians or nurses cannot be obtained, or if the program depends on an activity not permitted in law, then it cannot be implemented without changing the condition. Each of these qualifying factors is given a score of 0 or 1 and, since together they represent a product rather than a sum, if any one of them is rated a 0, it not only gives PEARL a 0 but makes the overall priority rating 0.

Implementation and evaluation. Before the program is implemented, the evaluation methodology has to be developed. As noted above, evaluation is linked to the definition of the problem, the objective, and the design of the intervention method. Once started, the program should return information, which enables progress and performance to be reviewed. The feedback continues throughout program operation, although it may be modified just as any other part of the program may be modified based on the feedback.

It is important to distinguish between activity reporting, performance reporting, and the reporting of results. It is also important to determine what is to be accomplished by the evaluation. Evaluation is similar to research. A hypothesis is postulated, the program (experiment) is run, and the results either confirm or deny the hypothesis. If the purpose of the evaluation is to study different treatment or intervention techniques to see which is best, it can be structured as a research project, in which case the production of the information is one of the end results of the project. Costs are usually high, and the research method is probably inappropriate to most ongoing programs. Evaluation as a management tool should be incorporated into the work of the program staff and not treated as a research project. In this case the data do not constitute an end product but are fed back into the iterative cycle as part of the program itself, helping the staff to correct the program. An evaluation should not become more rigorous than the program requires. A service program should not be implemented unless the staff is reasonably convinced that, properly run, it will accomplish the intended results.

Activity reporting is the most common form of feedback and is of little value for evaluation purposes. It counts the number of lab tests run, the number of home visits made, or the number of restaurants inspected. Performance reporting is more difficult but more useful. Performance enumerates results: deficiencies corrected, children immunized, full birth weight babies delivered. Performance is more directly related to objectives and serves as a better measurement of progress. Performance can be very difficult to measure. A reasonable objective for an alcoholism program would be to reduce the number of disability days caused by alcoholism, but keeping track of alcoholics is notoriously difficult. Follow-up without a very costly effort may be as low as 20% to 30%. Even if the effectiveness of the intervention program were as high as 70%, the overall "success rate" would be $0.20 \times 0.70 = 0.14$. With nothing known about the other 80%, no assumptions about their success or failure can be made.

Evaluation of a health education program is especially difficult. A campaign to increase the use of lap-and-shoulder restraints in cars could be measured by asking for police reports on the use of such devices by people stopped by the police for some reason, but such a sample would be heavily biased toward nonuse. The automobile accident fatality rate could be used, but it is so dependent on miles driven and speeding laws and their enforcement that no valid inferences can be drawn from such a measurement. When reliance on indirect measures such as these are necessary, it is helpful to select several different ones. If they form a consistent pattern, they have higher overall validity.

Cost has become a crucial variable in program evaluation. Cost-effectiveness analysis compares the ratio of cost to effectiveness for several different methods of achieving the same objective. *Effectiveness* is a relative term in cost-effectiveness analysis and may mean the attack rate for a disease, the fatality rate for those who get the disease, or the rate of secondary spread. Cost-benefit analyses attempt to quantify the benefits as well as the costs in monetary terms so that different types of programs and outcomes can be compared. The terms have become very popular and the procedures are arduous. The Office of Technology Assessment of the U.S. Congress has concluded that "CEA/CBA cannot serve as the sole or primary determinant of a health care decision. Decision making could be improved, however, by the process of identifying and considering all the relevant costs and benefits of a decision."[18]

One of the problems in evaluation is the difficulty of measuring something that can be accepted as an index of health or lack of health. Sackett and his colleagues[19] have developed and tested a survey approach that combines the necessary ingredients of comprehensiveness, a positive orientation, general applicability, sensitivity, simplicity, and precision that the authors required, but it basically measures health as the complement of ill health. Cochrane[20] has suggested a terse if irreverent measurement of ill health. He suggests that we define ill health for any condition as that point at which treatment does more good than harm.

Evaluation remains difficult and important. It is not impossible. It does require a thoughtful approach to objective setting and the use of evaluation criteria that are congruent with the scope of the program and the knowledge that exists about the program.

Legislative leaders will continue to ask that public efforts be evaluated and will continue to launch new programs without evaluation. The priorities listed by Congress for the National Health Planning and Resources Development Act of 1974 fail the test of good objective writing, and evaluation was not built into the law. That may just illustrate the difference between politics, or decision making, and planning.

REFERENCES

1. Bureau of Health Planning: Toward a better health care system, Annual report, fiscal 1979, U.S. De-

partment of Health and Human Services Pub. No.
(HRA) 80-14006, April 1980.

2. National Council on Health Planning and Development: Report on consumer participation in the health planning program, Feb. 6, 1981, U.S. Department of Health and Human Services.

3. Richmond, J.B.: Do we have a national health policy? The first annual Lester Breslow Distinguished Lectureship, Los Angeles, Oct. 6, 1980, University of California at Los Angeles School of Public Health Alumni Association.

4. The national guidelines for health planning: Standards regarding the appropriate supply, distribution, and organization of health resources, U.S. Department of Health, Education, and Welfare Pub. No. (HRA) 79-645, March 28, 1978.

5. Cooper, T.L.: The hidden price tag: participation costs and health planning, Am. J. Public Health **69:**368, April 1979.

6. Health systems plans: a poor framework for promoting health care improvements, U.S. General Accounting Office Pub. No. (HRD) 81-93, June 22, 1981.

7. Committee on Health Planning of the Institute of Medicine: Health planning in the United States: selected policy issues, Vol. 1, Washington, D.C., 1981, National Academy Press.

8. Gorham, W.: PPBS: its scope and limits, The Public Interest **8:**4, Summer 1967.

9. Levin, A.L.: Health planning and the U.S. federal government, Int. J. Health Serv. **2:**367, Aug. 1972.

10. Levy, S., and Loomba, N.P.: Health care administration: a managerial perspective, Philadelphia, 1973, J.B. Lippincott Co.

11. Mintzberg, H.: The structuring of organizations, Englewood Cliffs, N.J., 1979, Prentice-Hall, Inc.

12. Blum, H.: Planning for health, ed. 2, New York, 1981. Human Sciences Press.

13. Spiegel, A.D., and Hyman, H.H.: Basic health planning methods, Germantown, Md., 1978, Aspen Systems Corp.

14. Perlin, M.S., editor: Managing institutional planning: health facilities and P.L. 93-641, Germantown, Md., 1976, Aspen Systems Corp.

15. Hatry, H.P., and Cotton, J.F.: Program planning for state, county, and city, Washington, D.C., 1967, George Washington University Press.

16. Flagle, C.D.: Operational research in the health services, Ann. N.Y. Acad. Sci. **107:**748, May 22, 1963.

17. Merten, W.: PERT and planning for health programs, Public Health Rep. **81:**449, May 1966.

18. The implication of cost effectiveness analysis of medical technology, Congress of the United States, Office of Technology Assessment Pub. No. OTA-H-125, Aug. 1980.

19. Sackett, D.L., and others: The development and application of indices of health: general methods and a summary of results, Am. J. Public Health **67:**423, May 1977.

20. Cochrane, A.L.: The history of the measurement of ill health, Int. J. Epidemiol. **1:**89, 1972.

CHAPTER 12

Personnel management

If your company is run "by the book," If the job description is more important than the man, Your organization is in danger of creeping paralysis.

Clarence B. Randall

Health is a labor-intensive business. Even though the work has been heavily affected by technology, the advances are not usually labor saving, as is the case with manufacturing and some service industries, but rather labor consuming. For organized health systems, the need for effective personnel management is paramount.

Personnel management involves the administration of an organization's human resources in a manner that assures the best output with the least costly input while protecting and enhancing the welfare of the workers. Merit systems of personnel management attempt to base employment and career development on merit. They are organized systems that attempt to assure due process in the selection and advancement of personnel. Civil service systems are merit systems that serve the public sector—civil (as differentiated from private or military) employment. Civil service systems had one goal and three subsidiary objectives when they began:

GOAL: to remove personnel management from partisan politics

Objective 1: to afford everyone an equal opportunity for employment

Objective 2: to apply behavioral science to personnel management

Objective 3: to offer employees an opportunity for career development

These original goals and objectives have undergone considerable modification.

Many people think that the American civil service system is too dominated by faith in scientism—a belief that human beings can be "engineered" into job descriptions. Others assert that it is dominated by the self-declared systems of ethics of professional, clerical, and technical groups and that these self-declared roles have robbed the public of the opportunity to be served by a creative work force. To the extent that this is true, it raises fundamental questions about flexibility, motivation, and productivity in all organized personnel systems. Critics decry the rigidities of job specifications, minimum qualifications, and the lack of effective rewards and punishments. Many public health program managers fervently wish that they could do away with the system entirely. Such wishes are unrealistic. Without a well-managed personnel system, most public health program managers would spend a large part of their time in court defending their personnel management practices. A personnel system designed to assure equity and due process is necessary given the democratic heritage of the American governmental system. Personnel systems, like almost all systems, are compromises that attempt to satisfy often conflicting requirements but cannot maximize the satisfaction of any of them.

As previously noted, the original purpose of the civil service system was to remove employment and personnel management from the sphere of partisan politics. Human service workers generally attach a pejorative connotation to the word *politics*—a connotation that is both unwarranted and inappropriate. Politics is the way in which decisions get made when differing values are involved. When two or more people or groups have different views about a problem, the solution involves a political decision, no matter how much data and scientific analysis went into the process.

Management of public
health programs

HISTORY
The public health professions

Public health organizations in the United States
were not characterized by professionalism until the
1930s. There were some outstanding leaders in
public health in many parts of the country, but no
real training programs for the workers, nor were
many of the health professions generally recognized as distinct and requiring academic training.
The Johns Hopkins School of Public Health opened
in 1918 with a grant from the Rockefeller Foundation, and the Massachusetts Institute of Technology–Harvard program in public health (established in 1912) became the Harvard School of Public Health in 1922. By 1982 there were 22 schools
of public health. Even though they have provided
most of the leadership in public health, most public
health workers have received their training elsewhere—in nursing schools, engineering schools,
and medical schools or in undergraduate or graduate programs in public health that are not a part
of the schools of public health.

Improvements in the training and education of
public health workers in the United States have
been largely because of the work of the American
Public Health Association and its Committee on
Professional Education. Beginning in the 1930s,
the committee developed a series of model job descriptions with minimum qualifications that were
and still are used, with repeated modifications, by
civil service systems at the state and local level.
These descriptions were used by the Children's Bureau as it helped establish federally aided public
health programs in the states. However, job descriptions developed by professional groups have
their drawbacks. Those involved in drafting the descriptions are generally people with what at the
time is considered an acceptable graduate academic
education, and they insist that others who would
do their work must be similarly trained. When such
requirements become embodied in the official personnel practices of public agencies, professional
groups have effectively established control over the
work that is to be done, who shall do it, and how
they shall be trained. The civil rights movement of
the 1960s and subsequent reforms in the U.S. Civil
Service System have reduced the restrictive impact
of professional organizations on public service employment.

The civil service system

Beginning in the 1870s voluntary groups were
organized in several states to urge reform in public
hiring practices. The passage of the Pendleton Act,
the first national personnel legislation, is generally
attributed to the assassination of President Garfield
a half-year earlier by a disgruntled job seeker. That
dramatic event may have helped engender public
support for the act, but it is also apparent that the
Republicans anticipated considerable gains in
congressional seats by the Democrats in the 1884
elections and that they wanted to preserve the jobs
of those they had helped place in office. A new civil
service system would require that protected incum-
bents be removed only for cause, and it was Republican support that got the bill through Congress.
The first state civil service law was passed in New
York in 1883 (introduced by Theodore Roosevelt
and signed into law by Governor Grover Cleveland).

The civil service laws in the United States were
modeled after those in England, but there were and
are some significant differences. Competitive examinations are at the base of both systems, but the
English examinations tend to be of the essay type,
dealing with abstractions and suited for college
graduates with a liberal arts education. American
examinations are more objective in nature, dealing
with job-specific details and in some cases, designed more for a technical or vocational educational system graduate. The British system admits
new personnel only at the bottom of the career ladder and results in a closed service, with senior managers and policy makers coming up from the ranks.
The American system is more democratic in its origins and in its practices. In its original form it was
fervently Jacksonian in suggesting that participation in the government workforce should be representative in nature and even characterized by
turnover not dissimilar to that found in the patronage system. That has changed somewhat as job
security has become a more important feature of
public employment, and promotion from within the
ranks has been urged by employee groups.

Civil service systems usually are insulated from
partisan politics by placing them under the direction of an appointed commission. The commission
members serve staggered terms and cannot be removed except for cause. The commission hires the
personnel director and approves job classifications,
adopts rules of procedure, reviews employee appeals, and either recommends salary schedules to
the chief executive of the jurisdiction or in some

cases establishes such schedules on its own authority. Appointment of commissioners is usually by the mayor or governor and is often subject to review by the legislative body.

The Social Security Act of 1935 authorized grants to the states for human service programs. The act required that the states have an acceptable personnel management system but prohibited national program managers from prescribing what constituted acceptable personnel practices. Because of widespread abuse in the use of the new federal grants-in-aid, the law was amended in 1939 to require the adoption of a merit system covering all employees in any program that was established with federal funds. This was subsequently extended to all programs that had any reliance on federal dollars. The Hatch Act in 1940 prohibited political activities by civil service employees and this too was extended to state and local governments that were using federal grants-in-aid.

The work of the U.S. Civil Service System in developing standards and providing technical assistance to the states has been an outstanding feature of the national program. Although civil service systems are usually described in the plural, there is virtually only one such system—the national one—with modifications by states and local governments. The U.S. Civil Service System has substantial authority over state and local systems. Since its authority was tied to grants-in-aid in health and welfare programs, the System requested the agency that has since evolved into the Department of Health and Human Services to serve as the review and certification agency for state personnel programs. The Social Security Act resulted in the rapid proliferation of civil service systems at the state level, but extension to local governments has been slow and difficult. Local public health departments were common by the 1930s, which meant that public health was the vehicle for carrying civil service systems into local government. The operation of such systems is expensive, involving job classification, task analysis, recruitment, and testing. Many local governments cannot afford such systems and use their state system for personnel management. Because of that, local government civil service workers are often thought of as employees of the state civil service system rather than as employees of local government. The health programs are often thought of as state-mandated and state-controlled programs, less amenable to local control. When local government believes that it

has less control over some programs, it also believes that it is less responsible for them. This is one of the reasons that some analysts have claimed that civil service systems are too far removed from the politics of everyday life, and changes in recent years have made some program administrators more responsive to the day-to-day realities of local politics. Nationally, 55% of all local public employees are in education, 7% are in health programs, and 6% are in law enforcement. Both the law enforcement and the educational merit systems are different from the general civil service system and are usually under more direct local control, leaving only public health workers somewhat outside the sphere of influence of locally elected officials except in cities or counties large enough to maintain their own civil service systems.

The Civil Service Reform Act of 1978 was widely hailed as a progressive step. It separated the national civil service system into three agencies: (1) The Office of Personnel Management, which is responsible for administering the civil service system (seen as the voice of management); (2) the Merit System Protection Board, which is to adjudicate disputes, study the workings of the system, and conduct reviews of the effectiveness of policies and procedures (seen as the neutral guardian of merit); and (3) the Federal Labor Relations Authority, which is responsible for the designation of work units for collective bargaining, the supervision of elections by employees for representation in collective bargaining, and the resolution of unfair labor practices (seen as the voice of labor). The act also established the Senior Executive Service, which was intended to loosen some of the restrictive characteristics of civil service on senior-level managers as well as to offer them a wider opportunity for career development. The results have not lived up to expectations.[1]

Dissatisfaction with civil service systems is widespread. Managers and elected officials are dissatisfied with the system because it restricts their freedom to hire the person they think may be best for the job as well as their ability to move people around or to fire those whom they feel are not working effectively. Employees find the system rigid, restrictive in its rewards, and not sufficiently protective of their rights. The private sector has the same problems. Chief executive officers of large, established organizations function as satisficers rather than maximizers, trying to satisfy their boards, their employees, and their clients all at the same time to keep the organization functioning effectively. But satisfying for the sake of effective functioning does not necessarily foster creative management.

Collective bargaining and civil service

Collective bargaining emerged as the dominant public sector personnel issue of the 1970s and will likely remain so through the next 2 decades. The concept of unionization was not only foreign but was also objectionable to public health workers for many years. Patronage gave way to paternalism, not unionism, in the early days of civil service. In such a system, avuncular managers thrived on the reciprocal warmth of their employees, and the notion that unions might be necessary to protect the rights of employees was abhorrent. Beyond that, professional people (nurses and physicians especially) felt that unionization was antithetic to their code of ethics. As public health organizations grew beyond the original triad of physician, nurse, and sanitarian, it was inevitable that groups of workers with similar jobs and expectations would find it desirable to bargain collectively for their working conditions and their pay. Regardless of the law and the intentions, civil service systems were clearly the tools of management in their early days and very close to political control. Due process and employee rights were less often practiced than preached.

The central issue in the public sector is the right to strike—a right essential to the concept of collective bargaining. The right to withhold one's labor is widely assumed, but it is often denied in the public sector on the premise that the services— police protection, fire protection, hospital care—are essential and monopoly services; that is, the consumer has nowhere else to go for the needed, essential service. Contrary to popular opinion there generally are no statutes prohibiting collective bargaining by public employees; what is missing is a federal guarantee of the right to bargain collectively. Although the National Labor Relations Board has jurisdiction over the election of bargaining units in private industry, no such federal guarantees exist for public employees. From a legal standpoint local and state elected officials are free to ignore representations by employees, but from a

political standpoint it is very difficult to do so. To maintain the fiction that this is not really collective bargaining in the trade union sense of the term, local governments often call their agreements with employee groups "memoranda of understanding." Regardless of its title, once it exists and has been signed by both the government and the employee representatives it serves as a contract and forms the basis for the resolution of grievances.

The difference between a grievance and an appeal is subtle but real. A worker can appeal a personnel decision that is contrary to the rules of the civil service system. The appeal is usually through the layers of management to the Civil Service Commission and sometimes to the courts. A grievance is a complaint that a contract has not been honored and presupposes the existence of a contract. Grievances follow a different pathway than that of an appeal: through management, often to an arbitration panel, sometimes to the courts, but usually not to the Civil Service Commission.

There are four different processes that occur in collective bargaining[2]: (1) distributive bargaining in which there are only so many benefits to go around and what one group gains, some other party to the process must lose; (2) integrative bargaining in which both or all parties gain; (3) attitudinal structuring, a process in which the issues are structured into either the distributive or the integrative mold; and (4) intra-organizational bargaining in which the members of subgroups within the bargaining unit attempt to form a collective opinion about their bargaining objectives. Elected officials who have to ratify whatever agreements are reached may delegate responsibility for the bargaining process to their appointed representatives (sometimes a special consultant) but reserve final approval to themselves. Union leaders prefer to bargain with the final decision makers rather than the appointed representatives who can only make recommendations, and they often find a receptive ear because elected officials thrive on bargaining and want employee group support. Circumvention around the appointed bargainers by individual elected officials can make a shambles of management's bargaining strategy.

Because of the complex procedures for publicly reviewing and approving budgets, public sector elected officials have to meet privately to define the parameters of their bargaining position in detail and in advance of the actual bargaining sessions so their representatives can have a reasonable expectation that the agreements they reach with employee groups will be supported.

In collective bargaining, supervisors and supervisees are separated, the latter being covered by the collective bargaining statutes, and the former being considered management. In the National Labor Relations Act, a supervisor is

Any employee having the authority, in the interest of the employer, to hire, transfer, suspend, lay-off, recall, promote, discharge, assign, reward, or discipline other employees, or responsibility to direct them or to adjust their grievances, or effectively to recommend such action, if . . . the exercise of such authority is not of a merely routine or clerical nature, but requires the use of independent judgement.

This definition raises difficulties in classifying physicians and nurses as well as other professional and technical personnel. The act allows "professional employees" to bargain collectively and defines such employees.[3]

Regardless of the reluctance of elected and appointed officials, collective bargaining is a feature of public employment and will probably expand in its importance. The Health Care Amendments to the National Labor Relations Act and the Taft-Hartley Act (P.L.93-360 of 1974) permitted employees in both the not-for-profit as well as proprietary health care institutions to bargain collectively.

THE PUBLIC-PRIVATE DEBATE

It is commonly alleged that public sector employees are overpaid, unproductive, and only marginally ethical. The facts do not support the allegations.

The public sector is predominantly engaged in a service industry and is therefore labor intensive. Social work, venereal disease clinics, and good prenatal care do not lend themselves to automation. By contrast, the private sector has one overriding objective: to maximize profits. That can be done by increasing prices and decreasing costs, so long as one remains competitive, or by increasing the amount of product sold. The public sector has neither that overriding motivation nor implicit or explicit public support to use the tactics of the private sector. While it behooves the private business person to minimize personnel costs, the public sector has other objectives. In addition to the frankly political motivation to produce jobs for constituents, government is often urged to use its work force as a social instrument in times of unemployment or

to increase access to jobs by p
otherwise be employed. Whe
tomate to reduce costs and I
ment is reluctant to lay o'
ployment is a valid social purpo
not usually productive politically. Mor
more difficult to automate service functions u.
to automate manufacturing.

Ethics are another point of debate. Newspapers are replete with stories about some elected or appointed official who misused an office or the authority that went with it, but it appears that private sector abuses are both more common as well as more acceptable to the public. A double standard exists. Governments often become inefficient in their quest to prevent the embezzlement of nickels and dimes. To paraphrase an old English "rhyme:"

We punish the public man and woman
Who steals the goose from off the common,
Yet turn the private felon loose
Who steals the common from the goose.

Even though elected officials are prone to attack sloth and lapses of ethics in those known as bureaucrats, legislative investigations have generally concluded that there is less pilfering, embezzling, and cheating by public employees than by business leaders, managers, and private sector employees.

The private sector always has the option of excusing theft or misconduct in exchange for a resignation, an apology, or simply based on kinship or friendship. No such right exists in the public sector because it is not the manager's money that is being lost or stolen but the public's money for which the manager is legally accountable. The public sector manager never has the right to excuse dishonest behavior nor to make a personal decision that mitigating circumstances excuse the situation but has instead an obligation to turn the matter over to the appropriate legal representative and leave the pleadings about mitigating circumstances to the witness stand in court.

One admonition is consistently valid: personnel management is the most underrated essential skill for public health administrators. Until fairly recently most public health administrators were physicians, nurses, or sanitarians whose basic training was far removed from the study of administration. Personnel management got short shrift by people

...ho felt that their other skills equipped them to be effective managers of people. Given heavy reliance on the work of skilled people, it should be evident that the selection of capable people, their support and development, and sometimes their discharge are among the most important tasks that any public program manager has to perform. It is relatively easy to get along with an inadequate computer, typewriter, or building compared to the grief that can ensue from the wrong personnel choice. Most new managers are so anxious to learn the substance of their programs, the political milieu in which they must operate, and the nature of their constituents that they pay too little attention to the selection of new staff or the effective development of the existing workers. *Nothing* can be as costly as a personnel mistake. Failure to take the time to choose wisely in the first place or failure to admit a mistake and work as long and as patiently as it takes to help a miscast employee to move into a better role or out of the program altogether can result in more lost time, wasted money, and declining public and political support than virtually any other mistake. There are many good textbooks that explore public personnel systems in detail,[4-11] and anyone contemplating a career in public health administration, from a supervisory level to agency leadership, should study the subject thoroughly and decide at the outset to devote the time to personnel management that it deserves—it is an essential function.

THE PERSONNEL SYSTEM

There are several functions in a personnel system plus some special services that are highly desirable. The best personnel system should be considered a human resource development program and not simply a clerical function involving paper processing. That is true partly because the work to be done by public health is demanding and important, but it is also true because the growth and development of a worker's capabilities are synonymous with good public health practice within the agency and essential to the development of an effective and respected agency.

Job classification

Job classification lies at the heart of the attempt to make personnel work scientific and equitable. The first step is task analysis, a detailed description of the work that is required of the person expected to do the job. For a sanitarian this might involve driving a car, collecting specimens from the cooling vat at a dairy, recording the temperature of the wash water, examining the cleanliness of the milk-collection tubing, discussing results with the dairy manager, completing a report, and so forth. If this work is sufficiently distinct from the work done by an inspector of restaurants, then two separate job classifications might be prepared: dairy inspector and restaurant inspector. Since some dairies are more automated and complex than others, or because the employing agency might want to distinguish between a novice and someone with a year or more of experience, a series of dairy inspectors I and II might be developed in which the dairy inspector II would be required to be able to disassemble an automatic milking machine or evaluate the reliability of a computerized control system for the cooling and storage facility. Finally, if several dairy inspectors I and II worked for the same supervisor, and the supervisor's tasks involved training and supervision, a separate classification of dairy inspector III might be established for supervisors.

The classification description will attempt to distinguish between members of that class and some other class and between members of different grades of that general class, if a series is developed involving several grades. The job description will include examples of the typical work expected of members of that class.

For each classification there are a set of minimum qualifications that represent the effort by the personnel technicians, usually with the input of the health program managers, to estimate the kinds of prior training and experience required to carry out the tasks. The tendency of program managers is to set the minimum qualifications as high as they can to get only very well-qualified applicants, but this may result in over-qualified people in unsatisfying jobs. Excessive minimum qualifications also have the defect of denying job possibilities to those who have not had the opportunity to obtain graduate level or even undergraduate level education, but who may be qualified to run a complex piece of equipment. In recent years, the U.S. Civil Service Commission has stressed the *minimum* part of *minimum qualifications*. The test is job relatedness: if the laboratory testing can be done by a high school graduate, then a master's degree in microbiology cannot be required, since such a requirement would have the effect of denying an equal opportunity for employment to someone who has the skills to perform the necessary tasks. In part, this recent emphasis on minimum qualifications has had the salubrious effect of enabling people to enter the job market and have an opportunity for career development through on-the-job training and experience rather than placing over-qualified people in what for them will be dull jobs. The change in emphasis reflects the development of social policy from the civil rights movement of the 1960s, which rightly saw employment as a crucial ingredient in social stability and growth, particularly for minorities and women. This is one of many instances in which the governmental hiring apparatus has been used for some purpose in addition to its basic purpose of acquiring the human resources necessary to get a job done.

There are many ways in which the job classification process can be abused. If the nursing program director resigns or retires, it may be an opportune time to review a job description that is 20 or 30 years old. If there is a favored candidate in the program for the director's job or someone the agency director wants to exclude, the job description can be written so as to either tailor the job specifically for the preferred worker or to exclude the unwanted one. For example, if the director's choice had a teaching certificate before becoming a nursing supervisor, then an effort might be made to convince the Civil Service Commission that this particular job involves so much training that a nurse with a master's degree in education would be preferable to one with a master's degree in public health. When such efforts are thwarted, program managers complain about the civil service system. The efforts of civil service technicians to be objective about a job classification can reduce management's flexibility, but the idiosyncratic distortion of a job description to accomplish a desired appointment often means the denial of due process to a well-qualified individual. The manager's predilections may be both unfair and unfounded, and if the gambit is successful, the next time the job turns over, the manager may be back before the same Civil Service Commission pleading to reverse the arguments used during the previous revision.

Another common misuse of the classification process is the effort to reclassify a job to reward someone. A classification occupies a position or grade on a pay scale. Within that pay grade there may be as many as 15 steps. Although movement to a higher step within that grade is meant to be based on satisfactory performance, in most systems it becomes fairly automatic, and there is a step up each year until the incumbent reaches the top step of the grade. The top step usually pays about 25% to 30% more than the first step. After an employee reaches the top step, subsequent pay raises can only occur by the employee moving to a different classification with a higher pay-grade rating or when the governing body decides to move all steps and all grades up a notch to reflect cost-of-living increases. For example, a clerical worker in the director's office may be classified as a clerk II, may have done an outstanding job, may have reached the top step in the pay grade, and may have an opportunity to move somewhere else in the agency for a better paying job. If the office director does not want to lose a good worker, an effort may be made to reexamine the work done by the clerk to prove that it is not really a clerk II job, but a clerical supervisor's job or a secretary's job. The incumbent may have in fact acquired a number of duties over the years that placed de facto performance "out-of-class," and a new task analysis by a civil service technician will reveal that the job should be reclassified. The incumbent may, in some systems, have a right to that job without having to compete with others interested in the position if they can pass the test for the higher level position. In other cases, the job has not been expanded beyond the original duties, but the office director and others who do not wish to lose a colleague will join together in an effort to make the job appear more expansive or more demanding than it really is. If they wish to avoid competition with others who may be able to apply competitively for the job if it is reclassified as a supervisory job, they may conjure up a whole new description, such as clerical technician, and claim that they use some special equipment in that office, that requires that person's acquired skills.

Manipulative procedures such as these are common and reflect both the determination of managers to get what they want regardless of equity considerations as well as the rigidities of the civil service system. The manipulations, over time, result in a tangled web of classifications that makes effective personnel management very difficult. Rather than attempt to manipulate the system to achieve some preconceived notion, it is better to

meet with the personnel system director to review
the problem and see if the personnel experts can
help solve the problem without creating unnecessary distortions. It is sometimes best to let the system work. The clerical worker who was a good colleague may get a fresh start in a different work
environment, and a new worker in the director's
office may bring needed change and new capabilities.

Recruitment

Recruitment involves advertising the availability
of the job in an effort to attract qualified applicants.
Sometimes recruitment is carried out only when a
vacancy exists and it is the agency's intention to
fill the vacancy. This is particularly true for job
classifications in which there are few positions or
perhaps only one, such as the director of a maternal
and child health program. In other situations, advertising and recruiting is constant because there
are many positions in the classification, and turnover is such that the personnel agency needs to
have available a list of actively interested and eligible candidates.

One of the paternalistic abuses of the civil service
concept in the past was the tendency of managers
to tell a preferred candidate about an anticipated
vacancy so that there might be only the one applicant. In recent years, rules requiring that notice of
the vacancy be posted in a public place have been
more consistently honored. However, manipulation
still occurs. The rules under which the civil service
system operates generally require that the job possibility be displayed in a public place. This may
mean simply stacking it up with similar announcements on a bulletin board in the courthouse, where
it may go completely unnoticed by most of those
who might have the requisite qualifications. This
allows those who must fill the position to advertise
it where they think they will get suitable candidates. This has been a useful tactic for those involved in minority employment, either as a social
cause or because the work to be done requires
someone of the same cultural background as the
clients. In these instances, one job bulletin might
be posted in the required location, but hundreds of
more enticing announcements might be distributed
in churches, stores, and community centers in the
neighborhood where a high concentration of the
needed minority group live.

Jobs for which many people may be eligible can
be advertised locally. Jobs for which the minimum
qualifications reduce the pool of those who may be
eligible require wider distribution often in national
professional journals. The positions of director of
epidemiology for a large state health agency or a
new mental health center director require a wide
area search, as might a position that requires running a piece of esoteric lab equipment. Most agencies now include in the advertisement that they are
an equal employment opportunity employer to indicate that they operate under an approved minority
hiring plan (see section on Equal Employment Opportunity). It is important to determine whether the
civil service agency will do the recruitment as is
often the case for jobs common to several user
agencies, or whether the health agency is to conduct its own recruitment (for nurses or physicians,
for example) for which it will pay the advertising
costs.

The purposes of the recruitment process are (1)
to assure that all eligible people have an equal opportunity to apply for the job, (2) to be sure that
only those who truly meet the minimum qualifications for the job take the time needed to apply,
(3) to be sure that applicants know what they are
applying for (functions, location, salary, nature of
the agency), (4) to let prospective applicants know
how and when the applications will be reviewed
and an appointment made, and (5) to fill the position with a qualified individual.

The advertisement should indicate the last date
on which applications will be accepted, unless it is
a position for which open and continuous recruitment is appropriate. After the closing date, the applications are reviewed by personnel technicians
and sometimes by program staff to screen out any
applicants who do not meet the minimum qualifications for the job.

Testing

Those applicants found to be eligible for an advertised position will be sent a letter announcing
the date, time, and place as well as the nature of
the examination. Some examinations are objective
in nature, using written, machine-graded, and
standardized tests of ability and knowledge. Groups
of applicants are examined at the same time using
the same test. These are known as "assembled"
examinations because they are given once to all
applicants in an assembly. Other examinations are
open or unassembled, and the test can be taken by
individual applicants whenever they can demon-

strate their eligibility for the classification. Some examinations include a performance test, such as typing or the use of tools, whereas other examinations may consist of only an oral interview usually before a panel. This latter type of examination is particularly common for professional jobs. Some examinations consist of all three: a written test, a performance test, and an interview. Oral interview panels are usually briefed by the program manager about the kind of person the manager is looking for, which gives the examiners an opportunity to go beyond the confines of the written job specification to explore the nature of the work and the clientele.

When the examination process is completed, the eligible applicants are scored and rated. In some jurisdictions, two lists will be developed, ranked by test score; one list ranks all applicants, and the other separately lists a minority group, which has been identified by that jurisdiction as either underemployed or in need because of the nature of the task (usually the cultural or racial characteristics of the clientele).

The testing process has undergone considerable scrutiny in recent years because it has been demonstrated that commonly used tests discriminate against members of minority groups and rate more highly those with academic backgrounds that take them well past the minimum qualifications for the job. Again the basic requirement is job relatedness, but there is the added complexity of constructing tests that are not culturally biased, or conversely, deliberately constructing a test that is so biased culturally as to enable those with cultural assets for the job to score higher than those who may have had a stronger academic background but who know little of the culture in which they will need to work. The problem is not different from that faced by educators in the classroom, and it is every bit as difficult and important. This is one of the reasons why small communities can rarely afford to run their own civil service system. Good tests are expensive to develop and rarely go unchallenged.

Selection

In most civil service systems, the agency is sent the names of the three top candidates after the tests have been scored. The appointing authority is free to select from among those three, so long as the choice is not based on illegal discrimination (race, sex, religion, national origin, handicapping condition, or age, assuming that all apply in that jurisdiction). This is known as the "rule of three." Some

jurisdictions have a "rule of five" and some (Washington state, for example) have a "three plus three" rule, which provides the agency with the top three candidates among all applicants and a second list of the top three minority candidates. The appointing authority may choose from either list. In a few jurisdictions a "rule of one" operates, and either that candidate must be appointed or the appointing authority must show in writing why the individual would be inappropriate. The rule of one often operates when a closed competitive examination is used (that is, the list of eligibles is taken from those already employed within the Civil Service System of the jurisdiction who are seeking a promotion to the job). Open competitive examinations (open, that is, to both insiders and newcomers) usually offer the appointing authority a choice of the top three or more candidates.

Agencies have different ways of interviewing applicants who have passed the testing procedures. In some agencies and for some jobs, the working supervisor will do the interviewing, make the selection, and recommend the appointment to the nominal appointing authority, who may be the agency director or a subunit director. In other agencies, a panel may interview the applicants and rank them, sending their recommendations to the appointing authority. In other instances, particularly for clerical positions, the personnel director for the agency may do the interviewing and recommend appointment to the appointing authority.

Whether the interviewing and recommendation for appointment are done by an individual or a panel, the people involved need to be well versed in both the substance and the process. They need to know the requirements of the job and need to know how to elicit useful and pertinent information from the applicants about their abilities and motivation. The questions should be developed ahead of time and each applicant should be asked the same basic set of questions, although there should be an opportunity to probe the answers in the quest for additional insight into the applicant's suitability for the job. It is important that those doing the interviewing understand the sensitivity of certain questions. For example, they cannot ask a woman if her husband would object to any of her working conditions unless the male applicants are asked the same question with regard to their spouses. In either case, the question must be related to the job requirement or it is inappropriate. Any question that elicits useful information about the candidate's suitability for the job can be asked as long as it cannot be construed as a question that would enable the appointing authority to discriminate based on sex (unless there is a legally accepted reason for making such a distinction), race, religion, national origin, handicapping condition (unless it can be shown that the handicap directly interferes with the work to be done), or in many cases age.

The selection process offers both the opportunity to secure the future of the agency's programs by creative appointments of people with fresh insights and motivation as well as the chance to become entangled in both bad selections and improper practices. Sometimes the job seems so important and the qualified applicants so scarce that the appointing authority will accept someone who does not meet expectations and will not be able to carry out the job in the manner the agency expected. Sometimes there is no other choice, but it is worth considering whether or not the time should be taken to reexamine the job description, the minimum qualifications, and the recruitment process to see if a more useful pool of candidates can be obtained even at the cost of more time and money.

Occasionally the agency director has a preferred candidate, but that person is not among the top three or five sent to the agency for selection. If one or more of the referred candidates does not respond to the invitation to be interviewed for the job or declines the job, then the civil service system may replace that name with the next candidate on the list, and the appointing authority may ultimately get the preferred candidate into the list of the three under consideration. Some interviewers accomplish this by intimidation, describing brutal working conditions, long overnight travel requirements when it is known that the candidate has a need to spend more time at home, or even a physical impediment that would make the job impossible for a handicapped individual. The latter ploy is blatantly illegal and should result in the intimidator having to respond to charges of criminal misconduct. Other forms of intimidation, although less punishable in a legal sense, are nonetheless improper. All candidates need to be confronted by the same accurate portrayal of reality, and it must coincide with the reality

of the advertisement and the job description. Inability to reach a preferred candidate who is located too far down the list of those taking the test may be the best thing that can happen to a program; a preconceived notion of what or who is best (the worst kind of notions, generally) may get set aside and a fresh presence may have a welcome impact on the agency's programs. Some illegal personnel practices, particularly those involving discrimination, can result in personal charges being filed against an individual rather than a civil action against the agency, and monetary damages become the responsibility of the manipulative defendant if the plaintiff wins the case.

Appointment and probation

When the appointing authority and the selected candidate reach agreement about the appointment, the selection form is signed, usually placing the new employee in probationary status for 6 months. A common mistake is to negotiate salary with the prospective employee, something most appointing authorities are not in a position to do. Like most other features of civil service systems, there are rules governing placement within the steps of the appropriate pay grade, and appointing authorities often try to promise a little extra to get the person they want—a promise the civil service system may not be able to support. Some systems allow appointment above the entry level based on experience and others do not. The appointing authority, often sharing some of the same work background as the prospective employee, may count a few years of experience that the personnel managers will not recognize. After all the paperwork has been completed, the new employee may find the first paycheck less than anticipated, leading to some very hard feelings. The relevant salary range should be described to the recruit, but no figure agreed to before the appropriate personnel managers have reviewed the application and made a determination as to salary. In no case should the new employee be told to start work before the appointment has been officially completed.

If the new employee is an existing civil service system employee who is making either a lateral transfer (a move to another position in the same classification as previously held) or obtaining a promotion, the provisions for a probationary period may not apply, and the employee may have all the rights that an established worker has. If it is a new employee, the probationary period offers both the worker and the agency an opportunity to probe the correctness of the fit and to consider any changes that might need to be made, including discharge, before permanent status is obtained. A probationary employee usually can be discharged without cause so long as discrimination is not involved. Once the probationary period is over, the employee can be discharged only for cause, and termination becomes time consuming and frustrating, although neither impossible nor impractical as some have alleged.

During the early days of the probationary period, it is important that the supervisor and the new employee have a thorough discussion about what is expected on the job. This process is one of mutual negotiation and should be written down and signed so that the employee and the supervisor have something to review about halfway through the probationary period. They can then make any modifications either in the job or in the work plan that are both appropriate and permissible given the job description. It is this agreement of what is to be done that will be used to judge the abilities of the new worker, and this judgment should be scheduled to occur 2 or 3 weeks before the end of the probationary period. Most often, new employees slide into permanent status without this scheduled review, and it is that passive act that is later regretted by management when it finds itself encumbered with an incompetent worker without sufficient cause for discharge. Not infrequently, representatives of management may start to discuss the inadequacies of a new employee only to learn that the probation period has elapsed and they have a permanent employee who cannot do the job.

Evaluation

The evaluation of work is difficult and is usually done poorly if at all. Most agencies use forms that attempt to evaluate the worker either on the basis of traits (such as attendance or manner), performance (amount of work done), or results. Sometimes all three are rated, using rating scales. Employees usually are graded as poor, below average, average, above average, or outstanding. The scores are often summed and averaged in some way so as to arrive at an overall assessment. There is usually space for written comments by the supervisor about outstanding accomplishments or deficits that need attention. There also is a space for the employee to respond and to sign the document. The signature

usually means only that the employee has had an opportunity to read the form, not that he or she agrees with the evaluation. A more complex procedure uses behaviorally anchored rating scales that involve a series of expert panels defining first the kinds of situations in which the employee might be placed and the kinds of responses one might expect, usually involving mutually exclusive kinds of responses moving from those felt to be very poor to very good. The lists of the expert panel require considerable validation, which makes them very expensive and time consuming as well as difficult to work with when new job classifications are developed rapidly.

Overall, evaluation procedures are poor, but they should be used nonetheless. They should serve as a basis for discussion between a supervisor and an employee as to what is expected of each other and how well they measure up. Evaluations should be considered when promotions and pay raises are at stake and certainly when disciplinary action is being considered. Too often it is easier for a supervisor to use "good" and an occasional "outstanding" to fill out the form rather than have what might be an unpleasant but useful discussion with an employee. Once rated as good or outstanding on some trait or behavior, any subsequent rating that lowers that grade will be contested by the employee. It is easier for the supervisor to raise the score to its traditional level than to attempt to justify the reduction. When a new supervisor enters the picture and finds the work failing, or perhaps never up to standards, he or she may be confronted with 5 years of good to outstanding ratings and a Civil Service Commission that will not sustain a discharge or a demotion.

Supervisors need training in employee evaluation so that it will be done as consistently and thoughtfully as possible. While it is difficult to get traditional personnel managers and supervisors to accept the practice, it is helpful to initiate the process with the employee filling out a form asking about the job, how well it is understood, any problems the employee may have had with it, and how well the employee thinks the supervisor understands the nature of the job. This can form the basis of a discussion with the supervisor and an evaluation of both the job and the worker's performance as well as a new set of expectations for the upcoming year to which both the employee and the supervisor can agree.

Although some agencies can only afford or will only pay for a personnel office that processes papers, it is appropriate to consider the personnel function as a human resource development program. It is not the purpose of supervision or personnel management to force a particular worker to accept or keep an unsuitable position but rather to match people with jobs so that useful work is done for the agency by someone who takes pride in doing the work. Career development should be the objective for every employee. In enlightened organizations employee services include professional counseling that can help steer people in the right direction when they find themselves unable to get along with a supervisor, confronted with alcoholism or other health problems, or faced with financial dilemmas or difficult career choices. These services are often available from community agencies, some of which are paid by local government to provide such services. The normal life stresses as well as special problems that confront employees are costly to the agency as well as to the individual and the family. Corrective action not only is cost effective but also is appropriate for an agency that is concerned with public health.

Discipline

There is a constructive hierarchy to discipline that is both logical and often neglected. The basis for the hierarchy is fairness and a conviction that people would rather do a good job than a poor one. When a supervisor has reason to believe that an employee is either not performing up to the agreed expectations or has violated some rules of the organization, the first step is to discuss it with the employee. This obvious approach is frequently ignored even by rational people. If the violation is dangerous for the employee or others, immediate action should be taken up to and including suspension from work until the situation can be remedied. For example, a child welfare worker caught drinking on the job in an emergency shelter and molesting one of the children should be removed without hesitation and the situation reported to the police and the prosecuting attorney of the jurisdiction. Most problems are not as dramatic. The first discussion may clarify a misunderstanding on the

part of the employee or the supervisor about what was being done or what was supposed to be done. If that successful outcome does not occur, then the employee needs to be verbally warned about the problem (tardiness, for example) and the next time it occurs the verbal warning should be recorded in a memorandum to the employee, and a signed and dated copy whould be placed in the employee's file. The employee must be informed that the written reprimand is in the file and given an opportunity to place any explanations in the file that the employee thinks might mitigate the incident. If the employee believes that the written reprimand is erroneous, an appeal can be brought to have it expunged from the file. A written reprimand should contain a statement as to what is expected and precisely what will be the consequences if corrective action is not taken or if the violation is repeated. The nature of the threatened discipline should be in keeping with the rules of the personnel system. If in doubt, the supervisor should discuss the situation with the personnel manager before writing the reprimand.

In employment situations where collective bargaining agreements exist, the employee usually has the right to be accompanied by a representative or a witness of his or her own choosing in any such discussion with a supervisor. The supervisor should be sure that the employee knows of this right. Even without a collective bargaining agreement, it is good practice to allow the employee the help of an aid or an advocate, and it is equally advisable for the supervisor to have a witness to the exchange.

The next step in the process is usually a suspension from work without pay for a period of 1 to 30 days. Suspensions are appealable actions and may be immediately blocked until the matter can be reviewed by either the Civil Service Commission or some other panel. Alternatively, the suspension may go into effect with the possibility that a subsequent review will reinstate the employee with payment of back wages. In all such actions, the appointing authority must be sure that the employee is precisely informed of the rule that has been violated, the consequences of the violation, and the right to appeal as well as the nature of the appeals process and any time limits involved. The ultimate step in the disciplinary process is discharge. The same procedures to be followed in the written reprimand and in the suspension steps are applicable in a discharge action. Many people, especially in the national Civil Service System, complain that the procedures and the employee safe-guards are such that an incompetent or even dis-honest employee can never be discharged. The national Civil Service System does have some real problems with its procedures that make effective and fair personnel management difficult. At the state and local level, however, it is simply a matter of being fair, consistent, and persistent in the effort to secure good work.

Resignation and retirement

Resignation may occur at any time for a variety of reasons: dissatisfaction with the type of work, an opportunity for a better job elsewhere, a change in family circumstances that may necessitate a move and sometimes a decision to respond to the sug-gestion of the supervisor that resignation would be more helpful to the furtherance of the employee's career than continuing in the face of mounting and justifiable criticism of the employee's work. Most of those reasons must be honored, although some of them should be cause for reflection about the work environment and the treatment of the em-ployee. For example, has someone been concerned about rewards for good work, about career adv-ancement, about constructive criticism when ap-propriate, about equity among employees when promotions and pay raises were considered? It is useful to locate someone within the agency who can participate in an exit interview with a departing employee to review problems the employee may have had with the job and to be sure that manage-ment has not been overlooking poor supervision or inequitable treatment.

Resignations under pressure from management are a special case. They are a matter of judgment and ethics. An employee who cannot adequately perform a particular job may be offered a demotion to a less demanding task if such exists and if there is a vacancy. If that is not possible, the employee should be urged to seek other employment and giv-en a reasonable amount of time to do so before the supervisor has to complete the next employee eval-uation and the process of discharge. A problem aris-es when unethical or even illegal actions may be under review. As noted earlier, private sector man-agers have more leeway in considering whether they wish to condone unethical or illegal actions, since it is often their own businesses and reputa-tions that are at stake. The public sector manager does not have such latitude. If an action is thought to be unethical or dishonest, it becomes a matter

for the prosecuting attorney to decide because it is a public trust that may have been violated and only that individual who has been elected to uphold and protect that trust has the responsibility and the line of accountability to make such decisions. Moreover, unethical behavior that may not involve criminal or civil action against the employee ought not to be buried in the supervisor's memory in exchange for a voluntary resignation in good standing because a subsequent employer may thereby be denied im-portant information about the person he or she is considering for employment. There may be exten-uating circumstances in which professional judg-ment would argue for such a trade-off, but they should be considered exceptional cases and treated accordingly.

Retirements occur in accordance with the rules of the agency or the jurisdiction. Ordinarily retire-ment policies and their costs are not matters of direct concern to health agency administrators, but they become more important when disability re-tirements are considered. A worker not qualified for retirement based on years of service may be qual-ified for a disability retirement if it can be shown that he or she is no longer able to do the job or that the job carries some danger because of a health problem. Unfortunately some supervisors, when confronted with a marginal worker and the difficult task of either helping that worker improve produc-tivity or discharging the worker, will look for a health problem such as a bad back, high blood pres-sure, varicose veins, or chest pains to justify sug-gesting that the employee consider applying for a disability retirement. This may appear an easy way out, but disability retirements consume a large amount of the retirement funds that workers and management have contributed. Furthermore, as disability retirements increase in frequency, their costs exceed actuarial projections and erode the strength of the pension plan for all other partici-pants. An alleged disability calls for effective em-ployee counseling, possibly some job retraining and encouragement, and sometimes but not always an early retirement.

Most public employment systems pay for unused vacation time in some way. Good management en-courages employees to take earned vacation time on schedule as a way of maintaining their own health and welfare. If this is done, there will not be much unused vacation time at retirement or resignation. Sometimes the employee gets a severance check for the days still in the vacation bank. In other situations unused vacation time cannot be cashed out, and employees compensate by leaving the job an equal number of days before the official date of retirement or resignation. In some jurisdictions part of unused sick leave is payable. This is a very controversial point in personnel management. Some employees take every day of sick leave available as if it were a vacation day. This leaves the program chronically understaffed and creates morale problems. Such practices usually start because of bad morale, and instead of looking on them as labor problems that should be treated with disciplinary measures, they should be seen as management problems: why is it that the job is so unsatisfying that people prefer to stay home? If employees treat sick time as if it were vacation time, consuming it as fast as it is earned, when a serious illness does occur the worker and the dependent family may be left in a serious economic situation with no income available. As a compromise, some jurisdictions pay for part of the unused sick time at resignation or retirement, thus offering the employee an incentive not to waste it. On the other hand, if the cash value of an unused sick day is too high, it may provide an incentive to go to work when it would be to everyone's benefit for the employee to stay home. Most organizations now feel that it is desirable to provide some incentive to employees not to consume sick time capriciously, but the best method is debatable. The situation has become more confused in recent years by the advent of "personal leave days," which are added to vacation time and are usually a result of collective bargaining. In their origins they were related to the necessity for emergency time off when there was a death in the family or some other problem that required the time of the employee. However, they have since become used for mental health days, rest days, birthdays, or some other situations.

EQUAL EMPLOYMENT OPPORTUNITY

Title VII of the Civil Rights Act of 1964, as amended by the Equal Employment Opportunity Act of 1972 (P.L. 92-261), makes it illegal to discriminate against anyone in employment because of race, color, religion, sex, or national origin unless one or more of those attributes can be reasonably shown to be related to the normal operation of the business. The Rehabilitation Act of 1973 (P.L. 93-112) extended coverage to the handicapped by declaring that "No otherwise qualified handicapped individual . . . shall . . . be excluded from participation in, be deprived of the benefits of or be subjected to discrimination under any program or activity receiving Federal financial assistance." That includes virtually all health and health-related organizations. The 1978 Civil Service Reform Act also included a strong antidiscrimination clause, which, when coupled with executive orders, should have produced broad and complete protection for all minority groups and for women, but there has been much uncertainty and some unwillingness about the implementation of these acts.

Equal Employment Opportunity laws addressed the problem created by procedures that had the effect of discriminating against minority groups in hiring. It was clear that after a century or more of discrimination in education and employment, cessation of the practices would not redress the inequities. Affirmative action programs were developed to take positive steps to alter the imbalances created by past practices, and they sought, within the equal opportunity and due process dictates of the national constitution, to compare the size of the employed minority work force group with the size of the potentially avaiable minority work force and increase the penetration of minorities into all ranks of employment where an imbalance existed. Many procedures have been developed, such as targeted recruitment efforts, stratified lists of eligible candidates for jobs, and even quotas for employment. The situation has been made very complex by a series of court cases. It appears to be illegal to establish quotas for any minority group, but it is permissable and desirable to establish goals for employment and to shape recruiting, testing, and selection procedures so as to attain those goals. Two maxims can be reliably stated: (1) regardless of any manager's personal convictions about affirmative action, it is essential to employ minorities if minorities are to be well served, and (2) failure to institute a vigorous affirmative action program may well result in a successful court suit against the agency for discrimination. The result of a successful court suit is often a court order that controls hiring practices in such a way that effective management and program performance is no longer possible until the employment imbalance is corrected. For example, if it is found that there are too few black nurses, the court may rule that only black nurses can be hired until they constitute 30% of the nurses in the agency. Since there are not many black nurses readily available for employment (a function of past discrimination in employment and education), it may be impossible to fill vacancies for 3 or more years thus bringing the work of the nursing department to a standstill. The only way to avoid such situations is to develop a strong affirmative action policy and to pursue it vigorously and persistently.

MOTIVATION

Motivation theories are as common as are theorists. In the vernacular of the 1980s, theory "X" maintains that people find work enobling and that they are motivated by the self-gratification of doing good work. Theory "Y" has it that work is onerous, that people will shun it, and that only the need for money will provoke anyone to work. Discipline and control are necessary to be sure that the work gets done. Theory "Z" is a compromise: work may be enobling, but it takes attention to the work environment to get a day's work done for a day's wages.

The landmark studies in the United States began with the work at Western Electric's Hawthorne plant in Chicago in the late 1920s. When lighting was improved, productivity increased. After a little while the lighting was decreased, and productivity increased again. By today's standards the research was crude, but the lesson remains immutable: when one pays attention to the welfare of the work force and demonstrates genuine concern for what makes things happen, workers are well motivated.[12]

There is no doubt that people work for money, but many other factors are involved with different impacts on different people. The best known theories are those of Maslow, who postulated that people work for a hierarchy of motives: first, to satisfy physiologic needs for food, shelter, and clothing; then, when those needs are met, they work to protect themselves by developing a secure environment. Once security is assured, they strive for a sense of belonging or social ease. Next in the hierarchy is the quest for self-esteem and differentiation of self from other people, and finally, if all else has been attained, people will strive for self-actualization, a sense that their lives are important and fulfilled.[13]

Much of the research on motivation involves variations on the central themes of concern and

humanism. Although people vary in their devotion to their work, virtually everyone needs the self-gratification that comes with achievement, whether that be the acquisition of something they want with the money they earn or the esteem they receive from others. The sense that management cares about the well-being of the worker as well as the work output is essential to any theory or practice of motivation. How that is expressed may be a function of the job, the environment, the supervisor's personality, or interactions between all three with the worker. It is clear that lack of interest in the worker's welfare, whether real or perceived, is destructive to positive motivation and can be only partly overcome by other incentives such as wages.

In recent years, public agencies have paid much attention to motivation. Management by objectives became popular in the private sector in 1954 and became commonly used in the public sector in the 1970s. Simply put, it involves a group discussion of objectives so that they become internalized throughout the work force rather than known only to top management. By whatever title, it is sound practice. Organizational development is another type of group process, similar to group sensitivity training. It is meant to help people adjust to a changing environment. Change has been a marked feature of public sector employment in recent years, and organizational development efforts have been helpful so long as they do not become such a preoccupation that how workers and management feel about each other becomes more important than what gets done.

A variety of efforts have been undertaken to modify the conditions of work so as to improve morale and increase motivation and productivity. In addition to such obvious things as improving the physical environment, work-time alterations have been helpful. Many organizations now use "flexible time," which allows workers to start any time between 7 and 9 in the morning and finish anytime between 3 and 5 in the afternoon, so long as they work the standard number of hours for that agency. Other experiments have involved 4-day work weeks with 10 hours of work each day. This offers those who want them 3-day weekends on a regular basis. All of these changes and experiments have their benefits, and they all have their advocates and their critics. The principle to keep in mind is to get the job done efficiently. Within that requirement and allowing for any laws or rules that may control working hours or conditions, whatever a worker wants to do to get the work done should be seriously considered and allowed if it can be done in that setting. Supervisors and managers should be encouraged to avoid stereotypes of what works and to try to meet the needs of their employees, if that can be done while the work is still being accomplished without an increase in cost. In some typing pools, all workers are required to work the same 8-hour days, 5 days a week, even though that means that some will accomplish much more than others. There is no reason, save reluctance to struggle with change, that typists could not be employed to turn out some predetermined volume of work with some set error rate and allowed to do the work on their own schedule. If that is too much of a change for managers and personnel people to accept, then let those who wish to do so work their 40 hours whenever they want to so long as they get the work done when it is needed. There are no reasons other than tradition and laziness for failing to experiment with working arrangements that give the worker more control over the work. This is simply an extension of the concept of "job enlargement," a theory that is widely accepted if not widely practiced. Rather than each employee being given a small part of a big task to do, each worker is given as much of the total job as possible so that each may have the satisfaction of producing something recognizable. Civil service job descriptions make job enlargement difficult because they are seen as a restrictive list of tasks to be performed by anyone holding a particular job classification title, but this merely points the way to the arduous task of reform, not resigned acceptance. Public health agencies not only need managers who feel strongly about their employees' welfare, but they need personnel managers who take public health seriously and apply it within the agency to the well-being of the work force.

THE FUTURE

Personnel management is a difficult and underrated science and art. It has the attributes of a profession, and it requires professional attention in a public health agency. It is beset with a number of important problems. Collective bargaining and the right to strike will remain high on the list of issues for the public sector for years to come. The original purpose of the civil service movement has been largely accomplished. Many people are seeking new approaches to the problems of productivity and creativity, such as stronger executive leadership over the personnel system or even a return to the patronage system with some benefits from the experience with due process of recent years, or reliance on unionization and collective bargaining that would place some of the responsibility for personnel management on the work force.

The work of reforming and improving public personnel systems is made difficult by the size of the public work force and the resistance to change that size represents. In the present environment of budget cutting, the insistence of public employees on protectionist tactics makes consideration of reform even more difficult. Many governments have experimented with government by contract: discontinuing established public service agencies in favor of contracts with private agencies. New programs are often developed this way. Presumably this makes later cutbacks easier because government workers are not laid off directly. But private organizations have their own ways of lobbying legislative bodies, and they are often more direct and effective than are the traditional public employee organizations.

With the private sector largely unionized and the public sector under considerable stress because of budget cutbacks and tax revolts, strong efforts to form collective bargaining systems with more control over working conditions as well as program policies can be expected in state and local programs. When employees in the public sector begin to exercise control over the formation of policy—who gets what—serious problems of accountability confront the worker, the manager, and the community. The present personnel systems are scarcely up to the task.

REFERENCES

1. Lamourette, W.J.: SES: from civil service showpiece to incipient failure in two years, Nat. J. **13**(29):1296, July 18, 1981.
2. Walton, R.E., and McKersie, R.B.: A behavioral theory of labor relations: an analysis of a social interaction theory, New York, 1965, McGraw-Hill Book Co.
3. Munchus, G.: Collective bargaining: when is a supervisor a manager? Health Serv. Man. **13**(10):1, Oct. 1980.
4. Advisory Council on Intergovernmental Personnel Policy: More effective public service, first report, Jan.

1973, Washington, D.C., U.S. Civil Service Commission.

5. Advisory Council on Intergovernmental Personnel Policy: More effective public service, suppl. report, July 1974, Washington, D.C., U.S. Civil Service Commission.

6. Crouch, W.W., editor: Local governmental personnel administration ed. 7, Washington, D.C., 1976, International City Managers Association.

7. U.S. Civil Service Commission: Biography of an ideal, ed. 2, Washington, D.C., 1974, The Commission.

8. Stahl, O.G.: Public personnel administration, ed. 7, New York, 1976, Harper & Row, Publishers, Inc.

9. Shafritz, J.M., and others: Personnel management in government, New York, 1978, Marcel Dekker, Inc.

10. Nigro, F.A., and Nigro, L.G.: The new public personnel administration, Itasca, Illinois, 1976, F.E. Peacock Publishers, Inc.

11. Lee, R.D.: Public personnel systems, Baltimore, 1979, University Park Press.

12. Roethlisberger, F.J., and Dickson, W.J.: Management and the worker, Cambridge, Mass., 1939, Harvard University Press.

13. Maslow, A.H.: Motivation and personality, New York, 1954, Harper & Row, Publishers, Inc.

CHAPTER 13

Financial management

The rule is, jam tomorrow and jam yesterday—but never jam today.

Lewis Carroll

Public health programs are by definition public, although some of the activities may be purchased from private organizations. Many private organizations, profit making and not for profit, impinge on the health of the public both in a positive and in a negative way, but the administration of public health programs involves the use of public funds on behalf of the public's health. The management of those funds is a grant of a public trust. To assure that the conditions of the trust are met, public health agencies use financial management techniques that are a mixture of private sector practices and public sector traditions.

There has been a long history of distrust of governmental agencies in the United States—of both their honesty and their management skills. Many people have campaigned for office or for reform of government on a platform of better business management. There is a constant implication, often made vociferously explicit, that private industry is both more efficient and more effective than government. The generalization is undemonstrable and illogical. Efficiency is the ratio of outputs to inputs, and the value of the outputs of public health agencies (better health, less dependency, the continued prevention of polio) cannot be reduced easily to a dollar amount to satisfy economists or accountants (although the effort to do so by Cooper and Rice[1] is an important contribution to the literature). In a strictly fiscal sense, the value of certain human services is negative for society as a whole, and it is not the purpose of public health to do only those things that have a positive cash value. Effectiveness is the extent to which the actual output of an organization corresponds with its goals and objectives, but public agencies often have conflicting and ambivalent goals and objectives by virtue

of the statutes that authorize them. (The Comprehensive Health Planning Act of 1966 [see Chapter 11] was designed to reform health care but was prohibited from interfering with private practice traditions.)

In the private sector, the one dominant goal is the famous bottom line: the excess of revenues over costs. It is a goal that can be measured in a universally understood manner—money. In the public sector, the bottom line is the public's welfare. Revenues and costs are supposed to be equal (with some exceptions to be noted later), and the net gain in assets is supposed to be an improvement in the public's health, something that does not enter the balance sheet when the accountant is through with the audit. Anthony and Herzlinger[2] indicate that not-for-profit organizations differ from profit-making organizations in nine characteristics:

1. The profit measure is absent.
2. They tend to be service organizations rather than product oriented.
3. They tend to have legislative constraints on their goals and strategies.
4. They are less dependent on their clients for their revenue.
5. They tend to be dominated by professionals.
6. They have a different governance structure, often elected.
7. They are often lead by people not specifically trained for administrative leadership.
8. They (especially governmental agencies) are heavily influenced by the political process.
9. There has been a tradition of inadequate management controls in the public sector.

None of these characteristics are either absolute or as true now as they once may have been. The list has been developed by two eminent scholars of business administration, which for 500 years has derived its traditions from the private sector. This illustrates one of the problems of public administration and management—the short span of study and research and its dominance by techniques developed to suit a different world, the world of profits.

As recently as 1977, Anthony was asked by the Financial Accounting Standards Board to explore standards for nonbusiness accounting. His report[3] identifies a host of important questions that need attention. For example, who are the clients of accounting in the public sector? They are not the same as in a private enterprise. Anthony identifies five clients—investors and creditors (those who might buy bonds), resource providers (vendors with a large purchase order), oversight bodies (boards of health), and constituents—and asks if there are others. Other important questions have to do with measuring nonrevenue inflows, depreciating endowments, or capital assets, recording donated services and the time at which an expense is to be recognized (in the private sector, this occurs when a cost is consumed in the creation of revenue).

The study of public administration in the United States against a backdrop of private sector traditions leaves unnoticed the basic purpose of government, which is to assure the public welfare and to protect the rights of its citizens with adherence to the concepts of due process. A social and political structure established for such purposes is not easily adapted to the production of services or products, and due process is an expensive concept to preserve. For example, from a business standpoint, it would be far more efficient simply to close an offending restaurant or to sterilize an offending welfare recipient.

Public scrutiny of governmental programs results in a host of special accounts for separate programs and an account structure based on concern for accountability rather than good management. A health agency with three hospitals to manage usually cannot move funds from one hospital to another if problems arise in one institution during the year since statutory controls segregate the accounts for each of the cost centers (hospitals) and forbid transfers without legislative action.

The past 2 decades have witnessed a steady increase in stronger management practices in the public sector. Much more remains to be done to acquaint the public and the private sector with the differences and the challenges.

HISTORY

In private sector traditions there are two forms of accounting: managerial accounting and financial accounting. Financial accounting has to do with the presentation of the economic status of an organization to the outside world. It has given rise to the concept of the "certified public accountant" who expresses a professional opinion about the authenticity of the report. Managerial accounting is designed to provide timely information to management to improve effectiveness and efficiency. It is concerned with internal management information flow. Public sector management practices were established originally to provide a public accounting of the funds appropriated—similar to financial accounting in the private sector.

Budgeting is a fairly recent concept that began with the New York Bureau of Municipal Research in 1906. Budgeting became a common practice in the public sector before its development as a private sector planning device. During the 1930s and 1940s there was a broad move to bring better business practices into the public sector (the tradition of the Hoover Commission at the national level and the succession of "little Hoover Commissions" at the state level) with an increase in the use of accounting information to improve management. In the 1950s budgeting began to be seen as a planning tool, and planning was increasingly adopted as a management tool. Subsequent to the enormous investments of the so-called Great Society era of Lyndon Johnson, the concern for better resource allocation and program evaluation gave rise to the concepts of cost-effectiveness evaluation and cost-benefit analysis,[4] zero-base budgeting,[5] and social accounting.[6] (These terms are defined later in this chapter. Social accounting is the attempt to apply accounting techniques to the analysis of social costs and benefits.) Most of these techniques have had their fervent advocates, and all have fallen from their pedestals into a more realistic acceptance of their value. Concern for the effective use of tax dollars and the persistence of mixed motives in the support for most human service programs will continue to cause people to search for the "magic rule" that will enable them to measure the true worth of public programs. Public sector administrators need to remain conversant with the latest trends in financial management and skeptical about their universal applicability.

FISCAL POLICY

The fiscal policy of a governmental jurisdiction sets the structure for the financial management practices of the agencies involved. The tax policies of a jurisdiction are often set by the constitution of the state or the nation and extended by statutes. They state how taxes may be levied and their purpose. Revenue policies are usually set by statute and govern the management of both tax revenue and nontax revenue such as fees and duties. The policies governing revenue administration and treasury management are often set by statute, but most of the day-to-day procedures and policies are placed in the hands of the executive branch of government. Unlike the private sector, a state or local treasurer is frequently elected independently of the governor or the city or county officials in an effort to separate the power to spend from the responsibility for maintaining a strong revenue base. Governments, like private sector businesses, invest their tax revenues in a variety of forms designed to conserve the funds, increase their value through interest earned, and assure that enough cash is available to meet current obligations. Some jurisdictions permit the continued obligation of expenditures based on anticipated tax receipts, whereas others require that the full amount of money required for a period of time be in the bank before any obligation (for salaries, supplies, or equipment) is incurred.

Many important policies are devised by the chief executive officer or a strong budget or financial director. Even though a health agency administrator may have an approved appropriation for a program, the finance officer may require that all proposals to obligate any of the funds be approved by the finance director before the request can be acted on by the personnel system or the controller or the treasurer. Often these restraints imposed by agencies external to the operating agency lead to sharp conflict between them. The best way to avoid unreasonable external restraints (the "second-guessing" of the responsible administrator's decisions) is to maintain an effective and rigorous set of reliable controls internally so that the agency has a reputation for effective financial management. Occasionally there is a policy conflict when the finance director believes the purpose of the finance office is to save money by underspending the approved bugdet. The program director rightly holds that the funds were appropriated to be used to buy or produce services. The argument may be phrased in terms of the effective use of the appropriated funds, but the real goal of the finance director may be to reduce expenditures, allowing the unused funds to accumulate and thereby reducing the need for tax revenues in the next fiscal year.

Every jurisdiction has its own traditions, some of which are developed in the span of a few years. It is important to understand the reasons behind the traditions and the purposes to which they may be put by those in a position to control the flow of expenditures. One of the more important fiscal policy struggles in recent years has taken place at the national level as Congress sought to curtail President Nixon's ability to stop spending funds appropriated by Congress. The President attempted to impound funds for programs he did not approve of in his effort to restrain government outlays during the year. The Anti-Impoundment and Congressional Budget Act of 1974 (P.L. 94-344) attempted to restrict the President's power but subsequently had some unexpected consequences. The act requires that the President send a recision proposal to Congress and that, unless that recision proposal is specifically approved by both houses within 45 days, the President must make the expenditure. A presidential deferral, on the other hand, goes into effect unless one or both houses of Congress disapproves of the deferral.

Of less prominence when the act was passed was the new budget-making process that required Congress to build its own annual budget rather than just react to a Presidential budget. The act established a new budget committee in both the House and the Senate. The two committees develop a preliminary budget resolution in the spring that sets general spending and revenue goals. Then, after work by numerous committees on programs, taxes, and other revenue measures, a second resolution is adopted that establishes specific budget targets for major activities. The second resolution is binding on Congress and requires a reconciliation of revenue and expenditure laws to the targets specified in that resolution. This can result in specific assignments to committees to redraft numerous laws. The new budget act displaced the previously powerful heads of the appropriations committees and the House Ways and Means and Senate Finance Committees but was not used until the summer and fall of 1981 when Congress became obsessed with the budget-cutting pressures of President Reagan. Then the two budget committees were able to deal with dollar targets rather than program goals and activities to redirect a host of congressional committees. The result was the Omnibus Budget Reconciliation Act of 1981 (P.L. 97-35), which in 5 short weeks rewrote most of the important health legislation developed over the previous 48 years. It is difficult to predict just how the Budget Act will be used or amended in the future, but its recent impact has been a dramatic example of the effect of fiscal policy on health programs.

FISCAL OPERATIONS

The fiscal operations of government agencies vary somewhat in terminology from local to state to national government, but the essential concepts are the same. Most local governments must follow an accounting structure defined by the state. The major practices are accounting; budgeting; execution of the expenditure plan, including purchasing and personnel practices; and auditing.

Accounting. Accounting is a systematic means for recording the history of an organization in quantitative terms. A very elderly profession with its roots in the 1400s, there are numerous textbooks[7,8] on the subject, including do-it-yourself manuals and short courses for professionals as well as special accounting texts for hospitals and other enterprises. There are few texts specifically devoted to accounting in not-for-profit organizations and governmental agencies. Among those available and useful are Hay's *Governmental Accounting* text;[9] the Comptroller General's *Accounting Principles and Standards for Federal Agencies;*[10] *Auditing and Financial Reporting*[11] and *Governmental Accounting and Financial Reporting Principles,*[12] published by the Municipal Finance Officers Association; and the Anthony and Herzlinger text on the management of nonprofit organizations.[2] The reader may be confused by the phrase *not-for-profit* rather than the more commonly used phrase *nonprofit*. While the latter phrase has had a long history, many organizations with profit as their purpose are nonprofit organizations for a time. The term *not-for-profit* is of recent vintage but is literally more accurate since it deals with purpose rather than happenstance.

The invention of the double-entry concept was to accounting what the wheel was to locomotion. The accounting sheet has a left side that records assets and a right side that records liabilities. The two totals are at all times equal. The botton line, in a profit-oriented enterprise, is what the accountant calls *net income,* or income in excess of expenses. The liability side of the balance sheet usually shows an increase in the owner's equity to balance the increase in assets. Double-entry accounting is less often useful in the public sector, since revenue is usually appropriated, is known fully in advance, and is not dependent on sales or the production of services.

The amount of funds available by appropriation at the start of the fiscal year is distributed into a series of special funds, usually one for each major program, such as maternal and child health or a hospital, and further segregated into accounts for salaries, operating expenses (consummable supplies, phone service, heating and cooling), equipment, and "other." Each account and often each of many subaccounts is classified. Daily transactions are entered sequentially in a journal, then subsequently "posted" to the correct account classification ledger. The ledger is the record of the account, and each major fund usually has several accounts. The list of the fund accounts is known as the chart of accounts.

The multiplicity of funds is a unique characteristic of public sector accounting. Private businesses may have numerous accounts, but they are for management purposes, not for public scrutiny or disclosure, and they may be changed during the course of the accounting period if circumstances require assets or liabilities to be moved about. In the public sector, transfers between funds can rarely be made without going back through the legislative process, although transfers of funds between subcategories of an account (between office supplies and utility bills within a single fund, for example) can be made either within the agency or with the approval of a central budget or finance director.

The private sector has long used an accrual basis for counting its expenditures and its revenue, whereas the public sector has more often worked with cash accounting. In accrual systems, an expense is recognized when a cost is consumed, not when the money is obligated or disbursed, and revenue is recognized as a service is performed or a product is delivered to a customer. Cash may not be transferred until a later date and may be noted in the accounting balance sheet as an account receivable or liable until it is received. In the public sector, the distinction is less important except in programs that involve billing the client or a third party for services or products provided. The difference can be confusing. At the beginning of each payroll period, the public agency begins a new obligation to pay those people who are working. This obligates or encumbers the funds needed to make that payment at the end of the period, and the controller for that jurisdiction usually has to have some guarantee that (1) such an obligation is legal, based on the approved budget and (2) sufficient funds are available from the treasurer to meet the obligation. The agency administrator is responsible for adhering to the approved budget and may not obligate funds that have not been appropriated for that purpose. Current operating expenses are another matter. For example, the agency may have purchased enough antibiotics or contraceptives or reams of paper at the start of the fiscal year to last for several months. The expense is actually obligated when the purchase order is signed by the purchasing agent, even though the goods may not be received for several weeks and the bill may be paid by the treasurer even later. The goods received are then stockpiled and transferred into use as they are required by the workers in the program. When is the expense actually recognized in the public agency? In the accrual system, it is recognized as the costs (goods) are actually consumed. As an internal matter, the expense may be transferred to the appropriate program or fund account when it is withdrawn from the stockpile and placed at the disposal of the workers. If an agency shifts from a cash system to an accrual system during an accounting period, it can dramatically alter the appearance of the accounts by reducing the cash available to cover the costs obligated but not yet incurred or "expensed."

Public hospitals rely on accrual accounting since most of the external auditing and accounting structures used by third party payors recognize such systems. Unfortunately, some third party accounts have been known to linger as an account receivable

for an extended period of time, and this can jeopardize the treasurer's ability to vouch for the adequacy of funds to meet a payroll if the rest of the jurisdiction is on a cash basis. The move to accrual accounting is necessary but still slow. The problems in a cash-accounting system made it difficult to unravel the financial problems of New York City in the 1970s. The city had been urged to adopt accrual accounting in 1937 but had not done so as of 1980.

The enterprise account is unique to the public sector. Some public hospitals and other revenue-earning public programs do not begin each fiscal year with their anticipated total costs covered by appropriations of tax revenues. Rather they work against an enterprise fund that is built by revenue receipts for services rendered. The use of such funds allows a local government to operate its public hospital without tying up millions of dollars in tax anticipations and theoretically provides the program administrators with an incentive to be efficient and aggressive in their work and in their billing and collection practices.

The involvement of governmental agencies, particularly at the local level, in rendering services for a fee in hospitals and outpatient programs and in a host of national and state grant-in-aid programs has complicated governmental accounting enormously. The big revenue and expense accounts involved in hospital administration involve concepts and account structures not previously used by government. Grant programs, whether special project grants or more general block grants, usually require separate fund accounts, and the granting agency may have a different fiscal year from that of the recipient government. National grants to state and local agencies, which totaled only $5 million in 1915 (mostly for agricultural extension work, highways, and vocational rehabilitation),[13] amounted to approximately $83 billion by the late 1970s and involved 492 different programs, 78 of them in public health.[14] Many of these have matching requirements and unique provisions for transfers and carry-overs into subsequent fiscal periods. A strong accounting arm is necessary in most public health agencies, whether it is part of the agency or part of a central structure in smaller jurisdictions. It is necessary for good management to have timely and consistent accounting information.

Budgeting. Budgeting was a public sector invention. A budget is a plan that describes how much is to be spent during the fiscal year in each of several accounts. It may include a statement about outputs (activities) and the number of personnel that may be employed, but the essential and binding ingredients are the dollars appropriated.

Budgeting used to be a periodic exercise, beginning at some point in the fiscal year and continuing through the process of legislative review and adoption and final executive development of an approved plan of expenditures based on the legislative budget. In recent years, budgeting has become a nonstop process, with the development of a budget for one year overlapping the development of the next one, the management of the one for the year before, and the debate over recisions, deferrals, and impoundments. The dominance of the budget in the legislative process and in government generally is caused by its role as a planning vehicle. Although program managers think in terms of services and clients, elected leaders prefer to deal with dollars, even though they often talk of services. With the restraints placed on revenues in recent years, it has become necessary to deal more realistically with things that will not get done. Rather than talk of people who will not get food supplements, children who will not be immunized, or people with high blood pressure who will not be found and treated, it is far easier, perhaps necessary to preserve emotions, to reduce the arguments to a single common denominator, dollars, and allow the dollar targets for revenue and expenditure programs to force curtailments in the allocation of resources rather than services presumed to be vital.

Budgets are developed from the top down, from the bottom up, and from the middle out. Program managers count needs not met and the resources available to meet them. As these estimates of additional resources needed are aggregated, they begin to form the budget request first from the program, then from the agency, and finally from the governor, the president, or the mayor. At the same time, legislative budget committees, the President, governors, mayors, and county leaders are examining their revenue expectations and their tax policies in the light of program requirements and new initiatives they may wish to undertake. At some point, these two different approaches meet and a gap is recognized: the gap between what people want to do and the money available to do it. In most jurisdictions the revenue estimate, including any revenues to be gained or lost through tax changes, is used to set the budgeting process formally in motion. Each agency director is given instructions as to the assumptions to be used to form the agen-

cy's requested budget. One of the most productive approaches is to ask the agency to develop three budgets: (1) a budget that accepts a percent change in the cost of particular ingredients such as salaries, supplies, and utilities and builds a budget on the assumption that only 90% (or some other figure) of last year's appropriation will be made available for the next year (a reduced-level budget); (2) a budget that accepts all current programs, sets certain assumptions about cost increases, and aggregates what it would take, given those assumptions, to do the same things in the next fiscal year (a current-level budget); and (3) a budget that is built on the same assumptions about cost increases for the inputs, but asks the managers to describe what it would take to fully carry out what they believe needs to be done (an expansion, or optimal, budget).

The reduced-level budget forces the agency to take each program and ask, "What would we recommend if X% less money were available next year for this program?" Would it be altered in concept, reduced in size, or eliminated altogether in favor of maintaining or even expanding some other more essential program? It is a depressing but necessary process that requires each program manager to think through the efficiency and the effectiveness of the program and debate its essentiality with other program managers whose needs are competitive within the same fund. At each step up through the organization, the manager has the option of maintaining or even expanding some programs but at the expense of cutting or even eliminating other programs. Developing a reduced budget in this manner is similar to zero-base budgeting but is more practical given the time constraints placed on the budget planning process. In zero-base budgeting,[5] program managers start from an assumption that the program does not exist, and rather than add or subtract amounts from the prior appropriation, they have to justify the activity de novo and construct a whole new budget. Zero-base budgeting has been a valuable concept, but it has not proved practical as a regular exercise. Another budgeting technique is management by objectives. Missions and goals are stated for each program, followed by specific objectives to be attained during the budget period and the steps necessary to attain those objectives, whether they be steps to reduce costs, increase productivity, or expand services. The objectives become planning targets and take the place of a profit objective in private sector budgeting.

Effective managers are effective advocates. It is easy for an advocate to overstate expected revenues or grants and understate costs in an effort to gain support for a program or an activity, but it is important to keep wishful thinking to a minimum in budget planning. The credibility of program managers and agency directors is quickly eroded by budget planning that proves unrealistic. The figures developed should be reliable and realistic even if they reduce the salability of the idea.

What has been referred to above as the current-level budget is based on a series of guidelines about cost increases that may or may not prove to have been accurate. Those guidelines, usually developed by the chief budget officer of the jurisdiction, may actually represent reductions in expenditures if they involve curtailment of travel funds or arbitrary restraints on telephone costs that are known to be increasing. A current-level budget should allow realistic cost increases to be shown as well as work load changes that are based on externalities rather than internal decisions to change objectives or methods.

The expansion or optimal budget offers a rare opportunity to illustrate what managers feel would be needed to meet current statutory authorizations or requirements fully. It is not an occasion for irresponsible proposals but a chance to describe realistically what is needed, for example, to meet current fire and safety code requirements, to provide adequate patient care in the mental hospital, or to provide good prenatal care to all rather than just a fraction of the low-income, high-risk pregnant women in the community. As such, the optimal budget provides a rare glimpse at a community's real needs and the resources needed to meet them, even though the proposals have to be seen as reflecting a particular approach to public health interventions by their authors.

Budgets are usually developed in a series of hearings, first at the program level, then at ascending responsibility centers in the organization until the agency director decides on a final presentation. Those hearings, especially in the early stages of budget formation, should focus on needs, problems, programs, and activities as well as productivity, costs, and efficiency. Only after some of the proposals have been discussed in terms of their importance and acceptability should the staff begin the detailed process of developing complete budget displays. Staff of the jurisdiction's budget director or of the chief executive will often work intermittently with program staff in budget preparation and will be ready to make final recommendations to their superior about the agency's budget when it is under consideration along with the budgets of other agencies in that community. At some point, the chief executive decides on what will be put forward as a proposed budget for legislative consideration, whether that be by a county commission, a city council, the state legislature, or the Congress. Until recently, most legislative bodies then began a process of hearings and reviews as they attempted to wrestle with revenue expectations, taxes, and their own program preferences. In recent years more and more legislative bodies have acquired the staff necessary to build their own budgets, sometimes only using the chief executive's budget proposals as executive branch input to an essentially legislative process. Hearings are usually held before committees with jurisdiction over the programs of the agency. In complex legislative environments, this may involve several different committees. It is important that the agency's representatives have a clear understanding of their obligation to support the budget proposals of the chief executive. In some cases, the health director may work for a board of health and speak in opposition to the governor's proposed budget. In those jurisdictions in which the health agency director is appointed by the chief executive, the ground rules need to be worked out before the legislative hearings start. The chief executive may have cut the agency's proposed budget, and the agency representatives may be called on to support those cuts rather than their own proposals. In the best of worlds, the differences can be agreed to, and the agency director is free to discuss those differences so long as the discussion does not involve heavy-handed opposition to the chief executive's proposals. It can prove very difficult to support some recommendations without distorting facts and opinions. A proposal to close a public hospital cannot be unrealistically championed as an effort to maintain public sector employment, expand the provision of health services, and reduce public waste when the facts and the convictions of the hospital administrators do not confirm such claims.

It can be supported as a difficult, unpleasant, but necessary step, if the chief executive and the agency director can reach agreement on what is actually entailed and what the consequences will be.

Who represents the agency before the legislative committees is a matter of judgment. Often major division heads in the agency will be present at the budget hearings both to respond to questions and to obtain firsthand a sense of the committee's predilections and dislikes. Some program managers may be old hands at the process and well known to many of the legislators, and any attempt to restrain their input into the process may be greeted with suspicion by members of the committee. Nonetheless, it is better to keep the number of agency representatives to a minimum so that the legislators have some sense of consistency in approach and agency responsiveness as the process continues. It is not necessary that every question or suggestion be immediately answered. A prompt and accurate answer is necessary, but it is better to promise one tomorrow than offer an immediate but possibly inaccurate answer to an important question.

In a bicameral legislature (every state except Nebraska has a two-house legislature), both houses develop their own budgets, usually sufficiently different to require a joint conference committee to work out a single budget. In most states, and to some extent in Congress, the budgets are so lengthy and complex that the leaders of the budget committees and their staff have almost total control over the final product. House and Senate leaders will usually work to adopt rules of procedure that limit the attempts to amend the committee's budget on the floor. In the joint conference committee, members can and do bargain for their favorite eliminations and inclusions. The conference committee is not supposed to add items not a part of either house's budget, but it often happens anyway unless the house or senate leaders interfere for some reason.

The final budget, once agreed to and passed by both houses, goes to the chief executive officer (in states, in the national government, and in some cities), where a variety of outcomes can occur depending on the budget law of the jurisdiction: the budget can be signed as submitted, vetoed in its entirety, or any specific item in the budget may be reduced or eliminated, usually subject to an override by the legislature. The rules differ from place to place.

The budget is not the same as a statute. It amounts to a declaration of allocations of revenues to different programs. The budget bill obviously affects what can and cannot be done, but it is not technically a statute, and language that attempts to specify how appropriations shall be used is out of place; it belongs in the authorizing statutes. Once approved, the chief executive officer has to initiate the second phase of the budget process, which involves the development of expenditure plans for each separate fund in accord with the final figures in the approved budget. The general format for the budget display is best described as a series of columns:

1. The first column lists actual expenditures, line by line, for the immediately preceding completed fiscal year.
2. The second column shows the approved budget for the current fiscal year.
3. A third column may be used to list any changes made in the approved budget subsequent to its adoption.
4. A fourth column usually shows all expenditures in each category as of a certain date in the fiscal year.
5. The fifth column lists the agency's request.
6. The sixth column indicates the differences (plus or minus) for each category from the current year to the proposed budget.
7. The seventh column lists the chief executive officer's recommendations, line by line.
8. An eighth column may be left to record the details of the final approved budget.

Reference is often made to "program budgets" and "line-item" budgets. A program budget is one that describes the cost of a program and is made up of "X" activities (immunizations, clinic visits, or restaurant inspections) multiplied by the cost per activity. A line-item budget is built by aggregating the costs of the objects of expenditure (salaries, books, pencils, cars, or drugs). Most budget acts require that the final action be taken on a line-item budget, although whether the categories should be many and specific or few and broad is often a matter of legislative and executive discretion. Program managers need to have valid line-item budgets and accounts set up since they enable better cost finding and control. Program budgets are useful for public display and discussion. Activity costs often are difficult to deal with in a public forum. If a program spends $2 million to produce 40,000 clinic visits or to find 250 people with active tuberculosis, then the cost per activity is easily calculated to be $25 and $4,000 respectively. But the forty-thousand-and-first clinic visit produced or the two-hundred-fifty-first case of tuberculosis will not cost the same amount nor will a reduction of $100,000 result in a cut of 4,000 clinic visits or 25 cases of tuberculosis detected. Marginal costs are not the same as average costs: one more activity can often be accomplished for a fraction of the cost of the first activity, since the apparatus and the personnel are all in place and only have to adapt to one more visit. On the other hand, finding the first case of tuberculosis when tuberculosis is common is easy and inexpensive, but as tuberculosis becomes more rare, finding the last case can become unacceptably expensive. Most activities include ingredients that are fixed (an office building or a refrigerator) and ingredients that vary more or less directly with the number of activities carried out (the number of syringes of penicillin used). Cost accounting is an important activity in a public health agency, but it has been very difficult to get clinicians to understand the concepts of *fixed* and *variable* as well as *marginal costs*. Cost finding can be confusing as well when the purposes of the activity differ from time to time. In establishing a Medicaid cost report for a public hospital, it behooves the local managers to include as much of local government as possible in what they claim to be a part of the hospital: the motor pool, the buildings and grounds, the civil service system, the health agency staff if the hospital is part of a larger public health agency, and the associated outpatient clinics. By including these related costs or a part of them in the cost report, the agency may increase the revenue earned per inpatient day of care provided. The Medicaid auditors will try to reduce that universe as far as possible to reduce their payout. When the hospital's staff tries to compare its efficiency with that of other hospitals or clinics, it will reduce the universe of costs included in the display and come up with a very different figure. Neither figure may relate to the "true cost" of care, whatever that is. There are many different real or true costs for an activity, depending on what the question is and who is answering it.

The expenditure plan for a budget often allocates money to discrete parts of the year—a quarter or even 1 month. It is important to develop an expenditure plan that reflects actual pay outs, since they will not always occur uniformly over the year. Certain supplies are bought in large amounts once or twice a year; insurance premiums are due once, not monthly; and utility bills change depending on the season of the year. The director of the agency is usually required by law to spend no more than is appropriated. This necessitates careful planning and good information. Assuming that a particular account has $120,000 in it and that it requires steady pay out during the year, then $10,000 should be expended each month. If the accounting controls are not adequate and timely, $12,000 may be spent during each of the first three months, and those figures may not be available until the end of the sixth month. By that time, the figures will show that $36,000 was spent during the first quarter, and no one may know how much was spent during the next quarter. Assuming it was at a similar rate, then the estimate of expenditures to date may be $72,000 instead of the $60,000 that should have been spent. That $12,000 excess has to be saved during the next 6 months, and if it takes another month to figure out how to do it, that may involve saving $2,400 each month out of a budget of $10,000, which is a 24% reduction. Budget variances need to be detected as soon as possible and corrected swiftly. Most accounting systems are designed to start at a zero point at the beginning of each fiscal year so the information available in the first 3 months, even with an "on-line" rapid management information system, may be limited. It is better to have an accounting system that can display both the expenditures for the current fiscal year as well as the expenditures for the immediately preceding 12 months, even though that technically crosses over into the preceding fiscal year, so that variances from the expenditure plan are easier to detect. This is not possible with new programs.

Since overexpenditures are illegal and difficult to manage, most agencies have to control on the short side of a budget target. While a private business can operate within plus or minus 5% of its budget and borrow money if it runs over, public agencies cannot incur a deficit (except for the national government) and have to accomodate that same plus or minus 5% variance allowance under the budget total. They may work, unofficially, with a restraint aimed at spending only 95% of the budgeted amount, realizing that that may amount to a range between 90% and 100% of the approved budget. If they actually hit the 90% mark, they will have underspent the available appropriation, and people may have been denied services, or employees might have been denied the supplies and equipment they needed to do the job. Most public agencies underspend their budgets and are often critized for doing so. As noted above, some budget officers operate on the assumption that their job is to hold down expenditures and save money. Many people think of a budget as a device to save money. Unless the chief executive officer or some other compelling influence intervenes with contrary guidelines, the monies appropriated are there for a purpose, and it is the agency director's job to spend them—to spend them efficiently and effectively—but to spend them, that is, use them, for the purpose for which they were made available.

There are several external restraints on an agency that may curtail expenditures. The personnel system may or may not approve salary changes that were planned in the budget or the acquisition of the personnel needed to fill vacancies or newly created job slots. The budget director or director of finance may retard the rate of expenditure by reviewing each request for supplies, equipment, personnel, or contract approval. The purchasing officer has to obtain requests in an approved fashion, usually specifying what the equipment or supply item is to do, rather than the brand name or the vendor, then advertise for a specified period of time, review bids, and award a purchase order. Negotiations along the way between program managers and purchasing agents as well as the budget director may delay the process. The result is a retarded rate of expenditure that may be deliberate on the part of any of the people mentioned whether they have that explicit assignment or not. Such interagency tensions, which sometimes are created within the health agency between program staff and financial management staff, may get out of control, and the power to influence the agency's programs slips away to an external agency. The agency director and program managers have to walk a narrow line between insisting on an unreasonable degree of autonomy on the one hand and the collaborative effort to carry out some overall budget planning for the total jurisdiction.

Auditing. An audit is an evaluation, usually conducted by an external agency, of the management controls used by the health agency. It starts with the approved budget and attempts to find whether resources were expended in accordance with that budget and the general requirements of the jurisdiction. Auditors usually sample the transactions in an account and look at the nature of the controls used to account for cash receipts and the use of resources. Auditing is only one form of evaluation. "Sunset" laws are a form of agency evaluation in which the legislature periodically requires an agency to rejustify its continued existence. They have become common in recent years, but very few programs have been eliminated as a result.

Other evaluations are carried out as part of a cost-benefit analysis or cost-effectiveness evaluation (previously described). Such studies are arduous and rarely determinative of a program's future, but they are important efforts as public health professionals attempt to come to grips with the value of their efforts in real terms. Health care costs in the United States have increased as a percent of the gross national product from 6.1% in 1965 to nearly 10% by 1983. Public, or tax, funds have increased as a proportion of the total from 26% to 43%.[15] Health care expenditures, largely for medical care, intrude on all other areas of social investment and reduce the ability of government and private industry to support an expansion in employment, improved housing and educational systems, and other environmental conditions that have a greater impact on the public's health than medical care. Careful analysis of the cost-effectiveness and benefits of medical care and public health programs is needed, especially given the proclivity of the medical care system to acquire and use new, unproven, and expensive technology. The Office of Technology Assessment of the Congress has stated that "CEA/CBA [cost-effectiveness analysis/cost-benefit analysis] cannot serve as the sole or primary determinant of a health care decision. Decision making could be improved, however, by the process of identifying and considering all the relevant costs and benefits of a decision."[4]

REFERENCES

1. Cooper, B.S., and Rice, D.P.: The economic cost of illness revisited, Soc. Sec. Bull. **39:**21, 1976.
2. Anthony, R.N., and Herzlinger, R.E.: Management control in non-profit organizations, Homewood, Ill., 1980, Richard D. Irwin, Inc.

3. Anthony, R.N.: Financial accounting in non-business organizations: an overview of the research report, Stamford, Conn., 1978, Financial Accounting Standards Board.

4. The implications of cost effectiveness analysis of medical technology, Pub. No. OTA-H-125, Washington, D.C., August 1980, Congress of the United States, Office of Technology Assessment.

5. Cheek, L.M.: Zero-base budgeting comes of age, New York, 1977, AMACOM.

6. Melton, H.W., and Watson, D.J.A., editors: Interdisciplinary dimensions of accounting for social goals and social organizations: a conference of the department of accountancy, University of Illinois, Urbana, Ill., Columbus, Ohio, 1977, Grid, Inc.

7. Gordon, M.J., and Shillinglaw, G.: Accounting: a management approach, ed. 4, Homewood, Ill., 1969, Richard D. Irwin, Inc.

8. Granof, M.H.: Financial accounting: principles and issues, ed. 2, Englewood Cliffs, New Jersey, 1980, Prentice-Hall, Inc.

9. Hay, L.B.: Government accounting, ed. 6, Homewood, Ill., 1980, Richard D. Irwin, Inc.

10. Comptroller General of the United States: Accounting principles and standards for federal agencies, Washington, D.C., 1972, General Accounting Office.

11. National Committee on Governmental Accounting: Auditing and financial reporting, Chicago, 1968, Municipal Finance Officers Association.

12. National Council on Governmental Accounting: Statement 1: governmental accounting and financial reporting principles, Chicago, 1979, Municipal Finance Officers Association.

13. Reagan, M.D.: The new federalism, New York, 1972, Oxford University Press.

14. The federal role in federal systems: the new dynamics of growth, Advisory Committee on Intergovernmental Relations, Washington, D.C., December 1980.

15. Freeland, M.S., and Schendler, C.E.: National health expenditures: short-term outlook and long-term projections, Health Care Financing Rev. **2:**97, Winter, 1981.

CHAPTER 14

Health statistics and information systems

Familiarity breeds contempt—and children.

Mark Twain

THE IMPORTANCE OF DATA

Health statistics are not just the certificates of birth and death but all data that help describe life and those phenomena that affect it. An organized approach to the collection, analysis, and use of the information contained in health statistics is an essential activity of every public health agency. Epidemiology and biostatistics have been described as one of the three fundamental and generic fields of knowledge in public health.[1] It is impossible to imagine a sound program of maternal and child health, communicable disease control, environmental health, or laboratory services in the absence of health statistics. Its influence, if properly used, permeates every part of the organization. At one point it determines what visits should be made by staff nurses or sanitarians; at another it assists in deciding matters of policy for the top administrator. The principal applications of statistics in public health include (1) population estimation and forecasting; (2) surveys of population characteristics, health needs, and problems; (3) analysis of health trends; (4) epidemiologic research; (5) program evaluation; (6) program planning, (7) budget preparation and justification; (8) operational and administrative decision making; and (9) health education.[2]

It is difficult if not impossible for a public health worker to be either successful or satisfied without an intelligent and sympathetic appreciation of health data. The material of statistics, properly organized, leads to a critically important end product—a plan for disease prevention and health promotion.

ORIGINS OF HEALTH STATISTICS

The compilation of health statistics is of ancient origin. Enumerations of people were carried out long before the birth of Christ, notably in China, Egypt, Persia, Greece, and Rome, primarily for purposes of taxation and to determine military manpower. Data relating to births, deaths, and marriages were recorded in elementary form in the old church registers of England. The oldest known copy of these so-called "Bills of Mortality" can be seen in the British Museum and is dated November 1532. These bills were compiled by parish priests and clerks for more than a century before John Graunt in 1662 published his book *Natural and Political Observations Mentioned in a Following Index and Made Upon the Bills of Mortality*. Health statistics in the modern sense can be considered to have originated from the publication of this book.

The late eighteenth century saw the beginning of the modern national census. Priority is somewhat open to question. The outstanding claims are Canada, 1666; Sweden, 1749; and England and the United States, 1790. Regardless of the earliest claim, the U.S. Census had a significant influence on the spread of the idea throughout the rest of the world. The national census in the United States was the result of a political compromise that arose from conflict between the small and large states. The former demanded equal representation in the national legislature, whereas the latter considered that their larger populations justified more power. The compromise solution was to establish a bicameral legislature consisting of the Senate, in which states were equally represented, and the House of

Representatives, with representation in proportion to population. This compromise solution made necessary some provision for the periodic inventory of the population. As a result, the following was included in the Constitution: "Representatives shall be apportioned among the several States according to their respective numbers, counting the whole number of persons in each State, excluding Indians not taxed. The actual enumeration shall be made within three years after the first meeting of the Congress of the United States, and within every subsequent term of ten years, in such manner as they shall by law direct."*

All that was required was a simple count of people. From this basic purpose there has developed a national census of great complexity and detail that provides data of value far beyond what was envisioned by the framers of the Constitution. Few parts of the nation's social, political, economic, and industrial systems could possibly operate without it.

The collection and analysis of health statistics has always been considered one of the basic functions in public health. It is inconceivable that effective public health programs could be planned, implemented, monitored, and evaluated without a reasonably solid data base.

SOURCES OF PUBLIC HEALTH STATISTICS

Several different types of data are necessary to construct a useful health statistics system[3]:

Survival data
1. Births
2. Deaths
3. Population

Health status data
4. Morbidity data
5. Disability data
6. The growth and development of children
7. Data about social and economic conditions

Health services data
8. Service availability
9. Use
10. Health care financing
11. Effectiveness

The most fundamental information on which activities in public health must be predicated is a

*Article I, section 2, paragraph 3, modified by the Fourteenth Amendment.

knowledge of the quantitative and qualitative characteristics of the population to be served. This implies some form of a count or estimate of the people within a jurisdiction. On the surface it would appear that the decennial census, to which reference has been made, would supply whatever data are necessary. This was the case before paved highways, rapid transportation, and industrialization. Reasonably adequate intercensal populations could be estimated by means of simple projections. The situation changed drastically, however, as a result of World War II. In 1940 an extremely detailed census had been carried out. However, within little more than a year, the nation became engaged in an international conflict of great magnitude that required the enlistment and draft of several million citizens. In addition, new and old industries underwent spectacular expansion, necessitating the movement of additional millions of persons to serve them. Many communities within a short space of time found their populations doubled or trebled, whereas others were noticeably depleted. It soon became evident that neither the 1940 census data, which by this time had been released, nor any estimates based on them could serve much useful purpose.

Many attempts were made to find suitable substitutes in the form of school attendance records, work records, or food ration card applications. The latter was probably the most useful during the World War II years. Social Security registration provided some additional measure of the population, with the handicaps, however, of not including children and certain groups of the employable and not giving an indication of population movement. It was hoped that the confused situation would be temporary; but soon statisticians, economists, and public health workers were convinced that the national mode of life had been so deeply affected as to require some new form of population determination and analysis. During the same period of time, a new business and social study technique, the sample survey or poll, began to serve a valuable purpose in health and other fields especially during intercensal years and in obtaining answers to special questions. Intermittent population reports based on sample surveys are distributed by the Bureau of the Census.[4]

Next in importance to the population base are data obtained from administrative registration and reporting procedures. Responsibility for this function in the United States rests with the respective states. The most significant of these activities relate to the vital events of birth, death, and morbidity. Again, so that these data may be of value in the planning of public health programs, there must be some assurance of their qualitative and quantitative dependability. This need led to the establishment of birth and death registration areas by the Bureau of the Census. The death registration area was organized in 1900 and included the states of Connecticut, Indiana, Maine, Massachusetts, Michigan, New Hampshire, New Jersey, New York, Rhode Island, Vermont, and the District of Columbia. At that time these areas contained about 40% of the total population of the United States. The birth registration area was established in 1915 and originally included Connecticut, Maine, Massachusetts, Michigan, Minnesota, New Hampshire, New York, Pennsylvania, Rhode Island, Vermont, and the District of Columbia, accounting for 31% of the total population. By 1933 all states had become members of both the birth and the death registration areas. The program was included in the National Center for Health Statistics (P.L. 93-353) in 1974 along with other basic health data systems.

Part of the core research effort of the United States Department of Health and Human Services, the National Center for Health Statistics is the direct descendent of the National Office of Vital Statistics. It maintains 11 ongoing data systems, although budgetary constraints have caused the center staff to establish priorities for those systems and the periodicity of their operation. Those systems are[5]:

1. *Basic vital statistics.* "Basic vital statistics come from the records of livebirths, deaths, fetal deaths, induced terminations of pregnancy, marriages and divorces or dissolutions of marriages." These data are collected by each of the states, verified, coded, and transmitted periodically to the National Center.

2. *Vital statistics followback surveys.* Followback surveys are periodic surveys conducted by "following back" some item contained in a vital record to a local source to obtain additional information about natality or mortality not contained in the original vital record or to evaluate the quality of information in the vital record.

3. *National Survey of Family Growth.* The National Survey of Family Growth is a multipurpose survey of factors relating to fertility and family planning practices.

4. *National Health Interview Survey.* Initiated in 1957, the National Health Interview Survey is a continuous nationwide survey of the amount, distribution, and effects of illness and disability in the United States.

5. *National Medical Care Utilization and Expenditure Survey.* The National Medical Care Utilization and Expenditure Survey provides detailed national estimates of the use of and expenditures for medical services. First conducted in 1980 to 1981, it may be repeated in the mid-1980s.

6. *National Health and Nutrition Examination Survey.* The National Health and Nutrition Examination Survey is used to collect data from a national sample that is generally obtainable only by direct physical observation and examination. First carried out in the early 1970s, the study was repeated with modifications from 1976 to 1980. The third round is scheduled for 1987. A special survey of the Hispanic population began in 1982.

7. *National Hospital Discharge Survey.* The National Hospital Discharge Survey provides information about the characteristics of patients in civilian, short-stay hospitals: their length of stays, their diagnoses, surgical procedures performed, and patterns of patient use by size and ownership of the hospital.

8. *National Ambulatory Medical Care Survey.* The purpose of the survey of ambulatory medical care is to provide information about the location, setting, and frequency of ambulatory care encounters for different specialities and subgroups of the population.

9. *National Nursing Home Survey.* The National Nursing Home Survey is a series of sample surveys of the residents and staffs of nursing homes to provide information about need, costs, levels of care, and trends in the use of nursing homes.

10. *National Master Facility Inventory.* The National Master Facility Inventory attempts to identify and classify a broad array of facilities that provide 24-hour care, such as hospitals, nursing homes, and residential care facilities. In addition to serving as a statistical file of "beds" by type, it serves as a universe for sample surveys of special groups.

11. *National health professions inventories and surveys.* The primary purpose of surveys and inventories of health professions is to provide information about the distribution and training of people employed in the health labor force.

The reports of the National Center for Health Statistics are published in a variety of different series that continues to serve as a valuable source of information to health planners, analysts, administrators, and policymakers.[6]

Mental health statistics are developed separately by the National Institute of Mental Health.[7] They differ from National Center for Health Statistics data in that they are derived primarily from an encounter-reporting network rather than a population-based survey. This is based in part on the diffuse disagreement about diagnosis in mental health that makes population surveys difficult. The encounter-based system means that the mental health reporting system counts only those people who seek services, and for the most part who do so in the public sector of community mental health centers and public mental health hospitals.

ACCURACY OF HEALTH DATA

All data systems suffer from both systemic and random inaccuracies. Random inaccuracies, if not too frequent, do not generate bias in the data—that is, they do not disturb the data in an integral way. Systemic inaccuracies, unless they are understood and corrected through compensatory adjustments, can inject bias into a data set that may lead to invalid inferences. The registration of births and deaths is virtually complete in the United States. Some deaths are missed because a few people simply disappear. Although this may result in a slight underreporting of certain causes of death, it represents a very small proportion of the total number of events. As many as 30,000 births (out of 3.6 million births annually) may go unrecorded initially, but most of these are subsequently registered when the individual enters into the civil systems of society such as school, social security registration, or employment. Other problems are related to the inadequate reporting of stillbirths and babies born out of wedlock and to the known underenumeration of certain groups, especially minorities, in the census.

The assurance of prompt and adequate reporting of both live and stillbirths requires constant vigilance on the part of registrars and directors of vital statistics offices. Many different approaches have been used, and it would appear that no one approach alone is satisfactory. Education of the public, of attendants at birth, and of hospitals must be conducted constantly. In addition to this is the use of many types of checks such as entering school children in states that require a birth certificate for school attendance, and children attending well-baby or child health clinics. In many states hospitals prepare a birth certificate at the time the prospective mother enters the hospital, complete except for the date of birth, sex, and name of the child. These can be readily added after birth at the time the physician signs the certificate. In addition to producing highly satisfactory results, this procedure has added value in that the certificates are usually typed and therefore are more legible than they otherwise might be. Some states have made it possible for the hospital rather than the physician to report the birth. This helps produce more timely and accurate data.

The reporting of illegitimate births has been approached in three different ways by the various states. One is to make mandatory provision for the attendant at birth to file the birth certificate of an illegitimate child directly with the state office of vital statistics rather than to have it pass through the hands of the local registrar. Some believe that this weakens the local registration system and is therefore undesirable. Another approach is the provision that the certificate of an illegitimate child not differ from that of a legitimate child once the child in question has been adopted or legitimized. An objection to this is the necessity of preparing new certificates. A third method is to delete the item of legitimacy entirely. This has been successfully promoted in a few states by welfare agencies and certain other groups. What constitutes "illegitimate" conception and birth by the 1980s is a moot point. Births out of wedlock still have certain characteristics that are of importance to health planners and sociologists, but the term *illegitimate* has little functional value when an increasing number of women and even couples prefer child bearing outside of marriage and so many marriages end in divorce. The term creates other problems when illegitimacy rates are calculated for different racial groups. Single parenting in a black family has not carried the same social stigma as it has in white families, and "illegitimate" black children have not been participants in the types of abusive situations that frequently occur in white family environments. Whites have more often resorted to secrecy, forced marriages, abortions, relinquishments, and adoptions than have blacks, all of which feed into a syndrome of family breakdown. Publication of race-specific illegitimacy rates has served to perpetuate stereotypes that are the converse of reality. There are signs that this difference is changing as some white single women have begun to elect single parenthood. Many states have removed the item of legitimacy from the certificate proper and have placed it on a supplementary portion. Perhaps more satisfactory is the policy of a few states of including the item on the certificate but eliminating it on certified copies of the certificate, usually by the general use of an abbreviated copy of the certificate. Even though the basic demographic data on birth certificates are recorded accurately, information about years of education of the mother and congenital anomalies is often poorly recorded or, in the case of congenital anomalies, is dependent on the interest and training of the attending physician. Some may record every mole as a congenital anomaly, where others do not respond until an arm or a leg is missing.

One other phase of birth reporting that causes difficulty is delayed registration of births. Since routine court evaluation of the evidence is unwieldy, most states now have the evidence reviewed by the state registrar, with recourse to the courts in case of a rejection.

The value of death certificates is impaired not only by some inadequate reporting but also by the subjective nature of much of the data requested on the form. It is still not rare for the cause of a death to be misstated deliberately to circumvent potential social stigma. This occurs not only in relation to suicides and syphilis but also to some degree in tuberculosis, cancer, and some hereditary ailments. Incorrect diagnoses present a constant problem to the vital statistician. Numerous studies have been made regarding the degree of accuracy of the physician's statement of cause of death. The figure varies considerably by time, place, and cause of death. For cancer reporting, it appears that death certificates are fairly accurate for cancer of the lung, breast, prostate, pancreas, bladder, ovary, and for leukemia, but cancer of the colon may be over-reported in death certificates, whereas rectal cancer may be underreported.[8] The magnitude of this error is subject to steady reduction by virtue of improved medical education and the development and use of new laboratory and clinical diagnostic techniques. Even the most conscientious physician is faced with the difficult problem of deciding the primary cause of death as against contributing causes. This

problem has been partially solved by the publication and wide adoption of the World Health Organization's International Classification of Diseases, Injuries, and Causes of Death,[9] which presents primary and secondary causal preferences for all possible combinations of diseases.

The presentation of data and their interpretation present additional opportunities for mistakes. Health statistics are usually presented as rates or ratios. The rates are constructed by dividing a count of the events being studied by the number of possible events and multiplying the result by a constant (K) to convert the fraction to a whole number. There are several special-purpose rates, but the most common ones will be discussed here.

Most of the rates used in public health and demography are either crude rates, standardized rates, or specific rates. Crude rates count all of the events and all of the people. The *crude death rate* is a count of all deaths occurring in the jurisdiction (city, county, state, nation) during the year, divided by the total number of people in the population at the midpoint of the reporting period. This figure is usually multiplied by 1,000 and in the United States produces a rate of approximately nine deaths per 1,000 people.

Over time or between two different communities, the age distribution of a population may vary substantially. An older community with few children and many elderly people would be expected to have many more deaths per thousand people than a younger community with many children. The *age-standardized death rate* compensates for this difference. If the age and sex of each decedent is known and the population figures are also known for each age and sex group, *sex- and age-specific death rates* can be calculated. For example, if there were 25,000 white men aged 40 to 44 in the population, and there were 119 deaths of men aged 40 to 44 during the year, the sex- and age-specific death rate for that group would be $(119/25,000) \times 1,000$, or 4.76 per 1,000. If similar calculations are made for each age group of white men, each rate can be multiplied by the number of white men in the corresponding age group in a standard reference population. This yields the number of deaths that would have occurred in the standard reference group of white men if the age- and sex-specific rates of the study population prevailed in the standard population group. By dividing the theoretic number of deaths by the total population of white men in the standard reference population and multiplying by 1,000, the age-standardized death rate can be calculated. Similar calculations can be made in the study community for a different time or in another community, and if the age- and sex-specific death rates again are multiplied by the appropriate figures in the same standard reference population, another age-standardized death rate can be calculated, which can be compared to the first rate. The same sort of standardization process can be used to correct the rate for different sex or racial distributions, and multiple standardizations can be carried out on the same group. Age- or race- or sex-standardized rates have their uses, but they are summary indices of health status and should not be allowed to obscure the underlying differences that are found in the specific rates. A *case fatality rate* is calculated by dividing the number of deaths that occur from a specific cause by the total number of cases of the disease, condition, or injury. The number may be multiplied by 100 to yield a percentage figure that is an indication of the lethality of the condition.

A *maternal mortality rate* is calculated by dividing the number of deaths because of pregnancy occurring during the reporting period (usually a year) by the number of live births during that same time and multiplying the answer by 100,000. The result is about nine deaths per 100,000 live births in the United States at the present time. The *crude birth rate* is calculated by dividing the total number of live births occurring during the reporting period (usually a year) by the total population at the midpoint in the reporting period. This is obviously a crude rate. More useful is the *general fertility rate*, which is calculated by dividing the total number of live births during the reporting period by the population of women aged 15 to 44 and multiplying the answer by 1,000. It is currently expressed in the range of 65 births per 1,000 women aged 15 to 44 in the United States, with an international variation of about 58 to 205. The *age-specific fertility rate* is calculated by dividing the total number of live births to women in a particular age group by the total number of women in that age group during the reporting period.

The *infant mortality rate* is calculated by dividing the total number of deaths occurring between birth and 1 year of age by the total number of live births occurring during the reporting period and multiplying the answer by 1,000. It is currently expressed as about 13 deaths per 1,000 live births in the United States with an international range of about 8 to 200. The *fetal death rate* is more complex. It is usually calculated from some point in gestation that is assumed to represent the point of viability, but this is a controversial point in fetal development. Currently most states require reporting of fetal deaths past the twentieth week of gestation, although a few require reporting for any "product of conception." In the United States, the *fetal death rate I* is calculated by dividing the total number of fetal deaths occurring after the twenty-eighth week of gestation by the total number of live births plus the number of fetal deaths and multiplying the answer by 1,000. The current United States rate is about 6 to 7. The *fetal death rate II* is calculated by dividing the total number of fetal deaths occurring after the twentieth week of gestation by the total number of live births plus the number of fetal deaths. Because of the uncertainty attached to fetal age and the different reporting requirements, fetal death rates are less commonly used than are other indices of conceptual failure. The *perinatal mortality rate* is surrounded by the same confusion. The more common version in the United States is the total number of fetal deaths occurring after the twenty-eighth week of gestation plus the number of early neonatal deaths occurring before the end of the seventh day of life, divided by the total number of live births plus the number of fetal deaths with the answer multiplied by 1,000. Current United States perinatal mortality rates are about 14 with a range of 13 for whites to about 20 for blacks.

The *neonatal mortality rate* has two components: an *early neonatal mortality rate* and a *late neonatal mortality rate*. The early neonatal mortality rate is calculated by dividing the number of deaths from birth through the seventh day of life by the total number of live births multiplied by 1,000, and the late neonatal mortality rate is calculated by dividing the number of deaths before the twenty-eighth day of life by the total number of live births multiplied by 1,000. The late neonatal mortality rate includes the deaths counted in the early neonatal mortality rate. The *postneonatal mortality rate* is calculated by dividing the number of deaths occurring after the twenty-eighth day of life and before the end of the first year of life by the total number of live births minus the deaths occurring during the first 28 days. The result is multiplied by 1,000. Rates in the United States currently are about eight early neonatal deaths per 1,000 live births, nine late neonatal deaths per 1,000 live births, and four postneonatal deaths per 1,000 live births. Adding the late neonatal death rate and the postneonatal death rate results in the *infant mortality rate*. In a relatively stable health environment, partitioning the infant mortality rate into its two components, the neonatal mortality rate and the postneonatal mortality rate, can provide some indication as to the nature of a community's problems. If the neonatal mortality rate is comparable to the national average or better, but the postneonatal mortality rate is high, it suggests that the community is providing good hospital-based care from a technical standpoint but that environmental conditions in the community and its homes are not good or access to primary nursing and medical care for families is inadequate. On the other hand, if the component causing a high infant mortality rate is the neonatal mortality rate, it suggests that prenatal and delivery services are inadequate.

Two final rates commonly used in public health are the *incidence rate* and the *prevalence rate*. The incidence rate is the number of new events occurring during a reporting period (such as cases of measles) divided by the population at risk of the event. The prevalence rate is the number of cases existing at a particular time divided by the population at risk of the event. In both rates, the constant has to be selected based on the frequency of the event. For very rare diseases or conditions such as autism or leukemia the constant may be 100,000, whereas it might be 1,000 or 100 for more common conditions such as sinusitis or backache. Prevalence is usually referred to as point prevalence since it is calculated at a particular point in time. Incidence may be calculated for a week, a month, a year, or any period that is helpful in explaining the phenomenon. Prevalence equals the incidence of the disease multiplied by the duration of the disease, when incidence and duration are both expressed in the same units of time. If 15 new cases of a disease are diagnosed each month and each attack lasts 2 weeks (0.5 months), the prevalence will be 7.5.

More complete discussions of rates and their development may be found in the most current edition of *Vital Statistics of the United States,*[10] in most standard epidemiology textbooks, and in demography textbooks. Particular attention should be paid to techniques used for comparing rates between two different times or places, since the composition of the population groups studied may vary considerably. Kleinman[11] has discussed various indices for comparing age-adjusted mortality data between areas and has shown how each index, although essentially accurate, conveys a different perspective. Each of the indices has value, and the health administrator must have either a sufficient background in biostatistics or sufficient confidence in a staff biostatistician to avoid making incorrect inferences.

In addition to the mathematic problems involved in the analysis and understanding of vital statistics, there are a number of administrative and interpretive problems that can trap the unwary. Warshauer and Monk[12] found that New York City's reported suicide rate for blacks was almost identical to that determined by the medical examiner but that it underestimated the suicide rate for whites by 25% when the city's health department used the seventh revision of the International Statistical Classification of Diseases, Injuries, and Causes of Death. When the department switched to the eighth revision in 1969, suicides of blacks were underreported by 82% and suicides of whites by 66%! These marked changes occurred as a result of administrative procedures for closing out the reports at the end of the year, a change in classification practices, and differences in techniques used for suicide by blacks and whites. Such a marked change should cause the administrator of the suicide prevention program or the researcher to question the data, but lesser changes might well have been presented as real. A similar problem was found in Ohio when the recording of congenital anomalies was changed.[13] As a result of the change, the apparent rate increased from 8 or 9 per 1,000 live births in the period 1960 to 1967 to 18 per 1,000 in 1968.

Interpretive problems enter into the picture too. Morris and associates[14] studied the decline in infant mortality from 1965 to 1972 and concluded that 27% of the decline was caused by changes in the ages at which women had their babies. The infant mortality rate varies at different ages of the mother.

The rate is generally expressed as the number of deaths under the age of 1 year divided by the total number of live births, without regard to the age of the mother. So long as birthing patterns remained the same, changes in the rate represented changes in the mortality experience, but when the age at which a birth occurred began to shift in a systematic way, the composite risk of infant mortality shifted even though the rate for each individual age group might have remained the same. The same problem may occur with changes in abortion practices in the United States. Following the Supreme Court decision, making abortion legal on request, there was a marked increase in the number of legal abortions performed in some states and many of these were provided to low-income women through Medicaid. The impact of these changes on infant mortality has not been reported, but it seems likely that increased availability of abortions in some states reduced apparent infant mortality since many of the women requesting abortions are likely to be at higher risk of having a fetal or infant death experience than those who do not request an abortion. The result of the effort by Congress and the Secretary of the U.S. Department of Health and Human Services to limit abortions, especially for low-income women, is unknown although it should result in an increase in apparent infant mortality.

REPORTING PROCEDURES

Almost all states and territories place responsibility for vital records management in their state health department, and in the majority of instances the state health officer is designated by law as the state registrar of vital statistics. Actual collection is usually accomplished through local registrars who receive reports directly from attending physicians, midwives, undertakers, and others. The routing of reports of births and deaths is subject to much variation. In some states certificates are either filed with the county health officers, who transmit them to the state health departments, or are routed by the local registrars through the county health departments. More commonly, local registrars send the certificates directly to their state health departments. Some states have developed direct reporting systems wherein the state registrar serves as the only registrar. Whatever routing procedure

is followed, four basic principles should be adhered to:

1. Certificates should be completed promptly by medical or other attendants.

2. There should be a system of routine checking by registrars of all certificates for correctness and completeness.

3. Certificates should be forwarded to the state agency at intervals of not longer than 1 month.

4. Pertinent data on certificates should be made readily and promptly available to local health departments. If this is not provided for, much of the value of the reporting is lost.

Morbidity reporting, as distinct from morbidity surveys, presents an extremely difficult problem. There are two different reasons for morbidity reporting: (1) the analysis of trends and the study of the epidemiology of disease and (2) the need to implement public health control measures when cases of certain dangerous, usually communicable, disease occur. It is not particularly desirable to maintain a morbidity reporting program unless sufficient resources are available to make the system either fairly complete or one whose biases are known. This is true for cancer registries, studies of occupational diseases and accidents, as well as communicable disease reporting systems. Some states have developed especially good registries for one or more of these, and together with special surveys, their data can be studied by others. It would be expensive and unnecessary to replicate such registries in many states. It is possible to develop a good registry for one or a few diseases of special interest in a given area, but broad-scope morbidity reporting systems are too complex and expensive for most states. An underfunded registry is worse than useless—it is dangerous in that practitioners may draw incorrect conclusions from incomplete data and practice accordingly.

Public health agencies do need a reliable method of assuring that certain diseases will be reported promptly to institute control measures. Special procedures for reporting cases of venereal disease have been developed by the Centers for Disease Control in Atlanta, and most states use these to initiate case-finding activities, particularly when a new case of infectious syphilis is reported. It is essential that this effort to get prompt reporting by doctors, nurses, and health facility administrators continue. This is particularly true for cases of tuberculosis. With the advent of increasingly effective chemotherapy and the ability to rapidly convert the infectious patient to noninfectious status, some otherwise progressive medical practice communities have become nonchalant about tuberculosis. As the disease becomes increasingly rare, it becomes increasingly important to stress that this is a dangerous disease and that new cases must be investigated promptly and thoroughly by trained public health workers.

There are many reasons why physicians may not report communicable diseases to the health department: (1) it may be seen as a complicated nuisance, depending on the arrangements made to facilitate reporting; (2) it may be seen as an unimportant task; (3) the patient may attempt to interfere or block reporting; (4) the physician may see reporting as an infringement of confidentiality; or (5) there may be no real incentive for the physician to report. In a study of veneral disease–reporting practices, each of these phenomena was specifically addressed, and it was found that the single problem of most importance was the administrative complexity of reporting. When that problem was alleviated by making arrangements for a call to an office worker at regular intervals, reporting increased sharply.[15] The same reasoning may not affect reporting for other diseases because most physicians have some understanding of the health department's interest in case-contact investigation of venereal disease but may not be aware of the department's interest in many other diseases.

There is considerable variation among the states concerning the specific diseases included in the reporting requirement. All states require the reporting of conjunctivitis, diphtheria, measles, meningitis, poliomyelitis, scarlet fever, smallpox, syphilis, typhoid fever, tuberculosis, undulant fever, and whooping cough. Variation is noted with respect to morbidity reporting methods. Only two requirements are uniform in all the states. First, every state requires that cases of notifiable disease be reported by the attending physician or in the absence of a physician by the householder, head of the family, or person in charge of the patient. Second, the reports are to be made to the local health authority. Many states use report cards. Several use the same card for all diseases. Many states have a special card for cases of venereal diseases. Format varies from no regular form to single- and multiple-case report cards, stamped cards, and cards requiring postage.

The usual practice is to route morbidity reports through the local health department to the state health department. Some states require only that copies of daily, weekly, or monthly summaries be sent to the state health department. A few states follow the unreasonable practice of requiring physicians to send reports both to the local and to the state health departments.

PRACTICAL CONSIDERATIONS

Certain factors must be considered in regard to morbidity reports. Fundamental is the need to prepare and educate those in the community from whom reports are to be obtained. The most important of these are private physicians, hospitals, and schools. Two other sources worthy of mention are the dental profession and industry. Too often there is an inclination to require reports of too many diseases and in too much detail, whether or not any practical use is made of the information. Generally when this is done, physicians and other reporting agencies eventually question the practicality of the request and the use made of it. If they decide that the information is merely received and filed away, they soon become careless in their reporting. They can hardly be blamed if no one takes the trouble to explain the purpose of the items requested. An additional important factor is the amount of work involved in making the report. Busy practitioners are loath to spend much time in writing out details of cases for official agencies. The least that can be done is to standardize and simplify some of the forms and procedures insofar as possible.

In the case of morbidity reporting, requirements and methods should be reduced to the barest essentials. An increasing number of official health agencies accept reports of cases of communicable diseases in the form of telephone calls or preaddressed postcards, requiring only the diagnosis and the name, age, and address of the person affected. From there on it is the responsibility of the public health personnel to obtain what further details appear necessary for the adequate public health management of the case.

The purpose of the reporting requirement has to be considered when designing the reporting procedure. Where a case report is needed to initiate disease control actions, it may be possible to identify certain types of medical practice or health practice environments in which many new cases will be diagnosed and to concentrate services in those areas. This may be true for venereal disease. Urologists, family practitioners, and internists are more likely to see cases than are surgeons and psychiatrists. However, data collected in an effort that targets high-risk groups or practices cannot be reported as demonstrative of the incidence or changing patterns of the disease, since it is deliberately biased in an attempt to capture the greatest number of cases for control purposes. Clinics for sexually transmitted diseases are often established in inner-city areas where private medical care is not readily available. White patients are more likely to obtain treatment in a private office in the suburbs where reporting is uncommon, whereas black patients are more likely to use the available public clinic, which assures a high reporting rate. If incidence rates are reported by race or by neighborhood, blacks will appear to have a higher rate of sexually transmitted diseases than whites, which may or may not be true. When it is important to measure such differences or to monitor trends, special efforts have to be made to assure adequate reporting. In some cases special randomly selected panels of physicians may be called on for periodic reporting with greater effort on the part of the health department staff, which will assure more complete reporting.

In addition to reducing the amount of information requested, it is useful to review periodically the list of diseases that various people are supposed to report. Some disease reports are requested even though very little use has been made of the data, such as chickenpox reports. An important adjunct to the reporting process is an analysis of the data and the distribution of this analysis to those doing the reporting in such a manner that it has value for them. People who are required to report certain phenomena on a form on a regular basis maintain little regard for the accuracy of their reports if they never see any results. Analyses with written comments should be circulated regularly to those professional groups who do the reporting in such a manner that the information can be of help to them in the diagnosis and treatment of similar cases.

THE COOPERATIVE HEALTH STATISTICS SYSTEM

Since 1925 there have been many proposals for the establishment of a morbidity reporting area similar to the birth and death registration areas. The

American Public Health Association published the results of a symposium on morbidity surveys in 1949,[16] and the practicality and value of total community surveys have been established in Hagerstown (Md.), Tecumseh (Mich.), and Framingham (Mass.). The ongoing National Health Survey was described by Linder[17] in 1958, and the results of that program have been used by a growing number of public health analysts and legislators.

Langmuir[18] has stated the following viewpoint:

The morbidity survey is a particularly useful epidemiological tool in that data on both the sick and the well are obtained concurrently. The problems arising from underreporting of cases, from arbitrary classifications of causes of death, and from unknown shifts of population between census years are largely eliminated. . . . Its unique advantage lies in the detailed information that can be collected about the population. Frequency rates, specific for a wide variety of social and environmental factors, can be determined. Such comparisons are not obtainable by matching routine morbidity reports and death certificates with census figures.

He further points out the interrelationships between the simple survey and the special study:

The simple morbidity survey has one inherent limitation—only general data can be obtained. The questions asked by the interviewers must be simple and understandable to the informants. Few specific diseases can be adequately counted by this method. Special studies are necessary to collect such definitive epidemiological information.

To obtain health data for the nation as a whole, states routinely transmit the information they obtain to the National Center for Health Statistics in the Public Health Service for collation, analysis, and publication. Reports of communicable diseases are sent to the Centers for Disease Control in Atlanta. Numerous useful documents are prepared and made available. Among them are the annual *Vital Statistics of the United States*[10] and the *Morbidity and Mortality Weekly Report*,[19] which present data for the nation as a whole and for each state, including comparisons with the year before and indications of trends. In addition, the weekly report includes descriptions of unusual or particularly important epidemiologic occurrences. The National Center in its turn submits its data and analyses to the World Health Organization for inclusion in the development of the worldwide picture[20,21] and for epidemiologic intelligence purposes.

Brotherston[22] has commented that the reorganization of the National Health Service in Great Britain made possible the integration of hospital data, general practice data, and public health data into one system. The organization of such a system was described in a United States publication in 1969[23] and finally authorized by P.L. 93-353 in 1974: the Health Services Research, Health Statistics, and Medical Libraries Act. The National Center for Health Statistics (previously known as the National Office of Vital Statistics) was directed to establish a Cooperative Health Statistics System "to assist state and local health agencies and federal agencies involved in matters relating to health, in the design and implementation of a cooperative system."[24] The regulations identified seven components of the Cooperative Health Statistics System: vital statistics, health manpower statistics, health facilities statistics, hospital care statistics, long-term care statistics, ambulatory care statistics, and health interview statistics. The first four of these were selected for priority implementation. The National Center pulled together different units such as the birth and death registration unit, the National Health Survey unit, and the manpower unit, to develop new forms of contractual relationships with the states, including a multicomponent contract. In addition to technical assistance, substantially increased federal financial assistance was available through the contracts. In return, the National Center got back machine-ready computer tapes from the contract states, which reduced the center's lag time considerably. By 1980, 39 states had developed centers for health statistics and virtually all states had one or more of the seven components either in place or under development. The National Center obligated $10 million for Cooperative Health Statistics System contracts in fiscal year 1978. Of the 39 state-level centers for health statistics, 33 were managed by the state health agency in 1980. The others were run by either state financial offices or state development offices or as a special component of the governor's office. Almost all of the state agencies were engaged in multiple statistical collection and reporting activities, including health manpower, health facilities, hospital care, the development of health trend analyses, and population forecasts.

Among the principal weaknesses of the Cooperative Health Statistics System were the lack of a fiscal data base that could be meshed with the service and population data bases to produce expenditure estimates and the lack of environmental and social data. The shortcoming in environmental data was corrected by P.L. 95-623 in 1978, which authorized studies to determine the effects of employment and environmental conditions on public health. Unfortunately, as the National Center's programs have become stronger in conjunction with the state centers, fiscal support for the National Center has remained static or dwindled in recent years, making it increasingly difficult for the National Center to carry out its mission. Recent planning efforts within the National Center have been devoted to developing longer cycles and refined sampling procedures to maintain the major statistical systems currently in operation with reduced budgets. State support through contracts from the National Center has virtually disappeared, and many states are looking for other markets for their data to obtain enough money to keep their programs operating. That may be effective so long as new purchasers of state data do not force the states to alter their collection procedures to better suit the needs of the private interest groups. The Cooperative Health Statistics System has sharply upgraded the availability and quality of vital statistics in many states, but it cannot provide complete national data until it has progressed to all of the states and until all of the components are in place. This will take continued leadership, a hallmark of the National Center since its inception, as well as steady support from the President and Congress, who have been less reliable.

ADMINISTRATIVE USES OF VITAL STATISTICS

The collection and analysis of public health statistics are costly and difficult tasks. Certain records, such as certificates of birth, death, marriage, and divorce, are the result of ministerial acts and must be performed as a matter of governmental responsibility regardless of any public health use for the information contained on the certificates. Other data collection activities are more discretionary. They are of two types: (1) they are collected as a by-product of a service effort such as managing a clinic, an immunization program, or a water pollution control program or (2) they are primarily information-generating programs designed to produce data about the population, its health, the use of health resources, or the environment. The only real justification for collecting data is the use to which the resulting information may be put. Birth and death certificates are important legal records. Their personal value arises in connection with proof of citizenship, the right to attend school, to vote, to marry, to enter the armed services, and to draw benefits of many types. Records of births and deaths are of particular significance in the establishment of inheritance rights and in the prevention of capital crime. Beyond this ministerial function, which is not specifically a health-related function, is the use of the information contained in the records for the evaluation of the health of the community, the state, and the nation.

Statistics are the integers of information that constitute potential knowledge. Whether that potential becomes real depends on its management. In each case, it is essential to understand why the data are being collected and what the sources are. Data collected to answer specific questions about expenditures for the purchase of biologic supplies may not be particularly useful in determining the cost of immunizing children. Moreover, the people who collect or have access to that fiscal data may not have assembled it in a way that can be readily used by people in some other part of the organization who are interested in the costs and benefits of the overall program. At the same time, program managers may be collecting data that they believe will help them understand why and how people are using the program's services, but such data may not merge readily with budgetary or expenditure data kept elsewhere to produce a cost per unit of service.

Who collects the data, the purpose, and who manages the available computer resources for storage, retrieval, and analysis of the data have a great deal to do with the ability to use those data for planning and management purposes as well as the study of disease and disability patterns in the community. The fiscal officer of a public health agency has to have steady access to information about how much money has been spent on what and how much is left in each of the appropriated categories. This often results in competition for machine time, which can lead to the business office developing its own data system to maintain control of the budget. Since this tends to be the single most important control document in the agency, and usually the only agency "plan," the reporting and "inputting" of performance or activity data is often left to the individual program managers. This results in a lack

of linkage between activity data and fiscal data and makes it difficult to measure the cost of an activity or function. Then when special information needs arise, either to respond to an external question or an internal research inquiry, neither information program is adequate and the requester has to develop or find yet another data base. These conflicts are not just in the nature of the accountability each of the data users has to someone else but often rest in the very style or orientation of the people looking for information. The researcher, the fiscal manager, and the program manager usually come from different parts of the organization and have little interest in the others' questions, at least at the time they are pursuing their own. This can lead to some very difficult organizational problems. A health statistics center is not usually placed under the supervision of the fiscal officer. It is important that the center manager and the fiscal manager learn to cooperate in the use of computers. However, such cooperation may not be practical since the computers are usually under the control of one of the two managers whose programs will take precedence. It is now relatively inexpensive to acquire additional computer capability, and it is likely that most programs of any size will have an office computer before the mid-1980s. This can provide a significant increase in data management and evaluative capacity at an acceptable direct cost, but lack of coordinated planning may increase the indirect cost of information loss caused by idiosyncratic file development. It is essential that the program managers collaborate with the central office and the fiscal staff in the design of their data collection procedures and file construction so that cost and performance data can be linked without tedious and costly reconstruction in a third software program and file system.

It is not necessary to place the birth and death certificate registration process in the same management center with other statistical functions, although there are advantages in doing so in the use of microfilming equipment, computers, terminals, and printers. The management skills required to assure the continuity and accuracy of the certificate registration processes are those suited to a clearly defined line organization with fairly rigid practices and authority relationships. The health statistics center concept requires a more flexible approach to management and the challenge of irreverent questions. If these two management styles clash, it is possible to keep the certificate registration process as a clerical center in the business management area of the agency so long as the information contained in the certificates can be filmed or stored on tape in such a way that the health statistics center staff can have continuous access to it.

In any case, management of the health statistics center, whatever functions it includes, should be placed in a fairly prominent staff position close to the agency director or the director of planning. If the center has responsibility for handling a considerable volume of management data, care should be taken that sufficient time and resources are sequestered for the evaluation and analysis functions; hopefully, some will be left over for research inquiries. Administrators of smaller health agencies should not make the mistake of assuming that this advice is irrelevant to their needs. The director of such an agency may also function as the data center manager, but the requirements remain the same: keep the process close to the center of decision making; make sure that time is available for evaluation and that not all of it is used in balancing the budget; and keep a little left over for new inquiries.

The term *management information system* has become so common and popular in recent years that most health administrators with a few weeks of experience are comfortable with the term MIS. As this comfortable use of the term has increased, its value has decreased. Too many people have too many different ideas about what it means. Health administrators speak of a "mental health MIS", an "alcoholism MIS", a "drug abuse MIS," and even a "health systems MIS." There is no doubt that too many different information systems are requested by various officials and legislative bodies and that too many irrelevant questions are being asked at the expense of the few questions that should be asked and answered. Elected and appointed officials and their staffs rail against the forms and reports that they have to complete. This paperwork is all there because someone asked a question and someone else either had to answer it or believed that they had to. Statistics center managers and other administrators have to learn to curb their appetite for data in the interest of asking more penetrating questions. The question asked often has little relationship to what the questioner really wants to know. Recently a community mental health center director asked the director of the state statistics center for a printout of the names of all of the patients who had been discharged from the state hospital into the center's catchment area over the previous 5 years.

The community center director did not tell the state center director that his interest was not so much in the names as in calculating the percent of patients discharged into the service area who were subsequently included in the mental health center's programs over the 3 months following hospital discharge. Because the state data manager did not know the specific purpose, he could not help the community mental health center manager because the release of patient names was forbidden by agency policy on confidentiality. Had the two managers explored the question a little further, they would have found out what was really wanted and the state center manager could have produced the necessary information quite easily. Because information on discharged patients was regularly filed in the data system, as were patient data from the community center, the computer could have matched the two files. The manager of the health statistics center should never accept an inquiry as it is stated but should use that as a starting point to find out exactly what the inquirer is trying to understand. Once that has been accomplished, it may be found that (1) the information really needed is already available, (2) a different question will be more useful, or (3) the question being asked is not as important as some of the other questions pending in the center's work load and cannot be answered in the immediate future. This last point is important and should be more commonly considered. Questions can be costly. To answer them requires time and that represents an opportunity cost that has to be negotiated by the statistics center director, the agency director, and the inquirer. In cases where the latter two are one and the same, a particularly good working relationship is required if the agency's resources are to be used efficiently. Agency directors are just as prone as anyone else to ask whimsical or poorly formulated questions, and data center managers do not often feel that they have the ability to challenge such requests, which can lead to valuable time in the data center being used to answer relatively trivial questions of the agency director.

For statistical data to be of real value in the health program, efforts far beyond the strict legal responsibilities imposed on public health agencies are required. When all the statistics available to a health department are correlated, they become of fourfold value in that they make possible (1) the definition of the problem, (2) the development of a logical program for its control, (3) the planning of records and procedures for the administration and analysis of the program as it progresses, and (4) the evaluation of the results of the program.

PRESENTATION OF VITAL DATA

Of increasing importance in the planning and operation of modern public health programs is the use of fractionated data and of certain graphic devices. There is nothing particularly new or difficult about the breakdown of crude or general data into its component parts. The possible number and types of such breakdowns are practically infinite, and the public health worker must decide which are going to be most useful. With all statistical analyses, much depends on the form in which the material is arranged for study and presentation. A mass of numbers is generally incomprehensible. It is desirable, therefore, to depict the data in some manner that makes it possible for one to grasp the total picture and all of the details. One of the most common methods is the simple spot or pin map, which gives an instant overall answer to the question of where the problem is located.

By itself, a spot map of a disease or other single item is limited in that it does not indicate the extent to which population subgroups are affected. One general approach to this problem is to distribute the data on the basis of various personal characteristics such as age, race, sex, or economic status, calculating incidence or prevalence rates for geographic areas. This may help pinpoint high-risk groups. Information of this sort will largely determine the nature of the public health program of the area. The procedures described are obviously cumbersome, time consuming, and also easily subject to human error. Techniques have been developed in recent years to achieve the same visual and analytic ends by means of computer mapping printouts.[25]

In recent years public health administrators have come to realize that the health programs of large cities are best administered through decentralized neighborhood health centers. These centers are usually decentralized administrative units of the central health department and are often planned to serve populations of about 200,000. Merely to determine the best locations of the health centers, it is necessary to have detailed information concerning the various subdivisions of the jurisdiction. Although data have long been available for small villages and towns, this was not generally true of the neighborhood units of large cities until the 1940 census when the Bureau of the Census categorized and made available much of the enormous fund of information it gathered on the basis of census tracts.

A census tract is a small area with definite boundaries including a population of between 3,000 and 6,000. It is usually fairly homogeneous with respect to race, nativity, economic status, and general living conditions. This has made it worthwhile for public health administrators to tabulate the vital statistical data of their jurisdictions on the basis of similar administrative areas. The correlation of these two sources of information has two great advantages: (1) health statistics complied on a census tract basis serve to show the geographic distribution of health problems, and (2) health statistics compiled on a census tract basis may be related to other social and economic factors also available by census tracts. The ability to spot births, deaths, communicable disease cases, nurses' visits, and other pertinent data on a tract map shows the health administrator where the agency's business is. Prenatal programs should be ogranized in areas where high-risk births are most frequent. Well-baby clinics should be located in the areas where babies of low-income families live. Venereal disease and tuberculosis clinics should be located in the areas where venereal disease and tuberculosis cases are concentrated. Nurses' areas should be designed according to the distribution of demand for nurses' services. Housing inspections and inspections of food establishments are presumably made on a citywide basis. It is a good idea to design inspectors' areas by census tracts and to keep inspection records on this basis. Problem areas may be easily spotted, and special attention can be given to these areas.

It is not practical, of course, to establish a health center or clinic in each census tract. Furthermore, because of the small numbers of births, deaths, and cases of disease occurring in each tract, any rates computed in this relatively small population base are of doubtful significance. In using the information it is usually desirable to recombine the census tract data into larger areas. The usual practice is to form health or sanitary districts, the boundaries of which coincide with those of several census tracts. It may then be possible to compute statistically significant rates and ratios that are useful in identifying problems and in designing programs.

CONFIDENTIALITY

A number of technologic developments, political events, and social trends have come together in recent years and heightened the concern for confidentiality. The use of very large computers and the increase in the number of skilled technicians who know how to operate them make the linkage of separate records possible and probable. Burnett and his associates[26] have reported on the ease with which they were able to link family planning records in Georgia with official vital statistics documents to determine fertility rates in subgroups of the users of the family planning clinics. They found that black, young, and less educated users were more likely to have a baby after receiving services than were white, older, and better educated users. They regretted that they were not able to include all pregnancies but found that elective abortion records did not include sufficient patient identification data to make the matches possible. No doubt the information obtained from the study was useful (although neither surprising nor original), and it appears that they took pains to protect confidentiality, but the enthusiasm for such record linkage projects is disturbing. Similar concerns are raised by automating medical records in the Medicaid program in Alabama. Mesel and Writschafter[27] found that modern techniques allowed them to place information about 400,000 people, 10% of the state's population, into a computer system for about 12½¢ per year per person, and they rhapsodized over the ease of doing the same thing for 20 million Medicaid recipients nationwide. Although they spoke of the need to assure confidentiality, they acknowledged that the techniques for doing that were yet to be developed and suggested that the patients be reminded of the advantage they obtained by having their records available to physicians all over the state.

Concurrent with the ease of developing massive computer systems came the events of Watergate and the spector of an Orwellian government. The same Senator Ervin who chaired the Senate committee hearings on Watergate chaired hearings on confidentiality and expressed his concern about the loss of privacy in a computerized society. People are not only afraid that computer intrusions can occur,

they now know that such intrusions have occurred.

The desire to assimilate such data is ancient and seemingly unquenchable. Lunde[28] has reported on the history and current status of unique identifying numbers that can be universally used to link records. Many countries have developed extensive systems that link birth, death, marriage, and divorce data with medical records, income tax returns, employment history, Social Security benefits, family linkages, etc. The Social Security number in the United States was established by executive order in 1943, and its use had become so pervasive by the 1970s that a Department of Health, Education, and Welfare task force report recommended against any further expansion or the development of any other unique identifier system. But most states had already added a universal and unique identifier to birth certificates in 1968 for the express purpose of encouraging data system linkages.

The desire to learn more about health and the causes and treatment of disability leads many researchers into an omnivorous quest for data; and trading privacy for knowledge seems an easy bargain, especially when one is sure of one's own motives. The most conscientious researcher or administrator cannot forever protect information from an equally diligent intruder, however. The two conflicting values of privacy and freedom of information make the development of policy very complex.

A proposed "Model State Law for the Collection, Sharing and Confidentiality of Health Statistics"[29] makes the conflict apparent. In the "Model" no data can be divulged that will make it possible for the person described to be identified *unless:*

1. The individual described has consented. (In most cases it is not possible for the individual to know what is in the file and therefore what will be disclosed.)

2. The disclosure is to a governmental entity, and the recipient agency has a written agreement that it will protect the data.

3. The disclosure is for research purposes, and a written agrement to safeguard the data and allow it to go no further has been obtained.

4. The disclosure is to a governmental entity for the purpose of conducting an audit, evaluation, or investigation of the agency.

The "Model" notes that all of the disclosure exceptions are at the discretion of the agency except for the last one, which is mandatory and means that a government auditor can gain access to the records of clients in an alcohol detoxification program in the course of conducting a fiscal audit. Under this proposed "Model" possibilities for a breach of confidentiality will grow in direct proportion to the size of the data base.

The complex problems involved in balancing privacy and the need to know about things will not yield to polemics or statutes unless there is a better understanding of the ethics of both. For example, most applicants for a job or for college sign a consent form entitling the organization to gain access to the applicant's medical records. But since the applicant has not, in most cases, seen those records, it is not an informed consent. The applicant has no idea what opinions may have been recorded. Until the physician, nurse, or counselor has been taught to write records so that the client can read and understand them and discuss them, this will not change.

Some efforts to preserve confidentiality have been deleterious to the welfare of the person at risk. Mental health records are often so protected that it is technically illegal for a mental health worker in a community center to answer an inquiry from a psychiatrist in an emergency room as to whether anything is known about an overdosed patient. In most such cases the law is quickly violated in the interest of patient survival, but variations on the theme continue to occur with sufficient frequency to emphasize the point that the trade-off between privacy and the need to know cannot be settled by law or in electronics until the study of ethics has caught up with technology.

REFERENCES

1. Higher education for public health: a report of the Milbank Memorial Fund Commission, New York, 1976, Prodist.
2. Kraus, A.S.: Efficient utilization of statistical activities in public health, Am. J. Public Health **53:**1075, July 1963.
3. Murnaghan, J.H.: Health indicators and information systems for the year 2000. In Breslow, L., editor: Annual review of public health, vol. 2, Palo Alto, Calif., 1981, Annual Reviews, Inc.
4. Bureau of the Census: Current population reports (population estimates and projections), Ser. P-25, Washington, D.C. (issued intermittently), U.S. Government Printing Office.
5. National Center for Health Statistics: Data systems of the National Center for Health Statistics, Ser. 1(16), DHHS Pub. No. (PHS) 82-1318, Hyattsville, Md., 1981, U.S. Department of Health and Human Services.
6. Scientific and Technical Information Branch, National Center for Health Statistics, Public Health Service, Hyattsville, Md.
7. National Institute of Mental Health: Statistical notes, Publ No. (ADM) 159, (issued bimonthly), Department of Health and Human Services.
8. Percy, C., Stanek, E., and Glocekler, L.: Accuracy of cancer death certificates and its effect on cancer mortality statistics, Am. J. Public Health **71**(3):242, March 1981.
9. Manual of the international statistical classification of diseases, injuries, and causes of death, ed. 9, Geneva, 1977, World Health Organization.
10. Vital Statistics of the United States, Washington, D.C. (issued annually), U.S. Government Printing Office.
11. Kleinman, J.C.: Age adjusted mortality indexes or small areas: applications to health planning, Am. J. Public Health **67:**834, Sept. 1977.
12. Warshauer, M.E., and Monk, M.: Problems in suicide statistics for whites and blacks, Am. J. Public Health **68:**383, April 1978.
13. Naylor, A., and associates: Birth certificate revision and reporting of congenital malformations, Am. J. Public Health **64:**786, Aug. 1974.
14. Morris, N.M., Udry, J.C., and Chase, C.L.: Shifting age-parity distribution of births and the decrease in infant mortality, Am. J. Public Health **65:**359, April 1975.
15. Rothenberg, R., Bross, D.C., and Vernon, T.M.: Reporting gonorrhea by private physicians: a behavioral study, Am. J. Public Health **70**(9):893, Sept. 1980.
16. Morbidity surveys—a symposium, Am. J. Public Health **39:**737, June 1949.
17. Linder, F.E.: The national health survey, Science **127:**1275, May 30, 1958.
18. Langmuir, A.D.: The contributions of the survey method to epidemiology, Am. J. Public Health **39:**747, June 1949.
19. Morbidity and Mortality Weekly Report, Atlanta, Ga. (issued weekly), Centers for Disease Control.
20. Epidemiological and Vital Statistics Report, Geneva (issued monthly), World Health Organization.
21. Annual Epidemiological and Vital Statistics, Geneva (issued annually), World Health Organization.
22. Brotherston, J.H.F.: Health planning and statistics: an overview from Scotland, Int. J. Health Services **3:**35, Winter 1973.
23. National Center for Health Statistics: A state center for health statistics: an aid in planning, U.S. Department of Health, Education, and Welfare, Public Health Conference of Records and Statistics Document No. 626, rev. 1969.
24. The cooperative health statistics system: its mission

and program; final report from the Task Force on Definitions to the Cooperative Health Statistics Advisory Committee, Aug. 30, 1976, DHEW Pub. No. (HRA) 77-1456, 1977.

25. Lewis, R., and Chadzynski, L.: Evolutionary changes in the environment, population, and health affairs in Detroit, 1968-1971, Am. J. Public Health **64:**557, June 1974.

26. Burnett, C.A., and associates: Use of automated record linkage to measure patient fertility after family planning service, Am. J. Public Health **70**(3):246, March 1980.

27. Mesel, E., and Writschafter, D.D.: Automation of a patient medical profile from insurance claims data: a possible first step in automating ambulatory medical records on a national scale, Milbank Mem. Fund Q. **54:**29, Winter 1976.

28. Lunde, A.S.: The birth number concept and record linkage, Am. J. Public Health **65:**1165, Nov. 1975.

29. Expert Panel for the Development of the Model State Health Statistics Act: Model health statistics act: a model state law for the collection, sharing, and confidentiality of health statistics, Hyattsville, Md., 1978, U.S. Department of Health, Education, and Welfare, National Center for Health Statistics.

CHAPTER 15

Marketing public health

Public opinion is always in advance of the law.

John Galsworthy

DEFINITIONS AND PURPOSES

The concept of the market has become widespread in recent years partly as a result of the conservative shift that began in the late 1970s and the emphasis on "natural markets" or competition as a way to correct some of the problems of medical care. Yet it is a practice or a skill that is not routinely accepted in most public agencies. Marketing is the planned attempt to influence the characteristics of voluntary exchange transactions—exchanges of costs and benefits by buyers and sellers or providers and consumers. Marketing is considerably different from selling in that selling concentrates on the needs of the producer (to sell more products or to inject more vaccine), whereas marketing, which may have the same ultimate objective, concentrates necessarily on the needs of the buyer or the public. The sales force of an organization is one part of the marketing effort, which includes consideration of the product, its price or cost to the public or the consumer, its distribution and accessibility, and the information available to and used by the public, or the four "Ps" of McCarthy[1]: product, price, place, and promotion.

Social marketing, the use of marketing techniques to introduce or bring about social change, was first described in 1971 by Kotler and Zaltman.[2] That concept, as will be shown later, raises a number of important issues about the political structure of the United States and about the ethics of behavior-change strategies. Since the marketing of public health usually involves an effort to create social change, all such efforts are social marketing activities, and marketing will be used in that sense throughout this discussion.

Marketing is a relatively new business management practice, although some aspects of marketing have been carried out by public and private firms for centuries. When Benjamin Waterhouse persuaded Thomas Jefferson to be vaccinated, he was using one aspect of marketing, promotion, to gain wider acceptance of the product. Since marketing has traditionally been used to increase product sales, it has seemed irrelevant to the work of public health, which usually deals neither in profits nor in products. As it is applied in the business sector, the seeming irrelevance of marketing to public health is at least partly real, but adaptations of marketing concepts to the service environment and to not-for-profit enterprises has enhanced its attraction for public sector workers. There are several publications dealing with the subject,[3-7] although most efforts to date focus on hospital service marketing, which is often antithetic to the interests of public health. Most business marketing experts find it difficult to translate concepts from their customary environment to the unique world of the public agency with its legislatively derived mandates. Nonetheless, it would be a mistake for public agency personnel to ignore the subject and strategies of marketing. They can be very useful in enhancing the general credibility of the agency; in increasing protection against measles, rubella, and influenza; in improving environmental controls; and in reducing deaths caused by heart disease, stroke, and cancer. There are real ethical and political problems involved in the use of a public agency's resources to attempt to influence public opinion and behavior, but the fact remains that it is being done all the time, often by enterprises that seek to increase their market at the expense of the public's health, and there is no reason for public health workers to remain in self-righteous darkness about the strategies and purposes of marketing.

GENERAL CONSIDERATIONS AND CONSTRAINTS

Public sector marketing has a number of unique features. Consumers of services or products usually exercise some control over their market transactions through loyalty, exit, and voice.[8] Loyalty is a form of voting for the conditions that prevail in the market by staying with the "brand" or the policies of the business when other options are available. Exit is the ability to leave the market if one is dissatisfied with the conditions of the transactions. Voice is the ability to challenge the conditions of the market if one is dissatisfied with them, perhaps through a simple complaint or by organizing a citizen's group to protest the market's policies. These classic, democratic ways of influencing the market are not readily available to the consumer of public agency services. Loyalty cannot be demonstrated when there is no other agency from which to obtain a copy of a birth certificate or a burial permit. Exit is not practical for a restaurant owner who does not like the sanitary regulations or for many low-income people who cannot find a private physician who will accept Medicaid patients. Voice is usually left as the sole means of redress.

The service exchange. The concept of marketing developed to influence exchange transactions involving products. The health industry, public and private, is a service industry. Services are intangible and there is no transfer of ownership involved. Services cannot be transported or stored and recalled for later use. If the prenatal clinic has a surplus of supply (time for additional appointments) on Wednesday afternoon, it cannot be used when there is a surplus of demand on Thursday. Moreover, the buyer and seller (provider and consumer) are not exchanging the same thing. When one buys a toaster, the seller hands the buyer a toaster and the buyer gives the seller money. In a venereal disease clinic, the comsumer may obtain relief of symptoms and protection, whereas the clinic manager is engaged in exercising professional skills and controlling the spread of disease. In one sense, the consumer is only one of many consumers of the services provided. The cost to the consumer may be some discomfort, embarrassment, and time rather than money.

The not-for-profit environment. Not-for-profit organizations have not engaged in selling or marketing in the past, and their boards, even though they are often comprised of business people, are not accustomed to marketing what they believe to be a needed and valued service in their community. Not-for-profit organization managers are often professionals from the field of service, such as scouting or nursing, and marketing has never been part of their training or experience. Yet when attendance remains low in an immunization clinic and it is known that less than 80% of the children in elementary school have been protected against measles, the staff are likely to start talking in marketing terms: "Who are these folks?" "What do they know about measles?" "Are they afraid of shots?" "Is the price (waiting time or travel distance, etc.) too high?" Such problems should be recognized as marketing problems from the outset, and programs should be designed to contend with the problems inherent in the market.

Competition. The market is crowded with health messages from both profit-making and not-for-profit organizations. Many of the messages are confusing and conflicting, offering cautionary advice about things to do and not to do. Marketing is a consumer-oriented practice, but it is product based. To accomplish the goals of marketing, people have to be made aware of the product and then moved from awareness to action—the decision to obtain either the product or the service, or, as often happens in health promotion/disease prevention, the decision to stop doing something. In advertising it is often a case of describing the marginal advantages of one toothpaste over another, but in health promotion it often involves promoting doing something versus not doing something or vice versa. It is not a matter of brand preference so much as contrast preference in an environment that may make the alternative behavior (a fast car, a good martini, or a cool cigarette) an effective competitor. For example, car dealers are rarely faced with having to extol the virtues of driving versus walking.

Penetration. Penetration is a measure of the amount of the effective market captured by one provider or product. Ninety-three percent immunization of elementary school children is an effective degree of penetration: it will prevent epidemics of measles. In product or service marketing, 20% of the market may be a very good degree of penetration. Moving from 20% to 25% may require a costly marketing effort and may not return enough revenue to make the effort worthwhile. Unfortunately, in most public health efforts, it is the last percentage point rather than the first one that is most valuable. That is, the women who most readily accept the offer of a Pap smear to detect cancer of the cervix are least likely to have the disease. It is costly to get the interest and the action of 50% to 60% of women between the ages of 18 and 54, but that proportion, which would represent an extraordinary accomplishment in the marketing of a product, would represent failure in marketing Pap smears since the people at highest risk are in the last 5%. As a general rule, the most important people to reach in a health promotion/disease prevention effort are the hardest people to reach. There has been a marked decrease in the percentage of men smoking in the United States in the last 20 years, but the lung cancer death rate has not yet begun to decrease. This is because those most likely to quit smoking are the lightest smokers who have less excess risk than heavy smokers. In a statistical sense, the last recruit is known as the "last x," and the "last x" is always more difficult yet more important to get than the "first x."

Segmentation. Many health promotion/disease prevention efforts have focused indiscriminately on the entire population of a community rather than recognizing that there are many different facets of the public in even the smallest of towns. Identifying the different interest groups is known as market segmentation, and the segments may have geographic, demographic, socioeconomic, or behavioral characteristics that make them distinct. Each segment will respond to different marketing strategies. Families of alcoholics, alcoholics, judges, policemen, and employers will each have different perceptions of the nature of the alcoholism problem and what should be done about it. The family members will not respond to the same message that will interest a judge.

Most product or service enterprises have a relatively homogeneous product line, and it is not difficult to reach different segments with different but effective messages. But public health agencies have sponsoring clients (such as legislators and their "back-home" constituents), consumer clients (such as teen-agers), and competitive members of the community (such as physicians in private practice), each of which may see the public venereal disease clinic as serving a different purpose. It is very difficult for a public health agency to appeal

to all three at the same time with consistent yet effective messages. It would be difficult to expect the public to have equal regard for United Airlines, United Toasters, and United Home Health Services: what do they have in common? Yet the public health clinic may need to provide services to parents bringing schoolchildren in for required immunizations, teen-aged family planning clients who may know some of the parents in the clinic, other teen-agers with venereal disease, young women seeking public prenatal care because they cannot obtain access to private medical care, and mothers with infants seeking postdelivery checkups and well-child assessments. They all require the services of trained nursing, medical, and laboratory personnel, but their interests and commonality end there as do the reasons for public support of those different programs. The problems become more complex when one considers developers seeking variances to sewerage requirements, funeral directors who need a burial permit to arrange a ceremony for a bereaved family, restaurant owners who have to send their kitchen workers to a class in food handling, and the Association of Parents of Autistic Children who are demanding that the health officer require mainstream schooling plus special psychiatric care for their children. Market segmentation in a public health agency presents problems of diversity unknown to even the largest proprietary organizations, yet the agency has to think of those different market segments, formulate responses to their needs and promotional messages to bring about desired social change, yet never appear inconsistent to any of the different clienteles.

The governmental image. Even though many people have had one or more pleasing experiences with a governmental agency or know a public sector employee whom they respect and trust, most people do not have a high opinion of the creativity, productivity, and adaptability of government workers or programs. That perception does not appear to be justified, but a full discussion of the governmental image exceeds the confines of this book. Since such perceptions are relative, it may be that Americans have an unwarranted notion that private enterprise is efficient and creative, and the public sector image suffers in contrast. Mistrust of government was part of the origin of the United States as was private enterprise without governmental interference, and mistrust does have the advantage of keeping public programs under public scrutiny, but that mistrust also makes public sector tasks more difficult.

When a private enterprise has a negative image, it may resort to special tactics to change the environment, including a heavy dose of advertising, a name change, a product change, and a change in management. In the public sector many of those tactics are not available to counteract what seems to be a pervasive attitude. Yet many public health agencies have been able to develop and maintain a good public image. It is not an impossible task. Although multiple constituencies, purposes, and "products" make it difficult, respect can be earned and maintained by ability, behavior, and appearance, as noted later.

Decentralization. Many marketing strategies are dependent on macromarketing, which occurs at the national level and is sometimes individualized by local dealers, as in automobile advertising. Private, not-for-profit, national health agencies can engage in macromarketing by developing advertising and legislative programs to modify smoking behavior or nutrition, but public agencies are often mistrusted if they engage in the same efforts. The tobacco lobby or the milk producers may pressure key legislators to obstruct federal agency advertising campaigns. In their private capacity, citizens may object to the use of public funds to market a concept that they may not espouse, such as family planning. To avoid the perception that some anonymous "they" are trying to manipulate lives, public sector marketing efforts need to be decentralized so that local boards of health or legislative bodies can respond to such concerns. Lacking that intimacy, people who are mildly in favor of the particular effort or neutral on the matter may be aroused to opposition simply because the effort comes from afar under the auspices of a remote governmental agency. At the local level, if the opposition group is successful in blocking family planning services for teen-agers, it will only affect that community rather than the entire country.

Public health marketing needs to use well-developed, decentralized programs, even though this may be relatively inefficient compared to private sector marketing programs.

Honest marketing. No organization, private or public, can long endure if its service or product programs are dishonest—if the sponsors claim more than they can deliver. The effort to deinstitutionalize the mentally ill was marketed partly on the basis that it would save money, but the savings have not materialized because good community care of the mentally ill is not cheap. Legislators who were involved in the change process remain skeptical of the community mental health movement because they were promised more than could be delivered. The Secretary of the Department of Health, Education, and Welfare in 1976 promised that 95% of the American population should and could be immunized against swine flu despite the fact that most practicing public health workers knew it was not possible. The failure of that program was a serious though temporary setback to the credibility of public health.

Given the other problems faced by governmental agencies that have been discussed, public health workers need to be particularly careful not to promise results that cannot be reasonably anticipated. Many programs have been established on the basis that they would cost virtually nothing to implement and might even make money only to confront some of the same legislators a few years later with substantial budgetary requirements to continue a program that now had a vociferous constituency. The legislators may provide the money, but they may not forget the false claims made when another program is proposed by the same claimant.

THE POLITICS OF PUBLIC SECTOR MARKETING

Many of the special conditions that affect public sector marketing have been previously described, but the ubiquitous influence of the political decision-making process warrants special emphasis.

The generally negative image of governmental programs extends to legislators, elected executive officers, agency directors, and their employees as a class if not always as individuals. Legislative and executive branch sponsors of public health programs may surprise public health workers who thought they had an ally by asking very skeptical questions. Elected officials have many constituencies whose interests may clash on particular issues. Although the program manager and staff may think that they are running a model alcohol detoxification program, members of Alanon may be telling normally supportive county supervisors or state legislators that the manager doesn't know enough about alcoholism to be trusted with the program. Politicians have to listen to such information partly because they do not wish to unnecessarily lose votes and partly because they have learned that such allegations are not always incorrect. Occasionally, a knowledgeable manager may not be paying enough attention to what is going on and may have ignored the same complaint or been inaccessible to the complainants.

Beyond organizational or personal competition there exists a deep-seated ambivalence about many important social issues. Helping sexually active teenagers avoid pregnancy and protecting the concept of the family as a value-forming unit are examples of an issue about which many people have internal conflicts. The criminal justice system and public welfare are even better examples: is the purpose of the criminal justice system to punish or to rehabilitate? Is the purpose of the welfare system to seek out those who need help or to prevent people from becoming dependent? The answers vary not only between groups but within individuals, depending on the time the problem is considered and on whether a particular case or a class of cases is under consideration. Given that ambivalence, most elected officials would prefer not to take a clear position, especially if what is needed can be done without vote-losing position taking. An elected official who supported residential care for mentally retarded adults may be quick to investigate charges of mismanagement in the program when homeowners complain. Often those complaints come to the elected official because the program manager or the agency director has failed to pay attention to the need for constant program marketing both in the council chambers and in the neighborhood.

If a complaint is dismissed too often, it is easy to miss the signal that several people have begun to complain. Programs that are known to present such problems require constant marketing. Opponents to a program may well and correctly assume that the staff and managers will not listen to their complaints. Not hearing any complaints, the program director may forget marketing until it is too late. In the mid-1970s the residents of one community insisted on the establishment of programs to combat drug abuse, including detoxification and residential treatment. Many people think that any health problem can be solved by calling it a medical problem and assigning it to medical personnel. But drug abuse is a serious problem not always treatable and sometimes resulting in death. Most residential treatment programs for heroin users will experience violence from time to time. The manager of the program was concerned that the first such incident could result in allegations of mismanagement and even closure of a needed service. He took great pains to bring such problems to the attention of the community through contacts with newspeople and in public meetings, including the annual budget sessions in the county court house. When a fatal stabbing did occur, the reaction was temperate and understanding. Marketing is a constant effort and requires the same sort of careful attention given to other aspects of programs.

Even though it is true that marketing is a constant process, it is also true that the public may resent what appears to be an effort to sell services that cost tax dollars. The same community or legislature that approves money for prenatal care for high-risk, low-income women may disapprove of an organized effort to find all of the eligible clients. As previously mentioned, it is often the hardest-to-reach clients that are most important to reach, yet those same individuals may appear to be the least deserving clients in the eyes of the community. The family that is most splintered and least capable of providing effective support for its members may be thought to be so abnormal as not to merit the use of the public services available to less atypical citizens. Public programs are not established to support deviancy but because they are perceived as controlling it. The interests and the capabilities of the workers may lead them toward more constructive alternatives, but angry taxpayers may have a more conservative version of the purpose of the program. Although a dishonest representation of the methods and purposes of the program will not be tolerated, discretion in advertising program goals is often necessary.

The public arena is a competitive place. Success comes not from higher profits but from greater use, public support, and the attainment of objectives, which are often intangible. What might be an effective marketing effort in the private sector may be, or may seem to be, an unwarranted effort at personal aggrandizement either because of relative laxity on the part of other agency directors and elected officials or because of an overzealous effort by the director of the health agency. Other agency directors will not respond favorably when a peer is seen each evening on the local news, has frequent press conferences, and issues all of the news about all of the programs in that agency. Nor will most mayors or governors tolerate a health director who gets more press coverage than they do, even if they are at fault. It may be necessary to mute an otherwise effective marketing program if it appears overzealous by community standards.

Even with discretion, the marketing of a person rather than a program is never justified. It is often desirable and appropriate to feature an individual employee, including the agency director, to inform the public about a program or a problem, but repeated media exposure of the same person will generate adverse reactions. The public knows that no health director can be an expert on sewerage system design, skin rashes in schoolchildren, acid rain, the high cost of medical insurance, and alcoholism. Different messages are better conveyed by different spokespersons, provided they are knowledgeable and effective in a public setting. If not, it is better to obtain the help of people from the voluntary or private sector who may have those attributes.

PUBLIC RELATIONS

Public relations is the summation of many individual relations that go on in a complex agency. It is one part of a much broader effort to influence the public's health. In the private sector, public relations, good or bad, may be the result of a designated sales force, but in most public agencies there are few or no dedicated salespersons. This is not unique to the public sector. Commercial airlines generally have very effective marketing programs including an emphasis on good public relations. No one is totally dedicated to sales yet everyone does a bit of it, from the agent who handles computerized reservations on the phone (who is usually contacted through the automatic switching of what appears to be a local telephone number to a remote site), to the staff behind the desk at check in (often confronted with impatient customers who have confusing problems and heavy bags), to the flight attendants who may have to serve drinks and meals to a hundred or more passengers on a 45-minute trip. When a ticket or a child is lost, a customer can become a loyal fan when any one of those people solves the problem. Most of them are trained to do just that and do not simply refer the person with the problem to someone else located someplace else.

Good public relations are similar to good manners. They are developed from the appearance, behavior, and ability of the agency, collectively and individually.

Appearance. Dress codes are out of style and usually out of place, but effective communications are not. Appearance is an essential part of the ability to communicate effectively with people. An appearance that might be very effective in talking with teenagers about venereal disease could very well offend their parents at a civic meeting. It is fortunately difficult to discipline someone for eccentric dress in these litigious days, but it is quite appropriate to intervene when a worker's appearance is such as to offend or in some other way jeopardize his or her ability to communicate with someone who needs help. In most cases peer pressure will serve to normalize appearance. In cases where that does not work, provided the problem is real and not just a manifestation of intolerance on the part of one or two other workers, counseling and even reassignment may be in order.

Some agencies still use uniforms, particularly for nursing personnel. This necessitates some sort of dress code, but it should be interpreted liberally enough to allow individual personalization. Some people believe that a uniform adds an air of professionalism and identity to the interaction, whereas others think it indiscrete to have a uniformed worker knocking on the door of a family whom the neighbors believe to be in trouble. It is often tempting to discontinue the practice, but if it has been in existence for a long time, it may not be worth the effort especially if some of the community's leading citizens were initial sponsors of the agency.

Appearance is not just a personal matter, it extends to the appearance of the agency itself. For many years and still today in many communities, the health agency has been reconciled to the basement of the courthouse, often in quarters that a sanitarian might condemn for human use were it not a governmental program. The problem is complex. The national government and several of the larger state governments have made enlightened, at times even profligate, decisions about buildings and office space. Many states, however, and most local governments do not handle real estate transactions in the same matter-of-fact manner as they do other expenditures. The acquisition and construction of office space as well as its location and interior and exterior design are often highly politicized processes. Building design and construction are two of the areas in which patronage still operates, and it is important to recognize the competition that exists for such contracts. The temptation to purchase property that is of no use to anyone else is great, but marketing concepts of service distribution are too important to abandon just to avoid competition for a more useful or attractive site. Although the investment is relatively trivial as a part of the continuing cost of most public health programs, an unwise decision about location or design can exact a heavy toll over that same period of time. The concern and hesitancy may be a residue of an era when real estate manipulation was a more common source of corruption in local government. It is not only difficult for government at the local level to make sensible decisions about the location and design of buildings, but it is also difficult for elected officials to furnish and equip such buildings in the manner they would choose for their businesses. Whatever the causes, too many public agencies have to cope with a work environment that is improperly located and poorly designed. It need not be so. There are many examples of local health departments and clinics that were designed and equipped with both function and cost in mind. Even in these days of high property taxes and interest rates, capital investments for government are probably the least expensive decisions made.

Behavior. Although the first impression of an agency may be visual, the lasting impression has more to do with behavior. The essential ingredient is attitude: the clients of the agency are the reason for its existence. They are neither supplicants nor beneficiaries, but owners. To characterize the difference between good and bad public relations it is only necessary to compare the customary interaction in an office of the Postal Service (a private corporation, incidentally) to a similar encounter with a commercial airline. The difference is not innate, but acquired.

Most of the people who contact a health department would rather be doing something else: children come for shots, undertakers come for burial permits, some people come because they have been ordered to, some because they are not healthy, and others because they cannot afford to go elsewhere. There is no justification for making the contact more unpleasant. This begins with the ability to get to the facility, including bus service or parking convenience. Most governmental agencies reserve proximate parking for employees often stratified by their rank or tenure, and those with assigned places

are usually annoyed by interlopers. The most convenient parking should be reserved for clients, not employees. Parking is one of the most persistent problems in public agencies primarily because it is treated as an employee perquisite rather than as part of the marketing program.

Every agency needs a first-encounter process, either an information desk or someone near the entrances who can help guide visitors to the appropriate location and deter idle visitors. A common mistake is to place the most inexperienced person at the information desk, whereas common sense dictates that the most skillful and experienced people perform that function. Civil service systems unfortunately uphold the former alternative with pay rates to match. Handling a diversity of inquiries, some curious, some troubled, and a few angry, is difficult work and requires equanimity and a positive attitude toward the rights and needs of the people making the inquiries.

Another common mistake is to transfer inquirors from point to point, either on the phone or in person, leaving them with the burden of unraveling the bureaucracy. The reader should recall the airline representative who has been taught to take each problem through to a full resolution before ending the transaction. Phone callers should be transferred to the correct extension after making sure that there is someone there to handle the inquiry. Visitors should be carefully routed to the correct location, either in person or with well-placed signs. When they get to the correct extension or location, they warrant prompt and courteous attention. There is nothing wrong with the staff comparing notes about last night's party unless the comparison is done while a client waits.

The referral and problem-solving process highlights the need for initial and continuing orientation of employees and staff development. Many private agencies have very effective staff development programs and may be able to help establish similar programs in the public sector if the personnel system does not have the capability to do so. Complaint handling is particularly difficult. The recipient may think the complaint completely unjustified, but careful listening is important. It does little to enhance the agency's reputation to interrupt the complainant before the story has been told and begin to argue about the problem. Many warning signals about program problems are missed by defensive and premature arguments. Nor is it appropriate to become so empathetic as to leave the complainant with the impression that he or she has indeed been treated unfairly and that this is characteristic of the process or the person complained of: the defendent deserves an equally fair hearing before judgment. Skillful and attentive complaint handling may solve the problem at the first encounter or at least make the final resolution of the problem much simpler, whereas inept listening may make the problem worse.

Ability. Appearance and behavior help, but the reputation of the agency must rest on the ability of the staff. As previously noted, the public generally does not associate ability with its agencies despite evidence to the contrary. Public sector agencies do have a number of special problems associated with their mission and their environment, and they have not always been able to pay competitive wages for well-qualified people. Beginning with the development of major new human service programs in the 1930s, the public sector attracted outstanding planners, managers, theoreticians, and support staff, partly because private sector jobs were scarce and partly because of a sense of reformism in government programs. Those workers stayed in government service through World War II and began to retire in the 1960s, but they left a legacy of propriety and performance that has shaped the work of their successors.

During the 1960s and 1970s governmental jobs were opened up to people with minimal (as differentiated from maximal) qualifications as part of an overdue social concern about equal employment opportunity and affirmative action. As noted in Chapter 12, the practice of choosing the most highly qualified person from the eligible applicants gave way to choosing from a list of people who met the minimal established requirements for the job. Although civil service systems have been in a state of upheaval ever since, there is no indication that the quality of government work has been diminished. In fact, there is substantial evidence that those entering the management, professional, and technical ranks are better trained then ever before.

Program managers and agency directors should continue to insist on quality work and adequate training for public sector employment. Job classification descriptions warrant careful scrutiny to be sure that the skills necessary for increasingly complex work will be available. Competency needs to be rewarded by commendation, through regular personnel evaluations, and through attention to the reputation of the staff as it is protrayed to the community through the news media. Inadequate work requires the same attention through training, reassignment, demotion, or discharge when all else fails. The best safeguard of ability is diligence in recruitment and hiring and insistence on employee development as the principal objectives of the personnel office.

Private lives. Public employees, particularly those in visible and executive positions, do not have completely private lives away from work: their behavior is always associated with their public positions. As with public school teachers, double standards may be applied, with the community less tolerant of behavior by its officials than it would be of other neighbors in the private sector. Staff who participate in pot parties on the weekend can expect to be challenged even though others in the community may engage in the same activities. There is little point in complaining about such double standards: they are a fact of life and one of the conditions of public employment. Tolerance for atypical life styles follows a bell-shaped curve, with those who share the atypicality in one tail, those opposed in the other, and most people who are indifferent in the middle. Those opposed, whether in the "left" or the "right" tail, are often vociferous in their objections to atypicality. The tendency of the people in the middle is to be more tolerant of the objections of the "right" than of the "left," which results in not-so-subtle pressures to adopt a more conservative life-style.

In addition to this general caveat, public sector employees have other private lives in the social organizations of the community. Even people who are not inclined to join organizations need to make some sacrifices for their programs. If the Rotary Club is the leading service group in town, the director ought to consider joining. The chief medical officer of the public health agency needs to belong to the local and the state medical associations even if he or she does not join the American Medical Association, since the physicians of the community will consider not joining an affront. No employee should be urged to join an organization if he or she cannot afford it or if he or she is opposed to the organization's purpose or process, but program managers and executive officers especially should be supported in their participation in community organizations as part of the agency's overall marketing effort: that is why many of the other members of those organizations are there. Prudence is required to avoid joining the wrong group as it is in making the wrong friends, especially for newcomers. It is especially important to avoid joining an organization that continues to practice racial, ethnic, or religious segregation since that would compromise the very purpose of public health.

Residency is a sensitive issue, especially in major cities of the United States where "white flight" has resulted in a black inner city surrounded by white suburbs. Some states allow such jurisdictions to restrict employment to city residents, and the courts have been inconsistent in reviewing such restrictions. There are many reasons that justifiably enter into the selection of a family residence, but professional, technical, and senior management personnel can expect to continue to feel uneasy if they live outside the community that employs them. Research in recent years has reinforced what should not have been forgotten: the cop on the beat, the neighborhood school teacher, the local family practitioner, the visiting nurse, and the sanitarian can be far more effective when they are part of the community in which they work.

One final note about private lives: it is difficult for a public official to separate private gifts from public ones. Needless to say, employees should never accept gratuities, gifts, or favors of any value from clients or people whose lives or businesses are regulated in part by the health department. Some gifts may appear to be private expressions of gratitude, but employees should be taught to say, "No, thank you," politely, and to point out that while no offense is felt and surely not intended, agency policy forbids the acceptance of gifts. Some gifts are more overt in their intentions, such as the persistent attempts by a state milk producers association to entertain a health officer. It sometimes takes great ingenuity to avoid a gift.

Training. Much of what has been said is in the domain of common sense and good manners, but it is easy to overlook the development of bad public relations. As simple as it may sound, there is a great deal to be gained not only from regular orientation sessions for new employees, but from in-service training programs in telephone answering, correspondence management, complaint handling, and

reception techniques. It may be possible to use some particularly competent employees for some of the training programs, and other agencies, including private industry, are often willing to help. While it is difficult to arrange, it is useful to obtain the participation of the managers of the agency in similar training exercises—they too can forget.

THE MARKETING PROCESS

The marketing process depends on the ability of the organization to manage the four "Ps" of McCarthy[1]: product, price, place, and promotion. Without alliteration this translates to the ability to develop an acceptable service, the ability to offer it at a cost (in time, money, or effort) that will encourage those in need to make the necessary voluntary exchange, the ability to make the service accessible to those who need it (thereby reducing the cost), and the ability to inform or even teach the community and the high-risk segments particularly the value of the service. The development and implementation of a marketing plan is very similar to the planning that takes place for a program and should be a part of that same process.

The marketing plan begins with the effort to establish realistic marketing goals. The problem could be a simmering epidemic of measles or the fact that Americans have high death rates during their adult years. (Those who make it to age 65 are very durable, but a surprisingly large percentage of those who survive childhood never make it to retirement age). The goal may be to eliminate indigenous measles or to reduce the death rate between the ages of 17 and 64 by 15%.

Analysis of the goal may reveal a number of constraints, problems, and opportunities. For example, the number of cases of measles may have increased because immunization levels in schoolchildren have declined below 85% (ascertained through a survey of school records, which is a form of marketing research). The problems are information (not enough of the parents, teachers, or even pediatricians are aware of the severity of measles or the efficacy of the vaccine) and "cost" (it is difficult to get to the county health department offices during the one afternoon each week that immunizations are available, and a private office visit is too expensive compared to the benefits the parent expects to obtain). Even though many people are not impressed by the seriousness of measles, that is not as important as is access to a convenient source for the service, given the propensity of people to comply with school entrance requirements. Therefore more effort should be expended on distribution than on technical information. In the case of death rates in the 17- to 64-year age group, the difference between the United States experience and that of comparison countries in Western Europe is almost entirely because of violence and accidents, principally automobile accidents: speed and power were part of the advertising message for cars, drunk driving is far more common than most people realize, automobile safety is still poor, and very few people use seat belts. All of the known contributing factors need to be analyzed to determine their severity and frequency.

Once the factors have been identified and classified in terms of their overall importance, the various methods that might be used to modify their impact on the problem can be explored, and those most likely to have the biggest impact for the least investment per person can be selected. Simple changes may be attractive because of their simplicity, but if they are known to have little effect on the problem, resources should not be wasted on them. For example, a billboard campaign against drinking and driving may appear attractive, particularly if donated, but may accomplish very little and may even distract effort.

The techniques of change involve persuasion, legal controls, the use of technology, and economic strategies. Most complex problems cannot be solved using only one technique. In the case of seat belts, persuasion through advertising has had very little impact. Legal intervention to require the installation of seat belts on passenger cars has resulted in use by only about 15% of drivers and still fewer passengers. The use of technology and law to require warning buzzers or the installation of passive restraints such as airbags has been postponed or blocked by people who resent the intrusion of government into what they consider to be their private affairs. Economic tactics have not been used yet but might involve a sizable copayment for insurance claims in accidents in which the participants were not wearing seat belts. Surveys (market research) have indicated that a majority of citizens would not object to laws that required the wearing of seat belts. It is likely that a careful combination of several techniques together with well-designed information campaigns could result in a substantial increase in seat belt use and a reduction in motor vehicle death rates. An example of a multifaceted approach was reported by McLoughlin and her as-

sociates.[9] They found that burns in childhood were a serious problem but that educative messages alone were ineffective. She advocated product modification and environmental redesign in a more comprehensive effort to deal with a serious problem.

As in program planning, the next step in marketing planning is implementation. Efforts to achieve water fluoridation are excellent examples of implementation and indicate the kinds of communities in which the effort may be successful[10] and the failures that may nonetheless have some benefits for the agency.[11] In New Mexico, officials were concerned by what appeared to be overuse and misuse of rabies vaccine, which created certain risks for the victims and cost problems for the state health department. A thorough problem analysis verified the existence of the problem and the factors that maintained it, including ignorance by practicing physicians, lack of effective and prompt consultation, difficulty in obtaining rapid laboratory reports, and inadequate product information about the human cell vaccine. The marketing program was designed to cope with all of the problems, including an effective public relations effort with the state and county medical societies. Misuse of the vaccine declined dramatically.[12]

The feedback loop is just as important as in any other planning process. Manufacturers need timely information about their marketing objectives. Pretesting can provide valuable information before a program is begun, but with well-thought-out objectives and an information plan that is built into the implementation and management of the marketing program, the validity of the plan can be monitored and the effort modified quickly even after it has started. Expensive surveys are not always necessary: client response forms can provide useful information about the service, as can skilled community workers. An effort to reach deep into a Mexican-American ghetto that had been the source of several outbreaks of tuberculosis among school children was jeopardized by a raid by the Immigration and Naturalization Service. Community residents felt they had been betrayed by the public health nurses whom they had assisted in their efforts to trace contacts. The bicultural, bilingual community workers identified the problem promptly, and a few meetings in the homes of community leaders quickly reestablished the integrity of the public health nurses.

The ability to change a plan based on feedback is an important attribute and presents some difficult problems for governmental agencies. Occasionally, a governmental objective expressed in a statute may be considerably out-of-date, yet the agency may either mechanically continue performing the duty or be forced to do so by a community that does not understand the changing nature of prevention. A few health departments still require routine venereal disease tests for restaurant employees, and their communities are often surprised when told that it is a waste of time. An agency ought to routinely evaluate its services or products to be sure that they are still needed. Many laboratory services were introduced in an effort to market improvements in disease prevention such as rapid streptococcal testing. With the advent of easily managed office techniques and the proliferation of private laboratories, the agency may find that its resources could be better used in other efforts.

Governmental objectives are not always immutable: at times they are remarkably ephemeral. In the 1960s many states passed laws authorizing and directing the health department to engage in expensive multiphasic testing programs (see Chapter 16), including the use of mobile vans. They fell into disfavor shortly thereafter partly because those who had evaluated the programs found that they were of little use in preventing morbidity or reducing mortality, but many departments were still operating the units in the late 1970s. One mayor or governor may make a major issue out of alcoholism or child abuse only to be followed by a successor who is far more concerned about roads and industrial development. The environment can change quickly, leaving the agency with last year's organization and still older technology. Sometimes the change in the political environment occurs without regard to the importance or the continuation of the problem, and the agency needs to persist in its efforts often with a very different marketing strategy. If the need is not there or has been met, the program can be changed or discontinued, but if it persists, the marketing program has to be changed to fit the altered circumstances.

As noted at the outset, ethical concerns are close to the surface of any public health marketing effort.

Just how far can and should government go in trying to modify human behavior? The arguments over motorcycle helmets and seat belts have centered around individual responsibility, as have the arguments by legislators from tobacco-producing states. They argue that people have the facts and have the right to make up their own minds about their own lives. Dan Beauchamp argues to the contrary that the justice of the marketplace is not appropriate for most prevention efforts, that the goal of public health is to prevent hazards, not just to change behavior.[13] Not wearing a seat belt is a fairly safe practice for most individuals, since the probability of an accident for that individual is very small. Nonetheless, some people will be hurt, and some of that damage will result in a public tax burden of considerable magnitude. Is that a sufficient justification for intervention? Probably not in the American culture. Yet, since each individual action of nonuse may be rational in view of the probability of an accident even though many people will be hurt or killed and since each such loss diminishes the community in some way, the majority of the people who will not be hurt have an ethical obligation to reduce the probability that anyone will be hurt. This obligation can be fulfilled by developing and implementing a multifaceted marketing program to urge or even to require the use of seat belts and safety devices.

THE MEDIA

Good relationships with the press (newspapers, television, and radio) are an essential part of any marketing effort. Just as in other personal relationships, attitude is the key to good or bad media relationships. Many people regard the press with suspicion if not with outright hostility. Occasionally it is warranted. Some publishers and editors are every bit as capable of using the resources available to them to force their biases on the public as are some public health officials. More often than not, however, poor relationships are caused by a lack of understanding of the purposes and the problems of the news media. Most reporters are bright, well meaning, and literate. They have deadlines and an obligation to explore all sides of an issue, not just one side. They respond to candor, honesty, and courtesy with the same delight that others do.

Health agency directors and program managers may find certain reporters who are more favorable to their cause than others, but it is important to assure that all interested members of the press have equal access to public officials and to the information needed to write their stories. A new director should take the time to go to the offices of the community's papers and radio and television stations to meet the managers or editors to get to know something about their deadlines and any special interests they may have. Such contacts should be renewed periodically. The weekly newspapers that serve suburban and rural areas are an important part of that marketing effort since they are a major source of local news for many people. In some communities foreign language newspapers have an important role to play and may be instrumental in reaching certain high-risk groups with public health programs.

It is quite appropriate for the health agency director to suggest an editorial conference to deal with major issues in the community in which the agency or program director meets with the editor and other key reporters to describe the entire issue as the health department understands it and then respond to questions. Some questions may appear to be very skeptical yet require a thoughtful response, since skepticism is an essential technique in developing valid opinions about any major issue.

Most health departments have a policy, sometimes written and sometimes much less formal, about who is expected to talk to the press. It is important to avoid the impression that employees have been instructed not to talk to the press, yet it is equally important to demonstrate to the staff of any health agency that they must be sure of the facts and avoid speculating about rumors or gossip when talking to the press. Usually people who are not qualified to discuss an issue will refer the reporter to someone who is. Occasionally an employee will attempt to use the press to discredit a program or an individual. This sort of behavior should not be condoned but may be very difficult to correct. Reporters have old friends or "sources" and it is very difficult to locate them and intervene in the relationship without appearing to be repressive. There is no easy answer to the vindictive employee who may attempt to use the press in this manner except for an open and honest portrayal of the facts to other members of the press, including the editors and managers.

The health agency director's schedule is usually crowded, but the press have special needs for prompt access if that is at all possible. They have an important public information function to fulfill and it is enmeshed in deadlines. It is always ap-

propriate to ask if the matter can be postponed, but if it can not be, every effort should be made to find someone who can respond to the inquiry. Some stories may involve patients or other clients. Health officials have to be particularly careful about confidentiality: when in doubt, the health agency director should refuse to disclose the identity of any private citizen who may be involved in a public health problem until the matter can be discussed with the attorney for the agency.

Many people make the mistake of worrying about each error made by a reporter and sometimes insist on corrections of unimportant details. An official who may have been lauded one day may find a critical editorial the next about another matter. A thin skin is a liability in the public sector. News information should be reviewed in its totality and over time. Errors that are important should be corrected politely, but if the article or broadcast is generally accurate and does a reasonable job of informing the public, minor inaccuracies, personal criticisms, and matters of interpretation should be ignored.

Local radio and television stations often have feature stories that involve half-hour interviews or panel discussions. They can be important opportunities, but it is well to remember that such offerings are not aired during prime time. The audience is usually small and does not contain the high-risk target group of the agency. A panel discussion about alcoholism will not capture the attention of active alcoholics, but it may attract family members, and the session should be seen as a marketing effort targeted to a special segment of the public.

SUMMARY

Marketing techniques are not readily transferable from the private sector, where they were developed, to the public sector. The political nature of public health programs and the need to reach the most difficult segment of the public present some special problems. However, the basic concepts are still valid. Marketing is a comprehensive program involving the product or service, its cost, its distribution, and the education of the public to influence voluntary exchange transactions that will result in the prevention of disease and the promotion of health.

A successful marketing program in the public

sector requires skillful planning, careful attention to community attitudes and sensitivities, a thoughtful exploration of ethical issues, prudent balance between a campaign that is too zealous and one that is ineffective, constant feedback and concern, and consistency both in purpose and image in a very complex, multifaceted organization with a diverse product line.

REFERENCES

1. McCarthy, E.J.: Basic marketing: a managerial approach, ed. 6, Homewood, Ill., 1978, Richard D. Irwin, Inc.
2. Kotler, P., and Zaltman, G.: Social marketing: an approach to planned social change, J. Marketing **35:**3, July 1971.
3. Kotler, P.: Marketing for non-profit organizations, ed. 2, Englewood Cliffs, N.J., 1982, Prentice-Hall, Inc.
4. MacStravic, R.E.: Marketing health care, Germantown, Md., 1977, Aspen Systems Corp.
5. Tucker, S.L.: Introducing marketing as a planning and management tool, Hosp. Health Serv. Adm. **22:**37, Winter 1977.
6. Lovelock, C.H., and Weinberg, C.B., editors: Cases in public and nonprofit marketing, Palo Alto, Calif., 1977, The Scientific Press.
7. Robinson, L.M., and Cooper, P.D.: Health care marketing: an annotated bibliography, Atlanta, Ga., 1980, U.S. Department of Health, Education, and Welfare, Center for Disease Control.
8. Hirschman, A.O.: Exit, voice, and loyalty: further reflections and a survey of recent contributions, Milbank Mem. Fund Q. **58:**430, Summer 1980.
9. McLoughlin, E., and others: Project burn prevention: outcome and implications, Am. J. Public Health, **72:**241, March 1982.
10. Smith, R.A.: Community structural characteristics and the adoption of fluoridation, Am. J. Public Health **71:**24, January 1981.
11. Dolinsky, H.B., and others: A health systems agency and a fluoridation campaign, J. Public Health Policy **2:**158, June 1981.
12. Mann, J.M., Burkhart, M.J., and Rollag, O.J.: Antirabies treatments in New Mexico: impact of a comprehensive consultation-biologics supply system, Am. J. Public Health **70:**128, February 1980.
13. Beauchamp, D.: Public health as social justice, Inquiry **13:**3, March 1976.

PART FOUR

The control and prevention of disease

Epidemiology has been referred to as the "queen science of public health." In its broadest sense that is an apt description. Epidemiology is the study of the distribution of pathology within the population. That pathology may be mental, physical, or social. Combined with the basic natural and social sciences, epidemiology has helped define the principal problems of society and their causes. As a methodology, it enables researchers, planners, and administrators to develop and evaluate prevention efforts. Beyond that, the basic concepts of epidemiology are powerful tools in the administration of health programs on a day-to-day basis and play a leading role in the development of health policy.

Epidemiology is the basis for virtually all public health programs. It should be the basis on which sound therapeutic programs are developed as well. It has been instrumental in the analysis of the impact of nutrition on public health. Just as epidemiology is the key to the understanding of pathology and its prevention, nutrition is central to disease prevention and health promotion in all age groups and in virtually all public health programs. Even though many public health departments have developed organizational units to provide nutrition services, the concepts and practices properly belong in every public health program. It is significant that the United States with its enormous food-producing capacity and its high standard of living has not developed a national food and nutrition policy.

During the 1960s and 1970s the federal government in the United States embarked on a number of programs to provide more and better food to low-income families generally and to children particularly. The school lunch program was broadened and school breakfasts were added. The special supplemental programs for women, infants, and children grew rapidly, as did the food stamp program and community efforts to provide better nutrition for senior citizens. Yet attempts to evaluate the impact of such programs have produced equivocal results. Given the size of the investments in nutrition programs, the health status of the recipients has not always changed in a consistent and predictable fashion. Although the programs maintained their popularity with Congress and the citizens generally, the budget-cutting mood of Congress in 1981, forced by a President who felt social programs had extended too far at the expense of military efforts and private profits, resulted in sharp cutbacks in nutrition services in almost all areas. The results are not yet evident, but it is apparent that the United States needs to develop a more balanced nutrition policy to guide it in the future.

The third basic element of public health is education. Health education has been one of the consistent public health efforts since the beginning of the century, but its scientific base and its practice base have undergone a rapid transformation in recent years. The emphasis on disease prevention and health promotion that began to capture national attention in the 1970s stressed the need for a stronger research base in psychology and sociology. It became apparent that the relatively simple messages that had been so effective in reducing the prevalence of infectious diseases (except for sexually transmitted diseases) were ineffective in preventing cardiovascular disease, lung cancer, hypertension, and the other chronic diseases. Yet in spite of the relative ineffectiveness of the practice of health education, it is evident that many subgroups within the population have managed to make behavioral changes of considerable benefit. Research has begun to provide the information necessary to redevelop and strengthen the practice of health education. Organizational changes are necessary to accomodate the improvements.

These three "cross-cutting" fields of interest—
epidemiology, nutrition, and health education—
have applicability throughout public health and receive special attention in the chapters of Part 4.

CHAPTER 16

Epidemiology and disease control

In quenching the flames at one point, the good work is begun but not ended. Can infectious disease of all kinds never be quenched?

William Farr (1875)

BACKGROUND

There are many good textbooks dealing with epidemiology[1,2] and disease control.[3-5] The purpose of this chapter is neither to repeat nor to summarize that work but to provide an overview of epidemiology and disease control that will discuss administrative opportunities for disease prevention and health promotion.

All students of public health know that the profile of human disease has changed dramatically since the beginning of this century. Table 16-1 shows the number of lives theoretically "saved" as changes in occurrence and prevention have modified the human experience with communicable disease. Of course, even though these diseases have decreased in frequency and as causes of death, others have increased: homicide, lung cancer, heart disease, and the crippling, nonfatal diseases of an aging population. The patterns continue to change. One of the most important aspects of these changes is that no one really knows why they occurred. It is commonly stated that they were not caused by medical care, but it is also true that they were not caused solely by organized public health. Stallones[6] has said that "neither the proportion of doctors in a population, nor the clinical tools at their disposal, nor the number of hospital beds is a causal factor in the striking changes in overall patterns of disease. Morbidity and mortality are an integral part of the human environment and unrelated to efforts made to control specific diseases."

It is tempting to claim that the 20,799 lives "saved" from scarlet fever and streptococcal sore throat in 1976 were a result of public health laboratory screening, better understanding of the epidemiology of the disease, and better treatment by physicians. However, the nature of the human-streptococcal interaction has been changing for more than a hundred years, perhaps for thousands. In the 1860s the death rate from scarlet fever in England and Wales was 982 per million. In the 1920s, before penicillin or sulfa were invented, the death rate had dropped to 29 per million, and by the late 1940s, before penicillin was widely available, the death rate had dropped to less than 1 per million. The most common age of attack had shifted from young adults to young children. Since the streptococcus is spread by water and milk as well as through person-to-person contact, it is likely that much of this change occurred as a result of improved sanitation, but even that cannot explain such dramatic changes. The nature of a microorganism appears to change over time as does the human environment, the biologic nature of humans, and the behavior of individuals and of society. Heart attacks were almost unheard of before 1900. By the 1950s they had become the most common cause of death in the United States. Since then, the death rate has declined from 308 per 100,000 to 208 per 100,000.[7] Although surgeons, cardiologists, and public health workers would all like to take credit for this phenomenon, it seems likely that the reduction occurred because of a variety of diffuse, unorganized changes in the way people live.

It is commonly supposed that the communicable diseases have been conquered and the future of public health is in the control of chronic diseases. However, nothing ever stays the same. At the same time that smallpox was being eradicated from the earth in 1978, Legionnaire's disease frightened the nation, Reye's syndrome became the most famous new malady of children, and 2 years later, toxic shock syndrome provided new problems for epidemiologists. It seems quite likely that these three diseases, all related to microorganisms, had become important because of manufactured changes in the environment and the publicity they received. This is not a new phenomenon, just one of increasing importance and probably of increasing frequency. Centuries ago, when the Moors invaded Spain and changed the patterns of irrigation, they provided fresh breeding grounds for mosquitos, followed by the spread of malaria into Spain and the rapid increase of the sickle cell gene in the population, since the sickle cell trait provides some resistance to malaria. Perhaps the twenty-first century analog will come from space or from attempts to modify housing so as to consume less energy. The only thing certain is that it will not be the same. The etiology of change is human intervention, and hu-

mans are both the beneficiaries and the victims of the changes they create.

EPIDEMIOLOGY

Epidemiology is a "sequence of reasoning concerned with biological inferences derived from observations of disease occurrence and related phenomena in human population groups."[1] A quick review of the table of contents of any recent issue of the *American Journal of Public Health* shows the pervasive nature of the notion of epidemiology throughout public health: "Los Angeles airport noise and mortality," "Methodological issues in health care surveys of the Spanish heritage population," "Natural history of obesity in 6,946 women." "Changing trends in hypertension detection and control." However, although an epidemiologic notion may start with a statistical association between a characteristic and a disease, it is usually concluded with biologic relationships that can be demonstrated in the laboratory. The epidemiology of breast cancer is incomplete until the molecular changes are fully understood and prevention techniques are available, are in use, and are successful. There are three basic tools of research in health: clinical studies, basic science in the laboratory, and epidemiology—the queen science of public health.

TABLE 16-1. Estimated saving in lives during 1976 as a result of public health measures taken against certain diseases, United States*

Causes of death	Death rates†		Deaths		Lives saved
	1900	1976	Theoretic	Observed	
All causes	1,719.1	884.5	3,727,301	1,892,879	1,834,422
Infant mortality	99.9‡	16.0	315,024	50,525	264,499
Tuberculosis	194.4	1.6	421,492	3,333	418,159
Syphilis and its sequelae	17.7‡	0.1	38,377	272	38,105
Typhoid and paratyphoid	31.3	0.0	67,864	3	67,861
Dysentery	12.0	0.1	26,018	62	25,956
Diarrhea and enteritis	139.9	1.1	303,327	2,010	301,317
Smallpox	0.3	0.0	650	0	650
Measles	13.3	0.0	28,837	20	28,817
Diphtheria	40.3	0.0	87,377	5	87,372
Pertussis	12.2	0.0	26,452	8	26,444
Scarlet fever and streptococcal sore throat	9.6	0.0	20,814	15	20,799
Malaria	6.2	0.0	13,443	4	13,439

*Population 1976: 214 million.
†Per 100,000 population, except infant mortality, which is per 1,000 live births.
‡1915 rates.

In recent years epidemiology as a way of analyzing a problem has led to its incorporation in a wide variety of studies: the epidemiology of aging,[8] the epidemiology of obesity,[9] the epidemiology of mental illness,[10] the epidemiology of health services administration,[11,12] and epidemiology in health planning.[13] Some epidemiologists have fought back, claiming that the short-term interests of health policy makers are leading to a reduction in the training of epidemiologists who may unravel the causes of disability in favor of work on the causes of the cost of medical care. It is possible that government policy makers may shift training grants to favor one sort of worker over another, sometimes usefully, sometimes detrimentally, but the attempt to train more administrators in epidemiologic concepts and methodology can only have beneficial consequences. At the core of the epidemiologic concept is the rigorous and unbiased examination of a hypothesis, and all human service programs must have their underlying rationale challenged by such inquiry. That does not make an administrator an epidemiologist or vice versa. Epidemiology is an approach to a problem; an epidemiologist, whether in a local health department or in a university, is or should be a scientist.

One final introductory comment: it has always been assumed that the state has the right to intervene to prevent the spread of communicable diseases, but the notion that the state can intervene to prevent noncommunicable diseases has never been comfortably accepted, at least in the United States. Throughout this chapter, the acceptability of intervening will become an issue.

THE ETIOLOGY OF DISEASE

The period during the mid-1800s was a golden era for public health. Virchow combined pathology and social science, Lister discovered antisepsis, Pasteur discovered microorganisms and their link to disease, and Koch developed a set of postulates that laid the groundwork for the advances of public health over the next 100 years. In essence, Koch said that (1) the suspected microorganism should always be found in cases of the disease, (2) one should be able to recover the microorganism from the patient with the disease and grow it in the laboratory, and (3) when reintroduced from the laboratory, the microorganism should always cause the disease. John Snow had unraveled the mystery deductively 30 years before when he not only reasoned that the cholera vibrio was spread through the water supply but also deduced that cholera had to be caused by something that could grow in the human and that was excreted from the alimentary canal.

Koch's postulates and the work of Snow, Panum (measles), and Budd (typhoid)[14] set the stage for the work done in tuberculosis, syphilis, measles, polio, whooping cough, malaria, yellow fever, and a host of other diseases. However, the concept began to fail as it became apparent that diseases were multifactorial in nature. In the case of tuberculosis, when it was common, the notion that there was one and only one cause of the disease served well. But as the prevalence of the disease decreased, it became more important to understand why some got it and others did not. For less infectious diseases such as leprosy or noninfectious phenomena such as automobile accidents, Koch's postulates became a handicap. They caused people to think in simplistic terms. The tobacco industry asserted that since there were occasional cases of lung cancer in people who did not smoke and that many smokers did not get lung cancer, cigarettes could not be the cause of the disease. It took epidemiologists another 10 years to build a wall of evidence so high and so firm that the relationship between cigarette smoking and lung cancer became accepted. The National Rifle Association asserts that "guns don't kill people," people kill each other with guns and that outlawing guns will not get at the heart of the problem. However, from a rational epidemiologic viewpoint, reducing the number of guns in circulation certainly would decrease the number of homicides. In their very complexity, disease phenomena offer multiple options for intervention.

The single factor approach to the etiology (the science of causes) of disease is incomplete in the study of infectious diseases also. Some parasitic diseases go through a complex sequence to affect humans, and environmental factors (as in the colds of winter), behavioral factors (as in sexually transmitted diseases), and biological factors (as in tuberculosis in skid row alcoholics) play an important role in almost all diseases. The ecology of disease (the study of the interactive relationships between organisms and their environment) has been described very well by Marc Lalonde who, as Minister of National Health and Welfare in Canada, published *A New Perspective on the Health of Cana-*

dians in 1974.[15] The new perspective includes a review of biologic factors, the environment, lifestyle, and the organization of health services in dealing with important public health problems. For purposes of this discussion, environmental factors include both the physical and social environment and organizational factors include both the organization of direct health services and the organization of public policy generally. This is not a dramatic change from the more traditional view of epidemiology, which dealt with the agent (the bacteria or virus usually), the vector (nasal discharge or a mosquito), and the host (the susceptible human), but it expands the dimensions and opens the discussion to a greater awareness of variables not usually thought of as part of public health practice. Graphically, the older more traditional approach was linear with the agent (A) passing by means of a vector (V) to the host (H), causing the disease. It enabled epidemiologists to focus on eliminating the vector at its source (stagnant water as a breeding ground for mosquitos or the use of larvicides), interfering with the vector (window screens), or increasing the resistance of the host (with antimalarial drugs).

The more complete ecologic array is three dimensional with the human in the middle. Biologic factors may include such things as genetics, previous contact with the agent, immunization, general health status, sex, age, and many other conditions that might make the person either more or less vulnerable to the disease.

Environmental factors may include temperature, humidity, wind direction and velocity, the discharge of pollutants, sewage treatment, water monitoring, food protection, radiation control, highway design, and fire safety features in a home, office, or hotel.

Organizational issues may include such things as the location of hospital emergency rooms, the availability of services to low-income people, the school board's approach to health education, public support for family planning clinics, and public policy regarding social welfare benefits such as cash grants and nutrition supplements.

Life-style, or behavioral factors, may include smoking, drinking, exercise, weight control, and risk-taking generally.

One factor does not fit any of the four dimensions and overshadows all of them: poverty. The disad-

vantaged have more of virtually all health problems with higher rates of morbidity, mortality, and chronic disability.[16] Poverty and a lack of education affect the biologic dimension through malnutrition and a residue of diseases and injuries that accumulate over a lifetime. It has a powerful impact on the environmental dimension as it degrades the quality of housing, increases the risk of accidents, exposes people to excessive environmental hazards such as pollutants and animate vectors of disease, and subjects them to excessive crowding and noise pollution. Poverty alters the behavioral dimension: the poor smoke more than the nonpoor and are less likely to value prevention highly since day-to-day survival is more of a problem. Organizationally, although the poor have a number of official support systems, they generally have poorer transportation systems, poorer schools, and less effective access to necessary health and social services. The poverty problem is so ancient and so pervasive that it escapes the bounds of this discussion altogether and cannot be dealt with as a narrow public health issue, but it sets a persistent background for virtually all public health problems and programs and ultimately is the number one health problem.

None of the above is meant to support the notion that control of communicable disease is old fashioned. Health departments will always have an important role to play in preventing the spread of communicable disease, and many traditional methods are still effective and acceptable. However, a broader understanding of the disease or disability process is important if public health is to expand its array of options and its chances for success.

INTERVENTIONS

Most of the changes that have occurred in the prevalence of disease and disability have occurred without conscious planned intervention aimed directly at the disease. Urban sanitary reform was more often carried out for economic and aesthetic reasons than because of concern about a specific disease, and many efforts to intervene directly in the disease process ended in failure (consider the attempt to stop yellow fever in Philadelphia at the time of the constitutional convention[17] or the more recent attempt to head off a possible epidemic of swine flu[18]). In certain instances, however, intervention has worked extremely well, such as in smallpox eradication and the control of polio and measles, for example. The natural histories of many diseases are reasonably well understood, but the behavioral, environmental, and organizational factors are not as well developed. Success has been due to the dominance of the biologic factors and the public's acceptance of intervention. As interventions moved from such problems as measles and polio to such problems as coal worker's pneumoconiosis (black lung) or lead poisoning, the support for intervention changes. These latter diseases are not infectious, but they are spread to "innocent" people thus warranting the use of the police power of the state. However, the economy of an industry and of many communities is involved, which means that many people want to believe that the epidemiologic findings are not true. Because the diseases are multifactorial in origin and given the obdurate nature of science and of some scientists, there has been disagreement among the experts. This disagreement may be championed in disproportion to its significance because of the economic needs of the affected industry and communities. Intervention involves increased cost or the need for continued action or inaction. Intervention in such situations is often less acceptable. When the need to intervene involves something that is more truly a result of life-style or behavior, resistance to intervention can become formidable. For example, the evidence is conclusive that regulatory control of automobile safety has decreased the incidence of fatal highway accidents. The use of seat belts can reduce fatalities in crashes by up to 50% and in combination with shoulder harnesses by as much as 75%. However, the automobile industry resisted adding the cost to the purchase price, only about 15% of drivers use them regularly, and their use involves convincing adults to do something to themselves in their private cars repeatedly. Even though some countries and a few states have passed laws requiring the use of the installed seat belts with good results in terms of a reduction in fatal accidents, most Americans resist the notion of such interventions by government. Fluoridation for the prevention of dental caries is another example in which the condition is not communicable and the intervention involves doing something forever to adults as well as to children. There are unfortunately a few people who still claim that fluoride in the water at a concentration of one part per million is dangerous (there is still a flat earth society, too). The fluoridation debate has been slow and long, but the impact is noticeable in a 30% reduction in dental caries among schoolchildren during the last 20 years.[19]

Assuming that a proposed intervention is correctly designed to intervene in the etiology of the disease, it has a greater chance for acceptance if:

The victims are thought to be innocent rather than willful.

The intervention involves doing something once rather than repeatedly.

The decision makers do not have to give up much of their own freedom.

Not many people make their living contributing to the cause of the disease.

In spite of the obstacles, interventions are proposed more often than the facts would warrant. This will be discussed more fully later but it would be helpful to consider some of the questions that should be asked before undertaking any intervention effort.

1. Is the disease or disability important? That is, is it common enough or serious enough to be a legitimate cause of public concern?

2. Is the natural history of the disease well understood? That is, if one does what one proposes to do, will the desired result really be obtained? The natural history of the disease includes the interaction of the victim with the environment, including the intervention effort.

3. Is the intervention simple enough to use on the appropriate scale and are its effectiveness and efficiency known?

4. Is there good information (not wishful thinking) about the costs and benefits of the proposed intervention?

If the answers to any of the four questions are "no," then more investigation is usually necessary before a new program is implemented, although some interventions may be necessary because of public concern even if all the answers are not available.

Interventions, similar to the concept of prevention, may be categorized as primary, secondary, and tertiary. Primary interventions prevent the hazard altogether by eliminating it or preventing an encounter between a human and the agent or cause. Primary prevention may involve immunizing a child against measles, genetic screening to advise a couple of the possibility of having a baby with Tay-Sachs disease, or preventing someone from smoking cigarettes. Secondary prevention means preventing disability once the process has actually started. The detection and treatment of cancer in

The control and prevention
of disease

its earliest stages is an example of secondary prevention. So is a weight-loss program for young overweight adults. Tertiary prevention means preventing or retarding progression of the disability once it has occurred. Physical therapy for someone with arthritis is an example of tertiary prevention, as is the use of drugs to retard the growth of metastatic cancer of the prostate. From an organizational viewpoint, tertiary intervention could also involve the organization of rehabilitation services or a trauma center to minimize damage once the hazard has been encountered.

In the following sections, three common public health problems will be discussed in terms of the four dimensions of the new perspective (discussed previously) to illustrate the epidemiologic approach to intervention. The three health problems are streptococcal sore throat, a common bacterial disease with occasional severe complications; deaths from motor vehicle accidents, a problem of epidemic proportions that is not often thought of as a public health problem; and lung cancer, a chronic, usually fatal disease, the etiology of which is to be found in the environmental and life-style dimensions. The discussion is not meant to fully describe the problems or their solutions, but to illustrate the ways in which epidemiologic research can pinpoint likely areas for intervention.

Streptococcal disease[20]

There are many different types of streptococci. The ones of most common interest to public health are known as the beta hemolytic, group A streptococci. Among other things they commonly cause sore throats and scarlet fever. They are of special importance because in some people the acute illness is followed by rheumatic fever, which may cause permanent damage to the heart valves, or glomerulonephritis, which may cause permanent kidney damage. Scarlet fever has decreased in both frequency and severity in the United States, but strep throats are still very common among children. The treatment of choice is penicillin. The objective of treatment is not to terminate the sore throat but to prevent the occurrence of rheumatic fever. To do this means that treatment must be continued at a known level for 10 days. People who have had rheumatic fever remain susceptible to repeated episodes that can further damage the heart.

The biologic dimension of streptococcal disease includes the general health of the individual and prior experience with the disease. Some individuals develop effective resistance to the bacteria and others do not. It is not known why. Only a few of the people who get a strep throat develop rheumatic fever or glomerulonephritis, and no one knows the reason for that idiosyncrasy either. Some children have one sore throat after another all winter long, whereas others seem almost immune to the disease even though the same bacteria may be found in their throats. It is possible to increase resistance to certain strains of the bacteria with immunizing agents made from fractions of the microorganism, but it is not practical to do so, nor is it possible to know which children or adults need such protection.

The environmental dimension is just as complex although more amenable to intervention. Epidemics of strep throat appear to be more common in the Great Lakes region, in the Rocky Mountains, and in New England. They are particularly common in military recruits in training. The disease is commonly spread by direct contact, especially when the nasal discharges are still moist—dried room dust contains viable bacteria, but they appear to be noninfectious. The disease is readily transmitted through unpasteurized milk via udder infections, and explosive outbreaks have been associated with dairy products. The disease occurs most commonly in the late winter and spring months.

The life-style or behavioral dimension of streptococcal sore throat is poorly understood. Clearly there is something of importance in its high incidence among military recruits, and this is likely to be related to the life-style of the recruit during training, either the close living conditions or the intense physical and mental involvement in the training, or perhaps some combination of psychologic and somatic interaction common to young men under such conditions. Clearly people with a penchant for raw milk are more susceptible to the disease. Although it would stretch credulity to claim that behavior has something to do with the varying susceptibility among children in the same house, it is not inconceivable.

The organizational dimensions of the disease include the ability of the medical profession to stay abreast of new developments in the etiology of disease and its prevention and treatment. Not many years ago, many physicians did not understand the association of streptococcal disease with rheumatic fever and glomerulonephritis, nor did they understand the importance of a controlled dose of penicillin over 10 days or the need to protect people with rheumatic fever from repeated infections.

Given the nature of the process in all its dimensions (although the discussion has been too brief to do justice to the work of the streptococcal epidemiologists), what can be done to intervene in the process?

Primary prevention involves keeping the hazard from interacting with the host. In the biologic dimension, this might be accomplished by increasing the resistance of the host through immunization, but this has not proved to be practical with the streptococcus. Good health generally is a protective device against most diseases and injuries, so general health maintenance and promotion are worthwhile. If someone in the household is known to be susceptible to the bacteria, others might be examined and, if found to be harboring the microorganism, they might be treated so as to render them noninfectious, but the susceptible person would still be vulnerable to contact with outsiders in school, at work, or in transit. Secondary prevention in the biologic dimension involves truncating the infection once it has occurred, but before the sequelae have a chance to develop. This requires treatment of the disease early after the onset of symptoms and necessitates medical intervention. Tertiary prevention in the biologic dimension involves protection of individuals with rheumatic heart disease. They need to be protected from subsequent exacerbation of the problem by prompt treatment of infections. Some can benefit from surgery.

In the environmental dimension, primary prevention may be accomplished through effective sanitation of dairy herds and pasteurization or sterilization of milk and milk products. There is not much that can be done about the geographic propensity of the disease other than to exercise more diligent control techniques in those areas of the country. The problem in military recruits requires still more research, and it may prove to be practical to alter the training environment in some beneficial fashion. Secondary prevention in the environmental dimension is not practical. People with established rheumatic heart disease or glomerulonephritis may need special adaptations of their environment to make activities of daily living easier, given the physical limitations of the affected individual. This would constitute tertiary prevention.

In the life-style dimension, not much is known about the psychologic changes undergone by military recruits, nor why some children are more susceptible than their siblings. Individuals and groups with a strong conviction about the use of raw milk need continued attention and, if their convictions cannot be changed, then the environmental dimension warrants more vigorous scrutiny and intervention. Secondary prevention is effective to the extent that people's knowledge about their health can be increased to such an extent that they can monitor their own health and seek appropriate medical care promptly. Life-style changes may be necessary to live with chronic heart or kidney disease, and the psychologic trauma of heart surgery or ongoing kidney dialysis or kidney transplant requires special handling by specially trained people, including members of the family.

Organizationally, primary prevention of the consequences of streptococcal infections depends on increasing the spread of knowledge about the epidemiology of the disease, its sequelae, changes in the nature of the microorganism, and improvements in detection, surveillance, and drug protocols. Secondary prevention in the organizational dimension is dependent on continuing education of children, families, and health professionals. Some public health laboratories organized efficient streptococcal testing procedures in an effort to encourage more rapid identification and effective treatment of strep infections. This effort was very successful and the process has now been incorporated into many medical practice settings. Tertiary prevention of the consequences of streptococcal disease has required enormous investments in the management of "end-stage renal disease" and in cardiovascular surgery. Public payment supports are required for medical services as well as for disability payments and rehabilitation. Many health departments have established rheumatic fever registries that facilitate rapid intervention when strep infections occur or when other medical or dental interventions are contemplated. Some programs have absorbed the responsibility for continuing care for rheumatic fever patients, particularly low-income patients who may not have access to effective care otherwise. A system for detecting individuals in need of such support and maintaining an effective relationship with them often requires the intervention of public health nurses and social workers in local welfare agencies and the cooperation of the staff in a teaching hospital.

In summary, as shown in Table 16-2, primary prevention is most effective in the environmental dimension where regulatory controls have virtually eliminated milk-borne outbreaks. Otherwise, secondary and tertiary prevention efforts in the biologic dimension have to be used, even though they are relatively expensive. The bacteria are ubiquitous and have characteristics that, although well described, are poorly understood. Other than in milk, vectors do not play a significant role in the development of streptococcal disease or its unfortunate sequelae. Nonetheless, the incidence of scarlet fever is declining, its severity is lessening, and, as noted, the incidence of rheumatic heart disease is decreasing. In part this is because of better and earlier medical intervention supplemented by the efforts of public health to make physicians and other health professionals more aware of the epidemiology of the disease and its consequences. However, it should be remembered that the disease has been changing for a century or more and the experience of the last 30 years may be a continuation of that evolutionary process rather than the result of any organized intervention. No one knows where this evolution will lead.

It is important to note that the nature of the disease process is such as to confine its management almost exclusively to medical intervention. Once the sanitary control of dairy products is assured in all communities, the possibilities for organized intervention by government in any of the dimensions are very limited. The control of streptococcal disease has not become a public issue nor is its incidence commonly debated in public forums. If, on the other hand, further research were to suggest new avenues to control of the disease through interventions involving alterations of life-style or in the environmental dimension, controversy would spill over from the research arena into the political arena. It was not too long ago that many people vigorously fought pasteurization laws because they thought that pasteurization would destroy certain qualities attributed to dairy products. A few people still feel that way.

Deaths from motor vehicle accidents[21]

The subject of deaths from motor vehicle accidents is very complex and the discussion here will be brief, with the intention of illustrating the applicability of epidemiology to the possibilities for public health intervention.

Motor vehicle accidents have claimed more lives in the United States than all of the wars combined. More Americans are killed on the highways each year (about 50,000) than were killed in Vietnam throughout that long conflict. Motor vehicle accidents are the most common cause of death among teenagers and young adults between the ages of 15 and 24. They are responsible for more years of life lost than all other diseases and injuries except heart disease, cancer, and stroke.

In the biologic dimension, certain physical problems such as vision or hearing impairments increase the risk of a highway accident. People with uncontrolled epilepsy are at higher risk. Some individuals have better depth perception and hand-eye coordination than others, and some of that is surely genetically determined, although no one knows how. Children are particularly vulnerable since their smaller mass makes it easier for them to become projectiles inside the vehicle in a crash. Although people aged 15 to 24 contribute the largest number of deaths to the total, the fatality rate per number of miles driven is actually greater in the elderly, presumably because of the prevalence of infirmities associated with aging. The environmental dimension has a great deal to do with the incidence of motor vehicle accidents and the death rate in crashes. Highway design is an important factor and the rate of deaths per miles driven is decreased on the interstate highway system in comparison to the rate experienced on secondary roads. Weather obviously influences traffic accidents, as can air and noise pollution. The design of the car

TABLE 16-2. Opportunities for the prevention of strep throat and its complications*

Dimensions	Prevention		
	Primary	Secondary	Tertiary
Biologic	+	+ + + +	+ + +
Environmental	+ + + +	+	+
Life-style	+ +	+	+
Organizational	+	+	+ +

* +, least opportunity, + + + +, most opportunity.

itself is a major factor not only in the frequency of accidents but in the probability of dying in an accident. Some cars and trucks are inherently unstable, create vision problems, or have design flaws in their braking system or in the steering column. Some of these problems increase with the age of the vehicle. Passengers and to a lesser extent the driver become flying objects in a crash and are often injured or killed by an impact that is not absorbed over a large area. The behavioral dimension is particularly important in the etiology of motor vehicle accidents. The single most important behavioral factor is alcohol drinking. About 50% of drivers involved in fatal crashes have excessive blood alcohol levels. Other drugs are important as well—both legally used (but often abused) prescription drugs such as antihistamines (which cause somnolence) and illegally used drugs such as amphetamines and LSD. Risk taking, especially among young males, is an often described but poorly understood phenomenon. In addition, there is the aversion of most drivers to the use of seat belts and shoulder straps, presumably because they take an extra moment of effort to attach.

The organizational dimension has a great deal to do with the etiology of fatal motor vehicle accidents. For years ambulance driving was left to hearse drivers, and their training was minimal. Hospital emergency rooms were not well developed, nor were they in communication with any centralized dispatching system or with emergency vehicles. Many accident victims die because of such organizational deficits. Public policy toward drinking and driving has been a reflection of the social attitude, which seems to regard drunkeness as a humorous episode. The laws have been particularly lax and their enforcement even more so, virtually institutionalizing the parting lament, "Have one for the road."

Given the many aspects of the dimensions of motor vehicle accidents, the prevention of fatalities would seem to relatively easy compared to the prevention of the consequences of streptococcal disease.

Primary prevention in the biologic dimension is not especially productive. Although physical impairments are a factor in the etiology of motor vehicle accidents, they are not a common factor. The control of seizures in people with neurologic disorders has been an important accomplishment, but seizures are rarely the cause of motor vehicle accidents. Therefore even though effective management of certain biologic impairments is important

in its own right and may prevent an occasional accident, such efforts do not play an important role in preventing large numbers of fatalities. Secondary prevention in the biologic dimension is impractical since the time between initiation of the crash process and the crash leaves very little opportunity for any intervention. Tertiary prevention involves medical and surgical treatment and rehabilitation, which are very important.

Primary prevention is clearly possible in the environmental dimension, but resistance to intervention is strong. In many places, the car is a symbol of wealth, status, personal control, and power. Although driving on public roads is a privilege and not a right, the reverse describes the beliefs of the average driver. Intrusions into the environment of driving are generally resisted and often expensive. Even though a safer car is inexpensive in comparison to a lifetime of disability, the purchase price is an immediate problem, whereas the prospect of injury is more remote and its prevention a less attractive purchase option. Highway design has similar problems. Although good design and signage can reduce accidents and fatalities, it is expensive at least in the short run. The interstate highway system could afford it, but the system is not being maintained. Local governments do not have the money necessary to construct or modify roads appropriately or are unwilling to spend the money when faced with other more strident competing demands. Secondary prevention involves many of the same environmental controls, since steps taken to reduce the probability of a crash often reduce the intensity of a crash as well. Tertiary prevention, other than the same kinds of environmental design features that serve to make daily activities easier for people with physical handicaps, is an inappropriate notion in motor vehicle accidents.

In the behavioral dimension, primary prevention is simple in concept but difficult in practice. In the first place, since young people have most of the serious accidents, increasing the age at which people can drive should and does decrease accidents. However, as previously noted, the rate of accidents per mile driven is higher among the elderly. It might be appropriate to retest people past a certain age and restrict their driving, but it has not been possible to discriminate between someone at high risk and someone at normal risk. Therefore restrictions

The control and prevention
of disease

would have to be placed on a large number of people to prevent a few accidents. Such restrictions are vigorously resisted. Programs designed to reduce the use of both licit and illicit drugs while driving could have an effect on accidents, and the former effort is effective to some extent as people and their physicians become more cognizant of the dangers. Illicit drug use is similar to the problem of alcohol abuse and is very difficult to prevent. Since people exercise less control over their behavior when under the influence of alcohol and many other drugs, once the use begins it is difficult to intervene in the behavioral dimension. Efforts to encourage people not to drive when under the influence of drugs or alcohol is considered secondary prevention. Auto ignition interlocks have been designed that make it difficult for someone with a high blood alcohol level to start the car. Their effectiveness is untested since they have not been used in large numbers. It is difficult to imagine anyone purchasing such a device unless under a court order because of a prior arrest for drunk driving. Tertiary prevention is very complex and involves identifying people at high risk and then changing their behavior either to nondriving status or to non-drug-use status. Compulsory intervention programs for people with a drunk-driving conviction have had mixed success, but under certain circumstances (involving an aggressive court, effective probation work, and well-developed alcoholism treatment programs) they may be very effective.

Primary prevention in the organizational dimension offers some chance for success. More rigorous enforcement of strict laws regarding alcohol abuse and driving is needed and gaining in acceptability as affected family survivors form voluntary organizations such as Mothers Against Drunk Drivers. The organization of social policy both in the private and in the public arenas can help. Some states have required the wearing of seat belts, and in communities where that has been in effect, the evidence suggests that it can produce the desired change. It may be possible to void or reduce insurance protection for people who are involved in accidents but who are not using restraint systems, and some states have passed laws requiring the use of appropriate infant restraint systems. Primary prevention is also possible through the organization of better highway construction programs and the de-

velopment of safer cars. Although the automobile industry has claimed that additional safety features are expensive and not attractive options for the car buyer, other designers have suggested that safer cars are practical and no more expensive than unsafe ones. Moreover, there is evidence that many people will buy a safer car when given the option. More educational efforts are needed. Secondary prevention through organizational efforts could contribute to improved emergency response systems and a more useful distribution of graded emergency services in community hospitals. Tertiary prevention involves the better organization of rehabilitation services and disability payment systems.

It is apparent that traffic fatalities are theoretically as easy to prevent as are streptococcal infections—perhaps easier. It is also apparent that secondary and tertiary prevention efforts in all four dimensions are less effective than is primary prevention, as shown in Table 16-3. Primary prevention in the environmental and organizational dimensions could be very effective, and with more research the behavioral dimension could offer opportunities for more effective interventions. It is also apparent that primary prevention involves interventions that are customarily resisted. Most of the progress that can be made involves organized action in the public sector. The epidemiologic information is not fully developed, but it is compelling: traffic fatalities could be prevented in significant numbers by better highway and motor vehicle design and by the social organization of rewards, sanctions, and penalties to encourage the diffusion of such practices and their use. Given that automobile accidents are a leading cause of death and disability and that epidemiologic evidence indicates that primary prevention can be effective, preventive

TABLE 16-3. Opportunities for the prevention of deaths from motor vehicle accidents*

	Prevention		
Dimensions	Primary	Secondary	Tertiary
Biologic	+	+	+ + +
Environmental	+ + +	+ +	+
Life-style	+ + +	+ +	+
Organizational	+ + +	+ +	+

* +, least opportunity; + + + +, most opportunity.

actions in the life-style and organizational dimensions become proper areas of concern and action for public health workers. Public health workers are less likely to be immediately effective in highway and automobile design, although their analysis of the epidemiologic data can help convince legislators and others to take the necessary steps. They can be directly effective in working for better control of unsafe driving practices, principally alcohol and possibly drug abuse. Unlike streptococcal disease, primary prevention is practical, and the arena of action is in social policy and organizational efforts rather than in medical care.

Lung cancer[22]

The discussion of lung cancer can pertain to the epidemiology of many other lung diseases such as chronic bronchitis and emphysema. The cigarette is analogous to the streptococcus since it is so ubiquitous, its characteristics are a result of human intervention, and it can cause a wide variety of problems, some of which are relatively benign by themselves, but all of which can lead to more serious consequences.

Lung cancer was relatively unknown before the turn of the century. However, since World War I it has become the major cause of cancer deaths in men and is now the most rapidly increasing cause of cancer death in women. About 90,000 people die each year in the United States from lung cancer. There is some early evidence that the rate of increase in men has been leveling off since 1970, but, as noted, it is increasing very rapidly in women.

The evidence linking cigarette smoking to lung cancer has been the result of major epidemiologic studies in many countries. Since 1964, about 30 million Americans have quit smoking and the prevelence of smoking has decreased from 42% to 33%. Yet 54 million people still smoke, and the total cost of mortality, morbidity, lost productivity, and property damage has been estimated at $27 billion annually. According to the most recent comprehensive report, "smoking was the single most preventable environmental factor contributing to illness, disability, and death in the United States" in 1979.[22]

Cancer of the lung is a fast-growing tumor that usually has spread from its original site by the time a diagnosis is made. The only known treatment is surgery coupled with chemotherapy and radiation. All of these are debilitating and rarely successful. The 5-year survival rate is between 5% and 10%.

Most victims are dead within 6 months of the initial diagnosis.

Although there are other causes of lung cancer, the dominant cause is clearly cigarette smoking. Certain types of lung cancer occur with equal frequency in both smokers and nonsmokers, but those are rare kinds of lung cancer. The most common type almost never occurs in nonsmokers. Although there does not appear to be any threshold level below which smokers are not at greater risk than nonsmokers, the risk of lung cancer is directly related to the number of cigarettes smoked. Exsmokers have a lower lung cancer death rate than smokers but higher than nonsmokers. The longer the period of time since cessation, the better are the odds.

Although some rare types of lung cancer are the result of congenital abnormalities, there are no known causes of the common variety of lung cancer (squamous cell carcinoma) in the purely biologic dimension, which would make prevention possible. It seems likely that the cells lining the bronchi of some individuals may be unusually susceptible to the harmful effects of cigarette smoking, but this has not been demonstrated.

The environmental dimension is dominant. Some other pollutants may be associated with the etiology of lung cancer (chemicals such as benzo[a]pyrene or radiation), but cigarette smoke has such a powerful effect as to obliterate virtually all other causes. People who smoke and work in a polluted environment are more likely to get lung cancer than smokers in a rural, nonpolluted environment, but the impact of cigarette smoking still overshadows other causes by a substantial margin.

Even though cigarettes are an environmental hazard, the dimension that makes manifest the potential contained in the hazard is the behavioral dimension (see Chapter 28). The literature is profuse. Adolescents are a particularly vulnerable group, although preferences for risk taking change from year to year. Once again the poor are more vulnerable to the hazard than are the affluent. This pattern seems to parallel educational attainment and opportunity, but it is not clear why. Men have smoked more than women until about 1970 when it became apparent that men found it easier to quit. Younger women now acquire the habit in greater proportions than men. Children of smokers are more likely to be smokers than children of nonsmokers, and children whose peers smoke are more likely to smoke. In the organizational dimension, certain groups, especially the Seventh Day Adventists, smoke less than members of other groups, and their lung cancer mortality rates reflect the difference. Highly regimented environments such as military training camps and adolescent groups are associated with smoking, as are certain avocations.

Evaluators of prevention efforts offer discouraging reports and emphasize the need for more research, yet progress has been made. Little can be accomplished in the biologic dimension in primary, secondary, or tertiary prevention. In the environmental dimension, it seems likely that a reduction of air pollution levels will have a beneficial effect, although cigarette smoking is such a powerful and direct form of pollution that other sources must be considered minor in comparison. There has been much speculation about a "safer" cigarette, and the Surgeon General has recommended that smokers shift to a brand lower in tar and nicotine. That would be a form of partial secondary prevention. Cigarette labeling laws have required the publication of tar and nicotine content and risk warnings. Some of the changes in morbidity and mortality are suggestive of an association between the use of low-tar cigarettes with lower health risk, but none of the evidence is conclusive so far. It seems likely that such a change would have a beneficial effect similar to the lowered risk related to fewer cigarettes smoked per day. The evidence suggests that it is not possible to produce a safe cigarette, but they can be made less hazardous. This has occurred to some extent as a result of diffusion of information about the risks associated with smoking and competitive advertising that has been generated as a result of the labeling requirements. Environmental changes can have a beneficial effect on nonsmokers as well, particularly young nonsmokers. Children in the homes of smokers have more respiratory disease than children in the homes of nonsmokers. It is not known whether this difference extends to the incidence of lung cancer.

The life-style dimension has attracted the most attention in the effort to turn off the epidemic of lung cancer, since the tobacco hazard would be latent only, were it not for the penchant of people to ignite cigarettes and inhale the smoke. It is a very complex phenomenon, just as are drug and alcohol abuse, that makes intervention difficult. Teenagers are notorious risk takers, and intervention efforts have been disappointing at least in the short run. It seems likely, given the high rate of cessation by older smokers, that teenagers who have been exposed to valid information about cigarette smoking throughout their school careers will find it easier to quit as young adults than did their predecessors. Parental models are influential, and efforts to get parent-aged people to quit through stronger educative efforts may have the additional effect of influencing children not to start or to quit earlier. Peer group models are also quite influential, and efforts to reach "natural" leaders among teenagers have produced encouraging results in experimental programs. Although cigarette smoking is a specific hazard of known and significant risk, it is also part of an overall pattern of experimentation by young people, and in the long run the reduction of smoking may be partially accomplished by stronger efforts to incorporate health education into the fabric of the school curriculum.

Possible interventions in the organizational dimension are identifiable in the basic facts of the phenomenon. Efforts to organize effective and continuous health education programs as a part of all school curricula are of great importance not only in this effort but in the effort to improve health generally. Legislation affecting cigarette advertising has not produced detectable changes, but it seems likely that this is caused by difficulties in measuring what causes people to change their habits. Higher insurance rates for smokers may be effective, but this has not been demonstrated. The ultimate organizational effort would be prohibition, but that may be a matter of timing. It is alleged that it will never work, and unsuccessful efforts to prohibit the sale of alcohol are cited as evidence for that assertion. However, as the prevalence of smoking has declined, it has become increasingly possible for nonsmokers to expand smoke-free areas, and it is now more common for smokers to ask first before lighting up. If the prevalence of smoking continues to decline, it may become possible to ban smoking altogether. The gradual expansion of nonsmoking areas in the work place, in theaters, in restaurants, in public buildings, and in health facilities has a beneficial effect. In addition to protecting nonsmokers from cigarette smoke, it is a constant reenforcement to smokers (most of whom indicate that they would like to stop smoking), and it reduces the amount of time during the day in which they can smoke. It is important for public health workers to continue the process of expansion in multiple arenas.

The results of an epidemiologic analysis of lung cancer and cigarette smoking (Table 16-4) indicate that tertiary prevention (arresting progress after the damage has occurred) is essentially impossible. Secondary prevention is possible in the environmental arena, if the environment can be so managed as to discourage continuation of smoking or to reduce the hazard by modifying the final tar content of the smoke stream. It is more practical in the life-style and organizational dimensions since both can be used to support what appears to be a fairly pervasive desire to quit smoking. It is in primary prevention that intervention efforts may have their most powerful effect, in the environmental and life-style dimensions, supported by organizational changes. As in the case of motor vehicle accidents, prevention is possible principally through organized efforts in the public and private sectors, including the thoughtful use of the regulatory apparatus of government. Medical interventions are virtually useless in this, one of the commonest causes of death.

Common causes

The epidemiologic analysis of three common causes of death and disability is oversimplified yet remains complex. Although much useful research has been done, a great deal is still unknown. The list of problems is very long and the theoretic interventions would form a very long list. However, within the epidemiology of diseases certain patterns continue to emerge. Smoking is one. It is involved in heart disease, chronic lung disease, bladder cancer, deaths from fires, and several other disease or injury processes. Alcohol has a similar pattern. It is involved in liver disease, stomach and pancreas disorders, brain abnormalities, accidents, malnutrition, and severe social dysfunction. Other problems cut across a wide variety of human disorders and form what have been called "cross-cutting" issues. That is, it may not be necessary to deal with risk factors in the thousands: some of the most common causes of disability and premature death are related to just a few preventable phenomena. The evidence has come from careful epidemiologic investigation.

Prevention is possible through organized interventions, principally in the environmental, life-

TABLE 16-4. Opportunities for the prevention of lung cancer*

	Prevention		
Dimensions	**Primary**	**Secondary**	**Tertiary**
Biologic	0	0	+
Environmental	+ +	+	0
Life-style	+ + + +	+ +	0
Organizational	+ + +	+	0

*+, least opportunity; + + + +, most opportunity.

style, and organizational dimensions. The analysis of problems in industrialized nations is remarkably consistent. The Report of the Surgeon General[23] recommends action in 15 different areas:

1. Family planning
2. Pregnancy and infant care
3. Immunizations
4. Sexually transmissable diseases
5. The control of high blood pressure
6. The control of toxic agents
7. Occupational health and safety
8. The control of accidental injuries
9. Fluoridation of community water supplies
10. The control of infectious agents
11. Smoking cessation
12. Reducing the misuse of alcohol and drugs
13. Improved nutrition
14. Exercise and fitness
15. Stress control

Although a full discussion of all of these target areas would require a lengthy bibliography, much of which has not yet been written, enough is known to warrant a deliberate effort to incorporate such actions into the everyday practices of all public and private health organizations. The number of "cross-cutting" issues is manageable within the framework of prevention. It is important to point out that intervention across this broad panoply of human ecology involves medical care to some extent, but the principal efforts must be made in the environmental, life-style, and organizational dimensions. It is also important to point out that approaches to disease control in most of the world are very different since bacterial, viral, and parasitic diseases still head the list in most countries.

The control and prevention
of disease

ADMINISTRATION OF DISEASE CONTROL PROGRAMS
Legislation

Public health had its basis in law and the police power of the state. Public health was not established originally to provide services but to control the spread of dangerous diseases. The authority of the officially designated health officer is broader than that of virtually any other public official: under conditions that present a real and serious threat to the health and safety of the people, a health officer can enter private property, carry out inspections, and seize private property that is thought to present an imminent hazard.[24] In recent years some restraints have been placed on that authority by the courts, but thanks in part to the discriminating use of such authority in the past, it is still there when it is needed.

In addition to the authority to take reasonably necessary steps to neutralize an imminent threat to the health of the public, certain other tools are at the disposal of public health workers to (1) monitor the health status of the community, (2) establish a definitive diagnosis when certain kinds of problems appear to be present, and (3) in some cases to either remove the hazard or even treat a patient who may be a source of danger to others. Most states have reporting requirements for specified communicable diseases. Every physician and usually many other people, including hospital administrators, nurses, school teachers, embalmers, and hotel keepers, are required to notify the local or state health officer anytime a case of one of the diseases on the reporting list is encountered or reasonably suspected of being present. The lists generally refer to dangerous communicable diseases and vary somewhat from state to state. They fall into five categories[3]: (1) case reports universally required by international regulations, (2) case reports regularly required whenever the disease occurs, (3) certain selectively reported diseases in endemic areas, (4) obligatory reports in epidemics only with no individual case reporting required, and (5) diseases in which no official reporting is justified. Depending on the severity of the disease, reports may be made by telephone or by mail either as single reports or by weekly batching.

It is well known that most reportable diseases are underreported. Even though failure to report is a misdemeanor, physicians are not prosecuted because that would probably do more harm than good. The physician does have some liability, however, should a dangerous disease go unreported and others acquire a disease that might have been prevented by prompt reporting and early intervention by the health department.

The reports may go to the local health department where necessary action may be taken and the report forwarded to the state, or the report may go directly to the state health department where necessary action will be initiated. The reports are accumulated and are forwarded to the National Centers for Disease Control in Atlanta where nationwide surveillance is carried out with weekly reporting back to the states.[25] Providing timely and useful reports to those who must make out the case reports initially is essential if compliance is to be maintained.

Some states require that certain other diseases or injuries also be reported, such as occupational diseases or injuries, suspected child abuse, cancer, or traumatic injuries. In some instances the reporting requirements were established to aid in the development of a registry of the disease in question either for epidemiologic research or for control purposes. Occupational disease reporting can serve both purposes. Many states established cancer reporting requirements and cancer registries to study changing patterns of disease and the effectiveness of different treatment practices. Except in special circumstances, case registries are not particularly useful. In the first place, they require more resources to operate than are often available. An incomplete registry, or one with inaccurate information, is usually worse than none at all, because erroneous assumptions about treatment or incidence of a disease may stem from inaccurate or invalid registry data.[26] However, case management registries such as those established for tuberculosis or rheumatic fever control are useful administrative practices. From a public health standpoint, it is better to maintain a few well-supported, well-staffed research registries than many poorly supported ones.

Legislation usually requires the immunization of schoolchildren against certain common diseases such as polio, diphtheria, whooping cough, tetanus, measles and rubella, and sometimes mumps. The same or a different statute may require that all entering schoolchildren be tested for tuberculosis. Compulsory immunization is widely accepted in the United States and has had a demonstrably beneficial effect. Work done in measles control over the past 6 years has shown that where a good school immunization law is vigorously enforced, measles cases are less common. Indeed, although 300,000 to 400,000 cases occurred each year during the 1950s, only 1,697 cases were reported in 1982, an astonishing accomplishment for such a contagious disease. The principal administrative tool used was the compulsory immunization law. In some states, people with religious convictions opposed to immunization may be excluded, but in most states this does not make an appreciable difference. While the occasional unimmunized individual may get the disease, it is virtually impossible for most of the diseases for which immunizations are commonly available to spread in epidemic proportions when 85% to 95% of the community is resistent because of prior exposure or immunization. The level of protection needed varies from one disease to another based on the unique characteristics of each disease. For measles, 95% protection is needed to prevent outbreaks, whereas diphtheria is confined to the occasional micro-outbreak, usually in a skid row environment, at an 85% protection level. Most immunization laws affect children only and put the burden of enforcement on the school system, which is supposed to exclude any child without adequate proof of immunization. The health department should work closely with the school to establish standards for adequacy and to provide immunization services at convenient times and locations before the beginning of each school year. Reporting requirements are particularly important for the diseases commonly involved in immunization programs because rapid ascertainment of small outbreaks can enable prompt intervention and extinguishment of the outbreak by reexamining school records and correcting deficiencies in immunization quickly.

Quarantine and placarding laws are almost never used now, although they are still on the books in many states. When communicable diseases were more common, they enabled health departments to sequester individuals with a dangerous communicable disease until they were no longer infectious. Under certain fortunately rare circumstances quarantine must still be used. Occasionally a tuberculosis patient whose sputum is loaded with bacteria or a prostitute with infectious syphilis will refuse any treatment, and until or unless a treatment order can be obtained from the court, it may be necessary to sequester the individual to protect the public.

Compulsory treatment is sometimes possible, but it is rare. As a matter of law, it is often possible to prevent someone from infecting others by quarantining them, but it may not be legal to treat them without their consent. In some cases, a petition may be made to the court on the basis that the person is not competent to make such a decision, but such situations are rare except in mental institutions. It is difficult to substantiate the public necessity for compulsory treatment vis-à-vis personal rights.

Most of the disease control work of health departments and other agencies is carried out without compulsion but with a strong educational program often aided by a voluntary health association. Control programs may involve screening, testing, immunizing, and treating people for various diseases. Screening is the process of applying a simple test to a group of presumably well people to sort out those who may have the disease from those who probably do not. Most screening tests are presumptive only, indicating an increased probability of the disease, and must be followed up with more exact diagnostic procedures. Screening programs are not particularly useful, except possibly for educational purposes. Their advocates and practitioners are fervent in their support, but the evidence suggests that they have not been effective in preventing or controlling disease.[27,28] This is particularly true for diseases with a low prevalence. Most screening programs screen the people who are at lowest risk for the disease, do not use techniques of sufficient accuracy and reliability to warrant much confidence in the results, fail to link those with a positive screening test with someone who is interested in the problem and able to carry out the necessary diagnostic and treatment work, or cost more than the benefits realized. One exception to this interdiction of mass screening is phenylketonuria (PKU) screening in newborns and probably thyroid testing in newborns as well. An example of the problems with well-established screening programs has been described by Foltz and Kelsey.[29] In addition to examining the underlying premises that should be considered before embarking on any screening program, they illustrate the false positive problem. As an example, one might consider a disease that has a true prevalence of 5 per 1,000, and a screening test that is falsely positive in 5% of the cases (a modest assumption). If the test misses 1 out of 5 cases (a false negative rate of 20%—also a modest assumption) then only 8% of the 54 people screened as positive will actually have the disease. (Table 16-5). If the false positive rate is 20% and the prevalence is 2 per 1,000, then only 0.8% of those screened as positive will actually have the disease. This will occur even though some may claim that the test is "95% accurate" (the 4 positive-positives and the 945 negative-negatives divided by 1,000). This is the situation faced in many Pap smear and tuberculosis screening programs. It is very important that the natural history of the disease be well understood before embarking on any screening program, that the test be simple and reliable, that there be consensus on what needs to be done about follow-up and treatment, and that the resources are available to be sure it is done.

These are examples of the use of legislation in the biologic dimension. As described earlier, there is much that can be done in the environmental, life-style, and organizational dimensions to control disease. Auto safety regulations have substantially reduced deaths of occupants in car crashes—a savings of 37,000 lives between 1975 and 1978.[30] Legislation controlling hazardous substances, the use of alcohol, and the places where people may and may not smoke and requiring health education in the schools are examples of effective public health interventions in the legislative arena.

Program management

At the national level, the focal point for applied disease control programs is the Centers for Disease Control in Atlanta, a major component of the U.S. Department of Health and Human Services. Established as the Office of Malaria Control in War Areas in 1942, the Centers were concerned with certain communicable diseases until their present reorganization.[31] In addition to the epidemiology program office, which provides a rapidly mobile source of trained epidemiologists in outbreak situations, and the laboratory improvement program, there are six component centers in Atlanta: the Center for Prevention Services, the Center for Environmental Health, the National Institute for Occupational Safety and Health, the Center for Health Promotion and Education, the Center for Professional Development and Training, and the Center for Infectious Diseases. (The National Institute for

TABLE 16-5. Screening 1,000 people for a disease whose prevalence is 5 per 1,000. The screening test has a false positive rate of 5% and a false negative rate of 20%

Screening results	"True" diagnosis		
	Positive	Negative	Total
Positive	4	50	54
Negative	1	945	946
TOTAL	5	995	1000

Occupational Safety and Health may be moved to the National Institutes of Health in Bethesda, Maryland, by congressional action.) Historically the Centers have been a major source of support to state and local health departments in venereal disease control, tuberculosis control, immunization programs, epidemiology, and training and have played an important role in international disease control efforts. They also provide laboratory backup to assist in the identification of esoteric microorganisms.

It is at the state and local level that most of the day-to-day disease control programs are carried out. The pattern varies depending on the strength and competence of the local health departments. Most state health departments provide both leadership and epidemiologic service since only the largest urban areas can manage an effective disease control program. The health departments operate the surveillance programs through management and analysis of reports; epidemiologic investigations and studies, both in outbreak situations and to determine the patterns of morbidity and mortality in the community; educational programs both for the public and for professionals regarding new patterns of disease and their mangement; some screening services where indicated; and the development of recommended public policies and legislation. On a day-to-day basis, the largest disease control programs are the immunization programs, the venereal disease and tuberculosis control programs, and consulting with physicians and families about animal bites and rabies prevention.

Many state and local programs are unable to employ a full-time physician-epidemiologist. They are in short supply and in high demand. One alternative is to employ an epidemiologist with an M.P.H. from a school of public health as the manager of the program and assemble a panel of interested and knowledgeable experts from the geographic area. In many communities there are people with training in virology, microbiology, dermatology, occupational health, internal medicine, pediatrics, allergy, and psychiatry and psychology as well as a few graduates of the Epidemic Intelligence Service program (EIS) of the Centers for Disease Control. These people, sometimes in private practice and often in a nearby university medical school, are well trained, and the lure of an outbreak investigation is often enough to maintain their interest and involvement. The epidemiologist, trained at the master's level, can handle most of the day-to-day problems but can call on the panel of experts, often with good geographic distribution, to respond to any especially complex or sensitive problems. Sometimes the community or a family insists on having the advice of a physician even though a veterinarian or nonmedical epidemiologist knows as much or more about the problem. As a matter of good public relations, the involvement and interest of a select panel of physician-consultants can be quite helpful.

PUBLIC HEALTH LABORATORIES

It is now difficult to understand the role that public health laboratories once played in the development of disease control programs. At the present time laboratories can be found on virtually every street corner, and many previously complex tests can be done in a physician's offices, although often at an unnecessarily high price to the patient and without any real quality controls. From the time of the first public health laboratory in 1892 (in New York City during a severe cholera outbreak), laboratories have played a key role in public health advances. There were no private laboratories, and the limited clinical laboratory practice available was more interested in monitoring sick patients than unraveling complicated epidemics. Laboratories were the scientific cornerstone of modern epidemiology. The public health laboratory program in California did much to advance the field of virology and Valley fever. Grace Eldring and Pearl Kendrick in Michigan developed the whooping cough vaccine still in use today. The original Laboratory of the U.S. Marine Hospital at Staten Island was the forerunner of the National Institutes of Health.

For years public health laboratories have turned out enormous quantities of well-controlled work in syphilis serology, gonorrhea cultures and sensitivity testing, tuberculosis, salmonella and staphylococcus identification and typing, anaerobic analysis in food-borne outbreaks, streptococcus testing, rabies identification and control, milk analysis, and more recently the analysis of toxic chemicals, pollutants, mutagenic agents, and laboratory proficiency testing. Several state public health laboratories manufactured immunizing agents before they became commercial products, and six still make a few biologic products.

Their role has changed. Although they were once involved in sanitary bacteriology and disease outbreak investigation, they became overburdened with work in clinical medicine during the 1960s. In their interest to develop better and faster techniques to identify the gonococcus and the streptococcus, they made it possible for the procedures to be adapted to the small private laboratory. Then with the rapid expansion of fee-for-service medicine under Medicare and Medicaid beginning in 1965, private laboratories proliferated, including large mail-order laboratory services. The use of laboratory tests became still more common and there was little discrimination by physicians in ordering them where they were a public service. The pressures on public health laboratories for such clinically oriented work often precluded the basic work of public health that was not done by others—the examination of milk, water, food, etc. Then as budget restrictions began to become apparent during the 1970s, public health laboratories reexamined their services and found that much of what they were doing was available elsewhere. Many of them had become involved in screening for chronic diseases, testing for blood sugar levels or cholesterol levels, analysis of Pap smears, liver function tests, and routine stool examinations for blood. However, as noted earlier, such screening procedures, although popular, did little to increase health promotion or disease prevention.

Some local public health laboratories have closed entirely because of high cost and declining need, and the work has been consolidated into the larger state laboratories, which often have regional branches. Now, in turn, the state laboratories have begun to redesign their services, trying to work out more appropriate roles. Some of the emerging functions are proficiency testing of private and commercial laboratories, certification or licensing of laboratories for participation in third-party payment programs, standards development, training in new techniques, consultation to private and hospital-based laboratories, and research and development into new problems such as Legionnaire's disease and old problems such as anaerobic testing and the identification of new strains of bacteria under altered circumstances of human interaction. Problems occur that are not amenable to the efficient, highly organized but routine testing procedures of the service laboratories. They require investigation in laboratories whose job it is to unravel problems rather than to render a service for a fee.

All of the state and territorial health agencies operate laboratories. They spent a total of $161 million in 1980, about 40% of which was in support of patient care services.[32] Fifty-three of them provided analytic services for clinical, environmental, toxicologic, or forensic programs; 49 were involved in laboratory improvement programs; 40 provided reference services; 6 were still involved in the production of biologics; 11 operated poison control centers; and several were performing special work for occupational health and safety programs. Most state labs do PKU testing on newborn infants at an average cost of $3.00 per test. The cost of one untreated PKU victim may amount to $500,000 over a lifetime. Most states have now added thyroid testing to the neonatal testing process.

Some states operate a single central facility, whereas others have several specialized state-level laboratories, some serving strictly environmental programs, others serving the medical examiner program, still others involved in agricultural programs, which may include food and dairy testing as well as pesticide surveillance and analysis. A few states have attempted to build large multipurpose laboratories to serve as a central resource for numerous state agencies. The idea is attractive, but it remains to be seen whether the different purposes can be effectively accommodated under one management system. The savings in construction and heavy equipment costs may be substantial, but this could be offset by the time necessary to take a machine apart and restandardize it for another purpose.

About half the states have one or more regional laboratories that reduce the turn-around time on large-volume, routine testing of milk, water, and blood serologies. Regional laboratories are also useful in the distribution of testing supplies and biologics. In some states, certain local laboratories have become branch laboratories of the state and serve as a regional resource to surrounding counties, making the operation of a costly laboratory program in every local health department unnecessary. This was accomplished in the San Francisco Bay area in the late 1960s by several counties in an effort to make needed services available, which most of the counties felt they could not afford on their own.

Laboratories are expensive to build, equip, and operate. Some jurisdictions have attempted to consolidate the public health laboratory with a local hospital laboratory, but this rarely works well. Clinical laboratory managers and personnel are intensely involved in the immediate problems of acute patient care and not enthusiastic about a sample of stew brought in by a sanitarian who is trying to unravel the cause of an outbreak of gastrointestinal disease. The special objectives of a public health laboratory, involving epidemiologic investigation, are often incompatible with routine clinical laboratory programs. The development of a statewide system of public health laboratories with branch offices is preferable.

Laboratories have a life of their own, and most health department clinics will develop pressure to acquire on-site laboratory services to some degree. If physicians and nurses are involved who are providing direct patient care, especially soon after they have left the intensity of the medical school hospital, the pressure to acquire laboratory equipment is almost irresistible. Some of this may be warranted to make quick answers available for simple problems, but the pressures can quickly involve special construction, the acquisition of very expensive equipment, and the hiring of trained laboratory technicians to save physicians' and nurses' time. Such pressures have resulted in totally unnecessary and expensive replications of laboratory practice centers that suffer from high budgets, demanding personnel requirements, and all too often lack of adequate quality control. Indeed the whole problem of quality control has become very serious with the proliferation of laboratories in medical offices. It is important to develop guidelines for what can be done on site and why, and what has to be couriered to a more central laboratory.

Public health laboratory services are often confused with routine clinical laboratories. They do perform many clinical tests, but they should not be held to the same standards of performance. They have a more important role to play in standard setting, quality control, and the investigation of unusual events. For these purposes, the public health agencies need well-trained public health laboratory directors who have a strong background in epidemiology and biostatistics.

SUMMARY

Epidemiology, including sophisticated laboratory work, remains the queen science of public health. Epidemiology is the key to understanding not only the diffusion of disease and disability within a population but also the expansion of wellness and of disease prevention and health promotion. Moreover, what is sometimes called the epidemiologic method, which may simply mean a scientific method of inquiry, is applicable throughout the management of public health programs. The merger of epidemiology as one of the three principal methods of scientific investigation, with epidemiology as an approach to management, should not obscure the fact that epidemiologists and managers are different people who need to understand each other to get their jobs done, hopefully together. While epidemiologists continue to probe for answers to complex questions about the etiology and prevention of disease, managers have to respond to a climate in which decisions are demanded. Lalonde[15] pointed out that scientists must continue to inquire as to whether high salt intake causes high blood pressure, whether obesity and overweight mean two different things from an etiologic viewpoint, or whether synthetic vitamin A protects against certain cancers. However, from the point of view of the manager and the public, surely it is better to be thin than fat, to be a nonsmoker than a smoker, to drink moderately or not at all than to be an alcoholic, and to exercise and stay fit rather than become lethargic and inactive. The clues come from epidemiologic investigations. Their translation into the prevention of disease and the promotion of health requires epidemiologic management.

REFERENCES

1. Lilienfeld, A.M., and Lilienfeld, D.E.: Foundations of epidemiology, ed. 2, New York, 1980, Oxford University Press, Inc.
2. MacMahon, B., and Pugh, T.F.: Epidemiology: principles and methods, Boston, 1970, Little, Brown, & Co.
3. Benenson, A.S., editor: Control of communicable disease in man, ed. 13, Washington, 1980, American Public Health Association.
4. Last, J.M., editor: Maxcy-Rosenau's public health and preventive medicine, New York, 1980, Appleton-Century-Crofts.
5. Clark, D.W., and MacMahon, B., editors: Preventive and community medicine, ed. 2, Boston, 1981, Little, Brown, & Co.
6. Stallones, R.A.: Environment, ecology, and epidemiology, Sci. Pub. No. 231, Pan American Health Organization, 1971.
7. Office of Health Research, Statistics, and Technology: Health: United States, 1981, PHS Pub. No. 82-1232, December 1981, U.S. Department of Health and Human Services.
8. Haynes, S.G., and Feinleib, M., editors: Epidemiology of aging, NIH Publ. No. 80-969, Bethesda, Maryland, July 1980, U.S. Department of Health and Human Services.
9. Bray, G.A., editor: Obesity in America, NIH Pub. No. 79-359, Bethesda, Maryland, November 1979, U.S. Department of Health, Education, and Welfare.
10. Dohrenwend, B.P., and others: Mental illness in the United States: epidemiological estimates, New York, 1981, Praeger Publishers, Inc.
11. Thompson, J.D.: Epidemiology and health services administration: future relationships in practice and education, Milbank Mem. Fund Q. **56**(3), Summer 1978.
12. White, K.L., and Henderson, M.M., editors: Epidemiology as a fundamental science: its uses in health services planning, administration, and evaluation, New York, 1976, Oxford University Press, Inc.
13. Knox, E.G., editor: Epidemiology in health care planning, Oxford, 1979, Oxford University Press.
14. Winslow, C-E.A.: The conquest of epidemic disease: a chapter in the history of ideas, Princeton, N.J., 1943, Princeton University Press. Reprinted in Madison, Wisconsin, 1980, University of Wisconsin Press.
15. Lalonde, M.: A new perspective on the health of Canadians: a working document, Ottawa, 1974, Ministry of National Health and Welfare.
16. Rudov, M.H., and Santangelo, N.: Health status of minorities and low-income groups, Pub. No. (HRA) 79-627, Washington, D.C., 1979, U.S. Department of Health, Education, and Welfare.
17. Powell, J.H.: Bring out your dead, Oxford, 1949, Oxford University Press.
18. Neustadt, R.E., and Fineberg, H.V.: The swine flu affair, Washington, D.C., 1978, U.S. Department of Health, Education, and Welfare.
19. National Institute of Dental Research: The prevalence of dental caries in United States children, 1979-1980, NIH Pub. No. 82-2245, Bethesda, Maryland, 1981, U.S. Department of Health and Human Services.

20. Gordis, L.: Streptococcal disease. In Last, J.M., editor: Maxcy-Rosenau's public health and preventive medicine, New York, 1980, Appleton-Century-Crofts.
21. Haddon, W., and Baker, S.: Injury control. In Clark, D.W., and MacMahon, B., editors: Preventive and community medicine, ed. 2, Boston, 1981, Little, Brown, & Co.
22. Office of the Assistant Secretary for Health: Smoking and health: a report of the Surgeon General, Washington, D.C., 1979, U.S. Department of Health, Education, and Welfare.
23. Office of the Assistant Secretary for Health and the Surgeon General: Healthy people: the Surgeon General's report on health promotion and disease prevention, PHS Pub. No. 79-55071, Washington, D.C., 1979, U.S. Department of Health, Education, and Welfare.
24. Grad, F.P.: Public health law manual, Washington, D.C., 1976, American Public Health Association.
25. Centers for Disease Control: Morbidity and mortality weekly report, Atlanta, Georgia (weekly series), U.S. Department of Health and Human Services.
26. Goldberg, J., Gelfand, H.M., and Levy, P.H.: Registry evaluation methods: a review and case study. In Epidemiologic reviews, vol. 2, Baltimore, 1980, The Johns Hopkins University Press.
27. Holland, W.W.: Screening for disease: taking stock, Lancet 1:1494, December 21, 1974.
28. Reiser, S.J.: The emergence of the concept of screening for disease, Milbank Mem. Fund Q. 56(4):403, Fall 1978.
29. Foltz, A.M., and Kelsey, J.L.: The annual Pap test: a dubious policy success, Milbank Mem. Fund Q. 56(4):426, Fall 1978.
30. Robertson, L.S.: Automobile safety regulations and death reduction in the United States, Am. J. Public Health 71(8):818, August 1981.
31. Foegge, W.H.: Centers for Disease Control, J. Public Health Policy 2(1):8, March 1981.
32. National Public Health Program Reporting System: Public health agencies, 1980: a report of their expenditures and activities, Washington, D.C., 1981, Association of State and Territorial Health Officials.

CHAPTER 17

Nutrition services

A hungry man is not a free man

Adlai Stevenson

FOOD AND THE HEALTH OF NATIONS

In a dissertation written in 1851 on *Food and the Development of man,*[1] Ule stated:

Of all the influences which determine the life of the individual, and on which his weal and woe depend, undoubtedly the nature of his food is one of the weightiest. Every one has for himself experienced how not only the strength of his muscles, but also the course of his thought and his whole mental tone, is affected by the nature of his food. . . . The foods we use must contain the indispensable elements of nutrition in due proportion; our food must be mixed, varied, and alternating. And what is here said with regard to individuals, holds good also for nations.

The concern for national health and the political aspects of food and nutrition have been apparent for millenia. Much of human history and development can be understood in terms of the ability of people to obtain food. The evolution of modern society depended on its ability to reduce the amount of work that was needed to produce that food. Caesar, Napoleon, Hitler, and the military tacticians in the Vietnam war knew the power of food as a weapon, particularly the ability to destroy the opponent's supply.

The stupendous efforts of the allied nations during World War II to produce not only more food but also food of a better quality in the face of many difficulties is well known. Less well realized, however, is the effect on the general health of the countries involved. Not only did millions of young men and women of the allied nations who were in uniform get better meals than they otherwise would have obtained but civilians also benefited enormously, both in terms of education and in the substitution of nutritionally more desirable foods for some that were scarce and less beneficial.

The situation in Great Britain was summarized by Magee,[2] Consultant in Nutrition to the British Ministry of Health:

The war-time food policy was the first large-scale application of the science of nutrition to the population of the United Kindgom. . . . A diet more than ever before in conformity with physiological requirements became available to everyone, irrespective of income.

The other environmental factors which might influence the public health had, on the whole, deteriorated under the stress of war. The public health, far from deteriorating, was maintained and even in many respects improved. The rates of infantile, neonatal mortality, and the still-birth rate reached the lowest levels ever. The incidence of anemia declined, the growth-rate and the condition of the teeth of school children were improved, and the general state of nutrition of the population as a whole was up to or above prewar standards. We are therefore entitled to conclude that the new knowledge of nutrition can be applied to communities with the expectation that concrete benefit to their state of well-being will result.

The situation in the United States was much the same, although the immediate devastation of war was not as apparent as in Great Britain. So striking were the gains in nutrition since the years of the great depression that an ominous finding emerged from the Korean war: autopsies of young men showed very early evidence of coronary atherosclerosis. Americans had apparently become too well fed in some respects.

NUTRITION IN THE WORLD COMMUNITY

A measure of the importance of food to people other than its value in times of strife is the proportion of the productive resources that is devoted to providing it. The proportion of the labor force involved in farming has continued to drop in the United States, from 8% in 1960 to 2.8% in 1980. In less developed countries, the majority of the labor force is needed to produce food, leaving little energy for anything else. The differences depend on many factors, such as wealth, social constitution, the nature of the soil, the national economy, industrialization, scientific development, and transportation. Of great importance are habits, customs, and education. The international importance of these differences in capacity to produce food have become increasingly apparent as population growth, the ability to move farm product surpluses, and the speed with which modern telecommunications systems can portray the grim reality of starvation all make evident the importance of food as an instrument of peace or war.

Jelliffe[3] has defined malnutrition as a pathologic state caused by a relative or absolute deficiency or excess of one or more essential nutriments, the clinical results being detectable by physical examination or biochemical, anthropometric, or physiologic tests. Four types of malnutrition are distinguishable:

1. *Undernutrition,* which results from consumption of an inadequate quantity of food over an extended period of time. Marasmus and inanition are synonymous with severe undernutrition. Starvation implies the almost total elimination of food.

2. *Specific deficiency,* which results from the relative or absolute lack of a specific nutrient. With the exception of ascorbic acid and vitamin D deficiency in infants, specific deficiency conditions are uncommon in human malnutrition.

3. *Overnutrition,* which results from the ingestion of excess food over an extended period of time.

4. *Imbalance,* which results from a disproportion among essential nutrients, with or without the absolute deficiency of a particular nutrient required in a theoretically balanced diet.

It is difficult to determine the number of people in the world who are malnourished. The Third World Health Survey by the Food and Agriculture Organization concluded in 1963 that in the less developed countries at least 20% of the population was undernourished (insufficient calories) and about 60% had diets of inadequate nutritional quality. Overall it estimated that up to one half of the world's population (1 to 1.5 billion people) suffered from undernutrition or malnutrition or both.[4]

These figures and others similar to them are useful in dramatizing the impact of nutrition relative to other problems, but they cannot be accepted literally, since the politics of food and the clash of underdeveloped and developing nations with the more developed nations have resulted in rhetorical claims unsubstantiated by adequate definition or validation.

The most vulnerable group is young children. The World Health Organization estimates that about 100 million children under 5 years of age in developing countries are moderately or severely malnourished. Their malnourished state, complicated by disease, often leads to premature death. Measles, whooping cough, or chickenpox often become fatal. Studies by the Pan American Health Organization show that in the Americas malnutrition is directly or indirectly responsible for the deaths of children under 5 years of age in 53% of cases, and the situation in Asia is even more severe. In addition to increased susceptibility to illness and death, malnutrition has long been recognized to have a significant and long-lasting adverse effect on intellectual development and social behavior.[5,6]

Protein deficiency is one of the most severe forms of malnourishment in terms of its consequences. Since animal protein is the most expensive food, the extent of its availability and consumption is essentially a function of the economy of a family or nation. Whereas the proportion of protein from animal products in the North American diet reaches the exceptionally high figure of 40% and in the British diet nearly 30%, the figure for Latin America is only 17%, for Africa 11%, for the Near East 9%, and for the Far East 5%.[7] As the source of the protein varies, so does the amount needed. Scrimshaw[8] has estimated that Caucasians and the Japanese need to obtain only 9% to 10% of their calories from protein, whereas those who rely on predominantly vegetable sources of protein need to get 11% to 12% of their calories from protein; and in underdeveloped nations where much of the nutrition comes from roots and tubers, 13% to 14% of the calories needed should come from protein. Thus those countries with the poorest food supply have the compounding problem of needing a higher proportion of protein in their diet. Millions of children throughout the world are estimated to be stunted by protein deficiency. This condition is known in South America as *culebrilla;* in Africa, it is called *kwashiorkor*. It is characterized by retarded growth and development, apathy, gastrointestinal irritability, a reddish golden appearance of the skin and hair, edema resulting in a swollen abdomen, and fatty infiltration of the liver. Untreated, the mortality of this condition is high.

Food is the energy of people and, like the energy problem, it poses the same questions of production, acquisition, and distribution. In recent years it has become apparent that the United States can and will use its food-producing capabilities as a major instrument of foreign policy, whether dealing with the Soviet Union or bargaining for oil.

In view of the great advances in the science of nutrition, it is paradoxical that so much malnutrition still exists. In addition to ignorance, prejudice, and poverty, agricultural practices, economic policies, social values, and political factors play their part in the total picture of malnutrition.

In 1966 the President of the United States appointed a panel of technical experts to study world food problems. After a year of study these experts expressed the view that hunger and malnutrition are not primary diseases of the last half of the twentieth century. Rather, along with the so-called population explosion, "they are symptoms of a deeper malady—lagging economic development of the countries of Latin America, Asia and Africa in which nearly two-thirds of the people of the earth now live." The panel's deliberations led to four basic conclusions:

1. The scale, severity, and duration of the world food problem are so great that a massive, long-range, innovative effort unprecedented in human history will be required to master it.

2. The solution of the problem that will exist after about 1985 demands that programs of population control be initiated now (i.e., in the 1960s). For the immediate future the food supply is critical.

3. Food supply is directly related to agricultural development, and in turn agricultural development and overall economic development are critically interdependent in the hungry countries.

4. A strategy for attacking the world food problems will of necessity encompass the entire foreign economic assistance effort of the United States in concert with other developed countries, voluntary institutions, and international organizations.[9]

It is difficult to detect whether the circumstances have worsened in succeeding years or whether all of the efforts have resulted in no real change (which would be an accomplishment), but the target of having programs in place by 1985 certainly has not been attained.

THE DETERMINANTS OF DIET

Many practical problems remain to be solved by education, by agricultural and industrial production, by better food sanitation procedures, and by proper food storage. One of the most difficult problems is changing eating habits. Merrill[10] grouped the factors that shape diet into four headings: geographic factors, biotic factors, economic factors, and cultural factors. "Men eat," according to him, "not only what the soil and the climate allow them to eat, not only what the saleability and desirability of the products they grow allow them to purchase from their neighbors, but essentially they eat what they saw their parents and grandparents eat before them."

In addition to culturally derived preferences, food faddism has become a marked feature in American dietary habits in recent years. No other topic has had so much written about it with such a bewildering mixture of common sense and nonsense. Various forms of vegetarianism, a fetish for organically grown foods, and countless surefire formulas for weight loss have confused many. There are repeated articles in newspapers about a linkage of some food products to disease, most often cancer, usually produced in laboratory animals with excessive doses of the suspect ingredient. On the one hand, this ubiquitous interest in food and nutrition can augur well for the future nutritional status of Americans. However, the frenzied confusion that exists currently, in addition to endangering some, may cause many to treat the entire subject with increased skepticism. It is clear that there are a variety of ways to obtain a nutritious diet and that not all of them involve the kinds of balanced approaches commonly taught a few years ago. A diet of fruit and vegetables, whole-grain cereals, nuts, legumes, and seeds can be adequate, but it takes thoughtful effort to obtain that adequacy and it is difficult for most people to sort through all of the "how to" guides to find thoughtfulness. It seems likely that many people who are trying to attain a healthier diet lack the basic education necessary to design one, since most Americans know very little about nutrition. It is common for people to avoid bread when dieting and eat a piece of meat, even though the meat, ounce for ounce, has more calories and more fat than the bread. The concern about food additives has provoked many persons to reject any food product that lists an ingredient with a complicated chemical name on its label without knowing whether the questionable ingredient is beneficial, neutral, or harmful. Since there are so few recognized and acceptable authorities on the subject of nutrition, anyone can claim to be one and add to the confusion.

It is a rare person who can honestly deny having some food biases or idiosyncrasies. Some foods are shunned for fear that they might be fattening or poor chemical mixers or for other real or imagined physiologic reasons. Some foods are identified with low social or economic status (e.g., corned beef and cabbage); others are identified with affluence (e.g., lobster). Certain foods are symbols of hospitality, for example, wines and in some groups ice cream.

Because of some and in spite of other factors that influence dietary habits and customs, some remarkable changes have taken place in the types and amounts of foods consumed by the American public during this century. Except for World War I and during the middle of the depression in the 1930s, there has been a general increase in per capita consumption of dairy products, citrus fruits, vegetables, and animal protein from 1900 until the 1960s. Per capita caloric intake has slowly increased. The consumption of meat began to decline slightly in 1976. Dairy product consumption has declined sharply since 1960, while the consumption of fish has increased slightly.[11] The overall pattern, triggered partly by cost shifts particularly for beef and other meats, has been toward an improvement in the diet of Americans, although caloric intake remains too high and obesity is the most prevalent nutritional problem.

The increased use of dairy products between 1900 and 1960 resulted in considerable increases in calcium and riboflavin. The bread and flour enrichment program also contributed to the riboflavin increase, as it did to the increase in thiamin, niacin, and iron. With increased use of leafy, green, and yellow vegetables, considerable increase in the amount of vitamin A available has occurred. A similar change in the amount of ascorbic acid has resulted from the increased consumption of tomatoes and citrus fruits.

In 1980 the Food and Nutrition Board of the National Research Council issued its ninth revised edition of *Recommended Dietary Allowances*.[12] Because of decreasing physical activity and a corresponding tendency to overweight on the part of many Americans, the recommended daily calorie allowance for adults has been lowered in recent years. Other changes from the previous recommendations include a decrease in protein, vitamin E, ascorbic acid, and vitamin B_{12} for both sexes and a decrease in riboflavin and thiamin for women. Zinc has been added to the list. The definition of a Recommended Dietary Allowance (RDA) is difficult. The Food and Nutrition Board says, "Recommended dietary allowances (RDA) are the levels of intake of essential nutrients considered, in the judgement of the Committee on Dietary Allowances of the Food and Nutrition Board, on the basis of available scientific knowledge, to be adequate to meet the known nutritional needs of practically all healthy persons." The recommendations are for healthy population groups, not for individuals, and the Board states that most nutrients need not be dealt with equally each day but can be averaged over a 5- to 8-day period. Hegsted[13] suggests that recommended ingestion of nutrients should be higher than the RDA.

PUBLIC HEALTH NUTRITION IN THE UNITED STATES

During the years that have followed World War I, much fundamental research has been conducted and nutrition has become well established as a medical and public health specialty. But the profession is still in its infancy.

Changes in social organization in the United States have had far-reaching effects on national food habits. The process of "Americanization," involving the intermarriage of many nationalities, results in considerable interchange of dietary customs, ideas, and habits. Increased travel enables individuals to experience many new types of foods and methods of food preparation.

The increase in eating away from home has been the single most striking change in American dietary habits during the past 20 years. The implications for both harm and nutritional benefit are enormous. On the one hand, it should be possible to apply engineering technology to food processing so that more and more Americans will receive a well-balanced, sanitary, and palatable diet. So far, however, such efforts have not been a feature of the industry.

The massive processing and distribution systems now in use offer the potential for greater control over the safety of food, but they also mean that a breakdown in controls can lead to the rapid spread of contaminated products to hundreds of thousands of people. Some nutritionists think that as little as one third of the food eaten in the United States is being prepared at home. It seems unlikely that the phenomena responsible for this change will be reversed, and this creates a need for a major shift in the attempt to develop and implement an effective national food policy.

Until recently, educational efforts have focused on home economics courses in schools and the efforts of the agricultural extension service to teach rural housewives how to prepare nutritious meals economically. With fewer farm families and a smaller proportion of calories consumed from raw foodstuffs prepared in the home, educational efforts have to change. It is now as important to teach men about nutrition as it is women since they are as likely to buy processed or convenience foods. Labeling of prepared foods has become an important issue. The food industry has opposed governmental requirements for complete nutrition labeling, and some have claimed that the average person could not understand such complex information if it were available. In addition to underestimating the interest and intelligence of the average consumer, that assertion underscores the lack of good nutrition education in schools.

The ability of a family to obtain adequate nutrition has been described by Schorr[14]:

The portion of income that a family uses for food may be regarded as a rough indicator of its prosperity. That is, as total income goes up, a smaller and smaller percentage is devoted to food. The poorest families spend a third or more of their income on food; other families generally spend a smaller proportion. The point at which total income is less than three times the cost of the basic nutritional requirements of a family (of specific size and ages) may be viewed as the brink of poverty. . . . It is by this standard that almost one fourth of the children in the United States are counted as poor. The rapid increase in food prices during the 1970s has exacerbated the problem.

Food is a commodity and can be had only for a price. Those who are economically disadvantaged cannot afford expensive food habits. Furthermore, they cannot afford the auxiliary factors that influence dietary development, such as education and travel. As a result, large numbers of low-income people in the United States suffer from malnutrition, often in the face of food surplus.

In 1961 Congress enacted a 3-year pilot program to improve the nutritional status of low-income families by the provision of food stamps. The families who participated showed better diets than similar families who had not participated. "Findings showed food stamp families made significant increases in the value of food purchased with more than 80 percent of this increase accounted for by animal products—meat, poultry, fish, milk and eggs—and by fresh fruits and vegetables."[15]

In 1968 the Citizen's Board of Inquiry into Hunger and Malnutrition in the United States published its famous report, *Hunger, U.S.A.*[16] This was a passionate indictment of the circumstances that allowed poverty and malnutrition to exist so flagrantly in so wealthy a nation. The Citizen's Board was almost as concerned about the lack of knowledge of the problem. The report had a profound and continuing effect on federal programs. It also typified a sharp dichotomy between the ideologies of welfare and public health. The Citizen's Board found that the poor know how to use their food dollars but had too few of them. Its primary recommendation was for expansion of the food stamp program, making it available on the basis of need rather than a means test. It urged that the program be required in all states (this was done in 1974; in 1980 $8.7 billion in food stamps and food certificates were distributed to more than 21 million low-income people) and that those in need get the stamps free rather than have to pay varying amounts for them, as is currently the case. Public health workers, though grateful for the food stamp program, feel that it should be used in a more instructive fashion, with more controls placed on the nature of the products that can be purchased with the stamps. In short, public health workers would often prefer to limit the freedom of the recipient to obtain better nutrition, whereas welfare workers have preferred to provide cash (or the equivalent of cash) and leave the recipient free to choose. The food stamp program, like most other nationally supported public nutrition programs, is run by the U.S. Department of Agriculture's Food and Nutrition Service, not by the Department of Health and Human Services. It mixes the objectives of production supports for the industry, income expansion, and

The control and prevention of
disease

public health to the detriment of consistently comprehensible policy formation and good management.

The school lunch program began as a response to the needs of children, especially in urban areas. It was the largest of the child nutrition programs and served about 26.7 million children in more than 88,000 schools in 1980. The program was expanded in 1975 to serve children in other types of institutions. Although the school lunch program has generally been considered a joint enterprise of federal, state, and local authorities, it is of critical importance that the principal, teachers, parents, and school lunch managers be interested in and understand the program. On the federal level, information regarding the establishment and management of the program and the use of surplus foods has been available through the U.S. Department of Agriculture. On the state level, inquiry can be made through the state health department and through the state department of education. On the local level, health departments and school authorities can provide information necessary to the establishment and management of a school lunch program. However, the mere serving of food is not enough; the art of incorporating nutrition education into the entire curriculum so that the feeding experience is really a learning laboratory is essential if the aim of developing good food habits in children is to be achieved. Todhunter[17] has described some goals that must be attained if the school lunch is to contribute to the lifetime nutritional well-being of the child:

1. Educators and school administrators must understand the importance of nutrition for school children and recognize the value of the school lunch in nutrition education.

2. The school lunch must be a part of the total school program. Teachers need to have training which will provide sufficient background in nutrition to be able to give children adequate guidance in food selection and the development of desirable food habits.

3. The school lunch program must be managed by trained lunch managers, assisted by employees who have been given adequate training for their specific jobs.

4. The school lunch must be eaten by "trained" children—that is, children who are learning about foods in relation to nutrition and health as a laboratory for educational experiences.

5. The school lunch program must run on a nonprofit basis, financed in the same way that other school services are financed. The sale of nonessential foods and beverages at lunch times or at any other period of the school day should not be permitted.

6. There must be further research and study of the nutritional needs of children, of ways of developing new food habits, and of how to teach nutrition to boys and girls so that they will put into practice what they are taught.

7. Nutritionists, dieticians, public health workers, and health educators must be alert to the significance of the school lunch as a contribution to the nutritional well-being of the child and must direct their efforts to the fulfillment of such a program as has been described.

Nutrition education can and should be an integral part of the total school curriculum and be carefully planned as such. It should be developed to fit the student's level, beginning with kingergarten and progressing through secondary school and college. P.L.95-166 authorized the use of federal funds for nutrition education in the schools. Coates and co-workers[18] have shown that a comprehensive program can have an important effect on the knowledge and the eating habits of elementary school children that may influence the rest of the family. Glanz and Morris[19] have found that this can work in a college dormitory too.

RELATION OF NUTRITION TO SELECTED HEALTH PROBLEMS
Pregnancy

The most vigorous public nutrition activities center around the health of mothers and children. The first recognition of nutrition as a public concern came at the White House Conference on Child Health in 1930. The evidence relating nutritional habits to maternal and infant health has been confusing. It is widely believed that good maternal nutrition has a beneficial impact on the outcome of the pregnancy, but the few good studies carried out still have flaws in them that leave the answers in doubt. Except for situations involving extreme deprivation or the ingestion of toxic substances, the adverse effects of inadequate nutrition are subtle and difficult to establish in population-based studies. In spite of some study design problems, the most authoritative review of the supplemental nutrition program for women, infants, and children (WIC) supports the thesis that good nutrition (specifically, protein and iron augmentation) does increase the duration of pregnancy and birth weight and decreases the prevalence of anemia in high-risk women.[20] As noted elsewhere, these are all desirable outcomes. (See the section on *infancy* for a more complete discussion of the WIC program.) The study suggested that the WIC food supplements were actually serving as replacement rather than supplemental foods but still had the desired effect since they were replacing foods of less adequate nutritional quality. In women with a stronger educational background, higher socioeconomic status, and no known nutritional deficiency, it seems unlikely that added nutritional efforts will have any additive beneficial impact on the outcome of the pregnancy.

Many questions remain inadequately answered. For example, does maternal malnutrition play a role of the development of congenital anomalies? Can a woman poorly nourished all of her life compensate for long-term malnutrition by consuming adequate food during the pregnancy? What are the added risks for the woman who is malnourished when she conceives? Despite the fact that research groups have not yet been able to unravel many of the unknowns in this important aspect of preventive medicine, there exists adequate knowledge of the relation of nutrition to the health of both the mother and the baby to justify use of all resources at hand to encourage the best state of nutrition possible in all pregnant women. Furthermore, good nutrition throughout the entire prior life span, as well as during the period of pregnancy, is essential if optimal nutrition is desired in the off-spring. Nutritional status, good or bad, cannot be turned on and off like a faucet. Adequate nutrition during pregnancy must be based on adequate nutrition before pregnancy.

How should the pregnant woman's diet be managed? Although supplemental food programs are necessary for low-income families, circumstances place the responsibility fundamentally on the woman and the attendant to whom she goes for care. Her diet should be neither ignored nor considered merely in terms of a table of standards. Each woman is an individual and should be treated as such, and the physician who fails to study the pregnant patient's dietary problems as carefully as her blood pressure is clearly negligent. Public health nurses and nutritionists can help by interpreting the nutritional needs of pregnancy and lactation to women individually or in mothers' classes.

There is much misinformation about proper nutrition during pregnancy and during the period of lactation. The average pregnant woman in the United States obtains enough vitamins from her ordinary diet. On the other hand, there is no evidence that extra vitamins are harmful with the exception of vitamins A and D. Additional iron and folic acid are needed both during and after pregnancy, whether or not the infant is breast-fed. Ordinarily supplementary calcium is unnecessary, and it is not known whether prenatal fluoride will reduce the future incidence of dental caries in the child. The pregnant woman requires additional calories, and restriction of caloric intake as well as the routine use of diuretics can be dangerous. The average woman should gain 22 to 27 pounds during the course of her pregnancy.[21]

Infancy

The infant has certain nutritional requirements and dietary problems peculiar to early age. Many factors are involved, including the infant's lack of teeth, limited digestive powers, spectacular rate of growth, and need to acquire a taste for foods of a variety of flavors and textures. The mother also has nutritional needs peculiar to her own recovery from the physiologic strain of pregnancy and to the production of adequate breast milk for the feeding of her infant. The advantages of breast feeding are substantial.[22] The practice declined for several decades in the United States partly as a matter of fashion and partly because many women associated breast feeding with a less desirable social environment. That has changed since 1960 as public health workers, nutritionists, and physicians became more aware of the benefits of breast feeding and as attitudes towards breast feeding changed once more. Even so, only about 35% of mothers breast-fed their infants in 1975, and most stopped after 3 months.[23] Breast feeding became a matter of social advocacy in the 1970s as the American Public Health Association and other groups put pressure on manufacturers of processed infant food to modify their advertising to emphasize the importance of breast feeding. One of the unfortunate changes that occurred was the more aggressive marketing of the products to developing countries where they have compounded an already serious pattern of malnutrition.

In 1964 federal funds were made available to local and state groups for comprehensive maternity and infant care projects. By 1981, Maternity and Infant Care projects provided needed services, including nutrition services, to approximately 450,000 mothers and 300,000 infants.[23] The WIC program began with an appropriation of $40 million in 1974. Funded at a level of $934 million in 1982, the program served about 2 million pregnant women, mothers, and children but, along with most other human service programs, was under attack by a budget-cutting administration and Congress. This program differs from other public nutrition programs in that is is distinctively public health in its ideology. Food is treated as a prescription item following a professional evaluation of the pregnant or lactating woman or infant. The rules refer specifically to a "competent professional authority," which in practice means a physician, a nutritionist, or a nurse. If determined to be at nutritional risk because of inadequate nutrition and income, the woman or infant is provided specified amounts of certain foods: iron-fortified infant formula, iron-fortified cereal, fruits or vegetables high in vitamin C, fortified milk, cheese and eggs.[24] Unlike many other federal programs, nutrition education is an integral part of the WIC program and, as mentioned, the types of food included are specified. Although it might be pleasant for public health workers to contemplate congressional satisfaction with the WIC program as contrasted with the acrimony that persists concerning the programs oriented to the public welfare ideology, the differences may be based in the emotional responses to the two ideologies (one more authoritarian and the other more liberal) rather than an appraisal of the relative merits of the two approaches.

School nutrition

The school health program is perhaps the activity to which nutrition is next most closely allied. The relationship is threefold: (1) the attempt to assure adequate nutrition, (2) the imparting of good nutrition information, and (3) growing out of integration of the first two, the development of desirable nutrition habits.

Nutrition education should be a basic part of school studies for all socioeconomic groups, from kindergarten through the primary, secondary, and college levels. Major obstacles to the inclusion of more nutrition education in school curricula appear to be a combination of a lack of understanding of educational concepts on the part of nutrition specialists and a lack of workable information about nutrition on the part of the teachers. In the past, teachers' colleges have not provided their students with an adequate background in health, and nutrition has been particularly neglected. Consequently graduate in-service nutrition education is now being provided in many states. The training is offered by one or several agencies or institutions that employ personnel who are experienced in both the field of education and the field of nutrition. Included are county, city, and state health departments; colleges and universities, particularly those engaged in training home economics teachers; the American National Red Cross; and government agencies such as the Agricultural Extension Service.

Programs in nutrition education are now receiving increased attention, and both commercial and academic groups as well as official agencies have developed and made available helpful guides planned on graded levels. The use of tools appropriate to the age and interest of each grade level is an absolute necessity in this field, as in all health fields. In the primary grades the emphasis is best placed on food itself, that is, how it grows, how it tastes, and so on. In the upper elementary grades simplified technical information should be presented, such as the need of particular foods for growth. In secondary schools a more scientific approach will hold the student's interest, if earlier nutrition education has provided the information necessary for this more mature approach.

As has been mentioned, nutrition education that can accompany a well-managed school lunch or breakfast program holds great potentialities—potentialities that unfortunately are often ignored. Schools that feed but do not teach fall short of one of the aims of providing breakfast or lunch at school. Through the school feeding programs, children have an opportunity to become acquainted with foods not familiar to them and simultaneously to learn good patterns of eating by practicing them throughout their school years.

The school lunch program began in 1946 and remained fairly small until President Nixon pledged his support for the expansion of the program during the White House Conference on Food, Nutrition, and Health in 1969. By 1981, 23 million children were participants in the school lunch program, which had a total cost of about $3 billion. The program is unique in that its income requirements are high enough to permit almost all children to participate, making the federally guided program a major vehicle for improved nutrition. Only about half of the participants were categorized as "poor." Since the program subsidizes meals, it enables more families to use the school food service program, which in turn makes it possible for a school to maintain the program. During the budget-cutting frenzy of 1981 and 1982, most related programs were reduced, but the more pervasive use of the school lunch program meant that budget cuts were opposed by middle class families as well as the poor. This caused the President to focus budget cuts more exclusively on the low-income programs, giving credence to the assertion that he discriminated against the poor.

Although school nutrition programs are aimed at the problems of child development (intellectual, physical, social, and emotional), evaluation of the efforts to date have not produced significant evidence of improvement. Pollitt and associates[25] reviewed six studies of the short-term effects of the school breakfast program and found some suggestion of an improvement in very general terms, but they found all of the studies to be poor in design. These authors reviewed seven studies of the longer-term effects of school feeding programs and found only two that showed a beneficial effect. Again, the studies were poorly designed. Podell and associates[26] found that high school students reported a favorable change in knowledge and behavior after completing schoolwork on the relationship of diet to cardiovascular disease but reported that blood cholesterol value increases 1 year later were the same in the study group as in the control group. The experimental program described by Coates and others[18] suggests that a well-coordinated effort to integrate teaching programs with lunch activities and a general "ecologic" approach to good nutrition can have a significant impact. The evidence is neither overwhelming nor irrefutable. The flaws in each study design were such as to blunt the sharpness of any differences found between "treated" and "untreated" children. Given that most of the evidence is either positive or neutral, and that none of its suggests that good nutrition is bad for children, the programs warrant vigorous support and continuation.

Handicapped children

Children with special health problems, such as physical, mental, or economic handicaps, also need the services of a nutritionist. Mentally handicapped children are increasing in number and require special help in meeting their dietary needs. Nutritional factors are directly involved in retardation in conditions caused by inborn errors of metabolism, such as phenylketonuria and galactosemia. Severe brain damage will occur if these conditions are not detected early and medical and specific dietary treatment provided. Other cause-and-effect relationships linking nutritional problems to developmental disabilities will undoubtedly be found as research continues. The possibility that many of the children and adults presumably hopelessly disabled and housed permanently in public or private institutions may be there as a result of nutritional disorders, whether genetically or environmentally caused, should never be discounted.

Welfare departments and juvenile courts, migrant worker programs, and child care facilities all can use consultant services of nutritionists or dietitians, who need to be perceptive to programs that can incorporate their services and flexible enough to meet the variety of needs in children and youth programs to which they can offer valuable consultative service.

The aging population

Inadequate nutrition is one of the greatest concerns in an aging and an aged population. In many respects the former group is of more importance that the latter because there are many more people growing old than there are those already infirm by virtue of age. Far more can be accomplished for those who are still in the aging process than for those already advanced in years. Furthermore, the circumstances of middle life determine in large part whether the subsequent advanced years will be healthy or infirm. Arteriosclerosis, hypertension, arthritis, diabetes mellitus, degenerative conditions of the kidneys and liver, cancer, and various other disorders increasingly are becoming dominant challenges to the health professions. These are all conditions of as yet somewhat uncertain etiology. However, it is known that life-style has much to do with the development of all of them, and considerable research indicates a direct or indirect relationship with nutrition.

Certain facts about the older population should be borne in mind. In general, they tend to use fewer calories because of reduced physical activity.

The period of tissue and organ development is
largely past, and certain changes in food habits
have been enforced by virtue of impaired dental
function, elimination difficulties, various physiologic changes, boredom, or economic limitations.

The most common nutritional problem in the
United States is obesity. Obesity is defined as an
excess of body fat, whereas the term "overweight"
means an excess of pounds in relation to height.
Obesity is difficult to define in quantitative terms.
The prevalence of overweight (deviating by 20% or
more from desirable weight) increases with age in
women but not in men. Overall, about 14% of
American men and 20% of women are overweight.[27]
The problem is more common among the poor and
among black women. The causes are complex and
not fully understood, but they boil down to an excess of calorie consumption in comparison to the
number of calories burned up by physical activity.

Upper socioeconomic groups have made headway caused largely by unplanned and unorganized
social forces that focus on general well-being or,
sometimes, vanity. Public health workers need to
identify those forces and play on their impact, seeking ways to bring the same forces or others to bear
on lower socioeconomic groups as well. Studies
have consistently shown a higher death rate among
the overweight. Breslow and Enstrom[28] have shown
a positive relationship between weight control and
survival, and there is a positive correlation between
what are called good "health practice scores" and
education.[29]

In contrast with obesity in the middle and advanced years is the problem of underweight and
excessive leanness caused by caloric restriction.
The reasons may be impaired dental function, allergic difficulties, economics, disinterest in eating
because of living alone, or emotional reasons such
as anorexia nervosa. Significant underweight may
lower resistance to tuberculosis and various other
infections, and it may also cause serious disability
from ocular, vasomotor, endocrine, and skeletal
changes. In addition, there is the risk of mild to
full-blown avitaminoses. These in turn may aggravate further the underlying causes by bringing
about additional oral or psychic conditions.

Interest of Congress in the nutritional aspects of
aging is reflected in the Medicare amendments to
the Social Security Act. Written into the Conditions
of Participation for Extended Care Facilities are requirements for the dietary supervision and adequacy of meals. The Home Health Care section has
given the professional worker an obvious responsibility for the acute and chronic nutritional status
of the aged. Another important step has been the
inclusion in the Older American's Act of a program
to provide one hot meal each day to the elderly poor.
It became operational during 1972 and during its
first year served 212,000 people daily. By fiscal year
1977 approximately 338,000 meals were being
served each day at a cost of $204 million per year.
It was estimated that about 2.8 million elderly people received some of their meals from one of the
9,100 projects. Fifteen percent of those meals were
home delivered. In addition to the obvious nutritional advantage offered many low-income elderly
people, the programs provide a substantial opportunity for social interaction, which has an important
role to play in the health of the elderly. This is a
population particularly vulnerable to the hazards of
malnutrition since decreased mobility, income, and
ability to prepare meals as well as boredom, isolation, and dental problems may combine to produce
serious nutritional deprivation.

ORGANIZATION AND FUNCTIONS OF STATE NUTRITION PROGRAMS

The first states to employ nutritionists were Massachusetts and New York in 1917. The Sheppard-
Towner Act in 1921 supported the establishment
of state maternal and child health programs, and
nutrition services spread. The Social Security Act
of 1935 expanded federal support and established
guidelines for professional nutrition personnel. By
1980, 51 of the 57 reporting state and territorial
health agencies claimed that they had nutrition programs serving 3.37 million clients.[30] Most of this
was because of maternal and child health and WIC
activities. Work force estimates suggest that approximately 1,000 nutritionists or dietitians are
working at the state level and an equal number are
working in local health agencies, voluntary organizations, or local and regional WIC programs. At
the state level, 150 are performing administrative
and consultative activities, 55 are involved in facility licensure and certification programs, and the
other 850 are in direct service programs.[31]

"Public health nutritionists utilize a community
diagnostic approach in assessing needs of the general public and in applying the scientific knowledge
of nutrition to planning, implementing, and eval-

uating public health services."[31] Although licensure requirements are not yet in vogue (the profession seeks licensure to become eligible for fee-for-service reimbursement), most job descriptions require a master's degree. The roles and status of nutritionists and dietitians were controversial for years, but the two groups now appear to work cooperatively in the interest of pursuing common goals. There are no practically useful distinctions between a public health nutritionist and a community dietitian at this time. In some states nutrition has been organized as a separate division or as a staff agency responsible to the health department director. In others it has been placed in divisions of medical services, public health nursing, or local health services. Most commonly it has been allocated to the bureau or division of maternal and child health.

The major roles of a state-level nutrition program are to carryout nutritional surveillance; to develop standards for public nutrition programs, including Head Start, public schools, and similar activities; to provide consultation to local health agencies and other state agencies; and to carry out applied research in community nutrition. The ideal qualifications of the director of nutrition would include a medical education with special clinical experience in nutritional diseases, a basic background in biochemistry, and training and experience in public health. Such professionals are rare. The most important qualifications are the nutrition and public health backgrounds, which will enable the director of nutrition to give the necessary guidance and to integrate the program into the other activities of the health department.

The special 10-state nutrition survey carried out by the Public Health Service in 1968-1970[32] has been continued as a part of the Cooperative Health Statistics System known as the Health and Nutrition Examination Survey (HANES).[33,34] The data available, plus the data that can be obtained through WIC programs, through Maternal and Infant Care and other maternal and child health programs, and from the state agencies on aging should provide most state health departments with the ability to assess the special problems and needs of their states and the subgroups and areas within the state. Various techniques for incorporating nutritional assessment into health programs were described in a special supplement to the *American Journal of Public Health* in November 1973.[35] Continuing information is provided by the special bulletin *Nutrition Surveillance*, which is published by the Centers for Disease Control.[36]

LOCAL NUTRITION PROGRAMS

At the local level, the principal roles of nutritionists are assessment of dietary practices in the community and in subgroups of the community; nutrition education and counseling for selected groups such as pregnant women, mothers, and infants; the provision of referral services to needed food service programs; and the provision or securing of special equipment and food supplements. In an effort to further define the role of nutritionists in local health agencies, the California Conference of Local Health Department Nutritionists (a group related to the California Conference of Local Health Officers) developed *Guidelines for Nutrition Services in Local Health Jurisdictions*.[37] The standards cover nutrition in chronic disease control, children and youth programs, dental health services, environmental health programs (food and restaurant inspections), family planning, maternal and child health programs, communicable disease control, nursing, disaster relief, detention facilities, and laboratory services. Members of the Conference, with the support of the state nutrition staff, have formulated the following goal: "Local health jurisdictions will provide and/or assure community nutrition programming and articulated nutrition care services sufficient to meet the needs of the jurisdiction and administered by a designated and qualified person." The standards provide a comprehensive look at opportunities and also provide some insights into the ways in which professional groups define problems and solutions in terms of their own training and aspirations.

Planning community nutrition services is essential given the numerous needs and the scant resources in the official agency. Problem and program priorities must be established, otherwise nutritionists may find themselves spending all their time giving talks and providing one-on-one consultation with little impact on the community as a whole or any of its subgroups. There are many data sources available. Although nutrition surveillance can be highly sophisticated and expensive, Christakis[35] lists some of the kinds of data that may be available in one form or another in most communities to help a well-trained nutritionist formulate priorities: de-

The control and prevention of
disease

mographic information from the census, public utility companies and regional planning bodies; information about socioeconomic status developed by human service organizations; health statistics gathered by Health Systems Agencies and their predescessors between 1966 and 1981; information about cultural patterns from interested community organizations and local colleges; housing conditions from the housing agency; information about food supplies and costs from personal surveys; information about school nutrition programs from the office of the superintendent of schools; welfare data from the welfare agency; and information about transportation (particularly to and from low-income neighborhoods) and occupational patterns from regional planning and transit bodies.

There are many resources available to the nutritionist in most communities. It is a common mistake to look only at the one or two positions available in the local health department itself. Many local hospitals now encourage their dietary staff to become actively involved in community nutrition education and service efforts. Day care programs often have consultant nutritionists, as do Head Start Programs, local schools, and economic opportunity programs. The Extension Service in each state, supported by the federal and state Departments of Agriculture, has had a long-standing interest in nutrition. Local colleges and universities often have faculty and staff who are involved in nutrition. Federally funded migrant health centers and community health centers frequently have nutrition services available, and some churches and alcohol guidance centers have developed nutrition programs. (See Frankle and Owen[38] and Owen[39] for more complete information about the organization and management of community nutrition programs.)

Much of the function of the health department is that of a coordinator and catalyst for existing community resources. It is particularly important that programs that involve the actual distribution of food, or vouchers or certificates for food, be coupled with personal and group educational efforts. At one time the distribution of food was thought of as a function of a welfare program, and health departments were limited in their thinking and in their roles to that involving education and consultation. As noted before, health departments are in-

creasingly involved in the direct management of feeding programs and food distribution activities, and the linkage of supply to education must be established. Every effort should be made to work with other community agencies that have similar responsibilities, especially the public welfare office and those professionals who determine food stamp eligibility. Consultative service should be offered by well-qualified nutritionists to the various persons and agencies mentioned, the end in view being to demonstrate how nutrition education can be injected into daily routine without adding appreciably to the daily burden.

These phases of the work should be under the immediate supervision of a well-trained and experienced nutritionist with a knowledge of the area and its governmental and voluntary agencies. In the case of a state program, the state should be divided into regions. It is suggested that at first activities be restricted to counties or communities will full-time public health services, since their existence will facilitate public acquaintance and acceptance of the work of the nutritionist. The length of time to be spent in each local area, the frequency of visits, and the particular type of activity and approach should be worked out on the basis of cumulative experience in the locality by the regional nutritionist. At all times the nutritionist should keep in mind that efforts to render direct service to the public will reach only a few and that a real contribution is to promote the use of local talent and facilities for nutritional betterment by timely suggestions, correlation, and cooperation.

With the rapid expansion of the services of public health nutritionists, there is a critical need to evaluate the services they render and determine what services could be delegated to other personnel. The 6 or 7 years of training required is barely enough to provide all the many experiences needed to face the complex nutritional problems in urban and rural society in an age of advancing technology. The University of California has developed a 5-year program that produces graduates with a master's degree, an American Dietetics Association–approved internship, and some experience in public health. Various countries have developed other approaches suitable to their situations. Japan, for example, meets its personnel needs by graduating 2-year nutrition technologists. Just as the hospital dietitian has promoted the use of food service supervisors, so must the public health nutritionist look for ways of extending services through lesser trained workers. Underdeveloped nations have selected village workers, trained them for 1 year, and returned them to their homes to teach health and nutrition to their peers. Might not this principle be used to teach people in the ghetto areas of American cities, to saturate the neighborhoods with adequate nutrition information on food buying and budgeting, and to provide enough sound nutrition information so that people would not become vulnerable to fallacious practices and beliefs?

LEGISLATION AND THE NEED FOR FOOD AND NUTRITION POLICY

It is possible for a community, a state, or a nation to attack nutritional problems at their source, that is, the place of production or distribution of a product. Perhaps the earliest example of this was the addition of iodine in the form of sodium or potassium iodide to public water supplies, chocolate, and, more practically, to table salt.

On January 18, 1943, a government order known as War Food Order No. 1 went into effect in the United States. This order required that all white bread be enriched to meet the requirements of the order in thiamin, niacin, riboflavin, and iron. It remained in effect until October 18, 1946. Since then, a number of states have passed legislation for the continuance of a policy of enrichment of all white flour and bread within their borders.

In 1976 the West Virginia State Board of Education took the audacious step of banning the sale of all "junk foods" in vending machines in school buildings. Although various commercial groups have tried to weaken that ban it has remained in effect and is a clear example of the articulation of policy with practice. Many organizations have supported compulsory labeling to reveal nutrition information, but, as noted earlier, this has been successfully opposed by the industry so far, although some manufacturers have developed their own programs. During the Reagan administration the emphasis on deregulating rather than regulating will probably further postpone useful labeling practices.

Understanding food labeling is difficult because so many nutrients interact with each other in ways that make the process of simplifying daily needs and requirements complex. But it is no more complex than many other aspects of modern life that we are called on to handle. It may be possible to produce meat, dairy, and egg products with lower and more unsaturated fat content through altered animal breeding and feeding practices. To do so,

however, may take legislation both to finance the necessary research and perhaps to require that the changes be made, and it may be extremely difficult to effect such legislation in the United States.

Winikoff[40] has written a thoughtful comparison of attempts to develop a policy on food and nutrition in Norway and in the United States. The Norwegian government has produced a white paper that combines goals (which are very similar to those developed by the U.S. Senate Select Committee on Nutrition and Human Needs[41]) with a national policy on attainment. Implementation of the policies will involve interference with agricultural practices, manufacturing, processing, distribution, and even the purchase and use of foods. The goals and policies were developed by the Ministry of Agriculture and have the support of the government. By contrast, goals for the United States were developed by a Senate committee and never ratified by Congress or adopted by the President. The Senate Select Committee's goals are excellent. They call for reducing our fat intake from 42% of our total calories to 30%, for increasing carbohydrate intake from the present level of 46% of total calories to 58% with the complex carbohydrates increasing to 40% of the total and sugar declining to 15%, and for a concomitant reduction in cholesterol and salt intake. The balance of calories, 12%, should continue to come from protein. These goals were supported by the American Public Health Association in 1977,[42] but not by Congress, the President, the U.S. Department of Health, Education, and Welfare, or the U.S. Department of Agriculture. There is a deep-seated fear of the use of law to try to influence consumption practices in the United States. Actually, it may be more of a notion that is turned into a fear by the unflagging efforts of the food industry in much the same way that other special interest groups have been able to turn certain notions into catch phrases to effectively prevent the nation from considering an enlightened and progressive policy. The fact that special interest groups have been able to use legislation to influence purchasing and consumption habits goes unnoticed. Medicare and Medicaid restrictions on who can participate in the programs and how, federal subsidies for tobacco growers, and special interest group legislation dealing with virtually every edible product make it obvious that the power of law is

often used to influence behavior and restrict freedom on a broad scale. The use of these same procedures to create and implement a healthful policy
for food and nutrition must apparently await another time and other leaders.

REFERENCES

1. Ule, O.: Food and the development of man (translated
   from the German by J. Fitzgerald, from Die Natur,
   1851), Pop. Sci. Month. **5:**591, 1874.
2. Magee, H.E.: Application of nutrition to public
   health, some lessons from the war, Br. Med. J. **1:**475,
   March 1946.
3. Jelliffe, D.B.: The assessment of the nutritional status
   of the community, WHO Monogr. Ser. No. 53, Geneva, 1966, World Health Organization.
4. Third World Food Survey, FFHC Basic Study No. 11,
   Rome, 1963, Food and Agriculture Organization.
5. Scrimshaw, N.S., and Gordon, J.E., editors: Malnutrition, learning and behavior, Cambridge, 1968, Massachusetts Institute of Technology.
6. Birch, H.G.: Malnutrition, learning and intelligence,
   Am. J. Public Health **62:**773, June 1972.
7. Wolstenholm, G., and O'Connor, M., editors: Health
   of mankind, Boston, 1967, Little, Brown & Co.
8. Scrimshaw, N.S.: Through a glass darkly: discerning
   the practical implications of human dietary protein–
   energy relationships, Nutr. Rev. **35:**321, Dec. 1977.
9. President's Science Advisory Commission: The World
   food problem. Report of panel on the world food supply, Washington, D.C., 1967, U.S. Government Printing Office.
10. Merrill, M.H.: Meeting the challenges of the coming
    decades—the role of medicine in nutrition. Talk given
    at the Western Hemisphere Nutrition Conference,
    Chicago, Nov. 1965.
11. Bureau of the Census: Statistical abstracts of the
    United States, 1981, Tables 208, 209, Washington,
    D.C., 1981, U.S. Department of Commerce.
12. Committee on Dietary Allowances, Food and Nutri-
    tion Board: Recommended dietary allowances, ed. 9
    (revised), Washington, D.C., 1980, National Academy
    of Sciences.
13. Hegsted, D.M.: On dietary standards, Nutr. Rev.
    36:33, Feb. 1978.
14. Schorr, A.L.: Poor kids, New York, 1966, Basic Books,
    Inc.
15. Currents in public health, vol. 5, No. 2, Ross Labo-
    ratories, Feb. 1965.
16. Hunger U.S.A.; a report of the Citizen's Board of
    Inquiry into Hunger and Malnutrition in the United
    States, Washington, D.C., 1968, New Community
    Press.
17. Todhunter, E.N.: Child feeding problems and the
    school lunch program, J. Am. Diet. Assoc. **24:**422,
    May 1948.
18. Coates, T.J., Jeffrey, R.W., and Slinkard, L.A.: Heart,
    healthy eating, and exercise: introducing and main-
    taining changes in health and behavior, Am. J. Public
    Health **71**(1):15, Jan. 1981.
19. Glanz, K., and Morris, N.M.: Cafeteria nutrition ed-
    ucation for university students: an evaluation study,
    Paper presented to the School Health Section, Amer-
    ican Public Health Association, annual meeting, Los
    Angeles, November 1981.
20. Endozien, J.C., Switzer, B.R., and Bryan, R.B.: Med-
    ical evaluation of the special supplemental food pro-
    gram for women, infants, and children, Am. J. Clin.
    Nutr. **32:**677, Mar. 1979.
21. Committee on Maternal Nutrition, Food and Nutri-
    tion Board, National Research Council: Maternal nu-
    trition and the course of pregnancy, Washington,
    D.C., 1970, National Academy of Sciences.
22. Nutrition Committee of the Canadian Pediatric So-
    ciety and the Committee on Nutrition of the American
    Academy of Pediatrics: Breast feeding: a commentary
    in celebration of the International Year of the Child,
    1979, Pedes. **62:**591, Oct. 1978.
23. Select Panel for the Promotion of Child Health: Better
    health for our children: a national strategy, The Re-
    port of the Select Panel for the Promotion of Child
    Health, vol. 1., U.S. Department of Health and Hu-
    man Services, Pub. No. (PHS)79-55071, Washington,
    D.C., 1981.
24. Egan, M.C.: Federal nutrition support programs for
    children, Pediatr. Clin. North Am. **24:**229, Feb. 1977.
25. Pollitt, E., Gersovitz, M., and Gargiulo, M.: Educa-
    tional benefits of the United States school feeding
    program: a critical review of the literature, Am. J.
    Public Health **68:**477, May 1978.
26. Podell, R.N., and others: Evaluation of the effective-
    ness of a high school course in cardiovascular nutri-
    tion, Am. J. Public Health **68:**573, June 1978.
27. Bray, G.A., editor: Obesity in America, U.S. Depart-
    ment of Health, Education, and Welfare Pub. No.
    (NIH) 79-359, Bethesda, Md., Nov. 1979.
28. Breslow, L., and Enstrom, J.E.: Persistance of health
    habits and their relationship to mortality, Prev. Med.
    9:469, 1980.
29. Office of Health Research, Statistics, and Technolo-
    gy: Health, United States—1981, U.S. Department
    of Health and Human Services Pub. No. (PHS)82-
    1232, Hyattsville, Md., Dec. 1981.
30. National Public Health Program Reporting System:
    Public health agencies, 1980, Washington, D.C., Au-
    gust 1981, Association of State and Territorial Health
    Officials.
31. Bureau of Health Professions: Public health person-
    nel in the United States, 1980, U.S. Department of
    Health and Human Services Pub. No. (HRA)82-6,
    Jan. 1982.

32. Highlights: ten-state nutrition survey, 1968-1969, U.S. Department of Health, Education, and Welfare Pub. No. (HSM)72-8134, Washington, D.C., 1972.

33. U.S. Public Health Service: Forward plan for health, 1978-1982, Washington, D.C., 1976.

34. National Center for Health Statistics: Caloric and selected nutrient values for persons 1-74 years of age: first health and nutrition examination survey, United States, 1971-1974, U.S. Department of Health, Education, and Welfare Pub. No. (PHS)79-1657, Hyattsville, Md., June 1979.

35. Christakis, G., editor: Nutritional assessment in health programs, Am. J. Public Health **63**(suppl.), Nov. 1973.

36. Centers for Disease Control: Nutrition surveillance, U.S. Department of Health and Human Services (periodical).

37. California Conference of Local Health Department Nutritionists: Guidelines for nutrition services in local health jurisdictions, June 1980, Sacramento, Calif., Sept. 1981, Health and Welfare Agency.

38. Frankle, R.T., and Owen, A.Y.: Nutrition in the community: the art of delivering services, St. Louis, 1978, The C.V. Mosby Co.

39. Owen, A.Y.: Community nutrition in preventive health care services: a critical review of the literature, U.S. Department of Health, Education, and Welfare Pub. No. (HRA)78-14017, Washington, D.C., 1978.

40. Winikoff, B.: Nutrition and food policy: the approaches of Norway and the United States, Am. J. Public Health **67**:552, June 1977.

41. Report of the U.S. Senate Select Committee on Nutrition and Human Needs: Dietary goals for the United States, Pub. No. 052-070-03913-2, Washington, D.C., 1977, U.S. Government Printing Office.

42. Adoption of national dietary goals, Am. J. Public Health **68**:200, Feb. 1978.

CHAPTER 18

Health education and health maintenance

If you are planning for a year ahead, sow rice;
for ten years, plant trees;
for a hundred years, educate people.

Chinese proverb

THE GROWTH OF HEALTH EDUCATION

That remarkable universal man of American history, Thomas Jefferson, once observed, "Health is no more than learning." In considering the important subject of health education, the following statement written over a century ago is pertinent:

The time has gone by when people can be dragooned into cleanliness, or be made virtuous by police regulations, and hence it is that the most thoughtful among practical reformers of the present day base their hopes of sanitary progress on the education of the masses as the real groundwork of national health. The people must be taught that good conduct, personal cleanliness, and the avoidance of all excesses, are the first principles of health, hand-in-hand in the rearing and guidance of youth. . . . They must be interested systematically in the general results of sanitary progress, and become more intimately acquainted with the social and material causes by which it is impeded.[1]

This quotation from the first report of the Maryland State Board of Health, dated 1875, emphasized that the public's health is dependent on the public's convictions about health.

Health education in some form has always been an important activity of public health personnel. It was not until the second quarter of this century, however, that it became formally recognized as a specialty and as a major function in public health. The transition has been gradual. In the earlier eras of public health that focused on the sanitation of the environment and the control of communicable disease, public health activity was interpreted to consist of doing things *to* and *for* people, with great reliance on legislative and police power. With the development of the newer interpretation of public health as the summation of personal health, there developed an appreciation of the need to do things *with* people and to get people to accept an increasing responsibility for their own health.

Health education in the United States may be considered to have begun with the establishment in 1914 of the first Bureau of Health Education in the New York City Health Department. Soon after, the New York State Health Department and the Detroit Department of Health also formed designated organizational units. The field received its specialty name, health education, at a conference called in 1919 by the Child Health Organization of America, which also offered the first fellowship in health education the following year. It is interesting to note that this organization was formed by a pediatrician, L. Emmett Holt, and a nurse, Sally Lucas Jean, both of whom were convinced that emphasis on child health promotion through education and nutrition would accomplish much more than dogged, never-ending diagnosis and treatment of existing ills.[2] By 1922 there were sufficient numbers of people working in the field to merit the establishment of a separate specialty section in the American Public Health Association. Meanwhile, health education was recognized academically with the development of a specialized graduate curriculum by Clair E. Turner at the Massachusetts Institute of Technology.

During the ensuing period enthusiastic hopes were held for what health education might accomplish through targeted attacks on specific health problems such as infant mortality, diphtheria, and tuberculosis. Health education of that period has been described by Hochbaum[3] as

guided principally by the notions that its main goals were the prevention of certain categorical diseases, . . . the achievement of these goals depended on efforts to get people to carry out certain actions, . . . their failure to carry these out were due primarily if not totally to ignorance, and . . . therefore the mission of health education was first and foremost to remove such ignorance. Once done, it was assumed, the desired actions would be taken as a matter of course.

But, of course, the results did not meet these expectations; regression set in, and at the time the United States became involved in World War II, a mere 13 state and local health departments reported employment of health educators—44 persons in all. Wartime needs spurred renewed action, and special curricula were established in several of the accredited schools of public health. Several leaders in the field had been emphasizing the importance of community organization and the use of groups from the community itself in the health education and action process. This then became the principal method and function in health education.

The rapidity of response to the need and the acceptance of the approach influenced by the wartime effort were indicated by the fact that by 1947 over 300 persons, all of whom had completed graduate courses in recognized schools of public health, were employed as health educators in official and voluntary health agencies. Concurrent was an important change in attitude on the part of health officers and other more traditional health workers from one of skepticism and suspicion to welcome and professional acceptance.

This trend has continued, and although firm information is lacking, it has been estimated that about 25,000 individuals are currently employed in some aspect of health education in the United States.[4] However, this high figure appears to be based on some type of organization affiliation rather than on acceptable training and qualifications. More dependable but still inexact are the estimates that take into consideration training at the master's level in accredited institutions.[5] The lack of dependable worker data points to one of the most serious problems in the health education profession—self-engendered confusion. In 1979 the Bureau of Health Education of the Centers for Disease Control identified 252 training programs. In addition to curricula offered by some of the graduate schools of public health, health educators were enrolled elsewhere in 108 bachelor's, 83 master's and 31 doctoral level programs. These programs and degrees were offered by schools and colleges of education, health science, physical education and recreation, and other components of institutions of higher learning. Many of their graduates are employed as teachers in elementary and secondary schools, although a significant number work in community settings.

The confusion is further evidenced in accreditation and professional organization. The Council on Education for Public Health (CEPH) accredits programs in the schools of public health in addition to six of the graduate programs in other than schools of public health. The National Commission for Accreditation of Teacher Education (NCATE) accredits programs in colleges of education. This leaves an accreditation gap beyond the programs covered by CEPH and NCATE. With reference to professional organizations, health educators have a wide choice for affiliation: the Association for the Advancement of Health Education of the American Alliance for Health, Physical Education, Recreation, and Dance; the American School Health Association; two sections of the American Public Health Association (Public Health Education and School Health Education and Services); and the Society for Public Health Education. On the state level there are the Conference of State and Territorial Directors of Health Education and the State Directors of Health, Physical Education, and Recreation. In 1972 the Coalition of National Health Education Organizations was formed with the hope of finding some common ground. However, neither it nor any other organization can speak for the entire profession.[6] It should also be mentioned that on the global level there exists the quasi-official International Union for Health Education of the Public, which other organizations may join and help support.

SCHOOL AND HEALTH DEPARTMENT RELATIONS

The school represents a most important learning situation for a large and significant group of the population. What is learned as a child tends to have a deep and lasting influence on one's happiness, opinions, and behavior throughout life. A child is reached and influenced primarily through two channels, parents and teachers. Unfortunately the influence of some parents, chiefly because of limitations in their childhood, is not always of the best. In such cases the importance of the teacher in the development of desirable health knowledge and practices is doubly magnified and serves to emphasize the importance of teacher training in health and the maintenance of the personal well-being of those in this important relationship to children.

Today's schools contain all of tomorrow's "public" and affect most of today's. However, the President's Committee on Health Education[4] concluded that in most communities the next generation will be little better equipped to separate the basic facts concerning health and disease from the vast amount of misinformation that troubles the present generation. This emphasizes that not only is school health education a logical adjunct of a comprehensive community health program but should have high priority.

It is unfortunate that a certain amount of misunderstanding and self-defeating competition sometimes develops between public health agencies and departments of education because of their mutual interest in the transmission of health knowledge and behavior to children. No valid cause for conflict exists. In some areas both the health department and the school department reach for the school health education program with attitudes of equal proprietorship. The fact is that each has an important role to play.

The personnel of health departments must always remember that teaching is a professional specialty in itself and that in the final analysis it is the classroom teacher who does the teaching of the children. On the other hand, school personnel should bear in mind that the school health program and its educational component are merely parts of the larger total community health program. This does not necessarily imply a right for the official health department to usurp the activities of the schools in this field any more than this overall responsibility and concern entitles the health department to take over the private practice of medicine or the management of food industries.

The need is obvious. What is indicated is the coordination, in friendly, professional, and cooperative terms, of the contributions and abilities of those interested in health education, whether employed in a health agency, a school system, or elsewhere. The important fact to consider at this point is that the job that needs to be done is great, that neither group alone can accomplish it, and that much remains to be achieved. The conclusion is clear—greater resources, much better joint planning, and truly coordinated action are needed.

THE FOCUS OF HEALTH EDUCATION

The definition of health education has changed through time. One of the earliest was that of Wood,[7] who described it as the "sum of experiences which favorably influence habits, attitudes, and knowledge relating to individual, community, and racial health." As time passed, the philosophy, objectives, and methods of health education underwent significant change. This has been summarized by Rosen[8] as follows:

It has been recognized that it is not enough simply to present information; what counts is whether and how this knowledge is applied. Furthermore, it has been realized that the community is an organized structure, and that in health education, as in other health work, a coordinated program is needed which will touch each segment of the community in accordance with its nature and its needs. Finally, it is accepted in principle that when the members of a community have a chance to learn about their health problems and how they might deal with them, they will do so, but this was obscured during the early decades of the century by an excessive emphasis on tools and techniques.

More recently, another dimension has been added to the health education movement. Increasingly its members recognized that it was not enough to present fears or facts, and it was not enough to organize communities and groups for action. Something beyond this was needed—an understanding of how individuals, groups, and cultures viewed and interpreted conditions and events and, on the basis of this, how they might be motivated to apply, adapt, or even alter their views and interpretations for their own welfare. As a result, the current emphasis is on the role of the health educator as an agent of social change through the application of behavioral science.

All recent definitions emphasize the importance of methods to effect behavioral change. The most appropriate current definition of health education is the following, agreed on by the Society for Public

Health Education and the American Public Health
Association[9]:

a process with intellectual, psychological and social dimensions relating to activities which increase the abilities
of people to make informed decisions affecting their personal, family and community well being. This process
based on scientific principles facilitates learning and behavioral change in both health personnel and consumers
including children and youth.

To supplement this, the National Conference on
Preventive Medicine in 1975 developed a "working"
definition that is of practical value.[10] It said:

The term "consumer health education" subsumes a set
of activities which:
(1) inform people about health, illness, disability, and
    ways in which they can improve and protect their
    own health, including more efficient use of the
    delivery system;
(2) motivate people to want to change to more health-
    ful practices;
(3) help them to learn the necessary skills to adopt and
    maintain healthful practices and life-styles;
(4) foster teaching and communication skills in all
    those engaged in educating consumers about
    health;
(5) advocate changes in the environment that facilitate
    healthful conditions and healthful behavior; and
(6) add to knowledge via research and evaluation con-
    cerning the most effective ways of achieving the
    above objectives.

These sequential changes in the evolution of
health education are reflected in the various revisions of the statement on the educational qualifications of health educators first enunciated in
the 1920s. As summarized by Bowman,[11] the
"behavioral emphasis has supplanted for the most
part community organization and dissemination of
health emphases in health education. But it is interesting to note the continued attention given (1)
to community organization as a method for effect-
ing change . . . and (2) to the communication of
health knowledge and instructional technology."

FUNCTIONS IN HEALTH EDUCATION

In 1937 the American Public Health Association
began an attempt to set down the diverse functions
and activities of health educators. Many studies,
adaptations, and revisions have followed. In 1960
responsibility for statements of qualifications and
functions of health educators was passed to the
Society for Public Health Education. In its 1967
statement it attempted for the first time to differentiate the functions of community health educators with different degree levels of preparation—
baccalaureate and master's. The resultant document[12] also contains a section on the areas of knowledge, concepts, and skills that community health
educators on the two levels should have. The section on functions is presented here (Table 18-1) as
indicative of the variety of activities in which health
educators may engage. It should be kept in mind,
however, that these vary among types and levels of
agencies as well as through time.

THE SETTINGS OF HEALTH EDUCATION

Needs for health education are ubiquitous. Every
stage of life, every type of person or social group,
and all occupations and professions are appropriate
targets of programs for the prevention of illness and
disability, the control of disease, and the promotion
of wellness. Since the need is omnipresent, health
education must be provided in a wide variety of
settings that ideally blanket a community or soci-

TABLE 18-1. Functions of health educators

General functions	Specific activities for bachelor's degree level	Specific activities for master's degree level
Participate in formulation of agency goals and policies		Identify and analyze the educational implications to be considered in the formulation and modification of the agency's goals Help define the operational policy required to achieve the educational goals of the agency

Modified from Statement of functions of community health educators and minimum requirements for their professional preparation with recommendations for implementation, Society for Public Health Education, March 14, 1967.

Continued.

TABLE 18-1. Functions of health educators—cont'd

General functions	Specific activities for bachelor's degree level	Specific activities for master's degree level
Plan and direct continuous study and analysis of the community in relation to the educational objectives of the agency and the needs and goals of the community	Search out information about a specific problem in relation to knowledge, attitudes, and behavior of individuals, groups, and agencies Identify community resources and leaders for a specific problem, program, or geographic area; make a systematic record of this information	Identify community leadership and describe the distribution of power Maintain current information about the attitudes and behavior of key individuals and groups in relation to education and health Assess health education needs as they relate to various problems and target groups Identify the barriers that impinge on or create health problems, such as traditions, lack of knowledge, and cultural and geographic isolation Communicate with community agencies, representatives of the power structure, indigenous leaders, and others to determine the needs and effectiveness of programs
Provide leadership in development of educational aspects of agency programs	Establish health education objectives for specific activities Design, prepare, and test visual aids, such as flip charts, flannel boards, exhibits, and filmstrips Use appropriate audiovisual equipment, such as motion picture projectors, slide and filmstrip projectors, overhead projectors, and tape recorders	Define educational needs of the programs of the agency and the readiness of the community to act Set educational objectives and include an evaluation plan Plan a course of action to achieve the objectives, including identification of persons who need to act and what they need to do Select and develop needed educational methods, materials, and resources Determine strategic points in the agency's program for effective entry of specific educational activities
Implement the educational component of program plans	Implement health education activities Prepare materials, for example, releases, feature articles, reports, radio and television spot announcements and scripts, leaflets, brochures, and speeches Supervise assisting staff, for example, health education aides, clerical staff, and volunteers Use existing tools in the evaluation of activities	Locate, select, and develop resources needed for the implementation of the program, including personnel, facilities, and materials Organize and conduct training in health education for staff and volunteers on the basis of their contribution to the program Supervise and consult with persons carrying out the educational activities Conduct periodic evaluation of the progress of the program and adjust or modify the educational aspects of the plan accordingly Carry out a comprehensive evaluation of the educational aspects of the program to determine the effectiveness of the methods used and to provide a basis for planning future action: 1. Measure the extent to which educational objectives were achieved 2. Identify the barriers that were and were not overcome 3. Document the total program experience

TABLE 18-1. Functions of health educators—cont'd

General functions	Specific activities for bachelor's degree level	Specific activities for master's degree level
Provide leadership in the development of community-centered health education programs and initiate coordination of the agency's health education efforts with those of other groups and organizations	Work with community leaders and groups in the solution of health problems identified by them Inform community leaders about health problems and programs and encourage their participation in organized neighborhood groups, clubs, and civic organizations	Collect and keep current, data about the programs of other agencies that could be useful in furthering community health education efforts Maintain a current index of information about individual leaders, community groups, and organizations that includes areas of interest, methods of operating, points of conflict, previous involvement in programs, and positions on health and related issues Identify opportunities and ways in which the agency can collaborate effectively with other community agencies and organizations in the development of health education programs Relate the activities planned by the agency to other relevant community groups in such a way as to achieve greater impact on the community and avoid undesirable duplication and competition Serve as a bridge between school and community health education programs and alert health agency personnel to opportunities for using school health services as learning experiences for teachers, students, and parents Participate in school and community programs directed toward recruitment of manpower for service in the health fields Contribute educational knowledge and skills in the development of comprehensive community health planning
Provide leadership in the use of educational concepts, methods, and materials and serve as a resource on health education to the agency staff and the community	Work with other staff on the development of health education activities Assist in the planning of staff meetings and other activities to facilitate communication within the agency and between the agency and the community Involve other staff and community workers in the selection of audiovisual materials and provide instruction in their use Help professional coworkers select and use appropriate educational methods	Keep staff informed of new developments in educational technology and their potential Assist staff in analyzing educational problems and in defining educational goals, target groups, desired behavioral change, and communication methods Determine and recommend appropriate and effective methods and media for achieving the educational goals of the agency Develop and maintain an index of educational resources, personnel, and facilities Maintain a current inventory of sources of financial support for the educational efforts of the agency Keep abreast of relevant report literature and research findings

Continued.

The control and prevention of
disease

TABLE 18-1. Functions of health educators—cont'd

General functions	Specific activities for bachelor's degree level	Specific activities for master's degree level
	Maintain a collection of reference materials on health education and various health topics for use by agency staff and community groups Assist in developing orientation programs for new agency personnel Conduct orientation to health education for coworkers and volunteers	Identify communication patterns in the agency and between the agency and the community; assess their effectiveness and initiate action for their improvement
Design and initiate plans for professional development and training		Organize, plan, and implement the continuing education program for the health education staff Contribute to the professional development of other health personnel: 1. Plan, organize, and conduct continuing education in health education 2. Select educational methods most appropriate for use by others in continuing education and training; evaluate their effectiveness Evaluate these activities and their results
Identify health education problems requiring additional study and research		Identify problems encountered in achieving the educational goals of the agency that may be clarified or solved with the aid of social scientists or other specialists, and initiate a plan of action Pinpoint areas in which there is a need for further research or study as revealed by an analysis of the documented experiences of the agency in carrying out its educational efforts Obtain expert help in the design and conduct of research and studies related to health education problems Participate in the educational aspects of research, studies, and demonstrations in which the agency is involved Translate research and study findings into action directed toward improvement of community health education programs
Manage and direct the short- and long-range development of the agency's health education service		Perform administrative functions related to the operation of the health education service Supervise and direct the agency's health education services Recruit and train health education staff

TABLE 18-1. Functions of health educators—cont'd

General functions	Specific activities for bachelor s degree level	Specific activities for master's degree level
		Obtain and use funds required for training, research, and demonstration
Report and publish		Prepare for publication health education reports of program experiences, demonstrations, and other pertinent writings

ety: homes, schools, community agencies, voluntary and private organizations, governmental agencies, hospitals, professional schools, group practices, planning agencies, communications media, unions, business, and industry.

Preschool and school-aged children and their parents are especially important. This points to the importance of a carefully planned, comprehensive sequential program of health education for all students from kindergarten through secondary school aimed at the development of healthy life-styles and an understanding of the larger community aspects of health protection and promotion. Since parents provide role models in the establishment of good health practices, they should be assisted in fulfilling their role. Beyond this, college students, families, people in the occupationally productive years, and senior citizens also have special health education requirements.[13]

Germane to the selection of targets or settings for health education is the basis on which they are selected. In the instances just mentioned, special attention is justified because the individuals are actually or potentially at risk. Too often, however, as Galanter[14] has pointed out, health education and many other public health programs "focus attention exclusively on the victims of problems rather than on the problems themselves." As examples, she mentions workers exposed to carcinogens told not to smoke so as to reduce the risk, and mothers taught to stop children from eating lead-based paint. "Of course," she notes, "individual behavior influences health—and of course individuals can control some of their behavior. But many other behaviors and the problems with which they interlace are simply beyond the realm of individual action or

can be far more effectively tackled by societal or institutional action." As an example, Spiegel and Lindaman[15] focused attention on a significant but underrated cause of injury and death—falls of small children from high windows. As described in Chapter 19, in New York City such falls account for 12% of all accidental deaths in children under 15 years of age. This incidence in New York City alone, they indicate, is about equal to the annual number of aspirin poisonings nationwide, which has merited federal legislation. Although parental and neighborhood health education efforts are obviously important, more effective would be a housing code requiring window barriers.

With reference to the organizational setting of health education activities, especially in official health agencies, although each functional unit should be engaged in health education to some degree, there are certain overall aspects of the field that must be treated in a more central manner. Questions arise, therefore, concerning whether the work should be completely centralized in one health education unit or dispersed and whether such a unit should be line or staff. Every possible variation is seen in state and local health departments. Centralized health education units are organized sometimes as a separate line unit and sometimes as a staff agency close to the health officer. On the other hand, all activities for health education are often decentralized and dispersed throughout the organization. Beyond these are numerous expedient arrangements with health education placed in a division of vital statistics, of maternal and child health, or of communicable disease control. This has little to recommend it, since it usually results in provincialization of the service.

The control and prevention of
disease

Certain general conclusions may be drawn. It is impossible to centralize health education activities completely. Even if this could be accomplished, the rest of the health agency would lose most of its effectiveness. Therefore the functional units, augmented and supported by a central unit of health education staffed by specialists, should be encouraged to engage freely in these activities. In most circumstances, the central health education unit had best be a staff unit closely associated with the administrator, with whom overall community planning and programming may be effected.

One other aspect of the setting of health education merits emphasis—the relative importance of activities on the different levels of government. With health education, as with other health programs, one is apt to overemphasize the state and especially the federal role. Ogden,[16] speaking from the position of Director of the Federal Bureau of Health Education, has cautioned against this:

In a field like health education—with activities widely diffused within government and still more widely dispersed across the national scene—this foreshortened perspective can leave the false impression that government in general, and the Federal Government in particular, is "where the action is."

The truth, of course, is quite the reverse. Health education of individuals and families happens, or does not happen, where people live, in their home, workplaces, or communities. That is where people learn and practice, or do not learn and do not practice, means for keeping well, raising the quality of their lives, and how to use the services available to them. Government may, and often does, propose. Sometimes its proposals are sweetened by the offer of various forms of support. But local institutions and individual persons dispose. What they do determines whether or not health education fulfills its great potential for improving our national health status.

METHODS IN HEALTH EDUCATION

As the content of health education is difficult to define, so is its methodology. One problem is the variety of interpretations of intent and purpose of the field. Necessarily related to this are the different ways in which health educators are used by directors of health programs and others to whom health educators report and on whom they must depend for guidance and support. Another problem is the variety of knowledge and abilities a competent health educator must have—pedagogy, public

health, public relations, journalism, social science, and visual aids, to mention only some.

The term *health education,* or what might be regarded as the selling of sound health understanding and behavior,* usually gives consideration to at least five phases or types of activities: analysis, sensitization, publicity, education, and motivation. They are in no sense mutually exclusive but tend to be sequential, overlap generously, and be dependent on each other. The first, *analysis,* is, of course, fundamental. It involves a study of the problems of an area or a group, the factors that generated the problems and tend to maintain them, and the characteristics of the individuals or groups that may contribute to or hinder the application of sound knowledge or techniques toward the solution of the problems.

The next phase is *sensitization.* Here the intent or expected result is not an addition to health knowledge per se or an evident change in the health habits of a person or a community; rather, it is a process by which people are made aware of the existence of certain things: a health agency, a behaviorism, a disease, a service. Sensitizing techniques such as slogans, spot announcements on radio or television, and billboards are not expected to give the public more information about a subject or to make them do something they otherwise might not do. Examples are found in commercial advertising, where a manufacturer merely attempts to make potential customers aware of the existence of a product in competition with those of other manufacturers. The manufacturer may accomplish this by bombarding the public's eyes and ears with simple reminders of the product. In doing this, the manufacturer and advertising agent do not expect the public to rush to the nearest store to purchase the product. What is hoped for is that when people are in a situation where they must make a decision, "Shall I buy or not" or "Shall I buy this brand or that?" they will choose the product the name of which is now familiar as a result of the sensitizing process. Therefore when a health agency by any of the audiovisual methods asks, "Is your baby protected against diphtheria?" or states, "Diphtheria kills children," it is merely sensitizing the listeners or readers so that hopefully they will be receptive to subsequent more detailed information.

*The reader is referred to a charming essay, "The Pebble in the Bell," which deals with the application of advertising to health.[17]

One thing is certain—people cannot be sensitized by the term *health education*. It is not well understood by professionals, much less by laymen. The concept must be made meaningful by relating it to readily recognized problems and services that are already known to be practical and useful to the individual or the community.[18]

The third phase of health education is *publicity*. This is closely related to the foregoing and, like it, is of considerable importance in the public relations program of the organization. In one sense, publicity might be considered an elaboration of sensitizing procedures, presenting more details about the items that were mentioned in simple concise statements or exhortations. Examples of activities that might be included in this category are press releases that relate to the program of the health agency, announcements of clinics available for various purposes, and descriptive statements about the seriousness of certain conditions in the community.

The fourth phase of health education is *education* in the more usual sense. Usually this is accomplished in a rather intimate manner with personal contact between the one who imparts the information and those who receive it. It must be realized that education in health or in anything else is never something given by one person to another. The mere act of presenting information and knowledge accomplishes nothing. A gorilla, for example, might be exposed to the constant expostulations of the world's greatest philosophers, but it is doubtful that it would learn anything simply because of its inability to comprehend and interpret the sounds it heard. For many humans, the word *inability* might be changed to *unwillingness*. In other words, learning takes place only through the efforts of the learner. To impart information to increase the knowledge of others or to change concepts, personal discussions carried out in terms and circumstances familiar to the listener and related to the individual's personality and circumstances are required. This approach accounts for the success of certain companies that sell cosmetics and household products. It also explains why home visits by public health nurses are so often fruitful.

The fifth or final phase of health education is concerned with *motivation*. The mere transmission of information or knowledge, even if it is accepted, is not enough, since in itself it does not necessarily imply action or a change in habit or conduct. Among those who die each year from preventable diseases are many who have been exposed to much publicity relating to them and have even acquired considerable knowledge about them. Very few of the parents of children who needlessly acquire and even die from preventable conditions are completely ignorant of protective measures or opposed to them. They simply do not act on the information or knowledge. In other words, the acquisition of knowledge in itself is not an accomplishment; it is the extent to which that knowledge is translated into action that makes the difference. A note of caution is indicated with reference to motivation. It must be used cautiously or it might "backfire." An example was an intensive drug education program in a junior high school that apparently so stimulated curiosity that there resulted a sharp increase in the use of drugs.[19]

Various aspects of motivation are discussed in Chapter 3. It is recognized that for people to be motivated to use health knowledge, it must be presented to them in a manner comprehensible and acceptable to them. Their basic emotional needs and wants; their cultural attitudes, beliefs, and prejudices; their fears, ambitions, jealousies, determinations, pride, and malice; or any combination of these must all be taken into consideration. Rosenstock and colleagues[20] summarized the problem well: "It is known that human behavior is determined more by one's belief about reality than by reality itself, and that people vary markedly in their interpretations of reality." As a consequence, it has been pointed out that effective health education can be achieved only by linking what is taught to the endogenous motivation of the individual or group addressed.

Kost[21] points to the success of the advertising industry, which long ago found that one cannot reach everyone with the same message, so it selects specific audiences and talks in their terms to their interests. In the health field he says that if public health workers have a message for a certain group, they should write and promote the message for that group. If it is a low socioeconomic group with a low level of education, they should couch the message in terms different from those for a middle class, suburban population. The trouble, he adds, is that "those who would be heard also must be willing to listen. In public health, we haven't been listening enough. Only by listening can you find out what is important to the people you are trying to reach."

Whitehorn,[22] in seeking a working concept of human nature, has listed a basic set of motivational emotional needs and satisfactions that may be useful: (1) the desire for affection, (2) the desire for emotional security and trust, and (3) the desire for personal significance. He believes that since these sources of motivation are endogenous or arise from within, health education efforts based on them are more likely to strike a responsive chord and bring forth understanding and action.

In an interesting study of commercial advertising as a health education technique, inquiry was made with regard to the use of patent medicines. Of those interviewed, 60% said they used products of this nature before calling a physician. Although the majority recognized that the claims for the products often were not substantiated, the investigation indicated that the patent medicines resorted to most frequently were those for which the advertising played on emotions (especially fear), vanity, and desire for personal gain and those that promised or implied unequivocal cure and relief. Somewhat related to this, health educators and others in the health field should not be too ready to condemn the various "nonprofessionals" who provide question-and-answer columns in newspapers, in magazines, or on radio or television. Neither should the public be criticized for contacting them. The mere fact that such "nonprofessionals" are contacted by the public gives reason for professional introspection, and their advice and counsel is not necessarily bad. As Hemming[23] has pointed out in relation to the "Agony Aunties" in the British press, they apparently provide some commodities, such as reassurance and courage, that "professionals" so often ignore.

PROBLEMS IN HEALTH EDUCATION

It is paradoxical that despite extensive advances in literacy and education as well as vastly improved methods of communication, there still exists a great gap between existing medical and health protective knowledge and the public's acceptance and use of it. Professional journals are replete with reports of surveys of schoolchildren, college students, and the adult public that present discouraging and embarrasing evidence of failure in this field. Many parents still do not obtain immunization for their children, and many drivers still invite injury and death by

drinking and driving and by not using seat belts. The use of cigarettes and useless or harmful patent medicines is still widespread. One of the handicaps of public health work, of course, is the usual absence of pain and urgency (except when an epidemic occurs). Indeed, this is becoming even more true as the public health profession progresses from attacks on communicable diseases to an attempted control of chronic illnesses. There is little difficulty in motivating to prompt action an individual with a high fever from typhoid or a severe abdominal pain from acute appendicitis. To bring about a change in dietary or behavioral habits or to secure health maintenance examinations against possible future difficulty is something else. Results are less dramatic or rapid; cause and effect are less readily apparent.

Several reasons have been put forward to explain the inadequacies of health education at the present time. A practical starting point is Swinehart's[24] observation that "information presented through the channels commonly used by public health and voluntary associations is fairly easy for most potential audiences to avoid, since these audiences are not 'captive.' Even if they are exposed to communication, there is no guarantee that this will lead to learning and action." So in the field of health education, public health workers start with two handicaps.

In more detail, a committee of the New York Academy of Medicine presented the following points to consider.[25]

1. It is easier to sell symptomatic relief of illness or the promise of a cure than it is to sell health and prevention of disease.

2. Education is a catchall—a ready solution and means of disposition but one that is all too seldom put into action. Whenever there is a problem in a community, someone is sure to say, "The answer is education." And usually, that is where the problem rests.

3. Health education does not have high prestige. In the schools it is treated as a subordinate subject or as an additional chore to be passed out to a teacher whose main interest is not too remotely related. It is frequently made the responsibility of an athletic coach or physical training teacher.

4. In general, the people charged with health education programs lack special training and are not qualified.

5. Departments of education and health do not work together in programming, planning curricula, and raising standards of teaching health in the schools.

6. There is a lack of overall organization in the field of

health education with a unified program and a single-minded objective. An effective and dynamic program of health education must include: intercommunication of ideas, selection or priorities, formulation of program, and assignment of responsibility. As matters stand now, there is a great deal of shifting of responsibility from school to home to church to community organization.

Beyond this, it appears that health education has been regarded too much as a private preserve by the professionals in public health, medicine, and education. Actually, they often have tended to be stuffy, overly didactic, and lacking in understanding of what really concerns the average and less educated components of the population. This was forcefully brought out by an official of one of the most successful public relations and advertising companies in America in an address to a public health conference that he titled "Public Health is no Private Preserve (or things I never knew 'till now, no thanks to you)." This unusually well-educated man stated, "I was asked by your chairman to talk about selling public health. I, like most people, know very little about public health. I have no ready answers for your problems. I'm not even sure I understand the problems themselves. But I do know this: You are not communicating—you are not getting through to people. . . . I am amazed at the amount of effort, time, and money needed to safeguard my health and that of my family . . . yet the average citizen has no awareness of your efforts and actually impedes your work through ignorance."[26]

Concern over the foregoing reached a national focus in 1971, when a President's Committee on Health Education concluded that health education in America was "a neglected, underfinanced, unhealthily fragmented activity," and that "school health programs for 60 million American children are in disarray, and are scheduled for rainy days when children have nothing else to do."[4] The committee director, Victor Weingarten, president of the Institute of Public Affairs, pointed out that of the $75 billion spend on "health" in the United States during 1971, about 92% was spent after illness occurred and only 0.5% was spent on health education. And most of that, he complained, went into "packaged information" that was irrelevant and ineffective.

The President's Committee on Health Education produced three significant results: (1) the establishment of an extragovernmental health education consortium, the National Center for Health Edu-

cation; (2) the creation of a Bureau of Health Education within the Centers for Disease Control to serve as the Department of Health and Human Services' operating focus for health education activities; and (3) the formation of an Interdepartmental Panel on Health Education of the Public to assure effective coordination of federal resources devoted to health education. Accompanying these moves is significant congressional interest, evidenced by several bills to provide increased funding for training and project support.

Health educators are confronted by a group of formidable obstacles—so formidable that it is unrealistic to expect ready success. But obstacles are also challenges, and without challenges there can develop no grounds for some measures of satisfaction. When the Society of Public Health Educators met in 1971, it issued a statement that in its expanded horizon should give additional insight and courage to all in its profession:

Health education's effect on the quality of life can be broadened through political and social interventions as well as through the educational process, through interaction with consumers of all backgrounds—including labor and political office holders—and through a deeper understanding and sensitivity to the determinants of the quality of life.

In commenting on this, Dallas[27] noted three common threads that health educators would do well to bear in mind:

1. Quality of life implies choice—knowledge of all the available options, freedom to choose any option, and an understanding of the effects once a choice has been made.

2. Quality of life implies increased individual responsibility for health.

3. Quality of life implies the development of new skills and roles for health educators as well as the full use of existing strategies.

The evident inadequacy and ineffectiveness of health education up to the present obviously calls for continued evaluation and experimentation. Skillfully developed and properly used, health education can become a powerful force in social improvement and change. Its ultimate goal, of course, should be to encourage and assist the public in taking individual and group initiative to protect and improve its own health.

HEALTH HAZARD APPRAISAL: A HEALTH EDUCATION TOOL

Four health education approaches to the reduction or elimination of risks to health have been described as (1) educational, (2) preventive, (3) radical, and (4) self-empowerment.[28] The educational approach involves the exploration and clarification of beliefs and values in the hope that the individual will choose freely to avoid a health risk such as smoking. However, many find this difficult because of social pressures or parental examples. The preventive approach requires the persuasion or motivation of individuals on the basis that prevention is better than cure—that certain actions are involved in the etiology of eventual undesirable or fatal disease. The radical approach directs itself to the social, economic, and political roots of health problems, for example, poverty or subsidies or tax advantages to producers and disseminators of disease-causing materials such as tobacco, environmental pollutants, and the like. The self-empowerment approach attempts to avoid the passivity of the educational, the coercion of the preventive, and the posturing or subversive action of the radical approaches by creating a genuinely free and informed choice. It includes promoting attitudes for deferring present and immediate gratification (such as smoking) in favor of future benefit, challenging beliefs that life and health are controlled by others, and promoting self-esteem, which would help in responding to health education and in resisting pressures for unhealthy practices. The four approaches are by no means mutually exclusive and often overlap in practice.

The intent of self-empowerment programs is really to bring about a personal commitment for a change in life-style. By now the beneficial advantages of a healthful life-style are well documented. One example[29] that relates to the members of the Reorganized Church of Jesus Christ of Latter-Day Saints (Mormons) in Missouri will suffice. This group strictly avoids the use of tobacco, alcohol, and hot drinks such as tea and coffee. It emphasizes the importance of a well-balanced diet. A mortality study compared the 1972 to 1978 mortality of this group with three other groups. Missouri Mormons experienced age-adjusted death rates 22.6% lower than rates for Missouri non-Mormon whites; 19.6% lower than non-Mormon residents of Indepen-

dence, Missouri; and 14.4% lower than residents of Utah, 72% of whom belong to the Church of Jesus Christ of Latter-Day Saints. The Mormons experienced lower death rates than the other two Missouri groups for each of seven selected causes, especially for lung cancer, pneumonia and influenza, and violent deaths.

Risks to health are often multiple and interrelated. This is illustrated in Fig. 18-1 with reference to cumulative life-style risks in relation to motor vehicle accidents.[30] An actual example[31] was the recognition of multiple life-style hazards in persons convicted of improper driving. They were found to have a higher risk of death from diseases caused by smoking or alcohol, and they drove more miles and used seat belts less often than a control group. In general they had a more hazardous life-style and a diminished life expectancy.

During recent years there has been developed and increasingly refined a methodology that emphasizes prevention and does it by placing responsibility clearly on the individual. The basic tool used is referred to variously as health hazard appraisal or health risk assessment, and the overall approach is known as prospective medicine. The concept originated in 1958 with Dr. Lewis C. Robbins while he was chief of the cancer control program of the U.S. Public Health Service. Searching for some approach to primary prevention in place of secondary prevention or terminal care, he ignored the common doctrine that "you cannot apply group data to the individual."[32] Following an encouraging trial at the medical centers of Temple University and George Washington University, the method was adopted by the Graduate Medical Center of Methodist Hospital, Indianapolis, in its continued education curriculum. Dr. Robbins, who had joined Dr. Jack Hall at that institution, addressed the question of how to extend an individual's life expectancy. The important innovation was to approach the question prospectively on the basis of statistical actuarial probabilities rather than by postmortem retrospection.[33,34]

Briefly, the concept is based on the fact that whereas a given individual theoretically may be subject to a vast array of health risks that may lead to a large number of possible illnesses or injuries (i.e., potential causes of death), actually at any given point in life for a particular type of individual, a few conditions—perhaps about 10 or fewer—constitute most of the risk for the succeeding 10 years. This is a time span for which the usual person can comprehend and plan. For each type of person, categorized by age, sex, race, and perhaps occupation and location, the probability or risk of death from each of the predominant conditions during the next 10 years is provided by tables that are known as the Geller-Gesner Tables.[33,35] Similar tables have been produced for 1-year age intervals.[36] Gesner[37] has outlined the steps involved in a health hazard appraisal (see Fig. 18-2 for an example).

1. For each of the 10 to 12 leading causes of death for people of the individual's age, sex, and race, indicate the average risk of death during the next 10 years. These figures are obtained from the Gellner-Gesner Tables.

2. For each cause of death listed indicate the precursors or prognostic characteristics brought to light by the individual's medical history, life-style and, depending on the extensiveness of the program, physical examination, and laboratory and clinical tests. (Fig. 18-3 presents examples for several causes of death.) Decreases as well as increases in the group average risk are listed to refine the individual's risk for better or worse.

3. For each precursor listed indicate the positive or negative risk factor. A risk factor is a quantitative weight or multiplier that indicates the extent to which a precursor influences the risk of death. Risk factors are computed from mortality ratios and prevalence data and periodically reviewed and updated by groups of specialists knowledgeable with reference to particular diseases and causes of death.[38]

4. Compute the composite risk factor if there is more than one precursor for a given cause of death. Composite risk factors are determined by a formula similar to the credit-debit system used by the life insurance industry to determine total risk to the individual.

5. Obtain the present personal risk of the individual with reference to a particular potential cause of death by multiplying the average risk for the individual's population group by the individual's composite risk. The sum of all the

Text continued on p. 315.

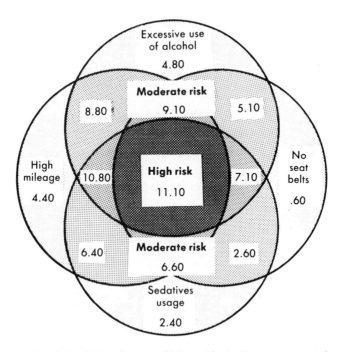

FIG. 18-1. Cumulative effect of risks of motor vehicle accidents. (Figures represent degree of risk for each behavioral factor.) (From Shires, D.B., editor: Bodycheck, Division of Family Medicine, Dalhousie University, Halifax, Nova Scotia)

HEALTH HAZARD APPRAISAL CHART

Quality control: Evaluate performance of a predetermined goal.

(Goal: "Get this patient safely through the next ten years.")

W M AGE 40-44		AVERAGE TO INDIVIDUAL RISK				
POPULATION AVERAGE 10 YEAR DEATHS PER 100,000		**INDIVIDUAL PROGNOSIS RISK APPRAISAL**				
Disease/Injury	Average Risk	Prognostic Characteristics	Risk Factor		Composite Risk Factor	Present Risk
From Manual	*From Manual*	*Listed in Manual Physician Select*	*From Manual*		*See Instructions*	*(2) x (5)*
			x	+		
(1)	(2)	(3)	(4)		(5)	(6)
1. ARTERIOSCLEROTIC HEART DISEASE	1,877	Blood pressure 108/70	.4		2.1	3941.7
		Cholesterol 214 mgs.%	.9			
		Diabetic No	1.0			
		Exercise Sedentary		2.5		
		Family history neg. over 60	.9			
		Smoking 3 pipes/day	1.0			
		Weight 69" 211# 39%ov.		1.3		
2. ACCIDENTS: MOTOR VEHICLE	285	Alcohol Mod. & Occ.	1.0		3.0	855
		Drugs & med. none	1.0			
		Mileage 32,000		3.2		
		Seat belt use 100%	.8			
3. SUICIDE	264	Depression no	1.0		1.0	264
		Family history neg.	1.0			
4. CIRRHOSIS OF LIVER	222	Alcohol Mod. & Occ.	1.0		1.0	222
5. VASCULAR LESIONS AFFECTING CNS	222	Blood pressure 108/70	.4		.4	88.8
		Cholesterol 214 mgs.%	.9			
		Diabetic No	1.0			
		Smoking 3 pipes/day	1.0			
6. CANCER OF LUNGS	202	Smoking 3 pipes/day	.3		.3	60.6
7. CHRONIC RHEUMATIC HEART DISEASE	167	Murmur No	1.0		.1	16.7
		Rheumatic fever No	1.0			
		Signs or symptoms None	.1			

FIG. 18-2. Example of a health hazard appraisal. (From Gesner, N.B.: The credit-debit system of health hazard appraisal, Proceedings of the Thirteenth Annual Meeting of the Society of Prospective Medicine, Indianapolis, 1977, Methodist Hospital of Indiana.)

Name _____John Doe_____ Patient No. _____ Birthdate_____

Street _____ Race, Sex, Age __WM 41__

City _____ State _____ Zip _____ Date _June 25_____19_71_

RISK REDUCTION FOR INDIVIDUAL

Prognostic Characteristics	Risk Factor		Composite Risk Factor	New Risk	Amount Reduction	Per Cent Reduction
PROGNOSIS AFTER INTERVENTION / **RISK REAPPRAISAL ***					**SURVIVAL ADVANTAGE**	
After Physician's Prescription	From Manual		See Instructions	(2) x (9)	(6) - (10)	**
	x	+				
(7)	(8)		(9)	(10)	(11)	(12)
	.4		.2	375.4	3566.3	46%
	.9					
	1.0					
Prescribed exercise	1.0					
	.9					
Stop Smoking	.7					
Reduce to desirable weight 150-154#	1.0					
None before driving	.5		2.6	741	114	2%
	1.0					
		3.2				
	.8					
	1.0		1.0	264	0	0
	1.0					
Stop before symptoms	.2		.2	44.4	177.6	2%
	.4		.4	88.8	0	0
	.9					
	1.0					
Stop Smoking	1.0					
Stop Smoking	.2		.2	40.4	20.2	.3%
	1.0		.1	16.7	0	0
	1.0					
	.1					

FIG. 18-2, cont'd. For legend see opposite page.

AVERAGE TO INDIVIDUAL RISK					
POPULATION AVERAGE **10 YEAR DEATHS PER 100,000**		**INDIVIDUAL PROGNOSIS** **RISK APPRAISAL**			
Disease/Injury	Average Risk	Prognostic Characteristics	Risk Factor		Composite Risk Factor	Present Risk
From Manual	From Manual	Listed in Manual Physician Select	From Manual x +		See Instructions	(2) x (5)
(1)	(2)	(3)	(4)		(5)	(6)
8. PNEUMONIA	111	Alcohol Mod. & Occ.	1.0		1.0	111
		Bacterial pneumonia No	1.0			
		Emphysema No	1.0			
		Smoking habits 3 pipes	1.0			
9. CANCER OF	111	Polyp No	1.0		1.0	111
INTESTINES &		Rectal bleeding No	1.0			
RECTUM		Ulcerative colitis No	1.0			
		Proctosigmoidoscopy No	x1.0			
10. LYMPHOSARCOMA &	76				1.0	76
HODGKINS DISEASE						
11. CANCER OF	56	Hypochlorhydria No	1.0		1.0	56
STOMACH &						
ESOPHAGUS						
12. HYPERTENSIVE	56	Blood pressure 108/70	.4		.7	39.2
HEART DISEASE		Weight 39% ovwt.		1.3		
13. TUBERCULOSIS	56	Current X-ray '67 neg.	1.0		1.0	56
		Econ. & soc. status Mid.	1.0			
		T B activity No	1.0			
Other Causes	1,855				1.0	1,855
Total	5,560					7,753

*Reappraise on assumption that physician's prescription is complied with.
Columns (7) through (10) same as columns (3) through (6) except where
the physician's prescription changed prognostic characteristics.
**Divide figures in column (11) by total of column (6).

Health appraisal age ___44½___

FIG. 18-2, cont'd. For legend see p. 310.

RISK REDUCTION FOR INDIVIDUAL

	PROGNOSIS AFTER INTERVENTION RISK REAPPRAISAL *				SURVIVAL ADVANTAGE	
Prognostic Characteristics	Risk Factor		Composite Risk Factor	New Risk	Amount Reduction	Per Cent Reduction
After Physician's Prescription	From Manual		See Instructions	(2) x (9)	(6) - (10)	**
	x	+				
(7)	(8)		(9)	(10)	(11)	(12)
Appropriate reduction	1.0		1.0	111	0	0
	1.0					
	1.0					
Stop Smoking	1.0					
	1.0		.3	33.3	77.7	1%
	1.0					
	1.0					
Annual Proctosigmoidoscopy	x0.3					
			1.0	76	0	0
	1.0		1.0	56	0	0
	.4		.4	22.4	16.8	.2%
Reduce to desirable weight	1.0					
Annual Chest X-ray	.2		.2	11.2	44.8	1%
	1.0					
	1.0					
			1.0	1,855	0	0
				3,736	4017	52%

Compliance age ___37___

Appraiser _Nancy Gilbert_ (SIGNATURE)

Physician _____ , M.D.

FIG. 18-2, cont'd. For legend see p. 310.

Risk factors — **Major disorder**

Risk factors	Major disorder
Depression Family history of suicide	Suicide
High annual mileage Seat belt nonusage Increased alcohol habits Drugs and medications (Influencing driving)	Motor vehicle accidents
Increased alcohol habits History of bacterial pneumonia Presence of emphysema/bronchitis Increased smoking habits	Pneumonia
Presence of crime record Weapons carried	Homicide
Increased alcohol habits	Cirrhosis of the liver
Increased smoking habits	Cancer of the lung
Increased smoking habits Blood cholesterol raised Blood pressure elevated Presence of diabetes Family history of diabetes	Cerebrovascular and peripheral arterial disease
Increased smoking habits Blood cholesterol raised Blood pressure elevated Diabetes Family history of diabetes Weight Lack of exercise Family history of ischemic heart disease	Arteriosclerotic heart disease

Risk factors	Major disorder
Rectal polyp Rectal bleeding Ulcerative colitis Protosigmoidoscopy not done	Cancer of the intestine and the rectum
Pap smear not done Early age of intercourse Poor economic and social status Jewish ethnic origin	Cancer of the cervix
Signs/symptoms or history treatment of rheumatic heart disease	Chronic rheumatic heart disease
Abnormal vaginal bleeding	Cancer of the body of the uterus
Family history of breast cancer or breast disease Late age of pregnancy or nulliparity Early age of menarche Late age of menopause Fibocystic breast disease Radiation exposure Upper socioeconomic class Above average height/weight	Cancer of the breast

FIG. 18-3. Precursors of selected causes of death.

disease-specific personal risks provides the total risk to the individual.

6. Apply intervention recommendations (e.g., stop smoking, use seat belts, exercise) and calculate the decreased risk possible, assuming compliance with recommendations. The difference between this potential risk figure and the existing risk represents the achievable survival advantage.

The use of the health hazard appraisal approach has been increasing rapidly during recent years. The purposes have included health education, behavior modification, health maintenance and disease prevention, and professional education. University populations, public and private health clinics, governmental and industrial groups, insurance companies, and many other groups and organizations have been adapting it to their special needs. An important landmark was its adoption in 1973 as a significant component of the national health program of Canada.[39,40] A very significant step has been the application of computer science to methodology.

As with all innovations, health hazard appraisal has its critics. This is by no means undesirable since it encourages further research and refinement. Furthermore, as Fielding[41] editoralizes, "Although health risk appraisal has many inherent problems compounded by some instances of misuse, concern with these problems should not lead us to overlook the number of actual and potential benefits which it can confer and the variety of other uses to which it can be put." Certainly for the purposes of health education and behavior modification it appears to provide an important tool with prospects of success in an area where so many other approaches have failed.

REFERENCES

1. Report of the Maryland State Board of Health, 1875. (Courtesy Clemens W. Gaines, Executive Office, 1965.)
2. Rosen, G.: A history of public health, New York, 1958, MD Publications.
3. Hochbaum, G.: At the threshold of a new era. Quoted in Ogden, H.: Health education: a federal overview, Public Health Rep. **91:**199, May-June 1976.
4. Report of the President's Committee on Health Education, Washington, D.C., U.S. Department of Health, Education, and Welfare, 1973.
5. Simonds, S.: Health education manpower in the United States, Health Educ. Monogr. **4**(3):208, Fall 1976.
6. Henderson, A.C., and others: The future of the health education profession, Public Health Rep. **96:**555, Nov.-Dec. 1981.
7. Wood, T.D.: In Fourth yearbook of the Department of Superintendent of the National Education Association, Washington, D.C., 1926, National Education Association.
8. Rosen, G.: Evolving trends in health education, Can. J. Public Health **52:**504, Dec. 1961.
9. New definitions; report of the 1972-73 Joint Committee on Health Education Terminology, Health Educ. Monogr. **3**(3):63, Spring 1973.
10. Preventive Medicine USA, New York, 1976, Prodist.
11. Bowman, R.: Changes in the activities, functions, and roles of public health educators, Health Educ. Monogr. **4**(3):226, Fall 1976.
12. Statement of functions of community health educators and minimum requirements for their professional preparation with recommendations for implementation, Society for Public Health Education, March 14, 1967.
13. Toward a policy on health education and public health: position paper of the American Public Health Association, Am. J. Public Health **68:**203, Feb. 1978.
14. Galanter, R.: To the victims belong the flaws, Am. J. Public Health **67:**1025, Nov. 1977.
15. Spiegel, C., and Lindaman, F.: Children can't fly: a program to prevent childhood morbidity and mortality from window falls, Am. J. Public Health **67:**1143, Dec. 1977.
16. Ogden, H.: Health education: a federal overview, Public Health Rep. **91:**199, May-June 1976.
17. Marti-Ibanez, F.: The pebble in the bell, MD **15:**13, July 1971.
18. Conant, R.K., DeLuca, A.J., and Levin, L.S.: Health education—a bridge to the community, Am. J. Public Health **62:**1239, Sept. 1972.
19. Am. Med. News, Dec. 11, 1972.
20. Rosenstock, I.M., Derryberry, M., and Carriger, B.K.: Why people fail to seek poliomyelitis vaccination, Public Health Rep. **74:**98, Feb. 1959.
21. Kost, K.: A communicator talks back. Environ. News Digest, Nov.-Dec. 1970.
22. Whitehorn, J.C.: Motivating pattern of the normal individual. In Psychological dynamics of health education, New York, 1951, Columbia University Press.
23. Hemming, J.: Agony Aunties and their contribution to health education, R. Soc. Health J. **5:**246, May 1972.
24. Swinehart, J.W.: Voluntary exposure to health communications, Am. J. Public Health **58:**1265, July 1968.
25. Health education: it present status: report by the Committee on Public Health, New York Academy of Medicine, Bull. N.Y. Acad. Med. **41:**1172, Nov. 1965.

26. Anderson, R.E.: Public health is no private preserve (or things I never knew till now, no thanks to you), Mich. Health, May-June 1965.
27. Dallas, J.L.: Health education, enabler for a higher quality of life, Health Services Rep. **87:**910, Dec. 1972.
28. Tones, B.K.: Health education: prevention or subversion? R. Soc. Health J. **101**(3):114, 1981.
29. McEvoy, L., and Land, G.: Life-style and death patterns of the Missouri RLDS church members, Am. J. Public Health **71:**1350, Dec. 1981.
30. Shires, D.B., editor: Bodycheck, Division of Family Medicine, Dalhousie University, Halifax, Nova Scotia.
31. Wilcock, A.R., and others: Evaluation of relative health-risk levels of a group of impaired drivers through health hazard appraisal, Can. J. Public Health **72:**264, July-Aug. 1981.
32. Robbins, L.C., and Petrakis, N.L.: Converting ratios to risks—a foundation for prospective medicine, Proceedings of the Twelfth Annual Meeting of the Society of Prospective Medicine, Bethesda, Md., 1977, Health and Education Resources.
33. Robbins, L.C., and Hall, J.H.: How to practice prospective medicine, Indianapolis, 1970, Department of Internal Medicine, Methodist Hospital of Indiana.
34. Hall, J.H., and Zwemer, J.D.: Prospective medicine, Indianapolis, 1979, Methodist Hospital Press.
35. Probability tables of dying in the next 10 years. Indianapolis, 1974, Methodist Hospital Press.
36. Althafer, C.: 1975, 1976, 1977 averaged probability of dying within the next 10 years of the 12 leading causes from 34 specific causes of death by age, race, and sex (1-year age groups), mimeographed paper, Atlanta, Bureau of Health Education, Centers for Disease Control.
37. Gesner, N.B.: The credit-debit system of health hazard appraisal, Proceedings of the Thirteenth Annual Meeting of the Society of Prospective Medicine, Indianapolis, 1977, Methodist Hospital of Indiana.
38. Gesner, N.B.: Derivation of risk factors from comparative data, Proceedings of the Seventh Annual Meeting of the Society of Prospective Medicine, Indianapolis, 1971, Methodist Hospital of Indiana.
39. Lalonde, M.: A new perspective in the health of Canadians: a working document, Ottawa, 1974, National Health and Welfare Ministry.
40. Lalonde, M.: Beyond a new perspective, Am. J. Public Health **67:**357, April 1977.
41. Fielding, J.F.: Appraising the health of health risk appraisal (editorial), Am. J. Public Health **72:**337, April 1982.

PART FIVE

Health and environment

"What is this thing called health?" once asked the journalist-commentator H.L. Mencken. "Simply a state in which the individual happens transiently to be perfectly adapted to his environment." But what is meant by the environment? Until recently, most people considered their environment limited to some of the visible, tangible, inanimate aspects of their surroundings. For long, public health workers' interpretation of environmental health did not go much beyond solving problems of insanitation. But a revolution has occurred, complete with speeches, marches, legal actions, and even occasional violence born of frustration. We have come to learn and understand the word and concept of *ecology*. The traditional egocentric concept that the planet and everything on it was ours to exploit and despoil without danger of repercussion has been set aside. Nature has begun to strike back.

The widening gap between technologic developments and the ability of our institutions to adapt is at the root of the multiplication of environmental problems that confront us—in our homes, at work, on the street, at play. Increasingly there seems to be no escape. And all of these environmental and institutional problems in turn are intertwined with and form a part of the social problems of the day. The situation is well put by C.P. Snow in his book *The Two Cultures and the Scientific Revolution:* "as history routinely and regularly records, because the engineering community and the political community could not get sufficiently on each other's wavelengths, one advanced civilization after another, sooner or later, collapsed." So now, our only recourse is to join the rest of the planet, to live on it with greater wisdom than before, and to anticipate and guard against those environmental forces, natural and man-made, that may mitigate against our health, well-being, and continued existence.

CHAPTER 19

Environmental hazards

I brought you into a plentiful country, to eat of the fruit thereof and the goodness thereof; but when ye entered, ye defiled my land, and made mine heritage an abomination.

Jeremiah 2:7

HUMANS AND ENVIRONMENT

Human health has always been dependent on our relationship with our environment. Humans, like other animals, are constantly transformed by natural forces in the environment that act on it, and they in turn continuously transform their environment. In company with all other life forms, from the whale to microscopic viruses, humans are part of a dynamic system in which they continuously interchange matter and energy with the world about them (their environments). The human being, for example, takes into its body solid, liquid, and gaseous matter from its environment and discharges solid, liquid, and gaseous waste into the environment. Beyond this, we even contrive machines that also exchange matter and energy with their environments. In the process of living, organisms may get into our bodies. Some act for our physiologic benefit, whereas others cause trouble. In addition, we both benefit from and become afflicted by the nonliving forces of our world. All of these interactions with the environment are involved in our relationship with our total environment. For those charged with the protection and enhancement of the environment, a broad concept of human-environment relationships is of critical importance. It must never be ignored that in the final analysis, concern for the public's health is the paramount reason for environmental action. This is often overlooked in the press for action for action's sake. On the other hand, public health workers themselves must be careful to avoid instituting or perpetuating actions or programs that are too narrow, environmentally ill-advised, or outdated, as if existing and potential external hazards to human health were fixed and isolated phenomena related to one or another specific environmental element, such as air, water, or waste. Admittedly such categoric approaches produced dramatic results in the past when people were confronted with widespread communicable diseases that superficially appeared to exhibit simple, specific cause-and-effect relationships. Unfortunately this viewpoint is dangerously unsuited to illnesses and disorders with multiple causes, which arise essentially out of an increasingly complex revolution in the environment. Such approaches ignore the convergent complexity of the relationship of the *total* person to the *total* environment.

As animals, humans are not particularly distinctive, except perhaps for certain physical and mental developments. Our environment in reality is a multifaceted system that encompasses the physical and biotic realms and the cultural setting fashioned by our unusual cerebral capabilities. Thus the human organism can be viewed relating simultaneously to the biophysical and to the sociocultural components of the environment. These interrelations between the *total* person and the *total* environment are dynamic. Each makes aggressions on the other. Each in turn responds to these aggressions. To support our biologic, cultural, and uniquely technologic needs, we boldly and continuously alter the naturally occurring environment and create ever new environments. Often this is done with inconsistency and without thought to the total or ultimate consequences.

An example of the complexity of such interrelationships was the experience of a mosquito control program in Borneo.[1] Extensive spraying of DDT proved very effective in reducing the mosquito population, hence the incidence of malaria. Soon after, however, the house roofs began to fall in because they were being eaten by the caterpillars, which did not absorb the DDT and so were unaffected by it. A species of predatory wasp, which had kept the caterpillars under control but which were susceptible to DDT, had been destroyed in large numbers. To compound the problem, indoor spraying was done to control the many houseflies. Until then, this function was performed by the small harmless gecko lizard that inhabited the houses. They continued to eat the heavily dosed houseflies and in turn began to sicken and die. The geckos were now easily caught by house cats, who in turn died from DDT, which had been ecologically concentrated many times over. As this occurred, the ubiquitous rat, now uncontrolled, underwent a population explosion, invaded the houses, consumed food, and brought a threat of plague. In a partial attempt to restore a balance, the government dropped fresh cats by parachute into badly affected areas. Obviously, this was a questionable solution.

Until the present, humans could respond successfully through biologic adaptation and evolution. This, of course, required long periods of time, but the pace of change was slow. Today the situation is different. Within recent decades there have been set in motion forces of such magnitude and rapidity as to challenge seriously our adaptive abilities. The ability of the human organism to maintain internal integrity in the face of changing external forces is one that is largely past oriented; that is, our internal integrating abilities evolved over many hundreds of thousands of years during which stimuli were occurring slowly and naturally. Thus the regulatory mechanisms to achieve homeostasis are genetically linked to a lengthy era in our evolutionary history unlike that which we face today.

In this era of burgeoning populations and rapid change, there is no longer time for leisurely adaptation and evolution. As a consequence, there can be no assurance that this limited natural adaptive capacity will suffice to carry us through all future experiences. Present human-induced drastic environmental alterations and disturbances are resulting in insults, excitants, and stresses that necessarily evoke responses from the human organism. Such responses may be physiologic, morphologic,

behavioral, or social, or a mixture of all of these. Through these responses the organism seeks to reach a modus vivendi, seeks to maintain or to regain homeostatic compatibility. The complexity of this adaptive effort is readily apparent, since it includes the *total* human organism and its whole nature as it relates to its *total* environment. Furthermore, simultaneous insults that arise out of both the biophysical and sociocultural components may exhibit synergism or potentiation, which can evoke human adaptive responses to threats that are so unequal, inadeqate, or inappropriate as to be disruptive in their own right. Thus an acceptable amount of water pollution, added to a tolerable amount of air pollution and combined with a bearable amount of noise and congestion, can produce a totally unacceptable health environment.[2]

The implications of this were dramatically emphasized several years ago by the so-called Club of Rome, an informal group of several hundred outstanding scientists, sociologists, industrial managers, and educators from several countries.[3] Because of shared concerns for the future of humanity, beginning in April 1968, they arranged to accumulate and analyze a large amount of data and attempted to develop predictive mathematical models. Five critical areas for measurement were chosen: population growth, rate of industrialization, ability to increase food supplies, rate of depletion of natural resources, and extent of environmental pollution. Obviously, these are all interrelated. They concluded that earlier individual warnings by population and agricultural specialists, ecologists, and students of natural resources fell short of the mark. They predicted that if the current course of continued growth and depletion of resources is followed, although conditions may appear favorable for some for a while, a sudden cataclysmic collapse of industrial civilization will eventually occur, accompanied by widespread famine, disease, and strife— probably within 100 years. They likened the situation to a spent light bulb that glows ever brighter before it suddenly blows out. The only hope they saw was the achievement as rapidly as possible of a "steady state society" on a worldwide partnership basis, in which there would be collective action to stabilize all five of the basic areas at the same time—population, food supply, industrialization, natural resource consumption, and pollution. That, of course, expects a great deal from human nature.

An attempt to illustrate the potential consequences of ecologic ignorance is provided by the work of Calhoun,[4,5] of the National Institute of Mental Health, with colonies of mice and rats. In a series of long-term studies he has illustrated the ultimate effects of uninhibited breeding and excessive crowding. He begins with a limited number of healthy laboratory animals provided with constantly ample supplies of food, water, and nesting material and unhampered opportunity to propagate in quarters carefully designed to be spatially adequate for 144 animals. Well before reaching the eventual naturally imposed ceiling not of 144 but of 2,500 animals, there develops a breakdown of almost all aspects of normal behavior. Laboratory mice are naturally clean about themselves and their environment. When limited in numbers, they typically avoid soiling each other or their nesting places. Under conditions such as those allowed in these experiments, however, gross insanitation from bodily discharges becomes ubiquitous, and the tendency for personal grooming is lost. Territorial prerogatives are ignored. The strong attack the weak, and groups of the strong drive off groups of the weak. As a result, in each large experimental pen, masses of essentially outcasts that Calhoun refers to as "behavioral sinks" appear. The members of the outcast behavioral sinks becomes excessively violent, but only among themselves—not with the strong overlords. Markedly aggressive behavior appears among many of the females. Scattered throughout may be seen individuals who clearly demonstrate various signs and symptoms of regression, confusion, and mental disturbance. Throughout, and even among the dominant animals, sexual desire and the ability to mate decline significantly. Homosexuality appears with males trying to copulate with males and females with females. Increasingly the group becomes nonproductive. Such normal mating as does occur becomes increasingly infertile; such cubs as are born are typically premature and weak and are typically ignored and cannibalized. It is physiologically significant that once arriving at this state, transfer of animals, even the few dominants, to more "normal" circumstances does not typically result in recovery. Permanent physiologic damage, probably through endocrine glandular change, has resulted.

One has only to read the newspapers of any large, crowded city to recognize that a reasonable amount of interpolation from such studies to humans, their numbers, concentration, living circumstances, and total environment may be valid. As cities become more densely crowded, as people pave over their farm lands and abuse and neglect the urban environment at an ever increasing rate—and as in the process people place ever more physical, chemical, biologic, and psychologic hazards and stresses on those who live in the cities—one has ample cause for concern about the immediate and long-range consequences.

These concepts have been crystallized by McCue and Ewald[6] into two basic forces of change: *macroimpacts* of the environment on the individual, including such factors as population, time, space, technology, and free-will expectations; and *microimpacts* of the individual on the environment, including physiologic, psychologic, cultural, social, and ecologic factors, plus spiritual free will. However, they emphasize that we do not necessarily have to accept a deterministic or fatalistic view. We find ourselves, therefore, with the uncomfortable understanding that human beings as individuals and in groups have their own impacts, therefore their own responsibilities, concerning the creation of the future environment through the proper application of the factors that make up the balancing micro-impacts. And the single most decisive factor in deciding the future is the will of people, not technology. The more aware, the more comprehensive this understanding, the greater will be the individual and group responsibility.

In the study of humanity in health and disease there has been much less interest shown in a better understanding of the *total* human organism's *total* response to the *total* environment than in the separate biochemical activities of its components. This narrow approach, although highly productive of detailed particles of knowledge and techniques, has not greatly increased our understanding of the interplay between the entire human organism and its environment. This caused Dubos[7] to observe that ". . . the time has come to give the study of the responses that the living organism makes to its environment the same dignity and support which is being given at present to the study of the component parts of the organism." And he predicts that "exclusive emphasis on the reductionist approach will otherwise lead biology and medicine into blind alleys."

A consequence of the inadequacy of the reductionist approach to environmental health hazards has been a gradually growing recognition of the need for a new conceptual framework to study and deal with the complex and ever-changing interface between *total* human beings and their *total* environment. Such a framework, growing out of a synthesis of many disciplines and fields, would include within its purview the study of cause-and-effect relationships on the bases that a human *is* a whole organism and reacts as a unit; that life *is* dynamic, and its infinite variations are primarily the result of reaction to specific and often compounded identifiable environmental factors, modified by individual tendencies of inheritance and qualities of resistance; and that disease or dysfunction, in any part, *is* the result of overall loss of ability to adapt successfully.

The emphasis that must be given to establish such a new basis for public health is in essence the application of the principles of ecology to the human circumstance. It is based on a recognition that our health status is the outcome of the interplay between and the integration of two ecologic universes: our internal environment and the external multienvironments in which we exist. As it is with the individual, so it is with the community. Human ecology is thus concerned with the broad setting of mankind in the total environment, that is, with all of our characteristics, our interpersonal and intergroup processes associated with culture, technology, and social organizations, and the basic personality drives that are expressed in behavior and emotion. It strives to develop a conceptual framework wherein the public health and medical needs of mankind, as individuals, in groups, and as communities, may be approached not merely in a reductionist fashion—that is, viewing only a disease entity of specific etiology affecting a special organ or system—but rather in a holistic manner wherein our integrated responses to environmental forces find expression on a *health-disease-death* continuum.

The human ecologic approach, of necessity and by definition, calls for an interdisciplinary effort wherein the natural, physical, and social sciences, in company with engineering, combine to study our adaptive responses, and especially the effects of unsuccessful adaptation on human health. Theologian Paul Tillich put it aptly when he said: "to speak of health one must speak of all dimensions of life which are united in man. And no one can be an expert in all of them."

If health and well-being are states in which we exhibit full adaptive capacity, the question arises as to the nature of the environment best suited to us. Increasingly one hears concern about the quality of the environment and the need to restore it. Restore it to what and for what purpose? Where is the blueprint for this restoration? Who drew it up and on what basis? Although there are many ideas and suggestions about the nature of a desirable or undesirable environment, there is little in the way of an intelligent comprehensive master plan. Indeed, for the most part environmental health is strangely underplayed if not ignored in most of the current so-called urban and national planning as well as in comprehensive health planning activities on all levels of government. One of the problems is that we simply do not know all the circumstances under which our adaptive capacity can be pushed beyond the norm of adequate response. This is a fertile and critical field for inquiry.

Perhaps the health worker can think of the human biosocial organism as an open-ended system through which the energy, resources, and influences of the environment flow, are transformed for good or ill, and transform us in the process. From many sources in the physical environment come hazards to health in the form of biologic organisms, toxic chemicals, radioactivity, noise, physical forces; they run the gamut of ecologic exposures. From the sociocultural component comes the never-ending stream of informational stimuli, which require correct decisions or adaptive strategies that too often pose a threat to psychologic and social integrity and trigger emotional and behavioral patterns inimical to self and others. In addition, the synergistic potential, the additive effect of these, elicits even greater maladaptive responses that manifest themselves as disease and disability. These become the clinical signs of an unsuccessful struggle.

How strange that we, who evolved as an integral part of the environment, by the development of our cultures have perversely adopted an attitude of environmental apartheid. The many terms that reflect our antagonistic attitude toward our environment are noteworthy. We *conquer* the environment. We *subdue* nature. We *push back* the frontier. We view the environment as a *threat,* as an *enemy,* instead of cherishing, protecting, and conserving it, instead of recognizing that we are in fact part of it, instead of saying "I am myself and my circumstance." Somehow the environment is seen as something to be shaped, molded, and transformed to meet our short-term preferences or merely as the stuff that through exploitation serves our transient needs in preparation for an anticipated "real" afterlife. That out of the manipulation and alteration of this natural bounty, and the societal institutions that make it possible, could come sickness and unhappiness is a thought foreign to an organism that has a Ptolemaic view of itself.

HAZARDS—AN OVERVIEW

Our relationship with our environment necessarily must be regarded in two contexts: (1) the elements of the natural environment that are hazardous to our health and safety and (2) our actions within our environment that themselves threaten our health.[8] Within the first context are biologic agents of disease or injury, including microorganisms, noxious plants, and toxic or physically harmful animals; weather, including violent storms, cold, and thermal stress; natural radiation from the soil or from the atmosphere; geologic perturbations such as earthquakes, volcanic eruptions, and floods; and certain naturally occurring chemical substances. The second context consists of hazards to our health that result from our own actions and maladaptations to the natural environment. This second context of human hazards brings the biologic scientists into a confrontation with conditions even more complex than those that comprise health threats of "natural" origins.

Self-induced hazards include such things as accidental injury; suicide and homicide (which are discussed elsewhere); injury and genetic damage from ionizing and nonionizing radiation; poisoning from industrial, agricultural, and therapeutic chemicals; noise-induced hearing loss; and health threats from polluted air, land, and water. These health problems are direct although unintended results of social and technologic advancement or aberrant human behavior or both.

The automobile is an outstanding example of a social and technologic advancement that has brought with it a staggering toll in accidental death and injury; pollution of air, water, and land; and unmeasured hearing loss from noise as well as some of the most hazardous occupational environments, such as oil drilling and highway construction. Elimination of the automobile as a threat to health and life cannot be achieved either by its removal from society or by "immunizing" society against its effects. Inevitably a trade-off must be reached when chosen systems of transportation provide sufficient benefits to justify whatever toll

results in terms of health effects. Similar cost-benefit decisions have to be made with respect to radiation, pesticides, drugs, industrial chemicals, and most other hazards in this category.

The unique nature of human and environmental hazards, especially those generated by ourselves, is such that many complex social, economic, and political factors bear heavily on them, their genesis, their study, and their solution. Although the net result of such hazards is an unwanted effect on our health and lives, the traditional training and experience of the life scientists is insufficient to cope with these problems single-handedly. By introducing the element of human action—either purposeful or by indirection—the health scientist finds it necessary to form an alliance with engineers, physical scientists, behavioral scientists, economists, educators, and political scientists if prevention or control of these human hazards is to be achieved.

If one accepts the conditions of trade-off improvements as opposed to absolute prevention and need for multidisciplinary involvement, it is necessary to reexamine the criteria by which program priorities are established. Eight such criteria may be listed: (1) mortality, (2) morbidity, (3) financial impact on national economy, (4) use of hospital space, (5) numbers and availability of health personnel, (6) types of control measures available for attacking the problem and the ease with which they can be attained, (7) available or obtainable human and financial resources, and (8) public receptivity to the idea and method of controlling the hazard.

None of the hazards to health considered here meets all of these criteria. Thus accidents and occupational injury and illness would receive high priorities in terms of the first four and possibly the fifth criteria but would probably be rated low on the last three.

With respect to scientific breakthroughs, the widest possible variance exists among the hazards considered.[9] They range from vast strides and control over many communicable diseases to meager beginnings on the subject of noise. In a real sense, accomplishments serve as a measurement of both society's concern for the problem and its willingness to invest in its solution. Even more specifically, progress in controlling human and environmental hazards reflect the extent to which political leaders are motivated by public health workers, scientists, and the general public, who may believe that a particular hazard can and must be controlled and eliminated.

THE CHANGING NATURE OF HAZARDS

Recent decades have brought great advances in medicine, science, engineering, and technology. In the United States varying degrees of affluence and high standards of living have been achieved for a large proportion of the population. The chief health problems of the past—yellow fever, plague, malaria, cholera, typhoid, dysenteries, and many others— have all succumbed to the application of new knowledge. Unfortunately many of the technologic advances have given rise to new and unfamiliar threats to human life. Population increase, road construction, and transportation improvement have led to grotesquely increased crowding and its accompanying stresses.

An ever-increasing barrage of new chemicals enters our bodies through food and water consumed, air breathed, and drugs taken therapeutically or otherwise. Streams and lakes have become contaminated with biologic, agricultural, industrial, and mining wastes. Increasing amounts of waste material and discarded vehicles multiply the opportunities for insect and rodent breeding. A crescendo cacophony is affecting the hearing of increasing numbers of people. Ionizing and nonionizing radiation are increasing in the environment. It is used not only in nuclear testing but also in industry, in laser and microwave technology, in electronic products in the home, and in devices for medical diagnosis and treatment. Not only is each of these environmental hazards becoming increasingly significant in its own right, but the implications in terms of total "body burden" are yet to be adequately comprehended.

Thus the modern environment is dangerous on two accounts: it contains elements that are clearly noxious and stressful, and it has been changing so rapidly that we appear unable to make proper adaptive responses to it. Since the rate of technologic change is constantly accelerating, a complex of physical, mental, and emotional stresses of human life are resulting from increasing urbanization. Small but long-term exposures to many environmental stresses, hazards, and contaminants cause many previously unrecognized and little understood chronic ailments, disabilities, and even death.

The various factors in the environment that may act together to reinforce each other (synergism) or to oppose each other (antagonism) are still subject to comprehension. It is important therefore that all concerned with human health must learn to assess the problems in their special areas of interest from an overall, holistic viewpoint. It will no longer do for the problems of one area to be considered separately from the problems of other areas.

Little has been learned about the interactions within the human body and mind of the various environmental stresses, although it is known, for example, that the intended effects of certain medications may be initiated, intensified, or otherwise transformed by certain other factors in the environment, including pollutants or other medications. Similarly, it is known that radiation, cigarette smoking, certain air pollutants, and various industrial chemicals can have a multiplying effect in the development of pulmonary cancer. The little that is know about multiple hazardous impacts merely highlights the vast amount still to be learned about human response to factors in the environment. Most of the vast and ever-increasing array of physical, chemical, biologic, and psychologic stresses to which modern urbanized humans are now subjected did not even exist in previous generations.

In the late nineteenth and early twentieth centuries, social and health pioneers were concerned primarily with malnutrition, overwork, filth, and microbial contamination. By contrast, the ailments characteristic of industrial societies result from economic affluence, chemical pollution, and high population densities. The increase in chronic and degenerative diseases is caused largely by these environmental and behavioral changes and not, as often supposed, by an increase in human life expectancy. Life expectancy after the age of 45 years has not increased significantly. A man now 45 years or older is little better off today than in 1900. It can be assumed that medical science will continue to develop useful techniques for ameliorating malignancies, vascular disease, and certain other degenerative disorders. Undoubtedly it will refine methods for organ transplants and for artificial prostheses. But most conditions that require treatment need not have occurred in the first place. Acquisition of more knowledge of environmental determinants is the path to prevention and control.[10]

The protection of the public from the newer hazards involves skills and knowledge far more extensive and complex than seemed sufficient even in the recent past. It requires sound scientific understanding based on intensive and extensive biologic and biochemical research. Fortunately there is a growing public awareness of the need for improved environmental quality. Increasingly, as environmental deterioration has affected more and more people, their uneasiness has produced demands for safer use of the environment and an increasing willingness to provide support for its restoration and preservation. This implies involvement, which in terms of universities and similar concentrations of expertise, brings one back to research. Without increased study of the effects of the newer environmental hazards on man, increases in disease rates and greater expenditures for avoidable therapy are inevitable.

Against this background two major breakthroughs during recent decades deserve special note. The first was the appreciation that small amounts of chemicals may become toxic after periods of accumulation or latency. Biologic and toxicologic research on beryllium, asbestos, benzene, and mercury exemplify this. Some of the fundamental enzyme systems involved have been defined and show that the rate at which the body acts on a chemical affects its toxicity. As a result, the basic mechanisms of toxicity are better understood. Safety evaluation techniques have been improved, and methods for studying the potential of chemical carcinogenesis, teratogenesis, and mutagenesis are being developed as a result of these research efforts.

The second major and concurrent breakthrough was that the scientific community became aware that there was inadequate information on the effects of these widespread chemicals (air pollutants, metals, persistent pesticides, additives, pharmaceuticals, and the like) in the biosphere. As a result, the research community is now aware that the total ecologic threat may in some instances be more important than any direct toxic effect on humans. In sum, the major breakthroughs have been an appreciation of the latent, insidious, and chronic effects of small amounts of chemicals in the environment, often over prolonged time periods, and their potential threat to future generations through their effects on the biosphere. Even this breakthrough is inadequate unless consideration goes beyond acute, easily recognized, clinical responses to consideration of genetic and mutagenic potentials.

TYPES OF ENVIRONMENTAL HAZARDS

The number of factors in the environment that may affect humans may be listed as follows:

Life support
  Food
  Water
  Oxygen
Physical factors
  Mechanical
  Acoustic
  Electrical
  Magnetic
  Thermal
  Particulate
  Ionizing radiation
Biologic factors
  Microorganisms
  Toxins
  Biologic wastes
  Biologic antagonists
    Animal
    Plant
  Allergens
Psychosocial factors
  Crowding
  Demands
  Physical time
  Biologic time
  Cultural time
Chemical factors
  Inorganic
    Light metals and their compounds
    Transitional and rare earth metals and their compounds
    Heavy metals and their compounds
    Nonmetallic elements and their compounds
  Organic
    Acyclic hydrocarbons including alkyl compounds
    Carbocyclic compounds
    Halogenated acyclic hydrocarbons
    Heterocyclic compounds
    Organic phosphorus compounds
    Organic sulfur compounds
  Product complexes
    Combustion products
    Macromolecular products
    Industrial wastes
    Agricultural wastes (including fertilizers, pesticides, and herbicides)

Some of these factors in proper form or amount are helpful or even necessary to life; others are hazardous. Consideration of several of them, with some consideration of significant breakthroughs and further needs, follows under three categories of hazards: biologic, chemical, and physical.

BIOLOGIC HAZARDS[11-15]

The biologic hazards to human health are mostly those posed by bacteria, viruses, and other microorganisms and parasites. Since the advances against them have been discussed in other chapters, they are considered here in a general way. Those microbiologic accomplishments directly related to human health include modifications of human susceptibility to disease or recuperative ability (improved diagnostic and immunizing methods and antimicrobial drugs) and modification of the environment or of the type of relationship to the environment (more knowledge of the agents that cause or induce infectious disease and how to control them; better methods of ensuring that food, milk, and water are free of disease-producing microorganisms; more aseptic homes, public institutions, and food distribution industries; better understanding of community health problems; and better control of disease in domestic and wild animals). Those accomplishments that have an indirect relationship to human health include, for example, improvement in worker productivity with consequent increase in plant and animal food production. During the past 30 years microbiologic research could have been even more effective had there been more complete communication between scientists, administrators, and agency representatives and less unnecessary duplication of research activities, whether funded by federal, local, or private sources.

Information exchange is vital to success and economy of applied research in the field of microbiology as related to health and disease. There has been little planned exchange of information other than through publication of scientific papers and presentations at scientific meetings. An exception is the Arbovirus Information Exchange, which is issued several times a year to scientists in 235 institutions. This plus an annual meeting in conjunction with the Society of Topical Medicine and Hygiene minimizes unnecessary duplication and directs attention toward critical problems. Progress in a much broader sense is now made possible by MEDLARS (Medical Literature Analysis and Retrieval System) and the National Center for Biomedical Communications, developed by the National Institutes of Health. Another deficient area of communication lies between the researcher and the tax-paying citizen, whose understanding of research activities and accomplishments is important to assure continued support.

The following achievements may be anticipated during the next decade in this fight against microbiologic hazards in the environment: (1) more effective and less expensive methods for disposing of human wastes, thereby reducing water pollution from this source and reducing the biologic usage of oxygen in rivers; (2) better methods of controlling disease caused by microbes in agricultural products (plants and livestock) leading to an increase in quality and quantity of food; (3) more specific drugs for use against microbes, fungi, and certain viruses that cause human disease and disorders; (4) more effective immunizing agents for human and animal use, including attenuated live virus vaccines administered orally or into the nose-throat region; (5) possible determination of viruses as causative agents of some types of cancer; (6) improvements in the control of those diseases transmitted from animals to humans—diseases such as Rocky Mountain spotted fever, plague, brucellosis, hemorrhagic fevers, encephalitis, and rabies; (7) more accurate and less expensive diagnostic microbiology by means of automation and reducing the size of clinical diagnostic samples; and (8) improved understanding of immune mechanisms in relation to certain diseases of the very young and the very old, such as multiple sclerosis, rheumatoid arthritis, and blood dyscrasias.

CHEMICAL HAZARDS
General[16-19]

Increasingly we live in a chemical environment. In addition to the many that exist in nature, an estimated 2 million chemical compounds with more than 30,000 chemical substances are man-made, and approximately 1,000 new ones are introduced each year.[10] Humans may be exposed to these through any of the components of the environment—air, water, and soil. Although a particular chemical hazard initially may be limited to one of these, dispersion to one or both of the others may occur. This is especially likely to be the case for persistent pollutants. Agricultural chemicals present a classic example. As a result, a fourth source of environmental chemical hazard should be considered in the form of food, in the sense that it may reflect concentrations from air, water, or soil. Chlorinated hydrocarbons have been widely used since 1945 to control agricultural and other insect pests. Unquestionably numerous instances of contamination of human food have occurred. Two episodes reported from the state of New York[20] clearly demonstrated the transmission of significant amounts of dieldrin to milk as a result of contaminated cattle feed. A somewhat more unfortunate example was the contamination of human breast milk throughout Michigan with the synthetic fire-retardant polychlorinated biphenyl (PCB), which in 1973 had been mixed accidentally with livestock feed.[21]

With reference to chemical hazards in relation to human disease, perhaps the major advance of the last three decades has been the realization that many apparently spontaneous diseases are in fact induced by environmental pollutants. Thus certain cancers and deformities may be largely explicable in terms of exposure to certain specific environmental pollutants. More recently there has been a growing realization of the importance of chemical induction of genetic changes.[22] Apart from preformed agents that may cause cancer (carcinogens), induce morphologic abnormalities (teratogens), or bring about genetic changes (mutagens), there is a growing interest in the possibility of their synthesis in the body from simpler chemical compounds normally present in the environment.

Although the term *pollutant* is often restricted to synthetic industrial chemicals, there are four broad categories of other important chemical pollutants. The first group consists of natural chemicals in excess. An example is found in nitrates that are normal dietary components. At high concentrations in food or water, they can cause a blood disorder (methemoglobinema) in infants. Also, nitrites, as reduction products of nitrates, may interact with secondary amines to form nitrosamines. Some of these are carcinogenic, teratogenic, or mutagenic.

Toxic chemicals in fungi on plants or in crop plant products comprise the second group, of which aflatoxins and cycasins are notable examples. The yields of these toxins can generally be considerably influenced by technologic factors, such as conditions of harvest, storage, and processing. A third group consists of complex organic and inorganic mixtures, such as air and water pollutants, which comprise a wide range of undefined and defined components.

Finally, there is the group of synthetic chemicals: agricultural chemicals, notably pesticides and fertilizers; food additives; fuel additives; household chemicals; industrial chemicals; and in a somewhat specialized class therapeutic and prophylatic pharmaceuticals, as well as synthetic habituating and addicting drugs.

Pollutants may have a wide range of adverse biologic effects, from mild sensory impairment to death. The possibility that chronic toxicity is also manifested in immunologic impairment or psychologic disorders has yet to be determined, although there is already suggestive evidence to incriminate carbon monoxide in these regards. Some pollutants produce any one or more of these types of reactions and may interact with one another outside as well as inside the body to produce otherwise unanticipated synergistic toxicity.

Naturally occurring chemicals[23]

There are many naturally occurring chemicals hazardous to humans. The toxicity of some, mercury and arsenic, for example, was known in ancient times. Recent research has indicated that many others play a role in human health and disease. Some trace elements are important in human nutrition and in many normal physiologic reactions. But excesses or deficiencies of certain metals such as cadmium, selenium, chromium, lead, copper, zinc, lithium (or of radiation) may be related to major degenerative diseases such as heart disease, muscular dystrophy, diabetes, multiple sclerosis, cancer, mental illness, or congenital malformations. There is growing awareness that many diseases have geographic patterns that seem to relate to the physical environment and its different geologic metal-containing areas. This awareness has led to a corresponding recognition of the need for interdisciplinary teamwork involving geochemists and medical scientists. Some of the observations that have resulted from this multipronged investigative effort are described briefly in the following discussion.

For a long time *arsenic* was believed to produce cancer, but recent research has dispelled this notion in the United States. Major sources of arsenic intake are food, especially crustacea, and beverages, particularly wines. Except for some isolated locations, the arsenic content of water supplies is extremely small. In Europe, however, there have been claims that arsenic induces cancer. Arsenic has long been known to counteract selenium toxicity, and it has been added to poultry and cattle feeds in areas where selenium content of soil and water is high. However, in hamsters selenium does not suppress the monster-forming effect of high levels of arsenic. It is possible that the different views of the United States and Europe concerning arsenic as a cancer-inducing agent may result from differences in exposures to these two antagonistic elements in the two regions of the world and to the quantities and chemical forms of these substances ingested.

Certain tumors (mesotheliomas) have been known for decades, but it was not until 1965 that *asbestos* was found to be a causative agent. Its carcinogenicity appears related to certain trace metals and certain chemical compounds such as benzpyrene.[24] Benzpyrene is a ubiquitous air pollutant, a prominent constituent of tobacco smoke and of charred and smoked foods. Asbestos workers who smoke cigarettes have up to 30 times greater risk of developing lung cancers than do nonsmoking fellow workers.[25] The trace metals (Ni, Cr, Fe) are associated with certain types of asbestos fiber (chrysotile). There is some indication that the cancerous growths are brought about by an interaction between benzypyrene or benzypyrene compounds, an enzyme, and the particular trace metals.

Asbestos is used extensively in shipbuilding. As a result as many as 50% of workers in some shipyards have been found to have asbestosis.[26] In addition, significant rates of asbestosis have been found in family members whose only exposure in many cases was by inhalation of particles from the clothing, skin, and hair of the shipyard workers.[27] Overall the U.S. Department of Labor estimates that about 8,200 excess cancer deaths occur each year among workers exposed to asbestos in various types of work.[28] A much lesser number of nonoccupational asbestosis occur, but their sources are unknown. Among possible sources suspected are asbestos water pipes, asbestos filters for beer, asbestos brake linings, asbestos household iron-holders, asbestos used in some cigars, and asbestos in water supplies (possibly the most continuous source). At the present time severe restrictions are placed on the use of asbestos.

Beryllium causes a serious disease, berylliosis, a name only about 40 years old. It is known to induce tumors in animals but has not been found to do so in humans. Beryllium poses no threat to health from water or food sources since it is poorly absorbed from the gastrointestinal tract and is insoluble in water either inside or outside the body. The potential environmental threat is from air and dust around beryllium production plants. The use of beryllium as an industrial material is increasing rapidly.

Another chemical hazard is the trace element *cadmium*. In 1965 it was shown that the kidneys of many persons dying from hypertensive complications had increased amounts of cadmium or increased ratios of cadmium to zinc, as compared with persons dying from other major diseases. This has been substantiated experimentally in animals. The chief sources of cadmium are believed to be drinking water and food grown in soils containing cadmium from certain fertilizers; beverages that have been in contact with galvanized zinc (container coatings), which contains small amounts of cadmium; and vegetables, coffee, and tea (all of which usually contain small amounts of cadmium). Drinking water is not thought to be a large source. Whether or not cadmium induces renal hypertension also seems to depend on the intake of zinc and selenium, antagonists to cadmium. In hamsters monster formation induced by cadmium is antagonized by selenium. The highly lethal effect of cadmium on fish is increased (synergized) by cyanide.

A significant finding was made in 1960 that in many locations in the United States, water with relatively more dissolved salts, so-called hard water, is associated with lower death rates from cardiovascular and coronary heart disease. The correlation was somewhat better for coronary heart disease in white men 45 to 64 years old in certain states and in the 163 largest cities, which had about 58% of the total national water supplies. Mortality from all other causes showed no such correlation. Before this discovery, state-to-state variations in cardiovascular deaths were unexplained on dietary, racial, or social bases. Evidently something in hard water, or the lack of something in soft water (relatively low in dissolved salts), influences the death rate. Of the various trace elements for which correlations have been worked out, only cadmium and *chromium* (Cr^{3+}) have been revealed as trace elements affecting cardiovascular disease. This raises the possibility that perhaps in time the prevalence of cardiovascular disease may be decreased by adding certain trace elements to water supplies.

Lead poisoning has been known from ancient times, but its clinical manifestations were classified only 110 years ago. Lead exists in many forms in the environment, and its industrial use is practically ubiquitous. Occupational safeguards have limited its harmful effects, but a special hazard is the use of tetraethyl lead as an antiknock and power-increasing agent in gasoline. Tetraethyl lead is highly toxic when inhaled or absorbed through the skin and predominantly causes cerebral or central nervous system symptoms. In addition, it pollutes the atmosphere. The use of toxic lead-bearing household paints has been largely eliminated, but still in the United States, thousands of small children eat dangerous amounts of flaked household lead paint, mostly in the older and poorer parts of large cities; some die and others develop mental retardation, cerebral palsy, convulsive seizures, blindness, and various other disorders. In 1980 more than 26,000 children in the United States were treated for possible lead toxicity.[29] Research is being directed toward safe and effective physiologic deleading procedures, and recently chromium as a trace element in food appears to decrease lead toxicity in some animals—and presumably in humans. Evidence suggests that trivalent chromium acts as an antidiabetic and antiatherosclerotic agent through its role in sugar and fat (glucose and lipid) metabolism.

Inorganic *nitrates* and *nitrites*, to which prior reference has been made, are a health concern because they contaminate drinking water. They are a special hazard to infants up to 6 weeks of age, to Alaskan Eskimos and Indians, and to those who have a genetically transferred methemoglobinemia. Young infants are susceptible because they have not yet developed certain metabolic enzymes, they have a more readily reactive hemoglobin level that decreases after birth, and they have a small blood volume relative to fluid intake. Milk from cows that drink nitrate-polluted water can be an added threat to children. Although nitrates are used in preservation of some meats and fish, such food is not a common part of infant diets. Continued intake of nitrates may result in death. Although in the United States community water supplies are monitored in accordance with standards set by the Public Health Service, well water on farms has no such surveillance. Any increase in the use of nitrate fertilizers and superphosphate wastes, both being sources of nitrites and produced by bacterial action, will necessitate even greater surveillance and increase the hazard of nitrates and nitrites in well water on farms.

Toxic chemicals in fungi and plants[30,31]

Substances produced in the process of growth and development of certain forms of fungi, more commonly called molds, represent another group of toxic chemicals. Molds cause economic loss through deterioration of food fiber, induce plant diseases, and cause certain pulmonary and invasive diseases in humans. Mold-damaged foods were once considered harmless and used as animal feeds. It is now known that a few molds of grain and other foodstuffs produce toxic chemical metabolites called mycotoxins.

The oldest mycotoxin is ergot, from a fungus that infects cereal grasses, especially rye. Ergot has been the cause of serious epidemics in Western Europe and parts of the USSR since the middle ages. The most recent outbreak of ergotism occurred in 1951 in southern France. Many were stricken and some died. Many showed central nervous system symptoms such as hallucinations, depression, and self-destructive manias.

Among the substances (alkaloids) identified in ergotized grain are some related to LSD (lysergic acid diethylamide). One, ergotine, causes contractions of blood vessels (arterioles) and smooth muscle fibers and is used medically to stop hemorrhage, especially after childbirth; to stimulate labor; to relieve spinal and cerebral congestion in treatment of paralysis of the bladder; and in diabetes (diabetes mellitus). Ergotamine tartrate inhibits certain sympathetic nerve endings and has been used to treat migraine.

Other mycotoxins include the aflatoxins, produced by molds on peanuts and other agricultural products. Even in low concentrations aflatoxins cause acute intoxication, liver damage, and cancer of the liver (hepatoma) in animals. Certain molds on wheat allowed to remain in the fields during the winter produce poisons that cause a blood disorder (alimentary toxic aleukia). In 1944, in a district of the USSR, this disorder affected about a tenth of the population. Another mold that grows on millet has caused epidemic polyuria (excessive urinary excretion). The paucity of knowledge regarding these types of hazards indicates the great need for future research efforts.

Complex organic and inorganic chemical mixtures

In addition to naturally occurring chemicals and plant and fungal poisons, complex organic and inorganic chemical mixtures make up a third group of environmental hazards, which arise as a result of the pollution of air and water by combinations of community and industrial wastes. We are now beginning to learn that the atmosphere and waters of this earth, although extensive, are not limitless and cannot with safety be used as sewers and disposal dumps. Air, water, and consequently food cannot continue to be mistreated in this way without rapidly increasing danger to a rapidly increasing population in a limited world. Most people do not realize that the average person in the United States takes into the body each day about 30 pounds of air, in contrast to only 4 pounds of water and 3.5 of food. The unused remains of these are returned to the environment as contaminants or as potential contaminants.

Air pollutants. There has been belated recognition of air polution as one of the most important sources of chemical hazards, especially in highly urbanized and industrialized societies. More than 200 million tons of toxic material are released into the air above the United States each year, about 1 ton per person. About 60% comes from approximately 100 million internal combustion engines, the other 40% from sources such as factories, power plants, municipal dumps, and private incinerators. The pollutants include carbon monoxide, sulfur oxides, nitrogen oxides, hydrocarbons, and particulates (Table 19-1). They produce ill effects in people

either by short-term, high-level or long-term, low-level exposures.[32-35]

Short, high-level exposures cause acute reactions with increased mortality, especially among the elderly and the chronically ill. There may be an increase in respiratory infections; irritation of the ears, nose, and throat; and impairment of physiologic functioning. The more serious effects that may lead to death include an increase in the severity of chronic illnesses such as bronchitis, emphysema, asthma, and heart attacks (myocardial infarction). In the United States more than 6,000 communities are considered affected by varying degrees of air pollution. Inhabitants who show asthma-like responses, the most frequent response to polluted air, tend to have an increase in β- and γ-globulins in their blood, and biochemical studies have shown that asthma patients also have increased γ-globulins.

The insidious long-term effects of low-level exposures to polluted air are perhaps even more significant, since they result in slowly developing symptoms difficult to define or measure. Chronic diseases of several kinds—including certain malignancies and genetic mutations—may be initiated, general body defense mechanisms impaired, and physiologic function interfered with. The protective cilia of the respiratory tract, for example, may be slowed down or destroyed by atmospheric sulfur oxides, nitrogen oxides, and ozone; and this injury may be associated with and followed by other respiratory disorders and diseases. In the United States chronic bronchitis and emphysema are among the most rapidly increasing causes of death. One out of 20 asthma patients is severely affected by air pollution.

A relationship between pulmonary carcinoma and air pollution has been determined with several pertinent socioeconomic variables taken into consideration, such as smoking habits, economic sta-

TABLE 19-1. Estimated atmospheric emissions, United States, 1968, 10^6 tons per year

Source	Carbon monoxide	Particulates	Oxides of sulfur	Hydrocarbons	Oxides of nitrogen
Transportation	63.8	1.2	0.8	16.6	8.1
Fuel combustion in stationary sources	1.9	8.9	24.4	0.7	10.0
Industrial processes	9.7	7.5	7.3	4.6	0.2
Solid waste disposal	7.8	1.1	0.1	1.6	0.6
Miscellaneous	16.9	9.6	0.6	8.5	1.7
TOTAL	100.1	28.3	33.2	32.0	20.6

tus, and degree of urbanity.[36-38] For example among English nonsmokers, a 10-fold difference was found between the death rates for cancer of the lungs for rural and urban areas. Adult British immigrants to New Zealand and to South Africa have been found to suffer a higher incidence of lung cancer than individuals of the same ethnic stock who were born in those two locations. Among Norwegians living in Norway, where air pollution is low, the lung cancer rate is also low. Among Americans living in the United States, where air pollution is heavy, the rate is twice as high. For Norwegian migrants to the United States, the rate is intermediate.

Correlations have also been found between air pollution and carcinomas other than pulmonary, such as the stomach. In addition, deaths from cirrhosis of the liver have been observed to be higher in heavily air-polluted areas, probably because livers already damaged by alcoholism decompensate when exposed to toxins of polluted air. In the laboratory, injection of animals with trace amounts of extracts of urban atmospheric pollutants from some cities, especially those using predominantly solid fuel, produced a high incidence of tumors of the liver, lymphatic system (lymphoma), and lung (multiple adenomas). Such amounts would be inhaled in about 3 to 4 months by a resident of the cities involved.

Apart from frankly evident air pollution and smog, specific gases may be harmful to health. A study in Chattanooga, Tenn., linked relatively low levels of nitrogen oxides to the susceptibility of children to Asian influenza. Evidence from California indicates that a concentration of carbon monoxide in the air of as little as 10 parts per million for about 8 hours may result in impaired performance because of reduction of ability of the blood to carry sufficient oxygen to the brain. Such levels are common in many cities around the world.

Elevated levels of carbon monoxide have also been associated with the increased probability of motor vehicle accidents and with the inability of individuals to survive myocardial infarctions. Although admittedly several other factors are involved, it is notable that death rates from coronary heart disease are 37% higher for men and 46% higher for women in metropolitan areas with high atmospheric pollution levels than they are in nonmetropolitan areas. Cardiovascular death rates are more than 25% higher for male Chicagoans between 25 and 34 years of age than for their counterparts in rural areas. The difference is 100% for men between 35 and 54 years old and nearly 200% for men between 55 and 64 years old.

Earlier, mention was made of the special problems presented by the addition of tetraethyl lead to gasoline for antiknock and extra power purposes. The consumption of leaded fuels has increased tremendously—from 100,000 pounds in 1940 to 450 million pounds in 1967, an increase of 4,500-fold in 27 years. With a uniform distribution throughout the country of its 90 million cars and trucks, the potential exposure to each individual (200 million) would approximate 2.25 pounds per year—certainly a frightening thought, particularly when lead distribution is not uniform but is concentrated in areas of heavy traffic. This has led to restrictions on the use of leaded gasoline and requirements for catalytic antipollution devices in automobiles. Blood lead values were found to be measurably higher in certain groups such as traffic police officers and persons living adjacent to busy highways. In none of these individuals, however, did lead values approach levels considered hazardous.

Measurable elevations in blood lead values found by regression analysis are interpreted as evidence of a measurable contribution to the body lead burden from the atmosphere, heretofore not considered of significance in comparison with the daily intake from food and beverage. The evidence is made plausible by the postulation of body absorption of up to 50% of atmospheric lead generated in submicron particle size from motor exhausts. Experiments with animals have suggested a need for larger cities to establish an air standard for lead. Several communities, including Philadelphia and New York City, have already established limits on atmospheric lead concentrations. However, these limits may be too liberal in light of the increased toxicity of lead in certain deficiency states observed in advanced age groups and the demonstration of the interference by lead in various endocrine functions.

Although many other examples of the relationship between general atmospheric pollution and ill health might be presented, the seriousness of the situation is perhaps most succinctly illustrated by the recommendation of the California Department of Health (1) that physicians should estimate the contribution that local air pollution conditions may make to the outcome of a patient's illness and (2) that in areas with high air pollution, some patients may benefit from a preoperative period in a clean-air room or chamber before receiving general anesthesia.

Water pollutants. Water is one of the prime necessities of life. Without it survival beyond a few days is impossible. In addition to oral consumption, water is used as a vehicle for the removal of human wastes and as a great cesspool for an ever-increasing complex mixture of industrial and related waste materials. As a result, waterborne epidemics of bacterial diseases, such as cholera and typhoid fever, have been frequent. In the late nineteenth and early twentieth centuries, technologic means were developed to remove these hazards from water, resulting in notable declines in incidence and death rates from infectious enteric diseases. However, it is estimated that 25 million rural Americans lack a safe and adequate supply of drinking water, and epidemics of enteric diseases still occur with alarming frequency.

The hazardous aspects of water have been complicated by the realization of its contamination by viruses. Thus current levels of bacterial purity of water must be maintained, improved practical methods of removing disease-producing viruses must be found, and effective means of surveillance and control of chemical pollution must be developed and put into practice.

We now realize that we live in an environment replete with agents that induce, promote, and accelerate malignancies and genetic mutations. Such substances contaminate our drinking water as well as urban air and other parts of the environment.[39,40] Water pollution with hazardous chemicals may be expected to increase as a result of the development of new industrial chemicals, including highly toxic and carcinogenic halogenated hydrocarbons and many other dangerous substances.[41] Many of these are unstable and may break down in water before they become a significant health hazard. Others will not. An additional threat may be posed, according to some epidemiologic evidence, by a combination of potentially mutagenic chemical agents with radioactivity in water sources.

The National Community Water Supply Study, completed in 1970, made many recommendations for the delivery of an adequate supply of potable and safe water. With specific reference to chemicals, inorganic and organic, the study clearly evidenced the need: (1) to simplify and lower the cost of removing excess chemicals known to be dangerous to the public health; (2) to improve systems to control undesirable concentrations of iron, manganese, hydrogen sulfide, and color as well as organic chemicals causing unpleasant taste and odor; and (3) to develop surveillance techniques or conditioning procedures to eliminate the deterioration in water quality between the time that the water leaves the community water treatment plant and the time it reaches the consumer's tap.

The study led to the enactment of the Safe Drinking Water Act of 1974, which, although an important step forward falls somewhat short of the need in its failure to address the problem of the many small public water supplies of poor quality and the many larger systems that obtain their water from sources polluted by numerous synthetic organic chemicals not affected by the treatment processes often used.[42] Better monitoring of water quality is needed. Instrumentation for routine continuous monitoring with computerized interpretation must be developed. The bacteriologic monitoring of drinking water in the United States employs satisfactory but inefficient methods. A tremendous investment will be necessary, however, if the proper tools and skilled personnel are to be provided so that the presence of potentially toxic materials in the environment can be identified. Only then can the epidemiologic studies necessary to identify the significance of various toxic substance in water be started.

An important breakthrough of recent years in instrumentation has been the development of membrane filters for the collection of microorganisms and large molecules. The membrane filter has permitted many research workers to adapt the filter to a wide range of problems, and the uses to which this type of membrane can be put are still being explored. A similar development might come from the application of other kinds of membranes, particularly the cellulose acetate membranes being used in desalination technology, which have possibilities for the concentration of microorganisms and other contaminants. There are numerous gaps in existing technology, however, that do not allow measurement of current procedures. Current drinking water standards do little more than mention viruses, neglect numerous inorganic chemicals, and identify only the index that is to cover the entire family of organic compounds. A breakthrough required in the next decade is the development of similar concentration and identification techniques for viruses, and particularly the ability to grow the infectious hepatitis viruses in vitro.

With the trend toward multiple use of water sources, plus the complex types of chemical contaminants, new methods of surveillance and treatment are required. Among the new contaminants that must be dealt with are fertilizers, herbicides, fungicides, and irrigation residues from agriculture; detergents from homes and industry; radioactive wastes from power plants and industrial and research installations; a spectrum of heavy metals; a wide variety of salts; and numerous other materials. Many of these are not readily biodegradable, are unaffected by conventional treatment methods, and build up in water supplies. This makes necessary continuous spot-testing techniques based on a variety of approaches, Some measure particular characteristics such as biologic or biochemical oxygen demand and acid concentration. Kits for determination of more than 100 different physical, chemical, or biologic characteristics or contaminants are now available. There are also more versatile instruments, such as the direct-reading colorimeter with which 20 or more different tests can be made. The gas-liquid chromatograph has proved its value in identifying traces of organic materials in water. Continuous water pollution monitoring of effluents from industrial plants can be carried out by ion-selective electrodes, consisting of an ion-selective membrane sealed onto the end of an insulating glass or plastic tube containing an internal reference electrode of silver chloride or calomel. The solution to be measured is placed in the tube, and a voltmeter measures the electric potential developed between it and an external reference electrode when both are immersed in a solution.

The need for knowledge about the health effects of waterborne contaminants will require thorough investigation. The concentration levels at which numerous contaminants, such as mercury, molybdenum, or selenium, cause adverse health effects must be determined. Similarly, the effect of the long-term ingestion of low-level concentrations of toxic, organic materials in water must soon be determined. Some of these toxic materials are carcinogenic, some teratogenic, and some have other toxicologic effects. Some of these effects are only identifiable after many years of exposure; and because the effects are little different from other types of exposure and deterioration, the cause-and-effect relationship is not easily established. This research will be very expensive.

Recognizing the relatively fixed amount of ground and surface water supply, the increasing water needs of the general population and industry, and the need to reuse the available supply to satisfy future demands, the public health and related professions can no longer afford to wait and see what happens. The types of research mentioned are essential and minimal, but this generation also bears a responsibility for the health and well-being of future generations. Realistically, answers to many of the currently identifiable research problems must be obtained quickly so that planners of the environment can formulate rational, economical, and effective plans for the continued growth, development, and survival of society.

Synthetic chemicals

A great achievement in recent decades has been the development of synthetic, longer lasting, more effective insecticides, a breakthrough the significance of which in terms of human health has been of the highest order. It was one of history's most spectacular advances in protecting and improving health; but in terms of certain problems engendered by insecticides, it has become a mixed blessing.[43] Although resistant strains of arthropods developed rather quickly, the several decades of effective use have dispelled the traditional acceptance of arthropod-borne diseases as normal conditions of life in many parts of the world. Ease of use has been important. Chemical control of flies, for example, is not as effective or as desirable as improved sanitation, but the latter had been difficult to accomplish in many places before the demonstrated benefits of flyless life through pesticides. The real impetus to the increased use of pesticides, of course, has been the tremendous benefits they have brought in production of food and fiber.

Researchers are now faced with the necessity of evaluating the unanticipated effects of the host of chemicals that have been in widespread use in ever-increasing amounts since World War II. These are not limited to pesticides, which comprise only a small part of the problem. Many more chemicals are used as food additives, drugs, other household materials, and a complex of industrial effluents that get into the air, food, and water on which we depend. The enormity of the task is not only beyond economic ability, but almost beyond comprehension, when it is known that hundreds of these substances have the potential for interaction with one or more other substances.[44-47] With limited talents and resources, problems must be selected that are representative of many others and attempts made at their solution.

An illustration is provided by the antibiotic griseofulvin. This pharmaceutical is administered by mouth over long periods to humans with certain fungal skin infections. In the laboratory, griseofulvin produces a high incidence of liver tumors in mice at proportionate doses less than these used therapeutically in humans. Meanwhile, a comparatively inert and nontoxic compound, piperonyl butoxide (PB), used in agricultural pesticide formulations to augment or synergize the effects of pyrethrums has been developed. The action of PB appears to inhibit detoxifying enzymes in the insect; thus the insect becomes more sensitive to the insecticidal effects of pyrethrum. Piperonyl butoxide administered alone to infant mice was neither toxic nor carcinogenic. However, when it was administered together with a variety of other agents at nontoxic levels, including griseofulvin, 3,4-benzypyrene (a polycyclic carcinogen widely distributed in the environment), and certain Freons (fluorocarbons with a wide range of domestic and industrial uses), the combination produced a significant synergistic toxicity. In addition, in the case of Freons, combined administrations with PB also produced liver tumors. These results suggest the need to consider interactions, synergistic and otherwise, between unrelated and related agents when testing for effects of environmental pollutants.

A serious problem not generally recognized concerns measuring long-term hazards. Pesticides, for instance, are usually evaluated for acute toxicity. The upper limit of tolerance is established in test animals by administration of high dosages over short time periods. Often, acute toxicity levels are far above exposures humans would ever encounter, but more and more chronic symptoms resulting from long-term exposure to low concentrations of these chemicals are being recognized. Thus acute or short-term effects are no accurate measure of chronic or long-term hazards. Methods of evaluating both acute and chronic hazards must be de-

veloped before irreparable damage is done to mankind or the environment.[48]

It may prove to be true that some substances are carcinogenic, irrespective of dosage, but since so many known carcinogens are widespread in the environment, investigators must develop means to assess the risks. The idea of identifying carcinogens by high dosages administered to exquisitely sensitive animals was predicated on the hope that if such substances were so identified, perhaps humans could avoid them and, furthermore, that unless a no-effect level could be identified, investigators should assume that none existed. Carcinogenic food additives and pesticides could be banned, and naturally occurring carcinogens could be avoided. The idea developed before human analytic capabilities had included a capacity to recognize the wide distribution of minute amounts of known carcinogens.

It is now known that carcinogens cannot be avoided entirely. The relative risks entailed must be assessed to guide future actions. Unless this is done, industrial research and development of pesticides, food additives, and other useful chemical compounds could be curtailed. The already high cost of such research is being driven to new heights. Many companies are sharply curtailing development of new products simply because their research resources are wholly engaged in defensive research to prove the safety of established products. This is the dilemma—not only benefit as opposed to cost but also benefit as opposed to risk. These companies are committed to the premise that products must be as safe as possible, that risks should be minimal. They believe that a long record of wide usage has proved the safety demanded.

The alternatives are not simple, but they suggest that federal funds must be spent either (1) to develop and test the safety of new compounds (after which companies will vie with each other in efficient production) or (2) to develop protocols for testing that are reliable and feasible for the companies to undertake. Otherwise, these extra costs will greatly increase product prices. Another approach might be legislation to permit industrial collaboration that otherwise could be viewed as industry-wide price fixing, outside the public interest. Science can study, but only the public can make such decisions. There is also a great need for reliable methods of extrapolating from animal experiments to humans. Although one could hardly expect this extrapolation to be either direct or simple, it would help tremendously if investigators could determine with repetitive reliability the dosage levels at which no chronic adverse effect can be expected. How this can be done is a subject of much discussion at present.

Meanwhile, it is reasonable to expect the following specific advances to take place:

1. Continued development of biologic pest control. Research on pest predators, radiation sterilization, and chemical sterilizants has increased the potential of control through means other than conventional pesticides and thus has reduced the risk that they offer to human health.

2. Continued development of specific pesticides. The development of agents that have control effects on specific pests permits more precise use of pesticides and reduces the necessity for widespread coverage of agricultural areas with a general purpose agent irrespective of local essential requirements.

3. Development of relatively safe, nonpersistent pesticides. The nonpersistent pesticides in current use are for the most part toxic to humans in the form in which they are used. Fatalities are not uncommon in children who have access to materials, and accidental poisonings occur in the applicators and other workers in recently treated crops. Safe forms of nonpersistent pesticides should be under development.

4. Development of integrated chemical and biologic control programs. The most effective and safest combinations of chemical and biologic control agents for various crops are under investigation and should lead to optimal combinations in the next decade.

5. Development of presently unavailable data on the more subtle and slowly produced effects of synthetic chemicals and pharmaceuticals individually and in combination on the basis of epidemiologic retrospective and prospective studies of large samples of humans.

6. Development of more effective and time-compressing methods of laboratory animal assays of synthetic chemicals and pharmaceuticals.

The principal effect of these developments would be reduction of the chances for the initiation or progression of long-term degenerative disease processes such as carcinogenesis. To this may be added a reduction of the risks of teratogenesis and mutagenesis from certain agricultural and household chemicals, as well as pharmaceuticals, on the human reproductive system.

Chemical hazards—summary

The overall picture of significant environmental chemical pollutants and the disease states that either have been proved or are highly suspected to be related to them has been summarized by Stokinger[16] (Table 19-2). It is noteworthy that several of these diseases are high on the list of causes of morbidity and death as well as the shortening of life expectancy. Stokinger draws the following conclusions with reference to chemical hazards:

1. Airborne pollutants possess greater potential for contributing to the deterioration of human health with age than do waterborne and foodborne contaminants together.

2. As a rule, pollutants express their effects only through interaction with other agents or with some preconditioning factor(s) within the host (a natural consequence of their extremely low ambient levels), be they infectious agents, trace-element deficiencies, or genetic defects of metabolism. Thus environmental pollutants must definitely be included among the multiple factors in the causality of chronic degenerative disease.

3. Acceleration of aging is the dominant characteristic of the effect of many of the top eight of the environmental pollutants. The imposition of such effects on the normal process of aging, whose complexities are only beginning to be understood, compounds the difficulties in either determining causal relationships or assessing the degree of contribution from environmental pollutants.

4. Finally, decidedly in the overall evaluation are the counteractants, the natural antagonists existing both in the environment and within the host. To measure only the pollutants without the counteractants can lead to an overestimation of the health problem. The homeostatic mechanisms leading to adaptation provide the balance to counteract the effects of pollutants at existing levels in the United States among the majority of the population. It is only when this balance is upset through predisposing disease or genetic fault that environmental pollutants exert effects on humans.

Major difficulties militating against the adequate solution of these environmentally induced disease problems include an inability to isolate the effects of any one chemical pollutant from others to which people are exposed; the long latent period for some cancers (e.g., 18 years for aromatic amine-induced bladder cancer); the longer latent period for genetic effects (e.g., more than one generation); grossly inadequate baseline data because of the lack of national registration systems for cancer, birth defects, genetic defects, occupational disease, and the like; and the gross insensitivity of animal testing procedures.

Realization of these concepts and also of the high total costs of human disease clearly indicates the need to strengthen anticipatory and preventive approaches, apart from improving techniques for testing, recognition, and measurement.

What is required is an adequately supported interdisciplinary investigation to determine the distribution of the respective chemical hazards in the environment and their availability to and effects on plants, animals, and humans; to consider ways and means of standardizing data collection and analysis and computer storage and retrieval; to establish avenues of communication and ways of disseminating information among the interdisciplinary groups; and to promote interdisciplinary national and international education in regard to the chemical environment and its effect on health and disease. The efforts of such an investigating group would provide an extremely important start toward the hoped-for identification on a statistically sound basis of those correlations between geochemical and disease patterns that do in fact exist.

PHYSICAL HAZARDS

Physical hazards in the environment were unquestionably the first recognized by humans. The impact of various geologic perturbations such as earthquakes, volcanic eruptions, floods, and tidal waves must have been dramatic. Yet, although natural disasters comprise one of the major areas of

TABLE 19-2. Disease states for which evidence points to environmental pollutants as either direct or contributing causes

Disease	Geographic distribution		Relative incidence index*	Etiologic pollutants and associated conditions	Direct	Contributing
	General	Localized				
Accelerated aging	+		High	Ozone and oxidant air pollutants	+	
Allergic asthma		+	High	Airborne denatured grain protein and other	+	
Cardiovascular and atherosclerotic heart disease	+		High	"Soft" waters and hereditary tendency, Cr-deficiency states, CO(?)		+
Berylliosis		+	Very low	Airborne Be compounds	+	
Bronchitis		+	High	Acid gases, particulates, respiratory infection, inclement climate		+
Cancer of gastrointestinal tract	+		Medium	Carcinogens in food, water, air and hereditary tendency		+
Cancer of respiratory tract	+		Medium	Airborne carcinogens and hereditary tendency		+
Dental caries		+	Low	Se	+	
Emphysema	+		Medium	Airborne respiratory irritants and familial tendency	+	
Mesotheliomas	+		Low	Asbestos and associated trace metals and carcinogens (air, water) (other fibers?)	+	
Methemoglobinemia infant death		+	Low	Waterborne nitrates and nitrites	+	
Renal hypertension		+	Low	Cd in water, food and beverage in As and Se-low areas(?)		+

From Stokinger, H.E.: Am. J. Industr. Hyg. Assoc. J. **30:**195, May-June 1969.
*A composite index derived from an estimate of incidence, geographic extent, and seriousness of effect.

threat to our existence, civilization and its resulting urbanization and industrialization have brought with them several physical threats that make the natural hazards appear minor. Three such outstanding threats are radiation, noise, and accidents.

Radiation[49]

Humans have always been exposed to radiant energy from the sun and from minerals. The extent of the role natural radiation has played in our evolution is a conjecture. The discovery of artificially produced x-rays by Roentgen in 1895 and successful nuclear fission in the 1940s significantly added to the problem.

New sources of radiant energy range from large-scale applications of nuclear energy, especially for electric-power generation, through lasers and microwave technology in industry, to the use of radionuclides and x-rays in the healing arts and the rapidly increasing use of microwaves by the communications industry and in electronic equipment in the home.[50,51] Scientific knowledge and protection against radiation are still at an early stage. The extensive use of x-ray and other devices based on radiant energy has added appreciable exposure loads to many patients. Between one third and one half of all critical medical and dental decisions depend on radiology.[52,53] However, only one sixth of the world's population has access to modern radiology. As a result, throughout the world, including the United States, many diagnostic x-ray films are inferior, uncertainly exposed, insufficiently collimated, poorly developed, and therefore difficult to interpret.

There are great disparities in the amount of radiation exposure used for comparable procedures and in the levels of genetic radiation doses.[54] Even one x-ray film taken during pregnancy may significantly increase the risk of a child developing cancer during the first 10 years of life. This risk is greatest during the first trimester but exists throughout the pregnancy of the mother. An example is provided by a study at the University of Oxford of 15,298 children born between 1943 and 1965, one half of whom died of malignancies before the age of 10 years, the remainder serving as matched controls. Almost twice as many of the children who developed cancer has been exposed to x-rays before birth, as had the children in the control group. If only one x-ray film had been taken, the increased cancer risk was 1.26 to 1. If five films had been taken, the increased risk was more than

double, 2.24 to 1. X-ray films taken during the first trimester of pregnancy led to more than an eightfold increase in risk of childhood cancer. Low doses of radiation for therapy may also involve risk. Thyroid cancer and salivary gland tumors have been associated with x-ray epilation of the scalp in children infected with tinea, a procedure fortunately no longer used. More important has been the repeated observation of leukemia resulting from cumulative doses of gamma radiation less than 50 rad.[55]

An Expert Committee of the World Health Organization found that "the types of cancer in man that are directly or indirectly due to extrinsic factors are thought to account for a large percent of the total cancer incidence." It concluded, "Therefore, the majority of human cancers are potentially preventable."

The rapidly expanding use of ionizing and nonionizing radiation for weapons manufacture, power development, industrial uses, communications, and other purposes introduces into air, water, and land long-lasting pollutants awesome in potentials and implications. Merely safe disposal of the large amounts of radioactive wastes is beginning to appear overwhelming. Also, there are the dangers of leakage from stored materials, of radioactivity transmitted to cooling waters, and the problem of thermal pollution of streams and lakes, possibly eventually of even the ocean itself. A dramatic demonstration of the potential for disaster was the breakdown of the Three Mile Island nuclear power plant near Harrisburg, Pa., in March 1979. The hazards of either or both explosion and core meltdown were averted only with great difficulty. Even so, many people had to be evacuated temporarily, air pollution with radioactive material did occur, and there were considerable economic consequences.

Of the total radiation exposure to which people in the United States are subject, 45% is from natural sources, such as from minerals and from the sky (cosmic); 55% is from man-made sources, most of which (45% of the total) is from medical equipment. Industrial and occupational sources account for 7% of the total; and television screens, luminous clock-watch dials, and fallout plus fission testing account for 1% each. It is important to remember that radiation cannot be directly detected by the senses and that the effects of radiation are irreversible. There is no immunity against radiation; parts of the body escaping damage from one exposure do not have an increased tolerance for future exposures.

Radioactive minerals provide serious radiation hazards for those who mine them. Among a group of 907 white uranium miners with more than 3 years of underground experience, death rates were 17.8 times the normal rate for heart disease, 5 times the normal for respiratory cancer, and 4.5 times the normal for nonautomotive accidents; of 6,000 men who have been uranium miners, it is estimated that 600 to 1,100 will die of lung cancer in the next 20 years.

Two outstanding achievements of recent decades in the field of radiologic health have been the development of an appreciation of the genetic effects of ionizing radiation and the development of a logical basis for standards in radiation protection. Standards in radiation protection have resulted from the cooperative efforts of many people and several organizations. Perhaps the best references are found in the published reports of the Federal Radiation Council, the National Committee on Radiation Protection and Measurements, the International Commission on Radiological Protection, the United Nations Scientific Committee on Atomic Radiation, and the standards hearings of the Joint Commission on Atomic Energy.

Research on the genetic effects of radiation provided an experimental basis for determining the limits of radiation exposure to large groups of people and for improving national and international standards. A nuclear test ban treaty was stimulated by the data accumulated. Although human health was not improved in the sense of curing radiation sickness, it was improved in a preventive sense. Undoubtedly the health of millions of people is more secure today because of the improved standards.

These research developments and higher standards have, from a preventive standpoint, led to a better basis of control in the nuclear industry, in military applications of nuclear energy, and in the medical use of radiation, as in x-ray machines. For the most part, the scientific community and government agencies deserve great credit for meeting this important problem in an orderly way. Yet even more could have been achieved more effectively if organized medicine had taken a more constructive approach toward a critical review of its practices and had encouraged a greater effort in establishing medical x-ray standards and techniques for compliance with them. Many physicians provided significant leadership in the effort, but more valuable human data could have been obtained if the medical profession had participated to a greater extent. Had it been possible earlier to have openly and freely discussed such things as plutonium, tritium, iodine, and krypton from the standpoint of radioactivity, problems involved in their use in the medical and bioscientific areas could have been recognized sooner.

Although some criticism of established standards continues, most knowledgeable scientists and organizations find them acceptable while continuing to reevaluate them. The adequacy of ionizing radiation standards could be improved if additional information were available on the long-term effects of the radiation on animals and humans, obtained through long-term animal studies and epidemiologic studies of human populations. Such studies, however, would require long-term investments, best assured as a national commitment.

Because of the extensive work already done in the field of ionizing radiation, further dramatic breakthroughs are not likely to occur in the near future. It is anticipated, rather, that painstaking research will produce new information in regard to such things as the genetic effects of radiation, the problem of radiation exposure during pregnancy, and radiation problems related to tritium. It is more likely that breakthroughs may occur in the field of nonionizing radiation (which has been investigated to a lesser extent) or perhaps in the area of sonic radiation (ultrasonics) and its biologic effects. Perhaps the achievements to date in ionizing radiation and standards relating to it will serve as a stimulus and model for advances in the more slowly developing field of nonionizing radiation.

Noise[56]

Another environmental physical hazard is noise. This immediately gives rise to perplexing questions: What is noise? Can it actually produce ill effects? If so, how, under what circumstances, and with what other factors? Are any ill effects reversible? How might they be prevented? These and other questions indicate noise to be the least understood of environmental hazards. Noise is more difficult to deal with than most other nuisances or environmental factors because it is partly subjective. In most societies each individual must necessarily accept a certain amount of auditory annoyance, inconvenience, and interference. The essential question is how much, and at what point may actual harm become a possibility.

There are three measurements of noise as a health hazard: intensity, frequency, and length of exposure. Depending on these, the environmental circumstances, and the individuals involved, the effects of noise fall into four general categories[57,58]: annoyance, disruption of activity, loss of hearing, and physical or mental deterioration. Annoyance is the most widespread response to noise. Some claim that annoyance is not related to health, but the issue is academic since noise abatement can be justified from either standpoint. An annoyance condition may aggravate existing physical disorders. Noise can disrupt sleep, lower the body's resistance to disease or physical stress, and generally disturb one's feelings of well-being. Excessive sound can lead to somatic manifestations such as gastric problems, including ulcers, and allergies such as hives. In certain instances excessive noise is thought to aggravate mental illness. Certain types of noise have been shown to cause constriction of the blood vessels near the skin surface, an effect that does not disappear with adaptation to the noise.

Noise can cause the blurring or masking of speech and other wanted sounds. Thus noise from machinery may interfere with instructions to a worker or awareness of safety signals.[59] Several hospitals, especially near airports, have noted an apparent effect on the ability of patients to convalesce.[60,61] In the field of education, noise disrupts attention and hinders concentrated mental effort.

The greatest physiologic effect of noise is temporary or permanent hearing loss. Temporary impairment of hearing, called auditory fatigue, occurs after short exposure to intense noise. Exposure to a continuous high level of sound with inadequate recovery time between exposures may lead to permanent hearing damage.

In terms of the measurements of intensity, frequency, and length of exposure, their effect on hearing loss is as follows. Intensity: exposure to sound pressure levels of over 80 decibels is hazardous, but there appears to be no permanent hearing hazard for levels below 80 decibels. Frequency: the inner ear is more susceptible to damage at middle and especially higher frequencies in the audible range than at low frequencies. Length of exposure: damage increases with increased exposure time. In addition, a fourth factor is the susceptibility of an individual's inner ear to noise-induced hearing loss. Individuals vary in this regard, but about 3% of the general population may be classified as highly susceptible. A survey between 1959 and 1961 by the Public Health Service of the population of the United States showed that the rate of hearing impairment per 1,000 persons was 7.6 for those under 25 years of age, 22.2 for those aged 25 to 44 years, and 51.2 for those between 45 and 64 years. Continued exposure to loud noise was believed to be the major cause of the increase as years of life passed. This agrees with the estimate that about 18 million Americans suffer total or partial deafness and that among working males two thirds of the hearing loss is caused by noise. The progressive loss of hearing as age progresses is known as presbycusis.

Research on hearing acuity has been carried out among the Nilotic tribes in the Sudanese desert.[62] These people live in probably the most noise-free area on earth. They have no musical instruments and apparently do not even sing. Remarkable hearing acuity has been observed, exemplified by their ability to communicate with a normal speaking voice over long distances and a sustained hearing acuity not only among the adults but also in the aged.

In the field of noise as an environmental health hazard, the progress made is the result of patient studies that often appear pedestrian but are necessary if realistic damage-risk criteria are to be established. To assess the physiologic effects of noise, one must either find a population whose necessary noise exposures can be measured in detail or expose experimental animals under controlled conditions. Because of individual differences in susceptibility to damage by noise, either course involves a large number of subjects and is therefore expensive.

Although no breakthroughs can be indicated, progress has been steady. It is now known how much steady 8-hour per day, 5-day per week noise can be endured with negligible risk to hearing. Scientists are on the way toward determining equally reliable damage-risk criteria for intermittent noise exposure and for impulsive noises such as gunfire. The quantification of the relations between the physical and temporal characteristics of intense sound and the degree of both temporary and permanent losses in hearing thus induced has been a significant accomplishment in the past 30 years. There is some agreement that impairment of hearing from exposure to noise can be predicted. As a result, it has been possible to set tolerable limits of noise exposure in both industry and in the community. This is important, since noise-induced deafness is a pervasive disease and social handicap that is suffered by millions.

Once it became possible to demonstrate that a level of 80 decibels or higher was hazardous, it was easier to convince workers to use ear protection devices. This, of course, is more of an educational achievement than a research one, but there now are many drop-forge operators, riveters, jet mechanics, and police officers who still have normal hearing because they use these ear protectors.

One of the most significant achievements has been to show that some of the effects attributed to noise on an anecdotal basis are not folklore. Research on the effects of noise on sleep and on the neurovegetative system should continue, even though results are ambiguous. Study of the physiologic changes in the cochlea associated with noise damage should also continue, even though there seems to be little hope for an ameliorative agent that will reduce significantly or partially restore the damage done by noise.

In the future some of the more subtle effects of noise on mental and physiologic stress may be discovered and measured. This would permit more useful specification of tolerable limits and noise control. Existing research data on the following are highly controversial and need clarification:

1. How much noise energy is tolerable as a daily dosage if the exposure is intermittent instead of continuous?

2. Are very young or very old people more susceptible than others to damage from noise?

3. In the case of persons with noise-induced hearing losses so severe as to cause trouble understanding ordinary conversation, how can the information in the speech signal be recoded so that understanding is restored?

4. Is hearing loss, as measured by changes in auditory threshold, really an adequate measure of the damage actually done by noise? (Recent animal research has indicated that extensive irreversible damage to the hair cells of the cochlea may occur without affecting threshold significantly; if this is

confirmed, it could be considered a genuine breakthrough.)

5. Is an ear that has already been moderately damaged more susceptible to further insult than one that is intact?

6. Are there any long-range consequences of repeated autonomic excitation by noise?

In addition to progress in the acquisition of physiologic and anatomic knowledge, there is need for significantly improved technology in noise abatement with reference to heavy industry, housing, streets, highways, and planes.

Accidents[63,64]

Although many people regard disease or disability fatalistically, this is most apt to be the case with accidents. In fact, even in sophisticated societies there is a tendency to attribute accidents to chance, to fate, or to the will of God, that is, something over which the individual has no control. This negative attitude explains in part why so little attention has been given to the problem until recent years. Yet this is a problem of prime importance. The National Safety Council[65] reported that in 1980 about 105,000 people were killed in accidents of all kinds in the United States. This represents over 12 deaths each hour. The number of nonfatal accidents is more difficult to determine. In 1980 there were also 360,000 permanent impairments and about 9,600,000 temporary total disabilities. About 52 million injuries each year require some medical care or at least 1 day of restricted activity. Injury victims occupy more general hospital beds than any other class of patient (about 20 million bed days per year) and require 80,000 to 100,000 man-years of professional care. The overall cost is a staggering $83 billion annually, consisting of $10.3 billion in medical and hospital expense, $16.6 billion in insurance, and $22.7 billion in wage loss.

Although three fifths of all accidents involve males, there is an interesting sex variation by age. Male accidental death rates exceed those in females of all ages except the most advanced. Accidental death rates for males are only slighly in excess of rates for females up to about the fifteenth year of life, after which male accidental death rates increase sharply and remain high from then on. By contrast, accidental death rates for women remain relatively low until about the sixty-fifth year, after which they rise sharply and exceed those in men at age 85 years. An unusual study[66] of 50,000 child-years of accidental injury in which 8,874 children were followed for 16 years showed that the rate for all medically attended nonfatal injuries was 246 per 1,000 children per year. Boys had more injuries than girls at all ages, and their injury rate increased with age, whereas for girls it went down. It was also noted that children with high rates at one age tended to have high rates in subsequent periods of childhood.

The carnage occurs in all parts of the environment—in automobiles, on the streets, in the home, at work, and on the farm as well as in the city. About five eighths of nonfatal accidents are urban, two eighths are rural nonfarm, and one eighth is rural farm. Because of their dramatic nature, accidents involving public or private vehicles tend to command public attention. These, however, are only a part of a much larger problem. Accidental injuries and deaths by place of occurrence present an interesting picture (Table 19-3).[65] Whereas the home is the most dangerous in terms of frequency of accidents, motor vehicles are most dangerous in terms of serious injury or death.

Motor vehicle accidents rose sharply after World War I and have continued high. Annual numbers of *deaths* from this cause were about 12,500 in 1920 but by 1930 had risen to about 33,000. They have continued to climb more slowly but constantly, except during the tire- and gasoline-rationing period of World War II. By 1973 motor vehicular deaths had reached a high of 55,511. The fuel shortage and establishment of a national speed limit of 55 miles per hour resulted in a drop of 17.4%, to 45,853 deaths in 1975. Since then the toll has begun to creep up again.

Despite the increase since World War I, however, the *death rate* from motor vehicle accidents per 10,000 motor vehicles registered has dropped significantly. Thus in 1920 it was about 13.5 deaths per 10,000 cars registered, whereas now it is only

about 3 deaths per 10,000 cars registered. Similarly, in terms of vehicular *deaths per 100 million miles traveled,* the rate dropped from about 14.0 in 1925 to 3.3 in 1976. Nevertheless, in terms of both absolute numbers of deaths and deaths per 1,000 injuries, motor vehicle accidents are by far the most serious part of the problem.

Occupational injuries and deaths have undergone a considerable reduction. For example, in terms of injuries per million man-hours, the frequency in 1926 was 32 injuries as against about 5 now. Work-related accidents do not appear to be as fatal as motor vehicle accidents, deaths per 1,000 injuries for the former being about one-sixth those of the latter.

Accidents in the home are particularly important because of their frequency, which approaches one half of all accidents. However, in terms of severity, they account for one third of disabling injuries, and as measured by deaths per 1,000 injuries, they exceed occupational accidents. In recent years there has been considerable study of home accidents that has brought out numerous facts of interest. Of social significance is the fact that among women the highest home injury rate is in the lowest income group, whereas among men it is just the opposite, with the home injury rate in the highest income group being twice the rate for men in the lowest income group. It is interesting that whereas the kitchen is the locale of the highest percent of all home accidents (26%), the bedroom is the most fatal place, accounting for 40% of all accidental deaths in the home. This is attributable to the many toxic drugs kept there plus the dangerous habit of some people of smoking in bed. Other fatal accidents in the home occur in living rooms (10%), in

TABLE 19-3. Distribution of accidental injuries and deaths by location, United States, 1980

| Location | Disabling injuries | | | Deaths | Deaths per 1,000 disabling injuries |
	Permanent	Temporary	Total		
Motor vehicle	150,000	1,850,000	2,000,000	52,600	26.3
Home	90,000	3,300,000	3,400,000	23,000	6.8
Work	80,000	2,100,000	2,200,000	13,000	5.9
Other, public	60,000	2,500,000	2,600,000	21,000	8.1
TOTAL	360,000	9,600,000	10,000,000	105,000	10.5

From Accident facts, Chicago, 1980, National Safety Council.

kitchens (12%), on stairs (4%), in dining rooms (3%), and in bathrooms (3%). By type of home accident, falls are the most frequent cause of death, accounting for 32% of accidental deaths. Fires account for 21%, poisons for 14%, suffocation for 10%, firearms for 5%, and gas for 4%.[65]

Accidents should also be considered from the viewpoint of their relative position as a cause of death. Although about 830 infants die accidentally each year, there are numerous other conditions that contribute more to infant mortality. Once the first birthday is approached and passed, however, the picture changes dramatically. Accidents constitute the leading cause of death in age groups 1 to 4, 5 to 14, 15 to 24, and 25 to 34 years. From 35 to 44 years and from 45 to 54 years, accidents are in second place; from 55 to 64 years, fourth place; and beyond 65 years, sixth place as a cause of death. Certainly a problem of this magnitude cannot be ignored. With specific reference to young children, although their death rates in general have declined remarkably in the United States during the past 50 years, largely as a result of control of communicable diseases and improved nutrition, deaths from accidents declined only slightly. In 1975, 70 per 100,000 children between 1 and 5 years died, but almost 40% of the deaths were caused by accidents.[66] Furthermore, it is estimated that there are about 200 severe nonfatal injuries and poisonings in this age group for each death.[67] An essentially overlooked cause of injury and death in children was brought into focus by a study by the New York City Department of Health. It found that 12% of all accidental deaths among children under 15 years of age were caused by falls from heights, with falls from windows representing a significant proportion. This resulted in landmark legislation in 1976 that requires owners of multiple dwellings to provide window guards in apartments where there are children 10 years old or younger. In addition, the health department has provided large numbers of window guards free to families otherwise unprotected. The results have been conclusive with no falls reported where window guards have been installed.[68]

During 1968, the Department of Health, Education, and Welfare conducted analyses of data from a wide variety of sources to obtain an estimate of the incidence of injuries from consumer prod-

ucts. It was not possible to refine the data in terms of severity of the events. The annual total for each broad source or type of injury is shown in the following list:

Household appliances	500,000
Cooking devices	150,000
Kitchen and serving devices	500,000
Home furnishings	500,000
Home fixtures	700,000
Home stairs—falls	1,800,000
Heating devices	175,000
Home tools—power	90,000
Home tools—other	785,000
Cleaning/polishing products	250,000
Garden equipment	500,000
Hobbies and toys	1,100,000
Mobile sports equipment	1,300,000
Camping and fishing	500,000
Other recreational	5,100,000
Flammable liquids	200,000
Clothing injuries (not burns)	200,000
Firearms and explosives	150,000
Cosmetics and toiletries	100,000
Pesticides	75,000
Containers	250,000
Estimated total injuries from consumer products	14,960,000

A special type of accident hazard is presented by the extensive and increasing number of toxic materials in the modern home. In recent years industrial chemists and pharmaceutic research have developed many wonderful products that have contributed greatly to the efficiency and enjoyment of life. Their widespread availability, however, has not been without danger. No longer is it possible to use a "universal antidote." The highly complex nature of many new pharmaceuticals and household products requires a knowledge of their chemical constitution so that a quick and effective remedy may be used in case of toxic ingestion.

It is estimated that each year between 1 and 2 million individuals in the United States, many of them children, accidentally ingest a wide variety of materials in the household; and about 4,700 die, including 115 children under 5 years of age. The total is over twice the annual deaths from tuberculosis and approaches the number of deaths from hypertension.

These substances, as listed by the National Safety Council, are summarized in Table 19-4.[69]

Particular attention should be called to poisonings from lead. Most of these occur in young children from low-income families who live in old hous-

TABLE 19-4. Accidentally ingested poisons, United States, 1975

Drugs and medicaments

Analgesics, antipyretics	1,275
Sedatives, hypnotics	557
Cardiovascular, gastrointestinal, hematologic	222
Psychotropics	215
Antibiotics, hormones, and other synthetics	59
Unspecified medicinal, including anesthetics	804
TOTAL	3,132

Household materials

Alcohol	391
Paints, varnishes, solvents	59
Pesticides, fertilizers, plant foods	30
Heavy metals, corrosives, caustics	29
Cleaning, polishing, disinfecting agents	18
Noxious foods and plants	6
Other unspecified	1,029
TOTAL	1,562

Modified from Accident facts, Chicago, 1977, National Safety Council.

ing, the interiors of which have been painted with many layers of lead-containing paint. The problem is complicated by the frequent casual attitude of many parents who accept pica as normal behavior in young children and by the frequent absence of supervision of children in such socioeconomic circumstances.[29] An estimated 600,000 children between 1 and 6 years of age, mostly in inner cities, have significant blood-lead levels from these sources. Lead paint has been banned for interior household use. Increased awareness and concern about this problem, hastened by the development of improvements in diagnosis and treatment, resulted in the Lead-Based Paint Poisoning Act of 1971, which provides for research, education, diagnosis, and treatment.

As a result of the growing concern over accidental poisoning, many communities in all of the states have developed poison control centers. In 1957 a National Clearinghouse for Poison Control Centers was established by the Surgeon General to (1) disseminate data to centers on ingredients and toxicity of household products and medicines, (2) collect and tabulate data regarding poisoning incidents, and (3) provide and assist public information and education programs on the subject. The poison control centers compile and keep up-to-date a readily usable file on pharmaceutic, household, industrial,

and other substances with data about their composition, toxicity, and antidotes; they provide laboratory analytic service and treatment; they answer telephone requests for first aid information and carry out educational activities for the professions and the public. Some provide follow-up by means of public health nurses or other types of investigators or educators.

An interesting question that calls for more study is the relationship of mental health to so-called accidental poisoning. Unquestionably a certain number of such "accidents" actually represent either conscious or subconscious attempts at suicide or homicide. With regard to the latter is the possible factor of withheld or avoided supervision, warning, or prompt treatment by some parents, older children, or spouses. The reader is referred to Chapters 28 and 29 for further discussion of this subject.

A significant reduction in the total number of accidents in the near future is unlikely, but recent developments may eventually bring improvements. Some of these are considered in detail in Chapter 21. New concepts from the fields of biostatistics, medicine, engineering, and behavioral science are providing impetus for experimental studies and the design of safety programs. Work is underway to determine injury thresholds of the human body relative to impact forces, data improvement to the design of protective devices. Neurosurgeons have studied head injuries from a variety of high-impact accidents. Public interest has increased somewhat, and there has been national legislative activity such as the Highway Safety Acts, the Occupational Safety and Health Act, and legislation relating to fabric flammability and other hazards to child safety, product safety, and consumer protection; these can provide impetus for increased attention to accident potentials in private and industrial sectors.

As discussed in Chapter 34, in terms of secondary prevention, health personnel and the medical profession seek to improve emergency medical services, but there is an urgent need for a strong, coordinated national accident prevention program to (1) conduct research, (2) provide technical assistance to states and communities, (3) train personnel, and (4) supply financial support. In the long run the savings could be enormous. An effective prevention and control program for accidents could result in (1) an annual prevention of 30,000 fatal injuries, (2) the saving of 60,000 human lives annually through prompt medical care, (3) the prevention of 10 million accidental injuries each year, (4) an annual savings of 2 million hospital bed days now required for accident victims, (5) an annual savings of 8,000 man-years of medical care services, and (6) an annual $3 billion reduction in direct costs to accident victims. Accidental death and disability truly represent the "neglected disease" of modern industralized society in this country.

CONCLUSION

Only some of the environmental hazards that confront modern society have been discussed in this chapter. These have given rise to the rapidly growing field of environmental medicine, which applies the principles and knowledge of biologic and epidemiologic research to an understanding of a complex of physical, physiologic, and psychologic disturbances. The results of these disturbances now constitute the major portion of conditions that come to the attention of the medical practitioner, unfortunately too often too late.

Patterns of morbidity and mortality are changing. Evidence from data obtained from past efforts may not be relevant to future events. People, their hazards, and their diseases are ever changing. The illnesses and injuries that will be experienced within a few decades will not be the same as those today, much less yesterday. Environmental factors certainly enter into their causation, but to what extent and in what manner is still largely to be determined, and only by means of research.

Several years ago the direct health effects of environmental hazards on humans were summarized by the President's Science Advisory Committee. Five categories of increasing severity were listed: (1) annoyance, irritation, and inconvenience, which although certainly real, produce effects that are uncertain and almost impossible to measure; (2) physiologic effects of unknown clinical significance, which occur on a transient basis and the cumulative effect of which is uncertain; (3) worsening of existing diseases or disability and an increase in the general level of sickness, the determination or evaluation of which is open; (4) a general increase in the death rate, again open; and (5)

initiation of specific progressive disease, an area also with many questions unanswered.

The general conclusion was that the human effects of environmental hazards were poorly understood, but because of the obvious importance of the effects, intensive and extensive study could not be delayed.

In any consideration of most needed research in this field, the following fundamental characteristics of environmental hazards stand out:

1. They tend to be ubiquitous.
2. They tend to be multifaceted as to sources and effects.
3. They are generally insidious in their action time frame.
4. Exposure to many is of a low level, insufficient to produce acute reactions.
5. They often act in concert and may potentiate one another.
6. By the time their effects are recognizable, they are often irreversible.

Despite these characteristics, it has been customary for science, industry, and government to study and deal with environmental hazards separately. For example, is mercury hazardous, in what physiologic way, at what levels, and with what effects? The same question is asked about lead, pesticides, individual pharmaceuticals, sulfur oxides, and so on, each separately, each usually in terms of acute effects, and each in terms of toxicity alone; possible carcinogenic, teratogenic, mutagenic, and psychic effects are ignored. This approach has led to the fallacious tendency to decide that X is the toxic or dangerous level of a particular substance or hazard and that to be conservative perhaps one tenth of that amount should be designated as the maximum permissible level. This ignores the fact that humans are not exposed to one substance alone but to an extensive and cumulative spectrum of hazards, each of which might even be minimal but the total burden or effect of which might be critical or overwhelming.

From an overall viewpoint present efforts for the study of environmental hazards to humans may be considered to fall into these categories: (1) the search for and application of new experimental and clinical methods of defining health risks for known or potential environmental contaminants and hazards; (2) more intensive studies of synergistic potentials of the innumerable combinations of environmental hazards with particular consideration of the development of toxicity, carcinogenicity, teratogenicity, mutagenicity, physical injuries, and psychic stress; and (3) the categorization of physiologic and biochemical hazards in terms of human populations at risk.

REFERENCES

1. Harrison, G., Gates, D., and Holling, C.S.: Ecology: the great chain of being, Ekistics **27:**161, March 1969.
2. U.S. Department of Health, Education, and Welfare: A strategy for a livable environment; report of the Task Force on Environmental Health and Related Problems, Washington, D.C., June 1967, U.S. Government Printing Office.
3. Meadows, D.H., Meadows, D.L., Randers, J., and others: The limits to growth, Washington, D.C., 1972, Potomac Associates.
4. Calhoun, J.B.: Population density and social pathology, Sci. Am **206:**139, Feb. 1962.
5. Calhoun, J.B.: Ecological factors in the development of behavioral anomalies. In Zubin, J., editor: Comparative psychopathology, New York, 1967, Grune & Stratton, Inc.
6. McCue, G.M., Ewald, W.R., Jr., and the Midwest Research Institute: Creating the human environment; report of the American Institute of Architects, Urbana, 1970, University of Illinois Press.
7. Dubos, R.: Environmental biology, BioScience **14:**11, Jan., 1964.
8. Health hazards of the human environment, Geneva, 1972, World Health Organization.
9. U.S. Department of Health, Education, and Welfare: Man's health and the environment—some research needs; report of the Task Force on Research Planning in Environmental Health Science, Washington, D.C., March 1970.
10. Harmison, L.T.: Toxic substances and health, Public Health Rep. **93:**3, Jan.-Feb. 1978.
11. Starr, M.P., editor: Global impacts of applied microbiology, New York, 1964, John Wiley & Sons, Inc.
12. Communicable Disease Center: Annual supplements, morbidity and mortality weekly reports, Atlanta; U.S. Department of Health, Education, and Welfare.
13. May, J.M., editor: Studies in disease ecology, New York, 1961, Hafner Publishing Co., Inc.
14. Sartwell, P.E., editor: Maxey-Rosenau preventive medicine and public health, New York, 1965. Appleton-Century-Crofts.
15. U.S. Department of Health, Education, and Welfare, National Center for Health Statistics: Vital statistics rates in the United States 1940-1960, Washington, D.C., 1968, U.S. Government Printing Office.
16. Stokinger, H.E.: The spectre of today's environmental pollution, Am. Ind. Hyg. Assoc. J. **30:**195, May-June 1969.
17. Epstein, S.S.: Control of chemical pollutants, Nature **228:**816, Nov. 28, 1970.
18. Singer, S.F., editor: Global effects of environmental pollution, New York, 1970. Springer-Verlag New York Inc.
19. Merck manual, ed. 13, Rahway, N.J., 1977, Merck Sharp and Dohme Research Laboratory.
20. Zaki, M.H., and others: Dieldrin in milk: the experience of Suffolk County, New York, Am. J. Public Health, **68:**260, March 1978.
21. Wickizer, T.M., and others: Polychlorinated biphenyl contamination of nursing mothers' milk in Michigan, Am. J. Public Health **71:**132, Feb. 1981.
22. Claxton, L.D., and Barry, P.Z.: Chemical mutagenesis: an emerging issue for public health, Am. J. Public Health **67:**1037, Nov. 1977.
23. Hemphill, D.D.: Trace substances in environmental health, Columbia, 1969, University of Missouri Press.
24. Dixon, J.R., Lowe, D.B., Richards, D.E., and others: The role of trace metals in chemical carcinogenesis—asbestos cancers, Cancer Res. **30:**1068, April 1970.
25. Selikoff, I.J., Hammond, E.C., and Churg, J.: Asbestos exposure, smoking and neoplasia, J.A.M.A. **204:**106, April 8, 1968.
26. Selikoff, I.J., and Hammond, E.C.: Asbestos-associated disease in United States shipyards, C.A. **28:**87, March-April 1978.
27. News item: High rate of asbestosis found in families of shipyard workers, Occupational Health and Safety Letter, Oct. 22, 1981.
28. News item: 8,200 excess cancer deaths due to asbestos exposure, Occupational Health and Safety Letter, June 22, 1982.
29. News item: Lead poisoning of children continues, Nation's Health, June 1982.
30. Wogan, G.N., editor: Mycotoxins in foodstuffs, Cambridge, 1964, The M.I.T. Press.
31. Russell, F.E., and Saunders, P.R., editors: Animal toxins, New York, 1967, Pergamon Press, Inc.
32. Goldsmith, J.R.: Effects of air pollution on human health. In Stern, A.C., editor, Air pollution, ed. 2, New York, 1968, Academic Press, Inc.
33. Anderson, D.O.: The effects of air contamination on health, Can. Med. Assoc. J. **97:**528, 585, 802, Sept. 23, 1967.
34. Borne, H.G.: Pathobiology of air pollutants, Environ. Res. **1:**178, Jan. 1967.
35. Toxicologic and epidemiologic bases for air quality criteria (special issue), J. Am. Pollution Control Assoc. **19:**629, 1969.
36. Kuschner, M.: The causes of lung cancer, Am. Rev. Respir. Dis. **98:**573, Oct. 1968.
37. Hartwell, J.L. (1951); Hartwell, J.L., and Shubik, P. (1957); Peters, J. (1969): Survey of compounds

which have been tested for carcinogenic activity, PHS Pub. No. 149, Washington, D.C., 1970.

38. Hanna, M.G., Jr., Nettesheim, P., and Gilbert, J.R., editors: Inhalation carcinogenesis; proceedings of the Biology Division Conference, 1970, Oak Ridge National Laboratory, Oak Ridge, Tenn.

39. Epstein, S.S., and Shafner, H.: Chemical mutagens in the human environment, Nature **219**:385, July 27, 1968.

40. Gruener, N., and Lockwood, M.: Mutagenic activity in drinking water, Am. J. Public Heatlh, **70**:277, March 1980.

41. Ibrahim, M.A., and Christman, R.F.: Drinking water and carcinogenesis: the dilemmas, Am. J. Public Health **67**:719, Aug. 1977.

42. Okun, D.: Drinking water for the future, Am. J. Public Health **66**:639, July 1976.

43. Report of the Secretary's Commission on Pesticides and Their Relationship to Environmental Health, Washington, D.C., 1969, U.S. Government Printing Office.

44. Moser, R.H.: Diseases of medical progress, ed. 3, Springfield, Ill., 1971, Charles C Thomas, Publisher.

45. Conney, A.H.: Drug metabolism and therapeutics, N. Engl. J. Med. **280**:653, March 20, 1969.

46. Jillette, J.R., editor: Proceedings of symposium on microsomes and drug oxidations, New York, 1969, Academic Press, Inc.

47. Selye, H.: Adaptive steroids—retrospect and prospect, Perspect. Biol. Med. **13**:343, Spring 1970.

48. Report of the NCI/Bionetics study of pesticides, J. Natl. Cancer Inst. **42**:1101, 1969.

49. Gitlin, J.N., and Lawrence, P.S.: Population exposures to x-rays, U.S., 1964; report on the Public Health Service x-ray exposure study, PHS Pub. No. 1519, Washington, D.C.

50. Moore, W.: Biological aspects of microwave radiation—a review of hazards, Washington, D.C., July 1968, U.S. Public Health Service.

51. U.S. Public Health Service: An annotated bibliography of regulations, standards, and guides for microwaves, ultraviolet radiation, and radiation from lasers and television receivers, Washington, D.C., April 1968.

52. U.S. Public Health Service: Report of the Medical X-ray Advisory Committee on Public Health Considerations in Medical Diagnostic Radiology, Washington, D.C., Oct. 1967.

53. U.S. Public Health Service: Radiation exposure overview: diagnostic dental x-rays and the patient, Washington, D.C., July 1968.

54. U.S. Public Health Service: Radiation bio-effects, summary report, Washington, D.C., 1968.

55. Dreyer, N., and Friedlander, E.: Identifying the health risks from very low-dose sparsely ionizing radiation, Am. J. Public Health, **72**:585, June 1982.

56. Ward, W.D., and Fricke, J.E., editors: Proceedings of the conference on noise as a public health hazard, Washington, D.C., June 13-14, 1968, Am. Speech Hearing Assoc. Rep. No. 4, Feb. 1969.

57. Kryter, K.D.: The effects of noise on man, New York, 1970, Academic Press, Inc.

58. Welch, B.E.: Physiological effects of noise, an overview, Fed. Proc. **32**:2091, Nov. 1972.

59. Cohen, A.: Noise effects on health, productivity and well-being, Trans. N.Y. Acad. Sci. **39**:910, 1968.

60. Farr, L.E.: Medical consequences of environmental home noises, J.A.M.A. **202**:171, Oct. 16, 1967.

61. Fife, D., and Rappaport, E.: Noise and hospital stay, Am. J. Public Health **66**:680, July 1976.

62. Rosen, S., and others: Presbycusis study of a relatively noise-free population in the Sudan, Ann. Otol. Rhinol. Laryngol. **71**:727, 1962.

63. McFarland, R.A.: Injury—a major environmental problem. Arch. Environ. Health **19**:244, Aug. 1969.

64. Marland, R.E.: Injury epidemiology, J. Safety Res. **1**(3):17, Sept. 1969.

65. Accident facts, Chicago, 1981, National Safety Council.

66. Manheimer, D., and others: Fifty thousand child-years of accidental injuries, Public Health Rep. **81**:519, June 1966.

67. Palmisano, P.A.: Targeted intervention in the control of accidental drug overdoses by children, Public Health Rep. **96**:150, March-April, 1981.

68. Spiegel, C.N., and Lindaman, F.C.: Children can't fly: a program to prevent childhood morbidity and mortality from window falls, Am. J. Public Health, **67**:1143, Dec. 1977.

69. Accident Facts, Chicago, 1977, National Safety Council.

CHAPTER 20

Occupational health

First ask, of what trade are you?

Ramazzini

HEALTH AND THE WORKPLACE

A joint committee of the International Labor Office and the World Health Organization has defined the objectives of occupational health as follows:

the promotion and maintenance of the highest degree of physical, mental and social well-being of workers in all occupations; the prevention among workers of departures from health caused by their working conditions; the protection of workers in their employment from risks resulting from factors adverse to health; the placing and maintenance of the worker in an occupational environment adapted to his physiological and psychological condition.[1]

Occupational health and safety has technical, legal, political, and economic aspects, but the World Health Organization definition is absolutist in tone: it indicates that worker health takes precedence over all other factors including the economic conditions of the worker, the family, and the community. That may not always be the case.

Occupational health and safety have been separate issues historically, legally, and technically. Safety preceded health as a social, economic, and legal concern because the etiology and cost of an injury could be immediately recognized. Compensation laws were written to deal with such issues, not with the illness that might occur 20 or 30 years after exposure to a toxic chemical. An effort has been made in law and in educational programs to combine the two aspects of worker health, but safety issues remain more in the province of the industrial hygienist, whereas occupational diseases are treated as medical problems. In this chapter the term *occupational health* will be used to refer to both occupational diseases and injuries.

The subject is of major importance to the public's health even though official health agencies are not always involved at the state or local level. A substantial proportion of the population spends about one quarter of its time either at work or in transit between home and work. Although the transit process and the home environment are the source of many hazards, the workplace has special significance: some of the hazards are unique and complex (such as radiation and chemicals that may affect a fetus); the problems have a direct economic impact on workers, their families, the workplace owners, and the entire community; and the voluntary exchange transaction that takes place between worker and manager (work for wages) is such that a contest can develop over fault. According to the National Safety Council, there were 10 million disabling injuries in the United States in 1980: 2 million caused by motor vehicle accidents, 2.2 million work related, 3.4 million in the home, and the remainder elsewhere.[2] In addition to the injuries, however, the work environment is laden with products and procedures that can cause disease and illness both in the unborn and in retirement. The magnitude of these problems is only beginning to become apparent. The working hypothesis of public health is that all of these injuries and illnesses can be prevented. Society will determine whether it is worth the price.

CONFLICTS OF FACT, PERCEPTION, AND VALUE

That an employer is responsible for the health of workers is a relatively recent concept in the Western world. Both workers and workplace owners have long assumed (1) that work is necessary, (2) that all work entails some risk, and (3) that people accept work knowing about the hazards and assuming them as part of the cost they must pay for the wages they receive. An individual worker finds it difficult to comprehend the importance of a potentially serious illness or injury when the probability of experiencing it is slight. If management points out the low probability of the problem and the high cost of preventing it (with the implied or explicit warning that prevention costs might result in a plant shutdown), the risks may be assumed without further challenge. However, society will pay for those inevitable events both directly and indirectly.

The direct costs of occupational disease and injury appear as higher product prices caused by absenteeism and worker's compensation payments. The indirect costs appear as welfare costs, unemployment costs, aid to families with dependent children, medical and rehabilitation costs, and a variety of other costs related to subsequent dependency. The total amounted to more than $30 billion in 1980.[2]

Owners have accepted some of the cost of injury through safety programs and worker's compensation plans. The adage, "safety pays," is true up to a point. An industry with high injury rates will have to pay more money into the worker's compensation fund, and these costs have to be added to product price or subtracted from profits. The costs appear fairly quickly after the accident occurs, and the fault is usually easy to determine. Moreover, the compensation laws of most states have set aside the right of an employee to sue an employer for damages if compensation payments are accepted, thus limiting the cost to management. Disease problems, however, tend to occur much later, often 20 or 30 years after exposure to the hazard. The worker may be killed in an automobile accident before the cancer develops or may be working in another industry in another part of the country. It is far more difficult to establish the cause of the disease since some people with the same exposure will not develop the disease and others without such exposure may develop an identical problem. Owners are inclined to avoid the costs of preventing such illnesses since they are not likely to accrue the benefits of their prevention efforts. The costs of preventing accidents may yield benefits through lower worker's compensation payment rates and less lost work time, but preventing illness 20 or 30 years later benefits the Social Security system, state welfare

programs, and families, not the business. Job injury victims average about 60% of their lost income through all sources of payment, while victims of occupational disease obtain only 40%, most of which comes from Social Security and welfare payments rather than from the compensation fund.[3] The courts have begun to hold businesses accountable for such problems, and to avoid the high cost of civil suits, some industries have favored inclusion of compensation for illness in the state-run compensation programs. Compensation after the fact may be less costly to the industry than prevention since the payments will occur much later at a discounted rate. Without the intervention of law, the costs of failing to prevent occupational disease can be externalized to other segments of society. Occupational health legislation seeks to internalize those costs to the business so that the product or the service will carry the full social costs of production or the cost of prevention. It is the job of public health to make the net cost of prevention less than the cost of compensation.

Conflicts occur because of different self-interests, a lack of knowledge, and different perceptions of what is fair. The worker is concerned about income; the manufacturer about price. The manufacturer will not add to labor costs unless some monetary benefit can be realized or unless forced to by law. Voluntary absorption of an additional labor cost to prevent a disease without any immediate benefit will make a single manufacturer less competitive. Legislation affecting all manufacturers can restore that balance but may make the industry less competitive with foreign manufacturers.

Some problems appear to occur more commonly in certain industries but cannot yet be linked to a specific hazard. Brain cancer has been found to be more common in certain petrochemical plants, but no cause has been identified. It is difficult to hold an owner accountable for a problem that cannot be prevented. Sometimes knowledge is adequate, but different values or ideas of what is fair result in a conflict about responsibility. For example, asbestos workers are at high risk of certain lung diseases. Asbestos workers who smoke are at greater risk. Should smoking asbestos workers be compensated at the same rate as nonsmoking workers or are they guilty of contributory negligence?

In addition to the economic importance of the work environment to the community, it has both direct and indirect spillover effects on the health of the community. In most instances, the work environment cannot be walled off: its effluents intermingle with the air, the water, the sewage, and the land-use problems of the surrounding community. The disposal of toxic wastes presents special problems—the same chemicals handled by workers in the plant can affect the community years later. Industrial accidents may cause a sudden spill of hazardous material into the community's water supply or air. Heavy trucks rumbling through residential streets present special hazards for young children. Workers do not leave the hazards in the workplace; asbestos fibers and toxic chemicals are carried into the house in clothing and have been shown to cause the same diseases at home as they do in the workplace.

There are indirect consequences as well: marginal companies that have avoided their responsibility for worker health in the short run eventually pay the price, which may involve shutdown and unemployment. Although local health departments do not often have the explicit authority or the resources to combat such problems and may accept them just as the rest of the community does, they can play an important role in surveillance, fact finding, planning, and correction.

Business associations constantly strive to reduce the scope of governmental intervention, and many business and political leaders believe that the forces of marketplace competition will serve to correct the health problems that may exist in the workplace, but even a cursory review of history since the industrial revolution shows that that is not the case. In the absence of regulatory controls, mine owners would not take steps to reduce the build-up of coal dust, nor would the asbestos industry adopt an adequate safety standard. The conflict that exists between wages and profits is such that governmental intervention is essential: the market does not internalize the costs of disability and dependency into the pricing of products and services. The cost of prevention does not always yield recognizable or sufficient benefits to the owners to prompt corrective or preventive action, and both direct and indirect spillover effects require that the community intervene with the force of law to establish an adequate program.

BACKGROUND

Ramazzini is usually considered to be the father of occupational health, based on the publication of *De morbis artificium diatriba* in 1700. Modern occupational health is an outcome of the Industrial Revolution in nineteenth-century England. As a result of the rapid development of deplorable work conditions in general and the exploitation of women and children in particular, numerous laws were passed for the protection of workers. During the first half of this century, America profited by the events, researches, and measures that had previously occurred in England, even to the extent of adoption by some states of some of the earlier English legislation. The Massachusetts Department of Factory Inspection was established in 1867, but further expansion of the role of the state was slow because of the three common-law notions that still affect occupational health programs: (1) that workers contribute through their own negligence to their problems, (2) that fellow workers share in the responsibility by creating or failing to correct unsafe conditions, and (3) that accepting a job means an assumption of the risks that go with it.[4]

In 1908 Congress passed the Federal Employers' Liability Act, which made railroads and other interstate carriers liable for industrial injuries sustained by their employees. At that time the Wainwright Commission in New York showed that only one out of every eight injured men was awarded any compensation and that he actually received only about a third of what was awarded. The other two thirds went for insurance adjusters, legal advice, and commissions. Various states had previously enacted workmen's compensation laws, but these early laws were declared unconstitutional by the courts. The year 1911, however, marked the beginning of the first valid state workmen's compensation laws, and no less than 10 states passed legislation in that year alone. By 1920 40 states had workmen's compensation laws, but interest waned after that until the 1960s when a broadened concern for environmental protection raised new questions about disease as well as injury and accidents. The principle had been established that the owners were responsible for the cost of medical care and the subsequent disability caused by accidents but that the worker gave up the right to sue the owners for additional damages when compensation payments were accepted. This allowed the owners to amortize their costs in a regular fashion, similar to other debts.

The whole subject of worker's compensation has become more complex and controversial in the

United States in recent years. Some compensation laws have been amended to remove the waiver of the right to sue and some court decisions have maintained that the owners were still susceptible to suit if they willfully exposed the workers to a hazardous situation. By 1979 approximately 78.6 million workers were covered by worker's compensation plans, and benefits paid totaled $11.9 billion, almost four times the amount paid out in 1970. As courts ruled that more and more disabilities were work related, business leaders and some economists began to attack the plans as too liberal. To some extent the systems have become a part of the general welfare system and thus are exposed to the same public ambivalence and, at times, hostility.

Compensation has become entangled in special interest group legislation or collective bargaining, which places certain problems in a separate category, such as black lung (coal workers' pneumoconiosis) or exposure to agent orange during the Vietnam War. Some disabilities are compensated more fully than are others. The administration of the programs has become very costly because of the expensive and extensive legal maneuvering that occurs. Certain categories of workers are treated as special risk categories and compensated differently than others, often obtaining compensation for total and permanent disability when they are perfectly capable of working in another occupation. These problems have caused many experts and legislators to urge a more uniform, national approach to compensation, but it seems unlikely that any basic reform in the nation's social insurance systems can occur in the immediate future that would both correct some of the abuse and bring about greater equity.

The period from 1910 to 1920 witnessed the establishment of occupational health as a medical specialty. The Department of Labor was established as a separate Cabinet entity and the Bureau of Mines of the Department of the Interior and the Office of Industrial Hygiene and Sanitation (later the Division of Occupational Health) of the Public Health Service came into existence. An Industrial Hygiene Section was established in the American Public Health Association (now called the Section on Occupational Health and Safety) and the National Safety Council was organized. The American Association of Industrial Physicians and Surgeons (now the Industrial Medical Association) was formed in 1915, and minimum standards for medical service in industry were adopted that same year by the Committee on Industrial Medicine and Traumatic Surgery of the American College of Surgeons. In 1937, the American Medical Association created the Council on Industrial Health to coordinate all medical efforts in the industrial health field. The *Journal of Industrial Hygiene* and the first specialized teaching of the subject appeared in schools of public health at about the same time.

Before the passage of the Social Security Act in 1935, little progress had been made by state health agencies in occupational health. Up to that time only five states engaged in any activities designed for the benefit of industrial workers. The first were instituted in 1913 in New York and Ohio. The Social Security Act made funds available for the expansion of state and local programs with the result that by 1950 all of the states and Alaska, Hawaii, Puerto Rico, and the District of Columbia were engaged in some type of activity to improve the health and safety of workers.

Since 1960 occupational diseases have drawn increasing attention partly as a result of continued research in toxicology and the rapid increase in production and use of complex chemical products. Reproductive research has heightened awareness of the special problems of women in the workplace. The subject has been surrounded by more mythology than fact until recent years. Even though women are on the average smaller and physically less powerful than men and have some unique considerations related to reproduction, there is little evidence that they have different risks because of occupational exposures. Many special risks have been alleged, such as greater susceptibility to lead poisoning, organic solvents, and carcinogens. The allegations have resulted in exclusion of women from certain work areas rather than an effort to alter the work environment, even though research has not substantiated important differences.[5] Generally those substances that may harm a fetus should be considered hazardous for men as well, and the objective should be to protect all workers from the hazards. In certain plants women who could become pregnant have been excluded from high-risk areas, which has resulted in legal challenges to a management policy that essentially required sterilization as a condition of employment. Problems can occur after giving birth as well because of contaminated clothing or toxic substances that may be discharged in breast milk.[6]

The epidemiology of occupational disease is an extremely complicated subject.[7] There is usually a long latent period during which time the worker may be exposed to a variety of agents in different plants and in different locations. Some exposures may have occurred because of a momentary accident that resulted in the unique combination of two or more products not intended by the manufacturer and never counted in the inventory of substances produced or used in the plant. There are rarely any adequate data about exposure levels, and lacking reliable, quantitative data about dosage, it is difficult to develop a dose-response hypothesis. Studies designed to demonstrate that there is no hazard from a particular product have to be very large and very sensitive, minimizing the random errors that are less important in studies of a positive relationship. Lacking that and quantitative data about exposure, such studies are only nonpositive, not negative.

The scientific study of occupational disease presents special problems to the lawyers, courts, politicians, and public health workers whose job it is to prevent the problems in the first place or to provide equitable compensation for those injured or made ill. The standards of evidence in science are higher than those in civil law with no necessity to conclude the debates. The courts and other public officials have to make decisions based on what is known at the time. Furthermore, they have the special problem of deciding whether to prohibit something until it can be proved safe or to allow something until it can be proved hazardous: an ethical question not subject to laboratory proof.

NATURE AND SCOPE OF THE PROBLEM

The hazards to the work force may be looked at in terms of injuries, illnesses and deaths from accidents, and occupational diseases caused by or occurring in the workplace. Valid national statistics on the nature and causes of occupational diseases and industrial accidents have not been available in the past. Detailed statistics have been compiled by several states, but these have not been usefully comparable because of different definitions and different reporting requirements. In recent years, as the programs of the Occupational Safety and Health Administration of the U.S. Department of Labor have become more extensive, reporting has improved. Even so, it is widely acknowledged that occupationally related deaths exceed the reported incidence by a factor of five and that job injuries are 10 times more frequent than official reports indicate.[8] The error factor for occupationally related diseases is unknown but probably exceeds 100.

For occupational injuries and deaths caused by work accidents, some data are available from the Bureau of Labor Statistics, the National Safety Council, the National Health Survey, and individual states. It should be pointed out, however, that not all of the states require reporting by employers. Because of increased emphasis placed on occupational safety since the Korean War, the number of deaths caused by accidents on the job has decreased from 14,200 in 1955 to 13,000 in 1980 despite a 63% increase in the number of workers (from 59.4 million to 96.8 million). This means a reduction in the death rate from 24 per 100,000 workers in 1955 to 13 per 100,000 workers in 1980.[2]

In 1979 11.3 million people reported that they had been injured on the job, but injury rates appear to be declining. Disabling injuries have remained at about 2.2 million per year since 1965 despite the increased size of the work force at risk. These figures, developed by the National Safety Council from a variety of sources, differ from the official figures of the Bureau of Labor Statistics, which reported 5.96 million occupational injuries in 1979 and only 4,950 deaths.[9]

Even though the accuracy of injury reporting is improving, the reported occupational illness incidence rate will vary as understanding of the relationship between the hazards of the work environment and illness improves. As the incidence of some occupational illnesses is reduced through education and prevention techniques, other linkages will be established through epidemiologic research, which should increase the reported incidence of occupational illness.

There are several reasons for poor occupational disease data. Nonrecognition and nonreporting of diseases are probably paramount. In addition, there are long development times before some occupational diseases become apparent. For example, silicosis does not occur usually until after about 15 years of exposure. Other dust diseases, such as byssinosis and asbestosis, also have prolonged developmental periods. In addition, there is a lag time between the onset of the disease process in the body and clinical evidence of frank disease. This holds true even though exposure may have long since ceased. Cases of mesothelioma, one type of lung cancer, have become manifest as long as 25 years after the last known exposure to asbestos.

Despite their inexactness, some examples of the incidence of various occupational diseases may be illustrative. It has been estimated that 12.8% of active coal miners and 21.2% of those retired, disabled, or unemployed have radiographic evidence of pneumoconiosis;[10] 173,000 may be disabled.[11] Three and a half million American workers are exposed to asbestos on the job. Significant numbers of them develop asbestosis, which often leads to mesothelioma, as previously mentioned. Studies of asbestos insulation workers indicate that half of the people who had worked in the trade for 20 years had x-ray evidence of asbestosis, and 1 in every 10 of their deaths was caused by mesothelioma, in contrast with 1 in 10,000 in the general public.[12] As many as 11 million American workers have been heavily exposed to asbestos and the possibility of suffering from a severe epidemic of disease related to that exposure hangs over their heads like Damocles' sword. Byssinosis, a lung disease caused by cotton mill dust, was long said not to occur in America. It is now known to be common. Talc, diatomite, sugarcane fiber, and dust from moldy silage all produce various forms of respiratory system diseases among workers. Of the 6,000 people who are or have been uranium miners, an estimated 600 to 1,100 will die of lung cancer within the next 20 years because of radiation exposure on the job. Large numbers of workers are exposed to heavy metals, each of which exacts its toll—lead, mercury, arsenic, and beryllium, to name only a few (see Key and associates,[13] and Clayton and Clayton[14] for details). Hundreds of thousands of workers each year suffer skin diseases from contact with materials used in their work. Dermatoses are the most common of all occupational diseases. An estimated 7 million industrial workers are exposed to noise levels that cause impaired hearing.

Another important aspect of occupational health and safety is the additive effect of mental stresses the worker brings from home to the workplace and vice versa. These may be domestic or neighborhood problems, concerns about economics or illness in the family, the use of drugs or alcohol, or other forms of delinquency. Such stresses cannot help but affect the worker's safety on the job, and it is reasonable to expect them to exacerbate work-generated stresses. In the same way, stresses in the work environment can affect an employee's health and safety off the job. Such terms as *ulcerogenic jobs, crawling up the wall,* and *the daily grind* or *rat race* are based on much more than apparent humor. Workers subjected to the stresses of noise, vibration, solvents, speed-ups, or overbearing supervisors can become occupational casualties just as much as if they inhaled dust or were exposed to toxic chemicals. Occupational health and safety programs are not complete without consideration of these psychologic considerations. Many authors have spoken and written of the problems of alienation and powerlessness as they affect workers in America.[16,17]

Toxicology has become one of the major "growth industries" in public health. There are over 12,000 products known to be toxic currently in use, and combinations of two or more of them run into the millions. New products are being introduced to the economy and the environment at a rate far greater than the rate of epidemiologic or toxicologic understanding of their nature. Given the long latent period for the development of many occupational diseases, it is necessary to use biologic systems that mature much faster and have a higher rate of cellular mitosis and meiosis, such as cultures of *Salmonella* or some types of fish. Although these systems are efficient and useful indicators of the teratogenic, mutagenic, and carcinogenic potential of chemicals, mammalian testing is a necessary second step, but it is very expensive and time consuming. It is necessary to determine several different levels: the maximum allowable concentration (MAC), a threshold limit value (TLV), a time-weighted average (TWA), short-term exposure limites (STEL), and emergency exposure limits (EEL).[15] Standards often use several different levels to specify what continuous background level is tolerable as well as the maximum exposure level for short periods. Even when such levels can be established with reasonable certainty, prudence as well as the law requires a margin of safety so that permissible levels are often set at one-tenth the level found to be acceptable in the experimental situation. Whereas some European countries specify pollutant limits in terms of their impact on the average person, the practice in the United States has been to set levels at such a point that even those with idiosyncratic responses are protected.

Serious attention to and support of occupational and public health activities carry with them many benefits to private enterprise. Three of the greatest items of loss to business and industry are labor turnover, absenteeism, and liability compensation for occupational illness and injury. (The National Safety Council has estimated the cost of work accidents at $30.2 billion in 1980.[2]) Among the tangible profits of good community and occupational health programs are remedies against these three sources of loss.

Manufacturing industries have gained the most through safety programs, with a reduction in their occupational death rate of about 60% during the past 45 years. The work-related death rate for manufacturing occupations in 1980 was 8 per 100,000 workers in contrast with 15 per 100,000 workers in nonmanufacturing employment. Time loss because of on-the-job accidents also has decreased.

Other benefits to business and industry are a diminution in employee grievances, improved employee relations, and consequently improved public relations. Health problems and responsibilities are always present in the plant or in the office, whether or not industry and business recognize them and whether or not they wish to do anything about them. If they do accept these responsibilities, they not only perform an important public service but may also turn that recognition and action to their own financial advantage. On the other hand, if they refuse to recognize their health problems and responsibilities, it becomes incumbent on official agencies acting in the public interest to step in and do something about the situation.

Sometimes the worker is his or her own worst enemy. All too frequently workers can be found circumventing safety devices because they are considered a nuisance or because they take extra time. However, management has the more serious problem. Ever since the Industrial Revolution the health of the work force has not been the primary concern of the businessman; rather, the concern has been how much productivity can be obtained per unit of investment. Many of the costs of occupationally related diseases and injuries are still so indirect as to have less bearing on the everyday decisions of plant managers and owners than the more direct and visible costs. It is rare for management to install a safety device or a disease or injury prevention program unless the cost of the installation can be offset by either a reduction in the direct costs of illness

or injury or by increased productivity. The only exception to this rule is when government intervenes to protect the health of the worker, and then it is often argued that the cost of the change required by government regulation will be either inflationary or may make the plant or the industry so noncompetitive as to jeopardize its survival. When faced with such a possibility, and denied access to the information necessary to verify such an assertion, workers often side with the managers and against their own health. There are instances where the real choice has been jobs or illness, but all too often the facts are obfuscated by propaganda and industrial secrecy.

Although business associations have argued that declining productivity in the United States has been caused by regulatory controls affecting occupational health and environmental pollution, studies by mixed groups of labor, management, and occupational health experts have concluded that, although they are inflationary, the negative impact of such efforts on the economy has been slight. There have been some plant closures because of environmental and worker protection programs, but they have been marginal plants at best, and the programs may be seen as a part of the competitive process that drives inefficient organizations out of the marketplace.

In some instances the nature of the work may be such that jobs and health are incompatible. When this occurs in a small community, the solution requires far more than the expertise of public health workers. The health of the entire community may be involved, and a thoughtful program of retraining, public assistance, economic development, and sometimes even relocation is required. As a result, the community may rather accept the risk they know "than fly to others they know not of."

OCCUPATIONAL HEALTH AND SAFETY PROGRAMS

It is appropriate to preface a discussion of the objectives and content of occupational health and safety programs with a pertinent comment made some years ago by the director of industrial hygiene of one of the world's largest corporations.[18] It is fairly representative of the basic approach and attitude of the private sector. "Business," this person pointed out, "is conducted on a practical, or profit and loss, basis and when losses equal or exceed profits, you do not stay in business long. Industrial hygiene programs that are not basically sound are not likely to survive the test of time."

Even though public health emphasis has been placed on education and the voluntary progress that can be made by an enlightened public and enlightened industry, many of the issues that have been raised have been settled only through confrontation. There is growing emphasis on educating workers to become more involved in protecting their own health through plant surveillance, reporting, worker education programs, the use of consultants, and the process of collective bargaining.[19] From the public health standpoint, the purposes of an occupational health program are the same as those of all other health programs: to promote the optimal growth and development of people and their capacities, to prevent illness and disability, and to reduce dependency that may result from social, mental, or physical insults. The inclusion of mental and social factors merits particular note. There are indications that up to 30% of absenteeism is caused by emotional disturbances resulting from interpersonal problems in the plant, in the home, and in the community.

Many factors influence the nature and extent of the occupational health program that a business may establish. Among these are the type of industry or business; the nature of its product and of the ingredients and equipment used in its manufacture; the disposition of the product; the size and location of the establishment; the complex attitudes and relationships among top management, labor unions, the community and its medical profession, the public health agency, and government; and the organizational status of the unit responsible for the activities. For these reasons, it is obvious that a detailed standard pattern is impossible. To the contrary, each program must be more or less tailored to fit the needs and circumstances of the particular situation.

Serafini[20] has shown how to apply the nursing process of assessment, diagnosis, planning, implementation, and evaluation to the design of an industrial health program in an orderly fashion. Webb[21] has adapted guidelines developed by the Council on Occupational Health of the American Medical Association and the Occupational Health

Institute as well as the work of Felton to describe a basic program of services, which he categorizes into two groups: those of economic benefit to the company (which he calls "short range") and those of benefit to the health of the worker ("long range" services):

Short range
Preplacement evaluations
Preplacement laboratory procedures
Personal protective devices as indicated by work environment
Periodic occupational health evaluations
Job transfer evaluations
Job termination health evaluations
Treatment for occupational illness or injury
Emergency treatment for nonoccupational illness or injury
Regular inspection of premises for potential hazards

Long range
Regular health evaluations
Health counseling
Special surveys for case finding
Retiree health program
Alcohol control program
Rehabilitation program
Liaison with personal family physicians
Liaison with community health insurance programs
Advice to management about health insurance programs

It is easy to debate the categorization of the different elements, but the listing, taken as a whole, seems reasonably complete. The concept of "counseling" should be expanded to include generalized health education programs with special emphasis on the hazards of each individual workplace.

In developing occupational health programs for different work settings, it is useful to consider the job classification system developed by Gamble and associates.[22] They found that the proliferation of chemicals and other environmental conditions together with the mobility of workers made it virtually impossible to categorize workers by their exposure to any particular element—chemical, physical, or biologic. They therefore developed occupational titles for workers in a rubber plant that were based not on exposure to any one element but on process, function, and product. With knowledge of when what worker did what task, it is often possible to use manufacturing or industrial information to reconstruct the work environment to develop and test hypotheses epidemiologically.

It would be helpful if manufacturers would post

information in every work location on the compounds and substances in use by their generic names; hazards should be listed, as well as first aid procedures to be used in the event of improper exposure and the extent of exposure in that setting.[23] The national Occupational Safety and Health Administration (discussed later) has been embroiled in the "right-to-know" issue for many years. Industry maintains that the information is too complex, that workers will not use it responsibly, and that it would disclose important trade secrets. Wegman and others[19] have demonstrated that workers can use the information quite capably, and courts have begun to rule in favor of "right-to-know" regulations so long as a reasonable effort is made to protect the secrecy of the manufacturing process.

In many parts of the country committees or health and safety teams have been formed to monitor the plant environment and make recommendations for improvements. Some teams or committees are combined labor and management groups with a carefully specified scope of action and authority. Others are comprised of labor but have management support. Lazes[23] has reported on his work on the shop floor with teams that have worked effectively to solve specific problems. Team members function during work hours and receive training from management. They function best when their activities carefully avoid issues that are a part of the regular contract or grievance process. Other more elaborate efforts have involved a consortium of unions, management, and a university, such as the agreement between the United Rubber Workers, B.F. Goodrich, and the Harvard School of Public Health.[24] Formed in 1971, the contract resulted in the formation of an Occupational Safety and Health Committee with three representatives from labor and three from management, which decides what issues require investigation and warrant research support. The Research Study Group consists of Harvard faculty. Results of the research efforts go to labor and management at the same time.

Several businesses have expanded their efforts into health promotion generally and provide help for those who want to lose weight, stop smoking, or exercise. Although this has been partly because of public relations efforts to improve morale, there are signs that some employee health promotion efforts are developing a more professional public health approach with impressive results in decreasing absenteeism and increasing productivity.[25,26]

Because of the numbers of employees involved, many of the larger business and industrial concerns find it practical to operate most or all of their employee health and safety programs themselves. Some industries have conducted genetic screening programs to detect employees or job applicants who might have a particular sensitivity to certain hazardous situations. Such efforts have been vigorously criticized by labor and civil rights groups as an unwarranted intrusion into the private affairs of an individual. Although a company may have the right to protect itself by excluding people from tasks that might harm them, genetic screening is not sufficiently well developed to support such exclusionary action in many cases, and resources might better be used in protecting all workers from such hazardous substances.

One of the greatest problems relates to small plants and businesses, which are in the majority and which taken together employ the major proportion, 60%, of workers. Individually they are usually too small to afford or justify the employment of even a single full-time nurse, much less a physician. Unfortunately they have been largely left out of the picture except for essentially token services rendered by state and occasionally local health departments. To overcome the problem, there has been a trend toward the joint employment, by groups of small industrial plants, of full-time health personnel who devote the necessary number of hours a week to each plant in the group. This plan has proved of value in several locations. For the supervision of the environmental hazards of small plants, various types of portable or mobile equipment have also been used to advantage.

ROLE OF GOVERNMENT

Reference has been made to the relatively slow growth of occupational health programs in government agencies, beginning with the initiation of activities in 1913 in New York and Ohio. Activity and interest accelerated with the passage of the Social Security Act in 1935 and again during the period of World War II. In 1940 more than one fourth of the state health agencies had no occupational health activities. In 1980 only 11 state health agencies reported lead agency responsibility in occupational safety and health. As is the case in environmental health, in many instances occupational safety and health at both the federal and state level has been separated from public health and placed in other agencies, such as a labor department or in an independent agency.

The new Director of the National Institute of Occupational Safety and Health, Dr. Millar, asked his division directors to rank what they believed were the most important occupational health problems. At a meeting of the National Advisory Committee on Occupational Safety and Health on March 31, 1982 he provided the Institute's list:[27]

1. Occupational lung disease
2. Musculoskeletal injuries
3. Occupational cancer
4. Traumatic deaths
5. Cardiovascular diseases
6. Reproductive problems
7. Neurotoxic illnesses
8. Noise-induced hearing loss
9. Dermatologic problems
10. Psychologic disorders

That list is a useful starting place for any organization at the state, local, or national level that is attempting to develop an occupational health program. In general, the function of government agencies on the state and local levels in occupational safety and health includes surveys and field investigations of environmental conditions in industry; the collection and analysis of data relating to occupational illness and injuries; the surveillance of atmospheric pollution and radiation in industrial plants; the development of techniques for the detection of occupational disease; methods of prevention and control; and consultation with labor and management. Health departments concentrate on the supervision of environmental conditions conducive to employment-related illness. They suggest measures for control, promote in-plant sanitation and medical services, provide advisory engineering and nursing services, and conduct health education activities.

The New Jersey State Health Department has reorganized its Division of Epidemiology and Disease Control and assigned four functions to it that are not customarily a part of such units: (1) response to environmental emergencies; (2) response to nonemergency environmental contamination problems, including clusters of disease that may be related to environmental exposure, (3) epidemio-

logic investigations based on the accumulation of data such as that contained in the state's cancer registry; and (4) epidemiologic study of occupational diseases.[28] Utah has developed a sophisticated computerized system for monitoring data potentially related to occupational exposures, including death certificate data (which include occupation), fetal deaths, and industrial accident and disease reports.[29]

Departments of labor and mines are primarily concerned with safety measures and the regulation of working conditions. The industrial or occupational health units of these agencies, in addition to their specific functions, coordinate their activities and services with those of units concerned with sanitation, health education, and preventable and chronic disease, thereby attempting to bring to industry a well-rounded health program. In addition, they usually maintain cooperative working relations with labor, management, and various pertinent professional societies.

To varying degrees state agencies are charged with the enforcement of laws relating to the field of occupational health. Whereas state health departments are frequently responsible for general occupational health and safety functions, labor departments are more often charged with enforcement powers.

The problem of occupational health and safety is large, complex, and destined to become even more complicated and to require the services of still more types of specialists. The availability of trained workers in the United States is thought to be a particularly serious problem. One of the principal recommendations of a national task force on prevention called for increased support for training programs for epidemiologists, engineers, chemists, and regulatory personnel.[30] The lack of trained personnel was made very clear when the cooling tower collapsed at a new power plant in Willow Island, W. Va., in 1978, killing 51 workers. The Occupational Safety and Health Administration did not have the work force necessary to carry out its mission, and the National Institute of Occupational Safety and Health has not been able to proceed rapidly with the enormous task of analyzing occupational hazards and developing appropriate and realistic standards. The problem is more political than technical; it became apparent in 1977 and 1978 that Congress was unwilling to support an aggressive occupational safety and health program while they were deluged with the problems of inflation, assertions that government regulation was a cause of inflation, and demonstrations that the taxpayers wanted less rather than more government, although the demand for services continued unabated. In spite of that general reaction and the marked conservative swing in the 1980 elections, public opinion polls show that such programs still have the support of a substantial majority in the United States, and Congress has not adopted legislation that would substantially reduce the programs. President Reagan did issue an executive order in February 1981 requiring agencies to carry out cost-benefit analyses on all proposed regulations, but the courts have ruled that such studies are not required under existing legislation. Even though presidential appointees have reduced the size of their work force and attempted to delay the issuance of regulations, the scientific base of concern is such that initially skeptical appointees have found themselves supporting regulatory efforts they had vowed to terminate before taking office. Although the President initially reduced or deleted funding for training programs, the 14 Occupational Safety and Health Educational Resource Centers established at universities to train industrial hygienists, occupational medicine and nursing specialists, and other needed categories of workers have been maintained by Congress.

The Coal Mine Health and Safety Act of 1969 (P.L. 91-173), placed significantly increased responsibilities on the Secretary of Health, Education, and Welfare and the Secretary of the Interior. For the first time in this country, a federal law recognized a specific disease, coal workers' pneumoconiosis or "black lung," required radiographic examination of all exposed workers, and provided federal funds to compensate its victims as well as survivors of deceased miners. In 1980, 480,000 beneficiaries were receiving more than $1.7 billion in payments. Because the review procedures in the original "black lung" bill enabled reluctant medical panels and eligibility workers to delay and deny benefits (the program is financed by a royalty on coal), Congress amended the law in 1978, requiring time limits for case review, allowing local radiologists to determine the degree of impairment, and extending benefits to other miners who were not directly involved at the coal face.

To date, no other categoric federal programs have been organized to deal specifically with other occupationally disabled workers, such as asbestos workers or those affected with byssinosis. The reasons for this are political, not medical or epidemiologic. The etiology and pathogenesis of the diseases differ, but the concept is fundamentally the same: exposure to toxic or hazardous substances on the job leads directly to severe and permanent disability, and such exposure could be reduced by control techniques. Therefore those who were and are in a position to implement control programs are held liable for the consequences (although the cost is ultimately passed along to consumers). The special attention given to pneumoconiosis is probably related to the interest in Appalachia generated by President Kennedy and to the effectiveness of the United Mine Workers and their occupational health program. This is in effect a special worker's compensation program to deal with one disease in one industry. It is likely that other disabled occupational groups will follow the same route and that eventually the pressures will result in reform of the worker's compensation laws at the federal level.

The Occupational Safety and Health Act (P.L. 91-596) of 1970 created a regulatory body (the Occupational Safety and Health Administration, OSHA) in the Department of Labor and regrouped the research activities of the Public Health Service into the National Institute for Occupational Safety and Health (NIOSH). The roles and relationships were confusing at first, with NIOSH serving as the research arm of the federal program and OSHA serving as the regulatory agency. The separation of functions was rationalized as logical and effective, but it was a compromise resulting from political battling for jurisdiction. The two agencies developed increasingly effective relationships during the last half of the 1970s as the work of OSHA was oriented more toward health, and NIOSH functioned more capably as a technical advisory group. Among the responsibilities of NIOSH are research on occupational safety and health problems, hazard evaluation, toxicity determinations, work force development and training, industry-wide studies of chronic or low-level exposures to hazardous substances, and research on psychologic, motivational, and behavioral factors as they relate to occupational safety and health. Field stations and research centers have been established in Cincinnati, Salt Lake City, and Morgantown, W. Va.

States can enter into an agreement with OSHA to administer a compliance program. The original agreements were funded on a 50-50 basis. By July 1982 only 21 states had approved programs. Many state occupational health authorities did not like the complaint-investigation orientation and the inspection requirements of OSHA, and the funding agreements were not particularly attractive. This severely impeded the implementation of the program, since OSHA could not acquire the resources to carry out the inspection programs adequately. In states without a federally approved program, OSHA is directly responsible for inspection and enforcement. The federal agency is prohibited from providing consultation services to businesses without triggering the enforcement provisions of the act, but states may provide such services. Federal reimbursement was increased to pay for 90% of the development of a state program and 50% of the maintenance costs, but no additional state plans have been submitted and approved since 1978, and some that had been approved or submitted have since been withdrawn. Since 1981 the administration has attempted to provide funds to the states in the form of block grants with a decreased regulatory overlay from the federal agency, and that may encourage more states to become active. Both industry and labor have been opposed to state assumption of the program: industry because they prefer not to have to deal with 50 different programs and labor because they believe that business interests are more influential at the state level and most state agencies lack the resources to carry out such complex programs of research, standards development, and enforcement. Even though the Occupational Safety and Health Act was a progressive national step, leadership historically has come from the states, with programs in Michigan, California, Minnesota, Oregon, and Washington providing especially good examples. State programs are amenable to change with changing governors and legislative leadership, perhaps more so than a national program, but that same malleability means that they can move more quickly and experiment with more creative approaches to problems. When hazards are universally understood and control technology is well developed and accepted, federal management of a program may assure better uniformity and equity across geographic lines, but when those conditions do not exist, as is the case for much of the occupational health field, state programs can produce more information in a shorter period of time.

In 1978 the Senate moved to exempt small businesses having 10 or fewer employees from OSHA regulations unless their injury and illness rate exceeded 7% per year (which could mean 0.7 workers). The injury-illness rate requirement would have applied to each individual business, a formidable task. The bill would have excluded the majority of American workers. It was not passed.

The Supreme Court ruled in May 1978 that OSHA inspectors would have to obtain warrants to enter a workplace if the owners refused entry. This was an extension of earlier Supreme Court rulings restricting the right of entry of health inspectors. In July 1980 the Court, in a confusing opinion, overturned an OSHA standard for benzene, a chemical known to cause leukemia. OSHA had attempted to lower the standard from 10 parts per million to 1 part per million. The industry had sought to block the regulation on the basis that (1) it was not based on scientific evidence and (2) it would be too costly to implement. The Court's ruling caused the agency to slow down the promulgation of other standards to do a more thorough risk assessment and to consider the need for cost-benefit analysis, but OSHA did not argue its case very effectively: the evidence it needed was already at hand.[31] In July 1981 the Court upheld the proposed cotton dust standard against a similar challenge and stated that OSHA was not required to carry out a cost-benefit analysis on its regulations.

It has been difficult for NIOSH to develop reasonable standards for toxic and hazardous substances. The research work has been tedious and costly; thousands of new compounds enter into the work environment each year. NIOSH has not had the resources required to conduct the necessary studies. In 1977 new regulations were proposed that would allow a generic classification system for carcinogens to be used so that they could be grouped. This change would help speed up the definition and promulgation of standards, but it has been vigorously opposed.

One of the more promising developments has been the agreement to support union educational efforts. Particularly strong programs have been underway in some unions, and OSHA supported those efforts with $4 million dollars in 1978; this was increased in subsequent years as part of the New Directions program.

THE FUTURE

The conservative tilt in 1980 has not eroded the basic support for the programs, and it seems likely that progressive legislation will continue to be adopted in the United States during the next decade.

Although the evidence suggests that occupational disease will prove to be at least as important as occupational injuries and far more complex both scientifically and ethically, lead agency responsibility for governmental programs will remain outside health departments for the most part. However, several aspects of the effort are very much a part of public health. Epidemiologic investigation will play an increasingly important role in elucidating cause-effect relationships in spite of the complexity of the interactions. The field of toxicology is growing rapidly and will continue to do so as industry, labor, and government agencies seek to learn more about the chemicals developed and used in modern society.

Technology will play a stronger role in control efforts. Finding the problems is only part of the process. Monitoring is increasingly important, and passive dosimeters are being developed for a wide variety of environmental conditions. These are badges or other devices worn by an employee and periodically tested in a laboratory. They will make it possible to carry out low-cost monitoring programs even in small businesses.

The biggest area of development over the next 2 decades will be risk assessment: the careful and painstaking attempt to differentiate between the hazards posed by a concentration of 10 parts per million and 1 part per million. The process will continue into the parts per billion range in an effort to determine what level of exposure, if any, is safe for most people. The issue was raised in the Supreme Court decision regarding the benzene standard. It is present again in considering ethylene oxide, ethylene dibromide, and formaldehyde, all known carcinogens, but presently uncontrolled pending the ability to demonstrate at what level they cease to be hazardous.

Labeling and right-to-know laws will continue to occupy the attention of labor and management forces and their lawyers for the next few years. They bring different interests into direct conflict: personal privacy, industrial secrecy, and the right to know what risks a worker is facing. To some degree, the conflict illustrates that the old common-law concept of the assumption of risk is still viable: if a worker is adequately informed about the hazards and still accepts the risk, the owners are not responsible. That concept appears moribund in a society that recognizes its responsibility to protect itself and its individual members from the grave consequences of an improbable event.

REFERENCES

1. Occupational health, WHO Tech. Rep. Ser. No. 66, Geneva, 1963, World Health Organization.
2. Statistics department: Accident facts, ed. 1981, Chicago, 1981, National Safety Council.
3. Des Jardins, R.S., Bigoness, W.J., and Harris, R.L.: Labor-management aspects of occupational risk, Ann. Rev. Public Health, **3:**201, 1982.
4. Ashford, N.A.: Crisis in the workplace: occupational disease and injury, Cambridge, Mass., 1976, The M.I.T. Press.
5. Messite, J., and Bond, M.B.: Occupational health considerations for women at work. In Zenz, C., editor: Developments in occupational medicine, Chicago, 1980, Year Book Medical Publishers, Inc.
6. Messite, J., and Bond, M.B.: reproductive toxicology and occupation exposure. In Zenz, C., editor: Developments in occupational medicine, Chicago, 1980, Year Book Medical Publishers, Inc.
7. Hernberg, S.: Epidemiology in occupational health. In Zenz, C., editor: Developments in occupational medicine, Chicago, 1980, Year Book Medical Publishers, Inc.
8. Gordon, J.B., Ackman, A., and Brooks, M.: Industrial safety statistics: a re-examination—a critical report prepared for the U.S. Department of Labor, New York, 1971, Praeger Publishers, Inc.
9. Bureau of Labor Statistics: Occupational injury and death statistics, Washington, D.C., 1980, Department of Labor.
10. American Public Health Association: Chart book: health and work in America, U.S. Department of Health, Education, and Welfare, Washington, D.C., 1975, U.S. Government Printing Office.
11. Bureau of the Census: Statistical abstract of the United States, ed. 102, Washington, D.C., 1981, U.S. Government Printing Office.
12. Selikoff, I.J., Churg, J., and Hammond, E.C.: Relation between exposure to asbestos and mesothelioma, N. Engl. J. Med. **272:**560, March 18, 1965.
13. Key, M.M., and others: Occupational diseases: a guide to their recognition, rev, ed., DHEW Pub. No. (NIOSH) 77-181, Washington, D.C., 1977.
14. Clayton, G.D., and Clayton, F,E.: Patty's industrial hygiene and toxicology, vol. IIa(1981), IIb(1981), and IIc(1982), New York, John Wiley & Sons, Inc.
15. Lauwerys, R.R.: Occupational toxicology. In Doull, J., Klaassen, C.D., and Amdur, M.O., editors: Casarett and Doull's toxicology: the basic science of poisons, ed. 2, New York, 1980, Macmillan Publishing Co., Inc.

16. Navarro, V.: The underdevelopment of health in working America: causes, consequences and possible solutions, Am. J. Public Health **66:**538, June 1976.

17. Work in America; report of a Special Task Force to the Secretary of HEW, Cambridge, Mass., 1973, The M.I.T. Press.

18. Patty, F.A.: The industrial hygiene program in industry, Am. J. Public Health **41:**971, Aug. 1951.

19. Wegman, D.H., Boden, L., and Levenstein, C.: Health hazard surveillance by industrial workers, Am. J. Public Health **65:**26, Jan. 1975.

20. Serafini, P.: Nursing assessment in industry, Am. J. Public Health **66:**755, Aug. 1976.

21. Webb, S.B.: Objective criteria for evaluating occupational health programs, Am. J. Public Health **65:**31, Jan. 1975.

22. Gamble, J.F., Spirtas, R., and Easter, P.: Applications of a job classification system in occupational epidemiology, Am. J. Public Health **66:**768, Aug. 1976.

23. Lazes, P.M.: Creating ways to solve health and safety problems on the shop floor, Paper presented at the annual meeting of the American Public Health Association, Los Angeles, Nov. 1981.

24. Spotlight: The rubber workers study: a model of industry-labor-university cooperation, Boston, 1980, Harvard School of Public Health.

25. Azarow, J., and Cardy, W.: Health on the job: change the worker or change the workplace, Paper presented at the annual meeting of the American Public Health Association, Los Angeles, Nov. 1981.

26. McGill, A.M., editor: Proceedings of the national conference on health promotion programs in occupations settings, Jan. 17 to 19, 1979, U.S. Department of Health and Human Services, Office of the Assistant Secretary for Health.

27. Bureau of National Affairs: Occupational Safety and Health Reporter **11**(45):957, April 15, 1982.

28. Koplin, A.N., Altman, R., and Finley, J.E.: The epidemiologic basis of environmental and occupational health policy: the New Jersey experience, J. Public Health Policy **3**(1):39, March, 1982.

29. Brockert, J.E., Levy, M.I., and Kan, S.H.: Utah occupational health surveillance system, Paper presented at the annual meeting of the American Public Health Association, Los Angeles, November 1981.

30. Peters, J.M.: Occupational safety and health. In Preventive medicine, U.S.A.: task force reports sponsored by the Fogarty International Center and the American College of Preventive Medicine, New York, 1976, Prodist.

31. Linet, M.S., and Bailey, P.E.: Benzene, leukemia, and the Supreme Court, J. Public Health Policy **2**(2):116-135, June 1981.

CHAPTER 21

Environmental health programs

Is ecology a phase of science of limited interest and utility? Or, if taken seriously for the long-run welfare of mankind, would it endanger the assumptions and practices accepted by modern societies, whatever their doctrinal commitments?

Paul B. Sears

SANITATION, SINE QUA NON

Activities aimed at the preservation and improvement of the environment will always represent a major part of community health programs. Chapter 2 discusses many sanitary installations that remain as evidences of the degree of sanitary consciousness attained by Minoan, Grecian, Roman, and other early civilizations. Reference also is made to the problems that concerned the early public health organizations of the United States. Most of them related to problems of the physical environment, particularly of the growing urban communities. The essential similarities among the sanitary concerns of ancient civilizations, those of the founding fathers, and those of the present time are striking.

Whatever the reason, activities in environmental health tend to be the most firmly established, readily supported, and vigorously demanded of the many parts of the community health program. Because of this, newly established local health departments have often begun operation with a sanitation program before proceeding to some of the other aspects of a well-rounded health program that might be less readily understood, less evident in results, or more controversial.

Many of the public health or epidemiologic accomplishments in the United States and certain other countries can be attributed to the sanitary measures that have been instituted. Included among these have been the spectacular reductions in typhoid fever, cholera, dysenteries, and summer diarrheas; the control of many of the milk-borne and food-borne infections; the control of malaria; and the elimination of yellow fever. It was not until the beginning of the present century that the

chains of events involved in the transmission and perpetuation of these diseases became unraveled. Prompt steps were taken to break links in these chains.

At first, activities in the field of sanitation were concerned primarily with the abatement of noisome nuisances. Gradually the provision and supervision of sanitary water supplies and sewage disposal facilities were added as the first well-defined and scientific measures. Meanwhile, the Rockefeller Sanitary Commission, established in 1909 to combat hookworm disease, led to programs by state health departments with emphasis on the eradication of hookworm and other enteric infections in the rural population. These activities laid the foundation for the eventual establishment and spread of many full-time county health departments in the United States.

In this regard the noteworthy surveys, demonstrations, and epidemiologic investigations of the Public Health Service, particularly those by Lumsden, should not go unmentioned. Throughout this formative era of the modern sanitation and public health program, much emphasis was placed on the construction and use of sanitary privies in rural areas and small towns as a practical means of preventing the spread of enteric disease.

CONTENT AND PURPOSE OF ENVIRONMENTAL CONTROL

It is essentially true that the initial phases of sanitation activities centered on keeping human excreta out of the diet. By comparison, the field today covers an imposing spectrum of responsibilities and activities, for most of which sound technical and scientific reasons have been demonstrated. This has been emphasized by numerous recent groups, particularly notable among which are the Task Force on Environmental Health of the National Commission on Community Health Services[1] and the Program Area Committee on Environmental Health of the American Public Health Association.[2]

In discussing the present definition and scope of the field, the latter group indicated that the administration of today's environmental health programs has become so complex that it must attend to situations involving air pollution; water pollution and surface-water and ground-water disposal; food and dairy product protection; occupational health and safety; solid waste management—its collection, transportation, disposal, and recycling; housing and neighborhood planning, conservation, and rehabilitation; noise abatement and prevention; radiation protection; insect and rodent control; institutional and hospital sanitation; accident prevention; sanitation and safety supervision of swimming pools; participation in planning and supervision of recreation, flood control, topography, highways, transportation, and traffic; and concerns about budgeting, tax jurisdictions, and neighboring communities and special districts. It must also place the economic, legal, sociologic, and political factors in their proper perspective in relation to the technical factors.

The trend has been to draw health agencies away as much as possible from activities that involve physical operation and correction toward programs of a positive or promotive nature. Until relatively recently, public health activities have been based on negative concepts, on definitions of environmental as well as human ills. This resulted in programs designed to attack things that have gone wrong. The public health profession has now reached the point in many areas, including environmental health, where it can think and act in positive terms. Increasingly, planning is based on a definition of good health rather than of illness, on the maintenance of cleanliness and salubrity instead of continually cleaning up an environment allowed to become insanitary.

This trend has led to the consideration of the human-environment relationship in both a positive and total sense.[3,4] In other words, it is a recognition of the fact that we can affect our environment and

our environment can affect us and that preventive and promotive measures may be applied to all aspects of our environment as well as to ourselves. Thus a task force[5] established by the Secretary of Health, Education, and Welfare in 1967 to consider the broad problem recommended that the purpose of environmental control be regarded as the assurance "that every American can thrive in an attractive, comfortable, convenient, and healthy environment by controlling pollution at its source, reducing hazards, converting waste to use, and improving the aesthetic value of man's surroundings."

It must also be recognized that we, our psyches as well as our physical beings, are inseparable from our total environment and that much more emphasis must be placed on our total ecology. For this reason, the task force, recognizing the multiplicity of environmental interests, authorities, and responsibilities, not only recommended some practical degree of consolidation but also urged that there be established a Council of Ecological Advisors on the federal level as a supracabinet organization to advise the President on all problems, proposals, or activities that relate to the complex interrelationship of people and their total environment.

Finally, the trend is a recognition of the synergistic and cumulative effects of a spectrum of environmental hazards. Because of the usually slow development of the consequences of environmental abuse, society has failed to recognize the full impact of environmental hazards on human health and welfare. This has led to sporadic and fragmentary efforts to meet only some of the most flagrant of environmental problems. Thus not only should the rate and direction of environmental pollution be changed but the citizenry also needs protection from a conglomerate total of environmental health threats. The threats include not only air and water pollutants but also combinations of these, plus noise and crowding, safety hazards, and other factors. It must be recognized that an individually acceptable amount of water pollution, added to a tolerable amount of air pollution, added to a bearable amount of noise and congestion can produce a totally unacceptable health environment.

It is entirely possible that the biologic effects of these environmental hazards, some of which reach us slowly and silently over decades or generations, will first begin to reveal themselves only after their impact has become irreversible. Because of this, the Task Force on Environmental Health and Related Problems insisted that an effectively coordinated environmental health protection system is necessary. It should be predicted on the premise that the environment may affect mental and physical health and welfare. Any approach toward environmental health protection that is limited to concern for less than the total range of hazards that do or may exist in the environment must be viewed as inadequate.

These recommendations bore fruit in the passage of the National Environmental Policy Act of 1969, which declared a national policy on the environment for the first time, established a Council on Environmental Quality, and prepared the way for the formation of the Environmental Protection Agency at the end of 1970. This consolidated in one agency the major federal programs dealing with air and water pollution, solid waste disposal, pesticide regulation, and radiation and noise control. Subsequently, some states and large municipalities followed suit, essentially removing many health agencies from the environmental scene. As will be discussed, however, health agencies still retain many environmental functions. Their roles, responsibilities, and relationships have merely changed.

The concept of a coordinated, total environmental health protection system has also been presented by Stead[6] in a three-dimensional manner. In the first dimension, he categorized the field into four basic sectors: water sanitation, food sanitation, air sanitation, and shelter sanitation.

Water sanitation includes consideration of the quantity, quality, and safety aspects of water from the stages of planning, development, transportation, storage, treatment, distribution, and use on through the stages of treatment and disposal or conservation, reclamation, and reuse of waste water or sewage. Public health concern must go beyond the provision of potable water. It must also extend to the use of water for recreation, irrigation, and food processing as well as the potential for vector breeding.

Food sanitation encompasses the entire chain of events from production of food on land or in the sea, its processing, distribution, storage, and marketing down to the actual preparation and serving of meals and the disposal of wastes. Stead summarizes this sector with the phrase that the food sanitation program must "follow the food" back to its source and forward to its ultimate consumption.

Air sanitation is concerned with the physical, chemical, and biologic quality of air as a natural resource. Problems vary from its clarity to its radioactivity and its pesticide and allergen content.

Programs should be alert to air quality at home, at work, during travel and recreation, and outdoors as well as indoors.

Shelter sanitation is regarded as encompassing not only the field of housing as related to separate dwelling units, apartments, hotels, public buildings, mobile homes and trailers, and camps but also the general artificial and natural environment for work, play, and general living. It includes the whole field of protection of human beings from rigors of the elements as well as the onslaught of insects, rodents, dust, dirt, odors, noise, radiation, accident hazards, and other detrimental impacts of the environment on people. The omission of any of the four sectors results in an unbalanced environmental health program.

In the second dimension Stead lists the four basic levels of concern with the environment in the order of program preference:

1. Ensuring the elements of simple survival
2. Prevention of disease and poisoning
3. Maintaining an environment suited to our efficient performance
4. Preservation of comfort and the enjoyment of living

Each of the four levels of concern necessitates programs in each of the four program sectors (water, food, air, and shelter). As the third dimension, each of these requires four program stages (research, field investigation, analysis and planning, and the action program).

To assist in the planning of broadly comprehensive environmental health programs, both the American Public Health Association and the Public Health Service have developed useful guides, the application of which can contribute to the improved development, performance, and evaluation of programs in this field.[7,8]

The American Public Health Association's policy statement[8] includes the following checklist of program areas, planning considerations, and methods for guidance:

I. *Environmental Program Area*
   Wastes
   　1) Air
   　2) Sewage and liquid
   　3) Solid
   Water Supply
   Housing and Residential Environment

Food and Drugs
Radiation
Noise
Accidents
Occupational and Institutional Hazards
Vectors
Recreation
II. *Planning Considerations*
Health
Economic
Demographic and Land Use
Social
Esthetic
Resource Conservation
III. *Methods and Techniques*
Research
Demonstration
Education
Standards
Legislation
Inspection
Enforcement
Planning
Evaluation
Incentives
Systems Analysis

The Association states that although environmental health programs were originally designed to protect against disease and disability, they should now, in addition, be designed to create surroundings

that will provide optimum health, safety and comfort for the present population; that will protect this generation, and coming generations as well, from hazards associated with the environment or any of its components; and that will result in maximum economic and cultural benefits for a healthy people. In attaining these objectives recognition must be given to the demands and expectations of the public and to esthetic requirements—not solely to morbidity and mortality rates.

REGIONAL DIFFERENCES

Although the basic objectives are universal, the details of the environmental health program have not developed uniformly throughout the communities and states of the nation. Furthermore, as will be discussed later, all activities in this field have not necessarily been centered in health departments. The more rural agricultural South and Midwest are faced with problems rather different from the urban industrialized Northeast, the fringe of

the lower Great Lakes, or the West Coast. As a result, certain activities are stressed more in one area than in the other, and dependence is placed on somewhat different categories of personnel. The congregation of large numbers of people in the many cities of the northeastern, western coastal, and Great Lakes states necessarily has led to their emphasis on the construction and operation of sanitary engineering facilities and to the employment of many sanitary and public health engineers.

In other more rural parts of the country, particularly in the southern states, the opportunity for centralized sanitary control has been limited essentially to the moderately sized towns and larger cities. Much emphasis therefore is placed on a somewhat simpler and more individualized approach. Here much more patient and persistent attention has had to be given to such matters as arrangements for the disposal of human and other wastes, well location and construction, dairy barn sanitation, and screening. To many health workers these may appear prosaic, elementary, and nontechnical. However, a background of technical knowledge is necessary for the solution of such environmental problems. These measures provide a degree of community health protection comparable to that resulting from the more complex and sophisticated structures of municipal sanitary engineering. Furthermore, they assume greater importance as increasing numbers of urban and suburban dwellers become more and more dependent on the smaller proportion of rural farm and dairy workers.

An administrative benefit for which the rural sanitation program may be given credit has been the development of a spirit of cooperation among the officials of the health agencies on the various levels of government. Thus it may be said with little exaggeration that it was in this field that the state health departments and the federal Public Health Service first learned to work together as did, to a considerable degree, the state and local health organizations. Furthermore, the successful pursuance of the program necessitated the integration of activities and therefore cooperation among public health departments and other agencies on the same governmental level, such as the agricultural and farm organizations.

SANITATION NEEDS

Although the United States is one of the most sanitized nations in the world, much unfinished business remains. Numerous surveys and evaluations of environmental health needs have been made by various organizations and agencies. They have resulted in a number of useful reports that have influenced public opinion, legislation, programming, and organization to a significant degree.

Although it is true that significant strides have been made during recent decades, the combination of population growth, continued urbanization and suburbanization, and industrial expansion has easily offset any additions and improvements in sanitary facilities. For example, there are still many communities, including some of large size, with inadequate or no sewage treatment facilities. The cost of remedying just this problem is estimated at many billions of dollars. Similarly, it is questionable whether the air and water pollution problems and the housing problem have improved to the extent they should have. With reference to dental health, there are still only about 103 million people, or 49% of the nation's population, who benefit from adequate natural or added fluoride in their public drinking water.

With this general background, a consideration of the most important present concerns in environmental health follows.

WATER SUPPLIES

Water is one of the prime necessities of human existence, so much so that, given dire enough circumstances, even the most educated individual will resort to the consumption of water from grossly polluted or dangerous sources. Beyond its importance for human consumption, water serves many purposes: as a source of fluid for animals; as a medium of transportation; as an agent for cleansing and cooling the body, objects, or the environment; as a means of recreation for swimming, boating, and fishing; as an agricultural irrigant; as an adjunct to innumerable industrial processes; as a conveyor for the disposal of human and industrial wastes; as a means of air conditioning; and as a fire extinguisher. In the United States per capita domestic use of water from public supplies has grown from about 90 gallons a day in 1890 to approximately 160 gallons a day at the present time. With regard to total use, it is estimated that in 1975 municipal water consumers used about 30 billion gallons of water each day; rural consumers, about 4.6 billion gallons; industry, about 65.5 billion gallons; electric utilities, about 157 billion gallons; and irrigation about 130 billion gallons.

The chief concern here is with the consumption of water by humans for domestic purposes. At the moment most of the other uses of water are of interest insofar as they affect the salubrity of the water that humans drink. Water supply systems may be classified as public and private. About three fourths of the American population are served by public water systems. However, about 10% of the families living in about 7 million homes in communities so served do not have water outlets readily available. In addition, there are still an estimated 2.5 million people living in communities of 200 to 500 population without a public water system. Federal assistance programs are under way to provide safe water for many of these. In fact, since 1963 the major area of improvement "has been the proliferation of small systems to serve small housing developments, mobile home parks, and the like, where the population served by each would be in the hundreds."[9] In rural areas about 27 million people need improved pure water facilities.

Public water supplies are derived from various sources—streams, lakes, deep wells, and springs—and their nature differs according to their source. Surface waters such as streams and lakes, which depend for replenishment on repeated runoffs, under most circumstances do not have as high a natural chemical content as do ground waters from deep wells and springs. On the other hand, increasingly surface waters are contaminated by dangerous industrial wastes and agricultural runoffs. Underground waters generally are clear, whereas surface waters ordinarily contain considerable amounts of suspended matter, which must be removed before they can be considered suitable for human consumption.

These differences in source, hence composition, necessarily give rise to differences in approach to administrative control. Streams and lakes in general do not lend themselves to adequate control of the watershed. On the other hand, some impounding reservoirs are subject to control from the standpoint of prevention of further pollution of the water. Increasing public pressure for recreational facilities is resulting in more liberal access to both the reservoir and the surrounding watershed. In any case, in view of the high factor of safety in relation to cost, surface waters should probably always be subjected to filtration and chlorination, and, preferably, also to fluoridation. Rapid sand filtration is the usual method of choice. Recent improvements in sanitary engineering have resulted in filters with rates up to 4 gallons per square foot per minute, about double the previous usual rate, and when properly operated do not sacrifice any safety.

The provision of a safe and satisfactory public water supply to a community involves the following procedures:

1. If a surface water, the watershed should be protected and controlled insofar as is practical.

2. The intake should be located properly with regard to all possible sources of contamination and pollution.

3. Provision should be made for primary sedimentation and clarification by means of storage reservoirs and exposure to air and light.

4. Bacteria, algae, and any residual turbidity should be removed by the addition of a coagulant (usually alum) and the settling out of the coagulated particles and then passage through a rapid sand filter.

5. Residual and subsequent bacterial contaminants are combated by the addition of a disinfectant, usually chlorine, to a concentration of from 0.2 to 0.5 parts per million. This is a most important procedure.

6. A concentration from 0.7 to 1.5 parts per million of fluoride should be achieved by the addition of sodium fluoride, sodium silicofluoride, or hydrofluosilicic acid for the prevention of dental caries. The ultimate concentration will depend on the average water consumption per individual.

7. Use of the water by all the population of the community should be assured by reasonable water rates, adequate distribution systems, and housing requirements.

8. Contamination of the purified water should be prevented by residual disinfection of the distribution system pipes and by prevention of cross connections and back siphonage.

To achieve these ends, the cooperative action of several community agencies is necessary. Among these are the health department, the department of public works or the water department, the tax or finance office, the plumbing department, the housing commission, and the dental society.

The assurance of safe water to the rural population poses a completely different set of problems.

The sources are usually relatively simple and primitive wells, often shallow and unprotected. Hence they are easily subject to pollution not only from the surface but also through seepage from poorly placed privies, improperly constructed septic tanks, or nearby barnyards. Contamination over greater distances may occur if fissures or other subterranean passages exist in the substrata. Offsetting these hazards is the fact that the use of each small rural water supply is usually limited to a small group of people, often one family.

The solution of this difficult problem lies essentially in persistent rural health education programs coupled with sanitary consultation from the local health department. The objectives of these efforts should be encouragement of proper locating of wells and excreta disposal facilities, proper construction of wells, and installation of a pump in a tightly sealed, curbed, and drained well top.

An important step was taken in 1974 in relation to the protection and improvement of the nation's drinking water resources. As a result of an extensive nationwide study by the Environmental Protection Agency, the Congress enacted the Safe Drinking Water Act of 1974. The act directed the Environmental Protection Agency to develop water standards and to assure their enforcement in cooperation with state and local agencies. It also appropriated significant funds to the Environmental Protection Agency for the financial support of state and local community drinking water programs and for the provision of technical assistance. The states may continue to enforce their own laws and regulations for the protection of their drinking water supplies provided they meet the following requirements: (1) adopt regulations at least as strict as the federal regulations, (2) adopt and implement adequate enforcement procedures, (3) make provision for adequate response to emergencies, and (4) keep adequate records and provide required reports to the Environmental Protection Agency.

STREAM POLLUTION CONTROL

Although pure water for drinking purposes is of paramount public health concern, the many other uses of this precious commodity make it desirable to regard the development, protection, and use of water resources as a unit. By now, 75% of the population in the United States lives and works in metropolitan centers with resultant concentration of tremendous burdens of human and industrial wastes on the bodies of water to which they are related. The magnitude of water pollution was first established on a systematic basis in 1950 by studies that covered 226 river basins in the United States, of which 146 were interstate. These studies[10] indicated that there were more than 22,000 sources of stream pollution in the country, including 11,800 municipal sewer systems and 10,400 industrial waste outlets. Of the latter, one half produced organic wastes that greatly increased the biologic oxygen demand and infectious material, whereas others discharged wastes that were toxic or gave rise to tastes and odors that detracted from the subsequent usefulness of the water by humans.

Concern with the problem led Congress to pass the Water Pollution Control Act of 1956. Although Congress recognized the primary responsibility of the states in the matter, the Water Pollution Control Act authorized and directed the Public Health Service to take the initiative in developing or adopting comprehensive programs for the solution of water pollution programs in cooperation with the states, interstate agencies, municipalities, and industries. The act stated that comprehensive programs were to be developed for surface and underground waters, giving due consideration to all water uses—public water supply, propagation of fish and aquatic life, recreation, and agricultural, industrial, and other legitimate uses.

The act provided federal grants to the states and interstate agencies to help them carry out industrial waste studies and loans to municipalities to assist in the construction of needed abatement work. It further provided federal research and technical and consultative assistance to state and interstate agencies, municipalities, and industries and the encouragement of uniform state laws, interstate compacts, and cooperative state activities in the field of water pollution control. Initial responsibility for enforcement of pollution control measures was left with the states; federal authority to be exercised only on interstate waters, only after the efforts of the states had been exhausted, and only with the consent of the states.

To carry out its responsibilities, the Public Health Service instituted a water pollution control program with field units in each of 10 large drainage basin areas, staffed with engineers and scientists to work closely with officials of the state governments. The Taft Sanitary Engineering Center in Cincinnati served as the research center for the work. In 1962 Congress further supplemented this program by providing for the establishment of a series of water pollution research laboratories throughout the nation.

As indication of its growing concern, Congress subsequently passed the Water Quality Act of 1965, the Water Resources Planning Act of 1965, the Public Works and Economic Development Act of 1965, and the Clean Water Act of 1966. In the process it established a Federal Water Pollution Control Administration in the Department of the Interior and transferred the water pollution control responsibilities of the Public Health Service to it. Subsequently in late 1970 the program became part of the newly established Environmental Protection Agency.

Despite the efforts made over the years, by 1970 there were still unfulfilled water pollution control needs in 1,008 communities with 89 million people. The remedial cost was estimated at about $20 billion.[11]

Congressional concern continues, and in 1976 Congress passed the Safe Drinking Water Act (P.L. 95-190). Of particular and growing concern are the ever-increasing numbers, types, and amounts of industrial chemicals that are discharged into sources of drinking water. Okun[9] has pointed out that "of 120 compounds (out of 496 organic chemicals) found in fresh water and examined for carcinogenicity in animals 22.5 percent were positive; of 32 compounds examined for teratogenicity in animals, 62.5 percent were positive; of 29 examined for mutagenicity all were found to be positive. . . ."

There are two particularly important conditions for successful control of stream pollution. The first is planning on a regional basis, since few situations involve only one state. Although it is important that each state develop its own programs based on its own legislation, it is fundamental to plan and coordinate the various state water pollution control programs and, insofar as possible, the laws on which they are based, to bring about a practical program that will serve the needs of the drainage basin in question.

The second condition is a recognition of the fact that although the chemical and physical characteristics of human wastes do not vary significantly, it is rare that industrial wastes, even those from similar enterprises, are the same. Hence each stream pollution problem, especially if it involves industrial wastes, is a case study in itself. Hunter[12] has pointed out that current policies on which water pollution control programs are based rest on (1) financial support for treatment plant construction and (2) the establishment of water quality standards. These policies are actually responsible in large part for the unsatisfactory rate of water quality improvement. They offer no economic incentives to institute satisfactory measures. In fact, they make it less costly or more economical for industries and municipalities to continue to pollute.

Added to this is the inability of current enforcement procedures to respond quickly enough because of inadequate monitoring staffs and usually overburdened and inefficient judicial procedures. One suggested approach is to levy "effluent charges." However, this is tantamount to a license to pollute, which could be tax deductable as well as passed on to the purchaser of the product made. Hunter suggested as more practical the combination of (1) the establishment of effluent standards, (2) the imposition of prorated fines, and (3) a thorough monitoring system. To these one must add a greatly improved judicial system, perhaps with special courts with built-in environmental expertise. Since its establishment, the Environmental Protection Agency has taken action to prohibit the discharge of mercury and other industrial wastes into lakes, rivers, and streams. It has also sponsored projects for new treatment methods of sewage and industrial effluents.

WASTE DISPOSAL

Closely related to the problems of water sanitation and stream sanitation is that of satisfactory waste disposal. The waste materials of present-day households consist of human excreta, garbage, and refuse. In urban areas there is also added an increasing amount of industrial wastes. Until recently each of these was considered to be a somewhat separate problem. In urban communities, however, they have become increasingly interrelated. In some instances garbage and refuse are collected and disposed of together. In addition, many households now grind garbage, which is disposed of with excreta and other household wastes through the plumbing and sewerage system. Industrial wastes may also be discharged into the sewerage system or directly into bodies of water that also receive raw or treated sewage.

There are various methods of disposal of waste

products of human societies. These may be listed as (1) discharge into bodies of water, with or without treatment; (2) discharge onto the surface of the ground in either a sanitary or insanitary manner; (3) burial in the ground; (4) incineration; (5) composting; and (6) recycling. No one of these offers the perfect solution, since each has some disadvantages or hazards and each may be more applicable than the others in specific situations. In general, the following principles should be applied to the choice of disposal methods:

1. There should be no contamination of ground water that may enter springs or wells.

2. There should be no contamination of surface water.

3. The surface soil should not be contaminated.

4. Excreta or other organic material should not be accessible to flies or animals.

5. There should be freedom from odors or unsightly conditions.

6. The method used should be simple, reasonable in cost, and require a minimum of maintenance.

It is not within the province of this book to describe and assess the various methods of waste disposal, since those details are readily available in several excellent books devoted specifically to the field of sanitation and sanitary engineering. An excellent overview of the complexities, needs, and methodologies in this field is available in a report by the National Academy of Sciences and the National Research Council.[13] The intent here is merely to present a general background picture of certain factors that must be considered with regard to a public health agency's interest and responsibility in the problem.

Social and environmental circumstances are of particular significance with regard to the disposal of human excreta, which is by far the potentially most dangerous type of waste material. The pertinent situations, hence the methods of approach, are three in kind. The simplest situation is that in which no water carriage is possible. Typically this applies particularly to rural and arid areas. Under such circumstances resort may be made to the pit privy, the bored hole latrine, the vault privy, the chemical toilet, the septic privy, or the box-and-can toilet. A second situation may be observed in suburban areas and some small communities where no public sewerage system exists. Under such circumstances individual cesspools or septic tanks are commonly used. (Increasingly, however, these systems are being replaced with small sewerage systems specially designed for such places.) Finally, there is the situation where both a public water supply and a public sewerage system make possible not only water carriage but also water disposal of human excreta. Here new problems arise in that there is a concentration of tremendous amounts of human wastes, the complication of plumbing hazards such as possible cross connections and back siphonage, and the frequent addition of garbage and industrial wastes. Some attempts have been made to dispose of sewage by using it for irrigation and agricultural purposes in so-called sewage farms. The success and practicability of this approach have been limited in the United States.

Generally speaking, therefore, and because of the large amount of water it contains, sewage is usually disposed of in a body of water. Unfortunately this is sometimes done without treatment. The dangers of discharge of raw sewage into streams or lakes are obvious, and increasingly it is important to treat sewage for the following reasons:

1. Public health reasons—to prevent the pollution of drinking water, fish and mollusks, and bathing places
2. Aesthetic reasons—to prevent the formation of foul odors and the development of streams and shorelines made unsightly by solid or suspended waste matter
3. Economic reasons—to prevent the killing of commercially valuable fish life, the infection of livestock and other animal life, and the deterioration of land values
4. Salvage reasons—to make possible the recovery of commercially valuable fertilizer, grease, gases, and other products

The objectives of the various methods of sewage treatment are:

1. To diminish the amount of solid materials discharged into a stream to lessen the demands on its purifying properties and to prevent the formation of sludge banks and the appearance of objectionable floating materials
2. To decompose by biologic methods the organic matter in sewage and to transform it into simpler organic compounds and into gases and liquids, thus greatly diminishing the burden of the final purification that takes place in a stream
3. To stabilize the organic matter in sewage by biologic methods operating under aerobic conditions so that the purifying proper-

ties of a stream into which the treated sewage is ultimately discharged will be taxed to a minimum

4. To diminish or destroy the bacteria present in sewage, particularly the pathogenic varieties capable of producing disease
5. To remove by chemical or other processes industrial or related wastes that may be toxic or otherwise affect the subsequent use of the receiving body of water

These objectives are accomplished in different situations by combinations of (1) screening and/or sedimentation; (2) anaerobic digestion of settleable solids in a septic tank, Imhoff tank, or separate sludge digestion tank; (3) oxidation of nonsettleable organic matter by filtration, activated sludge, or irrigation methods; (4) disinfection with chlorine or other disinfectants; and (5) chemical or other neutralizing procedures.

Although the operation of public sewerage as well as water systems is a local responsibility, the overall supervision of these facilities is largely a state concern. In most instances the state health department is the official agency with major responsibility, but in nearly three fourths of the states the responsibility is shared with other departments or special commissions.[14] Among these are departments of public works, labor, education, and industry; special state sewage, stream pollution, or sanitary boards or commissions; and state universities and laboratories. Currently there is an increasing trend for states to follow the federal lead and establish separate environmental control agencies with regulatory powers. In such instances, however, the state health departments usually retain authority for the establishment of hygienic criteria and standards. Among the functions for which the state commonly has responsibility are the promulgation and enforcement of laws, rules, and regulations; approval of plans and installations; examination and licensure of treatment plant operators; periodic inspection of installations; provision of consultation services to localities; provision of grants-in-aid to local sanitation units; and the promotion of satisfactory local facilities.

Authority for the supervision of semipublic waste disposal systems is more likely to be shared among several agencies than in the case of public supplies. Thus if the system involves educational institutions, parks, and/or industries, for example, the departments of education, parks, industry, and/or labor are almost certain to be involved in most instances. This shared responsibility and authority, however, does not alter the fact that the state health department must play the primary regulatory and supervisory role with respect to the sanitary aspects of the situation. Often, of course, these responsibilities are met in collaboration with or through the local public health structure if it is adequately staffed.

The weakest link exists in relation to supervision and control of individual private waste disposal systems in rural areas. In places where a local public health department exists, it almost invariably includes some form of activity in the field of human excreta control. The basis of the activity usually consists of a persistent health education approach on a personal visit basis, augmented by general educational measures, consultation from the state health department, and sometimes actual assistance in the financing and construction of private sanitary privies or septic tank systems.

REFUSE DISPOSAL

Each year about 3.5 billion tons of an incredible mixture of solid waste material is discarded in the United States. In consists of 165 million tons of household waste, 200 million tons of municipal and industrial waste, 2 billion tons of agricultural waste, and more than a billion tons of mining waste. Some of it provides a medium for the growth of pathogenic microorganisms as well as food and harborage for vermin and rodent vectors of disease. Other components contain a variety of toxic chemicals. Household and municipal waste material, much of which could be recycled, is composed of miscellaneous paper, 25%; newspaper, 14%; garbage, 12%; glass, stone, and ceramics, 10%; grass and dirt, 10%; metals, 8%; wood, 7%; cardboard, 7%; textiles, 3%; plastic film, 2%; and molded plastics, rubber, and leather, 2%.

Disposal of solid wastes is costly and difficult. A variety of methods have been used, most of them unsatisfactory. Simple open dumping accounts for 73% of waste disposal, and incineration essentially by open burning accounts for 15%. Only 8% is disposed of by sanitary landfill, only 3% by salvage, and only 1% is composted. Most urban communi-

ties are rapidly running out of places to dump or bury waste material, and if they incinerate it, the pollution of the atmosphere becomes worse. Meanwhile, much of its noxious contents runs off or seeps into and contaminates surface and ground waters.

New methods of waste disposal are being tried. One consists of grinding the total mass of waste and subjecting it to jets of air to separate paper from metals and plastics. Iron and steel can then be removed by magnets. A variation is coarse grinding of the material in a fluid state, followed by incineration at about 2,200° F. This produces a glasslike slag that can be used in the production of bottles, building materials, or highway aggregate. In another method the results of dry grinding are suspended in water and centrifuged into various components. Since a community's solid waste contains a significant amount of organic material, attempts at composting have been tried; but these methods have had limited results.

Approximately two thirds of the cost of solid waste disposal is represented by its pickup and transfer to a nearby collection vehicle. Partly with this in mind there have been developed garbage and trash compactors for installation in household kitchens. Material is compressed under high pressure into heavy-duty paper or plastic bags with provision for runoff of liquids into the kitchen drain. The result is a much smaller, more compact mass that is easier to handle and that requires less truck space, hence fewer trips by collection vehicles. Many communities and civic groups promote the separate collection of newspapers and aluminum cans, for which payment is sometimes made.

A special disposal problem is presented by discarded automobiles, which are increasing at an alarming rate. Several types of ingenious mechanisms have been developed. After removal of tires, the engine, and the differential gear, the chassis is subjected to high-temperature incineration to get rid of fabrics and plastic parts. The remainder is shredded and the metal shreds classified by magnetic means for resale. The economics are such that a plant that processes as few as 48 automobiles per day by means of hand dismantling, incineration, and shredding can yield a 20% annual return on the original investment including plant, equipment, and land costs.

A significant step forward in encouraging the development and use of techniques and mechanisms such as those mentioned was taken by Congress in

October 1976 when it passed the Resource Conservation and Recovery Act (P.L. 94-580). One of its chief purposes is to encourage recycling of natural resources. An additional goal is to promote the safe disposal of discarded materials and to regulate the management of hazardous waste. Authority and responsibility are placed within the Environmental Protection Agency. In commenting on the bill, Wands,[15] of the National Research Council, has observed that apart from its health and safety aspects, the intent to recycle natural resources "is a laudable goal since almost none of these resources are renewable in less than eons of time. Notable exceptions, of course, are forest products, manpower, water supplies, and fertile soil which are renewable in a generation or two."

FOOD AND MILK SANITATION

Food protection in urban communities is today one of the most challenging and probably least successful of all organized community health activities. The extent to which food protection can be improved depends largely on the interest of informed citizens, as reflected by their political representatives, as well as active support from industry, educational institutions, professional groups and the food control agencies at the local, state and federal levels.

The above statement by Walker and associates[16] epitomizes the whole field of food sanitation. Although their true incidence is unknown, unquestionably, food-borne infections and poisonings are outnumbered only by the common cold as causes of short-term illness. Estimates vary considerably, but 1 million cases or more are thought to occur annually in the United States. Their usual brevity and mild symptoms, treated commonly with home or proprietary remedies, result in poor reporting, making effective control difficult.

It is interesting to consider the changes that have occurred with reference to reported epidemics of enteric disease. The majority of the cases of epidemic gastrointestinal infections that occurred up through the first quarter of this century were attributable to impure water. Because of the remarkable strides that have been made since that time in providing safe water to concentrations of people in urban centers, water no longer plays an outstanding role as a transmitter of disease in the United States. Between 1938 and 1960 the Public Health Service compiled and analyzed reports of epidemics borne by water, milk, and food from data submitted by local and state health departments. An analysis of these data (Table 21-1)[17] is informative. Between 1938 and 1942, water not only caused many outbreaks but was most important in terms of persons affected. Although the average annual number of outbreaks caused by water and milk was about the same and in each case only about one fourth of the number caused by foods, the number of persons affected by waterborne epidemics was about 3½ times the number affected by other foods and about 11 times the number affected by milk and milk products.

However, when the data for the period since 1942 are considered, a significant shift is seen to have occurred. Comparing the two periods, although the average annual numbers of epidemics attributable to water and to milk and milk products have been cut in half, those caused by other foods have dou-

TABLE 21-1. Changes in food-borne and waterborne disease outbreaks, United States, 1938 to 1960

Time period	Water		Milk and milk products		Other foods	
	Outbreaks	Cases	Outbreaks	Cases	Outbreaks	Cases
1938-1942—Number	247	103,441	208	9,114	902	29,095
Annual average	49	20,688	42	1,823	181	5,819
1943-1951—Number	208	32,342	205	7,259	2,769	101,466
Annual average	23	3,594	23	806	308	11,274
1953-1957—Number	33	3,043	55	1,539	1,081	53,469
Annual average	7	609	11	308	216	10,694
1958-1960—Number	22	2,535	29	538	740	27,954
Annual average	7	845	10	179	247	9,318

From Dauer, C.C.: Public Health Rep. **76:**915, Oct. 1961.

bled in number. Furthermore, although the average annual number of persons affected in recent years by milk and milk products was one half of what it had been and for water only one sixth of what it had been, with regard to outbreaks caused by other foods, the number of persons affected doubled. The figures for the period 1953 to 1960 indicate a decline in all types of epidemics. However, the decline was greatest in the instances of waterborne and milk-borne epidemics, which declined both in number of epidemics and in number of persons affected. Indeed, although the average annual number of epidemics borne by foods was about one third less in the period from 1953 to 1957 than in the period from 1943 tq 1951, the number of persons affected remained essentially the same.

The figures, however, are deceptive and must be interpreted with caution. Whereas data for waterborne disease in the United States for the year 1971 is not available and would probably be low, there were reported to the federal Center for Disease Control 320 food-borne outbreaks, of which only 7 were attributed to milk and other dairy products. A total of 13,453 persons were affected. However, the center's report[18] makes this important observation: food poisoning in the United States is grossly underreported. In the state of Washington, where food-borne disease surveillance has been developed to a high degree, 57 outbreaks were reported to the Center for Disease Control in 1971. Projecting from this figure, the estimated number of outbreaks for the entire United States was about 3,100 in 1971 instead of the 320 reported. This serves to emphasize the need for improvement in both surveillance systems and investigations. In 1971, for the second time in 5 years, the number of reported outbreaks (320) decreased when compared with the number for the previous year (366). Such a decline probably does not reflect a decrease in the number of outbreaks of food-borne illness. Rather, it suggests that food-borne disease surveillance may occupy a position of low priority relative to competing health problems. Since 1971, the situation has not improved. During 1974, for example, 456 outbreaks of food-borne disease involving 15,489 persons were reported.

Despite their limitations, the figures illustrate two facts with regard to the present time: (1) foods are easily the most important and an increasing cause of gastrointestinal infections in the United States; and (2) although milk and milk products are potentially the most perishable and most dangerous foods and despite their ever-increasing use, they now are a relatively unimportant cause of disease when compared with other foods. This is explainable on the basis that their very perishability has focused so much attention on means of ensuring their safety.

To promote scientifically sound standards and uniform legislation, the Public Health Service in 1924 developed a recommended standard milk ordinance, which has since been revised numerous times. Representing the pooled opinions and experience of public health officials, the milk and dairy industry, veterinarians, agriculturists, scientists, consumer representatives, and others, by now this ordinance forms the basis for regulation and practice in all the states as well as in many counties and municipalities. The ordinance and its accompanying code now protect a majority of the urban and much of the nonurban population. It is recognized as the only fluid milk regulation approaching a national standard. For use in conjunction with it, procedures relating to the interstate shipment of milk and methods for rating milksheds have been developed. In addition, the Public Health Service has developed widely used standards for community infant formula services, automatic vending of foods and beverages, and food service sanitation. With specific reference to market milk, of special significance in the maintenance of the safety of milk and milk products is the widespread application of the pasteurization process. Pasteurization of all market milk is compulsory in almost all the states, counties, and municipalities of the nation. As a result, almost all of the fluid milk consumed by the urban population in the United States is protected by pasteurization.

Important in the successful supervision and control of the many complex factors involved in the production, processing, and sale of milk and milk products has been the cooperative action on the part of public health agencies, departments of agriculture, and representatives of the milk and dairy industry. The actual control programs are administered by sanitarians and veterinarians on the local level supported by the state departments of health and agriculture and by the industry. On the state level, authority may be vested in either the state health department or the department of agriculture and sometimes in both.[14]

From the analysis of epidemics presented, it is obvious that foods other than milk are a matter of considerable concern to public health agencies as an increasing source of preventable disease. The food-borne outbreaks during 1971 give a picture of the problem. Of those reported, the diseases involved were staphylococcal food poisoning, 92; salmonellosis, 30; shigellosis, 7; botulism, 9; noxious plant illness, 4; chemical poisoning, 30; trichinosis, 4; *Clostridium perfringens,* 51; streptococcal infection, 2; hepatitis, 4; others, 10; and unknown, 81. The types of establishments known to be involved were food service establishments, 96; schools, 22; homes, 123; camps and picnics, 13; and churches, 10. It is epidemiologically important to note that the last three types of situations that accounted for 146 (or 55%) of the outbreaks are of a private nature, as compared with 118 (or 45%) of the outbreaks attributable to public or semipublic food places that should be subject to control by health authorities.

The situation on the federal level is somewhat complicated by the retention of meat inspection responsibilities by the Department of Agriculture and by the obvious concern of the Department of Health and Human Services for all matters dealing with the salubrity of foods. Actually, these two federal agencies are concerned with different aspects of the food problem and work in close collaboration, each fulfilling certain responsibilities.

On the state level the situation is more confused. All states have some agency or agencies responsible for food control, but there is no uniformity. The agencies involved are departments of agriculture, 23 states; departments of health, 43 states; and others, 4 states. From the numbers it will be noted that in some states responsibility is shared.[14]

Almost all municipalities and a great many counties carry out some form of food control activities, usually by personnel of the local public health agency. The personnel vary in quality from untrained inspectors to well-qualified sanitarians and veterinarians. In general, the activities consist of inspection, rating, and certification of food processing and dispensing establishments, sampling of an analysis of foodstuffs, physical examination and training of food handlers, and local prosecution of infringements of food ordinances and laws. In carrying out these activities, the local personnel work closely with and are supported by personnel of the various interested state and federal agencies.

Particular attention is given by local public health

authorities to sanitary conditions in restaurants and taverns and bars. Many different types of inspection and rating forms have been developed, and many types of action such as certification, licensing, and awards of merit have been used. Since 1934 the Public Health Service has provided a *Food Service Sanitation Manual.* Included in the manual is a model food sanitation ordinance and code, which has been adopted widely.

Not infrequently, public health interests and private enterprise have found themselves in the same arena. Unfortunately, they sometimes act at cross-purposes. Sometimes business and industry have looked on public health workers as interfering, unrealistic, and restraining and have pointed with considerable justification to the maze of conflicting requirements, ordinances, codes, and standards with regard to the same article or process in different jurisdictions. Public health workers, on the other hand, have sometimes accused private enterprise of being completely mercenary and without social conscience. Fortunately in recent years industry and public health have worked to get together in an amiable and intelligent manner to arrive at mutually satisfactory conclusions and recommendations in the public's interest.

In the field of environmental health , and especially with regard to food sanitation, the National Restaurant Association and the National Automatic Merchandising Association have long supported the goals of the Public Health Service by preparing and promoting training classes and training materials. In 1944 the National Sanitation Foundation was established as an independent, nonprofit corporation financed entirely by business and industry and governed by a board of directors, which consists of individuals from private enterprise and public health. Its purposes are (1) to bring together representative industrialists, businessmen, and public health workers to define and outline mutual problems; (2) to finance research in fields of mutual concern and interest; (3) to promote a program of personal and community health to acquaint employees and the general public with the need for good sanitary practices and community cleanliness; (4) to provide a testing laboratory, similar to the Fire Underwriters Laboratory, for materials of sanitary and health-promoting value, and (5) to develop standards applicable to the food equipment and dispensing industries.

Somewhat similar are the increased activities on the part of business and industry toward "self-policing." Examples of this are the programs of the National Canners' Association, the Ice Cream Merchandising Institute, the Food Industries Sanitarian Association, the National Automatic Merchandising Association (food and beverage vending machines), and the American Institute of Baking. These point toward a more fruitful cooperative action from which the public may benefit. It conforms with one of the recommendations of the National Commission on Community Health Services,[1] which states, "Industry and commerce [should] assume more responsibility for self-policing and control of their products, services, and operations in relation to associated environmental health problems; and health agencies [should] encourage and assist them in so doing."

ATMOSPHERIC POLLUTION

The nature, magnitude, and biologic ill effects of atmospheric pollution are presented in the chapter on environmental hazards. Emphasis here is on what should be and is being done. During recent years the public and health officials have become increasingly aware of the atmosphere as the important medium in which we exist and of the possibility and consequences of overloading it with waste products of human activity. Increasingly it is recognized that the layer of air above the earth surface is thin, not limitless, and should not be used as an aerial sewer. Pound for pound, humans consume at least 10 times as much air as water. Although there has long been concern about the purity of the water used by human societies, little attention has been given to the quality of the air that constantly is breathed into the lungs and absorbed into the bloodstream. Even now, despite the mass of literature about the serious health effects of air pollution, most public reaction relates to the unaesthetic effects of smoke, dirt, and odor. This is clearly an area in which science and government together must provide not only the facts but, more important, the initiative and leadership to solve one of the world's most critical problems.

Historical records indicate concern with the problem and even legislation in earlier times. As a result of the widespread use of soft sea coal for fuel in English towns and cities, a smoke-abatement law was passed as early as 1273 by King Edward I. He banned the use of coal as prejudicial to the public health. Soon after, in 1306, Parliament formed a smoke-abatement group whose recommendations resulted in a royal proclamation that prohibited the use of coal in the furnaces of artificers. Records show that in 1307 one offender was actually executed for violating the regulations. In 1661 a report entitled *Fumifugium* claimed that almost one half of the deaths in London were "phthisical and pulmonic distempers" resulting from polluted air.[19]

The atmosphere may be polluted from many sources. Smoke results whenever fuel or other material is incompletely burned. Sources are industrial, commercial, or domestic heating facilities; incinerators; brush fires; dumps; and automobile motors. In urban areas especially, automobile motors are a major generator of toxic gases. In rural and suburban areas irritating pollens and toxic agricultural sprays and dusts are likely to be particularly prevalent. Industrial contaminants represent a particularly complex and important source of atmospheric pollution.

In general, air pollutants consist of particulate matter, aerosols, gases, and vapors. The most common forms are condensed organics such as fly ash and tar; oxides of sulfur, carbon, and nitrogen; metallic oxides and fumes; minerals such as asbestos; vegetable matter such as pollens; and mists and fogs. Carbon monoxide and sulfur dioxide are probably the most common of the gases. In addition, ozone produced by photochemical reactions can give rise to irritating proportions as well as aid in the development of additional irritants by its oxidizing action on other pollutants. The complexity of industrial, automotive, and other sources that may pollute air is illustrated by studies of smog samples from Los Angeles.[20] Among the contaminants found were the following:

Aerosols

Ether-soluble aerosols	Lead
Sulfuric acid mist	Aluminum
Carbon	Calcium
Silicon	Iron

Gases and vapors

Acetylene	Methyl chloride
Aromatics	Nitric oxide
Benzene	Nitrogen dioxide
Isobutane	Nitrous oxide

n-Butane	n-Pentane
Butenes	Phosgene
Carbon tetracholoride	Propane
Ethane	Propylene
Ethyl benzene and xylene	Sulfur dioxide
Formic acid	Toluene
Methyl cellosolve	Trichlorethylene

Unsaturated hydrocarbons ranging from C_5H_8 to $C_{12}H_{24}$

Products of oxidation of the above unsaturated hydrocarbons (aldehydes, peroxides, ketones, and organic acids)

This list is by no means inclusive in terms of the total possible pollutants that might occur in various locations or circumstances or that might be formed as a result of chemical interactions.

In addition to the discharge of contaminants into the atmosphere, certain fixed or variable meteorologic and topographic factors may determine whether or not an air pollution problem will develop, the degree of its concentration or extension, and the acuteness and severity of its result. If a community is situated within a topographic bowl, natural dispersal of atmospheric pollutants will be limited and concentrations of dangerous substances may result. In addition, depending on the location and nature of the emissions, localized or neighborhood areas at risk may develop.

Typically, insufficient attention is given to these factors until they combine under special circumstances to cause dramatic disastrous situations such as those that occurred at Donora, Penn., the Meuse Valley in Belgium, and elsewhere (discussed later). Any program relating to atmospheric pollution must take into account a study of winds, atmospheric stability, and precipitation as they are related to seasonal variation, diurnal variation, surface temperatures, and many other meteorologic factors. This accentuates the need to consider air pollution control measures from three viewpoints: (1) local or neighborhood problems that are only partly related to topographic and meteorologic factors and more related to proximity, nature, and concentration of the polluting source; (2) air conservation in an urban area; and (3) ecologic conservation of broad areas that might be affected by acid rains, atmospheric dissemination of lead, and the like, where even if the concentrations of such materials in urban areas may be low, their cumulative broadcast emission may become significant in the large, longer range context.

Pollution of the atmosphere may result in economic loss to individuals and to the general population in a variety of ways. Losses may take the form of damage to livestock and vegetation, corrosion of metals and structural materials, damage to clothing and other fabrics, damage to the finishes of automobiles and houses, disruption of communications and increased artificial lighting requirements, depreciated real estate values, and, last but most important, the acute and chronic harm done to humans. Not including the effect on humans, the national economic loss caused by atmospheric pollution has been estimated variously as between $4 billion and $10 billion annually. On the other hand, one can cite many examples of industrial establishments that by installation of control procedures, have actually netted from modest to substantial profits from the recovered materials. Furthermore, if permissible tax benefits are applied to pollution control equipment purchase and operation, the savings are even greater.

For health purposes, of course, the effects on human life are of greatest concern. The effect of air pollution on the health of people is usually so insidious that a cause-effect relationship is difficult to demonstrate. Nevertheless, it can be done, as in the case of cigarette smoking and cancer. Admittedly, base lines, standards, and methods of measurement necessary to determine adequately the physiologic or histologic effects of substances in the air still leave much to be desired. Even when a relatively severe short-term exposure occurs, such as that at Donora, conclusive answers are usually not obtained because the investigations take place after the fact and not before and during the incident. Nevertheless, much has been learned during recent years as a result of studying "epidemics" of air pollution, continuous smog situations, long-term effects on workers constantly exposed to certain substances, and laboratory experiments.[21]

The "epidemic" situation, of course, is the most dramatic, and severe facts of value have resulted from their investigation. Four of these occurrences merit special mention. During 1930 the heavily industrialized area in and around Liege in the Meuse Valley of Belgium was subjected to 4 days of continuous fog saturated with industrial smoke and fumes. Many thousands of people died. Although studies indicated significant amounts of sulfur dioxide, sulfuric acid, and other chemicals in the air, no single substance was found in a concentration sufficiently high to have caused the damage by itself.[22]

A similar tragedy occurred in 1948 in Donora, Pa., a small town of about 14,000 inhabitants. Because of its location in a valley and because of its industry, polluted fogs are extremely common in Donora. Usually the sun and wind dissipate the fog during the early hours of the day. Occasionally, however, it may remain throughout a day. On October 27, 1948, a thick fog settled down in the valley and remained for 4½ days, meanwhile becoming more and more polluted by the smoke, fumes, and gases from the town's industrial plants. During the period, 20 individuals died and about 6,000 others, or 43% of the population, became ill in varying degrees. The episode and the circumstances were studied exhaustively for a year by the Pennsylvania Department of Health assisted by the U.S. Public Health Service.[23,24]

As with the Meuse Valley disaster, although a large number of gases and fumes were identified in the atmosphere, it was concluded that no single contaminant was responsible. In both instances it was believed that a combination of irritating and toxic materials, of which sulfur dioxide undoubtedly was one, acted synergistically to produce the illnesses and deaths. In both instances the deleterious conditions were observed to affect the population selectively. Almost all the victims who died and many of those who became ill but did not die suffered from respiratory or cardiac difficulties. The intensive pollution of the air harmed the aged, the infirm, and enfeebled infants earlier than it affected the more vigorous fraction of the population. Among other things, this indicates the need for a completely different set of tolerance levels of toxic substances for a community as a whole as against those used heretofore. Most of the latter are based on the tolerance of industrial workers.

A third disaster of this type occurred on November 24, 1950, at Poza Rica, Mexico, where 320 persons were hospitalized, 22 of whom died.[25] This case differed from the Meuse and Donora episodes in that it was possible to point to a single toxic agent. A petroleum refinery at the site discharged a number of aerial contaminants, one of which was hydrogen sulfide. A combination of relatively localized unusual meteorologic phenomena, combined with an operational breakdown that caused more venting than usual, resulted in an extremely high concentration of hydrogen sulfide gas around the plant.

The city of London, England, has experienced several sudden increases in the death rate because of atmospheric pollution. Its situation is somewhat different from the others described in that the problem is not primarily related to industrial contaminants. Severe fogs with stasis and lethal concentration of atmospheric pollutants occurred particularly in 1873, 1880, 1892, 1948, 1952, and 1962. In the 1880 incident the death rate of 896 per million was about 50% above normal expectancy. In fact, it was significantly higher than the rate of 876 recorded for the worst week of the great London cholera epidemic of 1866. Despite this, the events of December 1952 and especially of the 5 days from December 5 to 9 were even more spectacular. It has been shown conclusively that during the total period of the first 3 weeks of December, about 4,000 deaths were caused by the polluted fog. Although the very young, the aged, and the infirm were affected most, it is interesting that all age groups contributed to the increased mortality. The mortality of infants doubled, deaths of children 10 to 13 years of age increased by one third, and deaths of young adults increased by almost two thirds. Deaths from bronchitis, which were eight times the normal, and deaths from pneumonia, which were three times the normal, accounted for about one half of the total increase in mortality. Other causes of death for which significant increases were observed were pulmonary tuberculosis and cancer, coronary disease, and myocardial degeneration.

The cause of the phenomenon in London was a prolonged absence of wind and a low temperature, which produced a low-altitude inversion whereby the normal upward air currents came to a stop. As a result, the usual air contaminants of the area accumulated to extremely high concentrations. For example, the concentration of smoke rose 36 times and the concentration of sulfur dioxide rose 19,000 times the summer daily average.[26] In December 1962 during 4 days, 1,000 persons were hospitalized and about 100 persons died from the effects of a similar but shorter episode.

More difficult than "epidemic" situations is the problem of determining the chronic effects of atmospheric contaminants. Attempts have been made to study this problem, but inherent difficulties have made them incomplete and inconclusive. Nevertheless, this is a highly active research field, some of the results of which are presented in the preceding chapter.

By its very nature, atmospheric pollution is difficult to control. Its causes are many and complex; adequate criteria, standards, and means of measurement have been developed only relatively recently; and an extensive number of public and private agencies, businesses, and industries have important interests in anything that is done. The atmosphere surrounding a present-day community is bound to be contaminated. A completely pure atmosphere is unattainable. Some trade-offs must be considered. It would seem that control must depend on legislation; public and industrial education; the further improvement of criteria, standards, and measurement techniques; the further development and application of practical devices for controlling automotive and industrial emissions; and the development and application of new sources of heat and power. Recognition of air pollution as a health and social problem has resulted in the enactment of legislation at all levels of government. Enabling legislation to permit local jurisdictions to act against specific problems was passed in California in 1947. This was followed in 1955 by legislation that permitted regional control programs. In addition to establishing a control authority and providing for continuous study and research, it placed a limit on the dusts, fumes, and sulfur that may be discharged by industry and required approval of plans for any installation that might add to the pollution of the atmosphere. Numerous states and local communities have since followed the example of Los Angeles and California.

In 1959 the California legislature required the promulgation of ambient air quality standards and emission standards for motor vehicles. This led to the California Motor Vehicle Pollution Control Act of 1960, which required the installation on motor vehicles of devices to reduce emissions. This affected the entire automobile industry, and exhaust control devices became applicable on all new cars in the United States beginning in September 1967.

Federal legislation in 1955 authorized and supported research and technical assistance on the federal and state level. The federal role was strengthened by the passage of a series of Clean Air Acts, beginning in 1963. These were administered by the National Air Pollution Control Administration of the Environmental Health Service, Department of Health, Education, and Welfare, until December 1970, when the program became one of the basic units of the new Environmental Protection Agency. The past few years have witnessed an acceleration of research and legislative and court action with the establishment and enforcement of increasingly exact and strict criteria and standards. On the basis of these, many large industries, especially those concerned with automobiles and energy sources, have been given tight time limits within which to comply. One leader in the field of air pollution control stated, "The automobile was recognized as a problem in 1950. We began to do something about it in 1960, the industry finally agreed that the problem existed in 1970. If we are lucky, we will have the technology for a true cleanup by 1980, and maybe there will be a 'clean car population' by 1990. Meanwhile the condition of the earth's atmosphere is getting more critical all the time." Among other beneficial steps have been the trend toward smaller automobiles, the increased use of lead-free gasoline, and attempts to develop a substitute for the internal combustion engine. Offsetting these is the increased use of coal by utilities because of the energy shortage and the high price of oil.

RADIOLOGIC HEALTH

One of the newest and very important aspects of environmental health relates to problems arising from the use of fissionable materials. Increasing amounts of radioactive isotopes are being used for medical diagnosis and treatment and for industrial research and materials testing. In addition, a number of ships and electrical power plants using nuclear energy have been constructed. The potential of fallout from nuclear weapons testing or attack compounds the situation. In several instances accidental spillage of fissionable material has presented health agencies with new challenges. The March 1979 incident at the Three Mile Island nuclear power plant near Harrisburg, Pa., provided a dramatic example of the potential danger.

The chief concern of the public health agency in this field is protection of the community and the nation from damaging radiations. These might arise not only from a military attack but also from misuse, accident, improper disposal of fissionable waste materials, or weapons testing. Understandably the last possibility mentioned is prominent in the public's mind, largely because of extensive discussion in the public information media. It is important to realize, however, that it does not represent a major threat. Bugher[27] pointed out that studies by the National Academy of Sciences and the National Research Council have shown that fallout in the atmosphere from weapons testing represents only a small fraction of the total radiation exposure of the public in contrast to the large part of the total exposure from the diagnostic and therapeutic uses of x-rays. He went on to predict that "with the rapid development of nuclear power and the expanding employment of radioactive materials and nuclear reactions in industry, agriculture, and medicine, we may anticipate that maintaining control over these potential hazards will become more complex rather than less."

Among the radiation control activities in which various health agencies have become involved are the determination of the amounts and effects of natural or background radiation; the prohibition of shoe-fitting fluoroscopic machines; the testing of x-ray and fluoroscopic equipment in medical and dental offices, hospitals, and clinics as well as industry; the use of collimators on such equipment; the surveillance of fluctuations in atmospheric radiation; the testing of milk, water, and other substances for levels of radioactive contamination; consultation in the construction of nuclear-powered ships and electric power plants; planning for civilian protection in case of nuclear attack; and the disposal of radioactive wastes.

These new responsibilities have made it necessary for increasing numbers of public health workers to familiarize themselves with totally new areas of knowledge. To facilitate this, the Division of Radiological Health of the Public Health Service, the Atomic Energy Commission, the Department of Defense, the Nuclear Regulatory Commission, and many universities have provided continued education and in-service training courses and have engaged in the development of various specialized technologists in this field. In addition, because of the extensive geographic, social, political, and biologic ramifications of this field, it has become increasingly necessary for public health workers to involve themselves in interdisciplinary, interorganizational, and intergovernmental relationships quite different from those of the past.

Governmental concern about radiation is not new. Its history in the United States began with the standardization by the National Bureau of Standards of radium for medical uses in 1913 and includes concerns in relation to radium poisoning of watch-dial painters as well as radium water tonics and rejuvenators, leading eventually to the formation in the late 1920s of the Advisory Committee on X-Ray and Radium Protection, later renamed the National Committee on Radiation Protection. In 1946 the Atomic Energy Act was passed, which provided for the distribution of radioactive isotopes on the basis of strict health and safety standards.

In the late 1950s the Public Health Service established a Division of Radiological Health and designated an Advisory Committee on Radiation. It cooperated with the Atomic Energy Commission, the Food and Drug Administration, the Department of Defense, and various other agencies. In the process it carried out many studies on the decontamination of radioactively contaminated waters, the treatment and disposal of radioactive wastes, the standards necessary in the industrial and transportation uses of atomic power, the evaluation of varying degrees of hazards associated with radioactive elements, and the biologic effects of radiation. These functions were subsequently transferred in 1970 to the then established Environmental Protection Agency.

In 1960 a further step forward was taken by the enactment of P.L. 86-373, which established the Federal Radiation Council. A major purpose has been to examine all scientific evidence as it develops regarding the biologic effects of radiation and leading to the development of broad guidelines for national policy. Federal efforts were later strengthened by the passage of the Radiation Control for Health and Safety Act of 1968, which provided, among other things, a practical measure of protection from unnecessary emissions from x-ray equipment, television sets, and other electronic devices.

Accompanying national action and greatly stimulated by it has been the development of programs of varying degrees of extensiveness throughout the states and major cities of the nation.[28] In the process of developing and carrying out these programs, one of the most difficult problems that confronts the public health worker is the maintenance of an appropriate balance between the benefits that may result from the use of radioactive materials and radiation-generating equipment and the risks that might possibly be entailed.[29] No one would suggest that the use of x-rays be ceased because of some measure of risk. Similarly, it would be ill-advised to deprive society of the tremendous benefits to be reaped from the application of radiation to industry, food preservation, power development, and the like. Bugher[27] has put the question well:

Nearly all of us of this scientific generation have been brought up on the concept that all changes produced by ionizing radiation are deleterious in general and that in the genetic sense any biologically beneficial effect is outweighed by the handicaps that are introduced. We find it difficult to conceive that absorption of radiation may not be followed by permanent cell changes. It is possible that we neglect to consider that all life on this earth has come to its present stage through continuous contact with a radioactive environment. There has been not a single living cell in all the history of life on this planet that has not been subjected to radiation from both without and within its substance.

The challenge, then, is for public health workers to deal with problems of radioactivity with a balance of respect and reason based on sound, proved scientific data and not emotion or fear of the unknown.

HOUSING AND COMMUNITY PLANNING

In discussing the need for public health interest in housing, Winslow[30] commented:

The filth epidemics of the Nineteenth Century have been conquered in civilized and relatively prosperous lands like ours. We can now think in terms of health rather than in terms of disease; and, from this standpoint, such problems as nutrition and housing come to the forefront. The slum of today is no longer a hot-bed of cholera and typhus fever as it was seventy-five years ago. It remains, however, one of the major obstacles to that physical and emotional and social vigor and efficiency and satisfaction which we conceive as the health objective of the future.

Many attempts have been made to establish a conclusive relationship between unsatisfactory housing and ill health. However, because the dwellers in poor housing are subjected to so many other undesirable factors, such as low economic income, malnutrition, and limited education, it is impossible to determine with exactness what is cause and what is effect. The difficulty and its proper interpretation was well summarized by Anderson:[31]

Of the many newer aspects of environmental sanitation, the standards of housing seem to rest on an especially insecure epidemiological foundation. I would not question the potential health significance of housing, and yet epidemiological data on which to base this belief are virtually nonexistent for poor housing cannot be separated from other attributes of poverty.

This inability to secure epidemiological support for housing standards should not discourage us from attempts to improve housing conditions or even to do so by regulation. Almost every community has houses that by no stretch of the imagination can be defended as desirable for human habitation. An appreciable fraction of our population lives under conditions that are undesirable socially, morally, and hygienically. Housing needs no defense nor need await epidemiological support.

In tracing the history of the housing movement, Bauer[32] suggested that it may be viewed not only as a significant chapter in scientific and public health history, "but also as a very lively and important chapter in political history." She points out that without exception "every major step in housing progress in the past century has involved some public action," and suggests that "political philosophy—the motivating forces behind public action and the application of scientific knowledge—is not secondary or incidental, but paramount." Of particular significance to our present consideration, she traces the gradual development of enlightened political philosophy, dating from the English Poor laws as far back as the early seventeenth century—with their expanding concepts of individual rights—to due process of law, to health, to education, to the more recent concept of the right of individuals to a decent home. She provides public health workers with a sound basis for future thought and action in proposing that henceforth their interest is "not just a question of 'minimum standards,' to allay disease or prevent divorce or save the taxpayers money, or of sporadic housing programs tied to one emergency kite or another, to provide employment or increase the birthrate or improve the physical qualities of soldiers or lessen the danger of revolution, but good housing for all, to be provided by public action where private enterprise could not do the job, on the fundamental democratic principle of equal opportunity."

The production of housing has depended essentially on the law of supply and demand. The demand, however, has been closely linked to the economic ability of individuals and families to afford the product. Budget experts believe that a family should not expend more than three to four times its annual income for housing purchase. An important consideration is that private housing is constructed largely during periods of economic upswing, when building costs are also going up. Furthermore, during periods of economic depression, the cost of houses does not go down to the extent that salaries and incomes decline.

In the United States, during the depression years of the 1930s, despite ever-growing needs because of population increase and continued movement toward cities, construction of homes lagged considerably. The postdepression spurt was then thrown off balance by the resource requirements of the war effort. By the end of World War II, a tremendous backlog of housing needs had developed. Since that time, the greatest building boom in U.S. history occurred. This, combined with extensive slum clearance and suburbanization, has resulted in only a small percentage of dwellings with basic health deficiencies. In 1970 out of almost 68 million occupied housing units, 94% had complete plumbing facilities including hot and cold piped water, flush toilet, and bathtub or shower. Less than 1% of vacant housing units were rated dilapidated. Overcrowding and deficient lighting, ventilation, and heating were not included among the criteria.

The components of healthful housing have been studied by the Committee on the Hygiene of Housing, which was established in 1937 by the American Public Health Association. In the course of its work the committee has issued a series of important documents on the subject that have filled an important need not only of public health but of other disciplines. Under four broad headings the committee has listed the following basic principles that must be considered with regard to healthful housing[30]:

Fundamental physiologic needs
1. Maintenance of a thermal environment that will avoid undue heat loss from the human body
2. Maintenance of a thermal environment that will permit adequate heat loss from the human body
3. Provision of an atmosphere of reasonable chemical purity
4. Provision of adequate daylight illumination and avoidance of undue daylight glare
5. Provision for admission of direct sunlight
6. Provision of adequate artificial illumination and avoidance of glare
7. Protection against excessive noise
8. Provision of adequate space for exercise and for play of children

Fundamental psychologic needs
1. Provision of adequate privacy for the individual
2. Provision of opportunities for normal family life

3. Provision of opportunities for normal community life
4. Provision of facilities that make possible the performance of tasks of the household without undue physical and mental fatigue
5. Provision of facilities for maintenance of cleanliness of the dwelling and of the person
6. Concordance with prevailing social standards of the local community

Protection against contagion
1. Provision of a water supply of safe, sanitary quality available to the dwelling
2. Protection of the water supply system against pollution within the dwelling
3. Provision of toilet facilities of such a character as to minimize the danger of transmitting disease
4. Protection against sewage contamination of the interior surfaces of the dwelling
5. Avoidance of insanitary conditions in the vicinity of the dwelling
6. Exclusion from the dwelling of vermin, which may play a part in the transmission of disease
7. Provision of facilities for keeping milk and food undecomposed
8. Provision of sufficient space in sleeping rooms, to minimize the danger of contact infection

Protection against accidents
1. Erection of the dwelling with such materials and methods of construction as to minimize danger of accidents because of collapse of any part of the structure
2. Control of conditions likely to cause fires or to promote their spread
3. Provision of adequate facilities for escape in case of fire
4. Protection against danger of electrical shocks and burns
5. Protection against falls and other mechanical injuries in the home
6. Protection of the neighborhood against the hazards of automobile traffic

An important addition with reference to public housing has been the inclusion of special structural considerations for the physically handicapped.

The achievement of these goals involves action on three fronts: first, *prevention* of accelerated rates of deterioration of dwellings and their environment, thereby forestalling the formation of new blighted and slum areas; second, *rehabilitation* of existing substandard housing, if salvage is economically feasible, and demolition—which is part of rehabilitation in its broader sense—of substandard dwellings that are beyond repair; and third, *production* of enough new housing to provide for population increase, for families now overcrowded, for replacement of demolished and decayed structures, and for the normal vacancy cushion.

Adequate housing is now considered to involve circumstances that extend beyond the physical structure of the dwelling. Many of the objectives are unattainable if the surrounding neighborhood or indeed the entire community is allowed to develop in a completely hit-or-miss fashion. Consideration should be given to the overall living needs of the neighborhood and to the planning of the community as a whole. This involves the development of long-range programs of neighborhood and community improvement, land use, and traffic planning, with attention to street and freeway layouts, parks and playgrounds, sites for schools and other public buildings, shopping centers, and the location of business and industrial enterprises. The following factors have been listed as important if an optimum residential environment is to be achieved.[33]

1. Space for light, air, and recreation
2. Adequate water supply
3. Proper sewage and waste disposal facilities
4. Drainage
5. Freedom from accident hazard
6. Clean air
7. Freedom from unnecessary noise and disturbances
8. Insect, rodent and nuisance control
9. Suitable recreational facilities
10. Building codes
11. A land use plan
12. Zoning

There is also a need for increased attention by public health workers and others to suburban areas that surround municipalities. Here, in addition to many structural signs of affluence, one can find some of the worst housing problems. Proper land use planning is very clearly a public health concern. As emphasized by Galanter,[34] "Nearly all governmental authority to regulate land use stems from a mandate to protect the public health, but this justification is often obscured for a variety of reasons, such as: (1) private investment decisions are the most crucial in determining land use; (2) land use regulation is fragmented by type of hazard and among different governmental agencies; (3) governments must balance many competing factors; and (4) office holders need funds in order to finance re-election campaigns."

Any reasonably adequate solution of the tremendous and complex problem of housing obviously requires the combined and coordinated efforts of private enterprise; the local, state, and federal governments; and various professional and civic groups. Governmental action on all levels involves participation by many different agencies and departments, including those concerned with health, building inspection, plumbing, water, legal counseling, schools, recreation, traffic engineering, fire protection, public works, tax enforcement, public welfare, public housing, and redevelopment. This is not a job for the offical health agency alone.

Several administrative approaches have been tried. Traditionally in the United States responsibility for the quality of new housing has been vested in housing officials who have been primarily concerned with protection against fire and structural collapse. Of somewhat secondary interest have been requirements relating to the water supply, plumbing, heating, lighting, and ventilation. Once housing is constructed and occupied, responsibility for the supervision of its quality is generally transferred to the local health department. This is perhaps because the health department is in the best position to use effectively the police power and other legislative measures[35] and because of the multiplicity of interests of public health agencies. Thus many local health departments have long been active in various aspects of housing. Among these are the enforcement of requirements with regard to heating, lighting, and ventilation; control of atmospheric pollution; supervision of water supplies and of plumbing and sewerage systems; rodent and vermin control; nuisance abatement; accident prevention; and sanitary education.

The contributions of the local health department to the solution of the broad problem of housing may be of several types:

1. Development and promotion of the acceptance of local desirable housing and neighborhood standards
2. Participation in the enactment and enforcement of proper building codes and housing ordinances
3. Measurement of the quality of existing housing and neighborhoods
4. Participation in the remedying of existing housing deficiencies through rehabilitation and slum clearance
5. Participation in the proper control and direction of new housing through zoning, city planning, and the issuance of various permits and licenses

6. Education of the public in the hygiene of housing

Mood[36] has cautioned, however, that in assuming a leadership role, public health officials should realize that the involvement of health agencies in housing programs is not revolutionary in nature; rather, it is evolutionary. In this regard it should always be remembered that whereas laws and regulations may provide a basis and a legal means of requiring conformance to housing standards, they have never in themselves provided or maintained a decent dwelling. One of the greatest areas of neglect has been in health education as it relates to housing. If adequately pursued, it would undoubtedly correct more housing deficiencies than could ever be accomplished by laws.

Mention should be made of the roles of the state and federal governments. They may provide types of assistance and service that individuals, communities, and organizations are unable to provide for themselves. State governments may provide funds and consultation for the planning and construction of public housing, for slum clearance and redevelopment, and for regional planning. In a few instances statewide housing legislation has been enacted and enforced. The federal government through legislation may assist by the insurance of mortgages and of deposits in home loan banks, by the subsidization of slum clearance, redevelopment and low-rent public housing, by rent controls, by grants for farm housing, by research, and by the collection of statistics on housing, labor, and materials.

In 1949 Congress passed the Federal Housing Act, which established a Housing and Home Finance Agency as part of a major national housing instrument, the Federal Housing Administration. The functions of the Federal Housing Administration were gradually expanded by subsequent amendment and in 1965 given cabinet status as the Department of Housing and Urban Development. The Department establishes standards and requirements that qualify local governments for grants and loans for surveying, planning, and correcting substandard housing and environmental living conditions. To qualify, the local government must submit a plan of action designated as the "workable program." It should give consideration to seven basic elements:

1. Enforcement of sound local housing and building codes; an end to tolerating thousands of illegal, degrading, unhealthy, substandard structures and areas where many people have to live

2. A general master plan for the community's development; an end to haphazard, thoughtless planning and growth; a road map for the city's future in a planned framework for the region, metropolitan, or intercity urbanization of which it is a part

3. Basic analysis of neighborhoods and the kind of treatment needed; an inventory of blighted and threatened areas to form the basis of a plan of treatment to stop blight in its tracks

4. An effective administrative organization to run the program; coordinated activity toward a common purpose by all officers and arms of the local government

5. Financial capacity to carry out the program, using community revenues and resources to build a better city for the future instead of continuing to pay heavily for past mistakes

6. Rehousing of displaced families; expanding the supply of good housing for all income groups through new construction and rehabilitation so that families paying premium prices for slums can be rehoused

7. Full communitywide participation and support; public demand for a better community and public backing for the steps needed to get it

ACCIDENT PREVENTION PROGRAMS

There are many reasons why public health agencies and workers should be concerned with the problem of accidents. The absolute and proportionate magnitude of the problem that has been described in Chapter 19 is of course one reason, as is also its economic significance. Beyond these, however, there are actually a great many activities of public health agencies that do or could impinge on the problem. Emphasizing this are several useful manuals and other materials to assist the public health worker and others in the development of accident control and consumer protection programs. The Department of Health and Human Services, the American Public Health Association, the National Safety Council, and the Departments of Transportation, Agriculture, and Housing and Urban Development are all useful sources.

In 1960, the American Public Health Association issued a policy statement[37] that expressed its growing concern about accidents as a public health problem and challenge equal in scope to infectious and chronic diseases. It recommended that

Accident prevention be recognized as a major public health problem and that all component units of the American Public Health Association cooperate to improve accident prevention activities at the local, state and national level;

State and local health departments and the Public Health Service increase the size and scope of their accident prevention activities to be more commensurate with the magnitude of the problem and with the level of activity that has been or is being achieved in the field of infectious and chronic disease;

All state health departments and large local health departments provide that:

Their accident prevention programs be headed by a full-time administrator qualified by training and experience to discharge this responsibility adequately and that a wide range of consultant services be made available to the administrator and

Active educational efforts be designed to dispel ignorance about the basic causes of accidents and the role people play in their causation, devised and carried out in cooperation with other interested agencies and organizations, and

Research efforts be significantly increased in number, scope, and depth and embrace the study and control of all types of accidents regardless of their place of occurrence, and

Greater attention be directed to identifying the human factors involved in accidents, and to developing active methods of coping with them, and that in this concern full consideration be given to the structures, implements, and conditions created by man himself which make accidents more likely to occur, and

Increased efforts be made to enlist the cooperation of physicians and state and local medical societies in accident prevention activities;

Increased cooperation be promoted by official agencies with the National Safety Council and state and local safety councils, which have played so important a role in accident prevention; and

Additional funds be provided for the Public Health Service to encourage and support additional research efforts and to assist state and local health departments in developing more effective accident prevention programs.

Among the activities of public health agencies that may make significant contributions are public health statistics, health surveys and studies, community health and safety education, child health, occupational health and safety, housing, and mental health. The latter is mentioned specifically in view of the growing body of knowledge about accident proneness and the development of techniques for its determination. Increasingly public health and preventive medicine personnel have been relating their activities to accident prevention. In several communities accidental injuries and deaths are reported to the public health agency for study and analysis to determine improved and more fruitful avenues of attack. In many other communities surveys have been carried out for the same reason. In still others the recording of and educational activities about home accidents have been incorporated as part of the public health nursing function. Some excellent epidemiologic studies have been made of the problem.[38,39] Much of this has been made possible by research grants from various federal agencies.

Of particular interest are some studies on program analysis and cost benefits carried out by the Public Health Service.[40] One of these relates to motor vehicle and passenger injury prevention. The problem was examined exclusively in terms of human factors. Three major factors in the vehicular accident complex—law enforcement, road design, and traffic engineering—were for the most part excluded. Thus the problem was limited to considerations traditionally within the purview of health agencies. Six alternative programs were examined in terms of the program cost per death anticipated to be averted if an effective program were adequately financed and carried out. The results were as follows:

Program	Cost per death averted
1. Seat belt use—to encourage people to use seat belts	$ 87
2. Restraint devices—to educate people to obtain and use additional safety restraining devices	103
3. Pedestrian injury—to educate accident-prone pedestrians on how to cross the street	666
4. Motorcycle injury—to encourage motorcyclists to use helmets and eye shields	3,336
5. Reduce driver drinking—to educate people not to drink and drive	5,824
6. Driver licensing—to establish a medical screening program for licensing and to exclude drivers with certain conditions	13,801

Reference has been made to the significant decline in occupational accidents. This has largely resulted from activities in industrial health and safety programs involving inspections and surveys, improved plant and machine design, development and use of safety devices, preemployment examinations, and worker education.

Through the efforts of workers in the field of environmental health, more and more accident prevention measures are being included in the standards, specifications, and requirements for dwelling and city plans. Such measures, coupled with persistent public educational measures, have until recently formed the core of the attack on home accidents. Educational efforts, however, have been found to have limited effectiveness. Therefore increasing dependence is being placed on "passive" measures, such as safety caps on medicine bottles and legislation for mandatory product safety standards.[41-43]

Unfortunately no single government agency has general authority to prohibit, supervise, control, or conduct programs with reference to the ever-increasing number of products that do or may present risks to the consuming public. Federal product safety legislation consists of a series of isolated acts that deal with specific hazards in generally narrow product categories. Usually legislation follows some unfortunate occurrence. Among other faults, this approach results in both gaps and overlaps. The Department of Health and Human Services, for example, operates under certain general provisions of the Public Health Service Act as well as a long list of specific legislative acts, such as the Food, Drug, and Cosmetic Acts of 1938 and 1959; the Hazardous Substances Acts of 1962 and 1966; the Consumer Product Safety Act of 1966; the Child Protection and Toy Safety Acts of 1966 and 1969; The Fair Packaging and Labeling Act of 1967; the Flammable Fabrics Act of 1968; and the Electronic Products Act of 1969. This is only a partial list. Other departments have similar diffused categoric responsibilities and authorities.

Such limited federal authority as does exist, therefore, is incomplete and scattered among many agencies. In fact, jurisdiction over a single category of products, of which pesticides is an excellent example, may be shared by as many as four or more different agencies. Moreover, as the National Commission on Product Safety observed, where it exists, federal product safety regulation is burdened by unnecessary procedural obstacles, circumscribed investigational powers, inadequate and ill-fitting sanctions, meager budgets, distorted priorities, and misdirected technical resources. Data collection and processing programs and early warning systems, to the extent they exist, leave much to be accomplished. In recent years there have been repeated attempts to establish a national consumer protection agency, but in view of the magnitude and complexity of the problems, combined with the confused uncoordinated arrangements to deal with them, such efforts have all been doomed to ineffectiveness. This will continue to be the case until proper and comprehensive organizational and legislative coordination occurs. The states have done somewhat better, but they too have similar complexities and inadequacies.

Many state health agencies engage in some activities relating to accident prevention at the present time. Accident prevention educational activities are carried on by the majority. In addition, many attempt to stimulate local accident prevention programs. Special conferences, short courses, and workshops are held for local health department personnel and for representatives of other official and nonofficial local agencies. Also, many state health agencies cooperate with other official state agencies, such as those concerned with mines, industry, labor, and traffic safety, in carrying out cooperative programs in those areas.

In the final analysis, of course, the prevention of accidents depends on the individual, and if efforts are to be fruitful, they must take place especially on the local level.

Public apathy to the mounting toll from accidents must be transformed into an action program under strong leadership. This can be accomplished by the methods employed to bring poliomyelitis and other epidemics under control, and to make frontal attacks to conquer cancer, heart disease and mental disease. . . . Basic to this unified approach is identification of the individual citizen with a means by which he can satisfy the inherent desire to serve his fellow man.[1]

No single satisfactory pattern has yet been devised or adopted. It is certain, however, that there must be involved some of the basic epidemiologic approaches and techniques that have proved to be effective in many diverse fields. Among these are (1) development and improvement of data on the prevalence and incidence of accidents through reporting, surveys, and studies; (2) education of the public through effective pertinent channels; (3) improvement and extension of safety devices in the home, public buildings, industry, vehicles, and farm machinery; (4) inclusion of training in accident prevention in schools of public health, public administration, and architecture; (5) improvement of structural safety through the general inclusion of accident prevention factors in building codes; (6) improvement of city planning, traffic studies, and highway design; (7) improved driver training, education, and supervision with consideration given to physical and mental factors that may indicate accident proneness; and (8) improvement of the functional design of toys, household equipment, dispensers, and furniture with particular attention to the peculiar needs and behavior habits of the very young, the handicapped, and the elderly.

Only through the cooperative efforts of many community agencies—one of the most important being the health agency—in attacking along all of these and many other fronts will the toll of accidents be lessened eventually. In the process, because of its all-embracing interest in all aspects of safe and healthful living, it is the official public health agency that is best fitted to serve as a catalyst and rallying point.

VECTOR CONTROL

Pathogenic organisms that involve nonhuman hosts or vectors at any stage of their life cycles offer an additional point of potential control. The number of such diseases is substantial, and the numbers and types of vectors are impressive. Vectors of public health concern are rodents and arthropods. Increasingly, wild rodents have been found to be the true reservoirs of plague and widespread epizootics with commensal rodents being merely side or incidental aspects of the particular biologic cycles. Among rodent vectors, rats, ground squirrels, and prairie dogs are most important, especially in view of their role in the spread of plague. Among the innumerable arthropods, certain mosquitoes, flies, fleas, roaches, lice, mites, and ticks are of impressive significance. It is all too easily overlooked by residents of the United States that insects exact a far greater toll on health and life than any other thing. Malaria is still one of the world's leading causes of death, and other insect-borne diseases are far from rare. Furthermore, considerable numbers of the insect vectors of many of those diseases are present in certain areas of the United States. Accordingly, the control of insect vectors of disease is

still and will long continue to be an important phase of environmental health programs.

The possibility of controlling disease-transmitting insects became a reality at about the turn of the century. Life cycles of many organisms and of many vectors became known. Experiments and demonstrations of various methods of control of breeding places and of protection against adult insects were carried out. The use of courageous administrative procedures for the widespread use of these methods established Havana and Panama as famous landmarks in public health history. Elimination of mosquito breeding places was accomplished by drainage and fillings; larvae were killed by fish and by the spreading of oils; adult insects were destroyed or repelled by fumigants and smudges and were excluded from living and sleeping quarters by screening and bed nets. Subsequent decades brought cheaper and easier larviciding with Paris green; and pyrethrum became widely used as an insect adulticide.

However, it was not until World War II presented the terrible risk of action in far-flung disease-ridden areas that insect control really came into its own. Some of the older materials like pyrethrum were made more effective by refining their insecticidal principles and applying them with aerosols as the medium. Remarkably efficient new repellents were also developed. It was the development of DDT, dieldrin, and other potent insecticides and their widespread use against mosquitoes, lice, and other disease vectors, however, that really opened a new epidemiologic era. Offsetting this, however, is the disturbing combination of pesticide-resistant strains of insects and the undesirable side effects of pesticides on humans and the ecosystem. One of the most interesting and potentially important approaches to the solution of these problems is the large-scale breeding and dissemination of insects that have been sterilized artificially.

The control and destruction of rodents is of importance because of two diseases in particular, plague and murine typhus. In the United States, plague-infected wild rodents appear to have been spreading eastward from the West Coast at a rapid rate, necessitating intensified control procedures to prevent epidemics. However, the ecologic distribution of plague is inadequately understood. The density of positive recovery sites seems to represent the degree of intensity of surveys as much as geographic involvement of rodents and fleas in nature. Murine typhus is endemic in several southeastern and some western states. In this instance rats and mice that infest households are the carriers of consequence. Other mammalian hosts of diseases dangerous to man in certain areas are wild monkeys and some ruminants (in relation to yellow fever) and dogs, wolves, foxes, and bats (in relation to rabies).

Many urban and rural local health departments, as well as state health departments, have established vector control activities, usually in conjunction with their environmental health programs. Activities included are educational and promotional programs; vector surveys; research with regard to vectors, materials, and control measures; direct application of insecticides and rodenticides; licensure and supervision of pest eradicators; studies on or supervision of garbage collection, storage, and disposal; rat proofing in relation to the housing program; and elimination of mosquito breeding by spraying, drainage, filling, or variation of impounded water levels. Some communities have achieved notable success through the participation of trained neighborhood citizens and groups. These various functions require a variety of types of personnel, including sanitary engineers, laboratorians, sanitarians, sanitary inspectors, and sometimes biologists, zoologists, and chemists. Of particular importance are entomologists and ecologists, to whose services and abilities increasing attention is being given by public health agencies.

MISCELLANEOUS SANITATION ACTIVITIES

In addition to the areas of environmental health already discussed, a variety of miscellaneous activities and programs may be carried out by health agencies. No more than passing mention will be made of them here, since most are of specialized or limited importance, interest, and responsibility.

Of specific federal concern is the supervision of the salubrity of vehicles of interstate and international traffic, that is, buses, trains, boats, and airplanes. The Public Health Service, which is responsible for these activities, has long since developed standards for each. The maintenance of a sanitary environment in connection with parks, recreation areas, and trailer camps may be a concern of a local, state, or federal health agency, depending on governmental jurisdiction. Usually the responsibility is shared with another branch of government, such as those concerned with highways, recreation, or conservation. Related to these problems but more exclusively the responsibility of the public health agency is the supervision of the quality of swimming pools and bathing places.

ENVIRONMENTAL HEALTH PERSONNEL

The exact number of people employed in some aspect of environmental protection in the United States is unknown. About 300,000 would be a fair estimate. What is known is their diversity. They represent a wide range of the physical, biologic, and social sciences. In the physical sciences, representation extends from classic physics and chemistry through meteorology and radiation physics to hydrology, oceanography, and engineering. In the biomedical sciences, requirements extend from molecular biology, botany, and microbiology through biochemistry, pharmacology, and radiology to ecology, epidemiology, veterinary medicine, toxicology, genetics, and several clinical medical specialities. To these may be added individuals versed in mathematics, statistics, law, sociology, anthropology, political science, management, and economics. The roles and functions of the specific professional and allied environmental health occupations have been evolving, and for some occupations clear definition is still lacking.

The foregoing list of specialties and professions is subject to some simplification. It consists of some who are concerned with environmental health technology development, and with environmental health policy, and finally those involved in what might be termed applied environmental health. This last and largest group is the chief concern here and includes essentially individuals employed by public health or environmental protection agencies on the several levels of government. Aside from veterinarians, who play extremely important but somewhat specialized roles in epidemiology and food and milk control, the majority of those involved in "action" programs are engineers, sanitarians, and environmental technologists.

Because of regional differences with regard to types of problems, degree of urbanity, and availability of funds, facilities, and trained personnel, there is some difference of opinion concerning the type of training needed to direct and conduct environmental control programs. Not infrequently, rural areas and small towns have found it necessary to depend on nonengineering personnel, sometimes with no training except perhaps for a few weeks' indoctrination and orientation provided by the state health departments. In contrast, because of the complexity of their problems, urban centers have characteristically employed civil or sanitary engineers to provide the leadership for their environmental control programs. These, of course, must be augmented by a cadre of qualified sanitarians and other types of environmentalists. Engineering is concerned essentially with design, construction, operation, and maintenance of a water treatment system, a sewage treatment plant, air pollution control equipment, or an incinerator.

Sanitary inspection antedated sanitary engineering by a considerable period. Its efforts have been directed toward more local and personal environmental factors that were thought to exert a deleterious effect on living. During much of its development, sanitary inspection was based on supposition rather than scientific knowledge and may still be regarded as concerned with aesthetics to a significant degree. For a period this concern was downgraded, but interestingly both the public and health professionals in recent years are again giving it more attention on the bases of mental health and the quality of life. During recent decades the horizon of sanitarians has been extended in many ways. Substantial qualifications and detailed curricula have been developed that have been accepted and used widely by educational institutions, health agencies, and industry.[44] Increasingly the unqualified have been either upgraded or winnowed out. A certification system has been established, and sanitarians now represent a large and growing cadre of important health professionals who may be found making significant contributions to all aspects of environmental health work. It is difficult to visualize a viable public health program without them.

Under either rural or urban circumstances, local health departments that provide direct service must for economy and efficiency supplement their professional engineers, veterinarians, and sanitarians with auxiliary workers, commonly referred to as environmental technologists and environmental aides. They perform specific tasks under supervision. Such tasks may include obtaining samples of air, water, food, or other materials; assisting in the operation of various environmental protective facilities; and determining compliance through inspection and evaluation. As in medicine, dentistry, and nursing, such individuals in significant numbers serve as valuable professional extenders. Originally trained "on the job," in recent years these workers have had well-designed training programs developed to improve their ability and status.[45,46]

The question of supervision in environmental health is sometimes raised. Much depends on the size and nature of the community and its health program, the responsibilities placed on the latter, the availability of personnel, and sometimes custom. Smaller jurisdictions often cannot afford or make efficient use of an engineer. In such circumstances, when needed, assistance may be sought from the state. Larger jurisdictions with problems involving water and sewage treatment, air pollution, and the like, must have engineering competence, but they also need sanitarians. The questions of who supervises what should depend on the program. On the national and state levels this does not usually present a problem, since most environmental advisory and policy-making functions on those levels imply the employment of engineers. The difficulty arises chiefly on the local level.

Many municipalities of significant size employ engineers who may plan and supervise the total environmental control program, including its inspectional phases as well as those of a more complex engineering nature. Some municipalities, on the other hand, divide the functions and responsibilities into those of a true engineering nature and those that deal with sanitary standards, surveillance, and enforcement. In small communities and rural areas that are served by the usual county health department, the employment of engineering personnel is relatively rare. As a result, the environmental health program depends entirely on sanitary inspectors, or increasingly and far better, on sanitarians who have received formal training to qualify them as registered sanitarians.

In areas where needed professional personnel does not exist on the local level, supervision, planning, and direction should be provided by the state health department. This makes possible a more comprehensive program in the field and enables the local sanitarian to assist with certain difficult and technical activities that formerly were handled exclusively by the state. This acknowledgement by the state of the responsibility to provide the local personnel with technical assistance and direction also expands their usefulness and makes it possible for small local health department to provide much more adequate service to the public than would otherwise be possible.

Theoretically some of the need for supervision of the local environmental control personnel should be met by the local health officer who, after all, is ultimately responsible for all phases of the community health program. In some instances, however, this is neither attempted nor possible, since some local health officers unfortunately appear to lack the inclination, interest, or professional background to assist their environmental control staffs with their problems.

PRESENT ORGANIZATION OF ENVIRONMENTAL CONTROL PROGRAMS

As has been indicated, responsibilities and functions in environmental health are divided among the different levels of government in a variety of patterns. Generally speaking, the supervision of public water supplies and sewerage systems and the prevention of stream pollution are responsibilities of the federal and state governments. The federal concern, until recently through the Public Health Service and now through the Environmental Protection Agency, is based largely on responsibility for interstate sanitation and for interstate and international public carriers, watersheds, and air sheds. In recent decades federal grants-in-aid to states and localities have become a factor of great potential significance. State precedence over local communities in these matters results from legislative direction, the potentiality of intercommunity problems, and the availability of professionally qualified personnel in the state health department.

In general, federal interests are concerned with research, the development of criteria and standards, and the promulgation and enforcement of various national laws relating to foods, wastes, pollution, and the like. The states in turn are responsible for the establishment of state laws, policies, and regulations; and the promotion and general supervision of local programs. In some instances state agencies engage in the field inspection activities necessary for the implementation of the standards and regulations, but more often this is left to the local health department.

The developmental history of local health units in a state has much to do with the functional relationship that exists between the state and local agencies in matters of environmental control. Those states that were slow to promote the establishment of local health units still tend toward the centralization of environmental health activities in the state, even though there may not exist capable city and county health departments.

In contrast with public water and sewerage systems, those private facilities that are designed to serve single or small groups of families are almost always left to the supervision of the local health department. In many instances these small private facilities are inspected only on request or complaint or when they are related to epidemiologically significant circumstances such as dairies or food processing or handling establishments. Between these two types of facilities, public and private, are some that are called semipublic facilities. These are found in tourist camps, roadside parks, comfort stations, rural schools, hospitals, and other institutions. Since they serve a number of unrelated persons of diverse origins, they constitute an obvious public health responsibility. In some areas this is met primarily by the state, whereas in other areas the local health departments provide most of the supervision.

Aside from the variations in responsibilities for environmental health that relate to the different levels of government, the organizational and administrative picture is further complicated by dispersion of health functions, and especially those relating to environmental health, throughout several agencies of government. This has been most evident in the states. Usually the state health department has been designated as the regulatory agency responsible for public water and sewerage systems, although in some instances other departments of government—particularly state universities and special sanitary authorities, commissions, or boards—enter into certain phases of the program. Similar variation is found in connection with most other sanitary activities, including the control of stream pollution, industrial safety and health, insect and pest control, resort sanitation, and many others.

A common complaint, therefore, among public health workers today is that environmental health concerns and authorities are being bled away by other agencies. Areas of particular concern are air pollution control, radiologic health, solid waste management, occupational health and safety, water hygiene, food and milk sanitation, housing, vector and rodent control, injury control, recreation safety or sanitation, pesticides, and hazardous product and drug surveillance. The extent of jurisdictional confusion was illustrated by a study in 1969[47] (Table 21-2). In cases where no information was provided there is probably no program activity in a particular category. Several exceptions to that assumption may exist, such as in drug surveillance and food and milk sanitation.

The data show that health agencies at the time were still for the most part the responsible or lead agency in the various problem areas considered. Areas where primary responsibility appeared most diffused were air pollution control, solid waste management, water hygiene, food and milk processing, sanitation, and pharmaceutical surveillance. In these areas special pollution control authorities; departments of public works, public service, or sanitation; water departments or water development boards; departments of agriculture; and boards of pharmacy played significant roles. It is notable, however, that even in these instances, health agencies tended to be the most common responsible or lead agency.

The confusion and diffusion in the face of accelerating and mounting environmental problems has brought about the beginning of a much needed trend toward consolidation of environmental planning and effort. Several references have been made to actions on the national level that resulted in the consolidation of many of the responsibilities, authorities, and resources of several previously separated agencies in the Environmental Protection Agency. Since then, a number of state governments and many municipalities have followed suit. This trend has been disturbing to many in the field of public health. Some of the concern is justified and some is not. The problems are so great that all help possible is needed. What is disturbing, however, is a dangerous tendency in some reorganizations to underestimate the important partnership role that public health must be allowed to play in all aspects of this broader approach. Although it is certainly true that the environment has many facets, of which public health is only one, nevertheless in the final analysis it is the effect of environmental abuse and mismanagement on the health and well-being of people that constitutes the ultimate concern.

This has been recognized officially by the Environmental Protection Agency, which in a policy report for 1979-1980 reemphasizes the top priority it now accords to the protection of the public health.[48]

In summary, the organization of environmental protection activities in the United States is obviously disorganized. It is difficult to find any agency of government that does not have some concern or involvement. The remarkable extent to which this is true has been well documented, and this, of course, cannot begin to convey the complexities of the interagency-intergovernmental relationships required to solve a problem or to activate a program. As indicated by Sargent,[49] the problems of environmental health are really "adisciplinary;" that is, they relate to no particular discipline yet at the same time involve many disciplines, as noted in the brief discussion on personnel. The major problems of the sciences concerned with environment, Sargent says, make meaningless the traditional boundaries that have compartmentalized knowledge and methodology. To paraphrase his thoughts, because the problems are adisciplinary, it is necessary to develop institutions wherein problem-oriented configurations can be brought together to work effectively and efficiently. Such institutional formulations, he notes, are being explored in government at the federal and state levels, in professional organizations, and in educational institutions. Progress is slow, however, because innovation disturbs traditional values and alignments and creates insecurity in established federal barónies. What is disturbing is that the field of public health, and its environmental health component, appears to be included in this last category. Instead of anticipating and preparing to react to problems that are essentially of a public health nature, there seems to have transpired a period of nonresponsiveness based on jurisdictional protectionism.

In observing this with distress, Sargent concludes: "The essence of the challenge to public health is to establish itself as a significant force in planning for and in implementing meaningful action-oriented programs aimed at solving important environmental problems. To achieve such a goal, public health must develop unifying concepts that allow identification of the real problems and operationally-meaningful approaches to the solution of those problems."

TABLE 21-2. Agencies with sole or primary responsibilities in environmental health management in 53 states

Agencies with sole or primary responsibility	Air pollution control	Radiologic health	Solid waste management	Occupational health	Water hygiene	Food service sanitation
53 states and territories						
Health agencies	37	48	44	23	37	46
Health plus other agencies (see footnote)		1[c]	4[d]	4[e]	8[a]	
		1[m]			7[b]	
Other agencies (see footnote)	14[a]	2[c]	3[a]	5[e]	1[a]	5[g]
	1[b]		1[b]			1[i]
Reported no activity	1	1	1	10		
No information				11		1
45 major cities						
Health agencies	23	22	11	8	16	37
Health plus other agencies (see footnote)			5[d]	1[e]	12[f]	7[g]
					14[d,k,m]	
Other agencies (see footnote)	14[a]	1[c]	23[d]	1[e]	7[f]	
	4[m,r]				2[a]	
Reported no activity	4	22		19		
No information			6	16	4	1

Key: a, Special Pollution Control Authority; b, Department of Natural Resources; c, Nuclear Energy Agency; d, Depart- Compensation Board; f, Water Department or Water Department Board; g, Department of Agriculture; h, Consumer Pro- tion; I, Department of Housing; m, Department of Licenses and Inspection; n, Department of Community Affairs; o, Department; s, Department of Neighborhood Improvement; t, Safety Council.

UNITED NATIONS CONFERENCE ON THE HUMAN ENVIRONMENT

It is appropriate to close this chapter with a few words about the international conference held in Stockholm by the United Nations in June 1972. By the end of the 1960s concerns about the ecologic consequences of environmental abuse had reached the point where several nations suggested that a large meeting be called to discuss the problem and hopefully lay the groundwork for an international effort. The proposal was overwhelmingly approved. Meticulous planning took place through a prepa- ratory committee, which sponsored four prelimi- nary regional meetings that developed reports and recommendations to form the agenda for the larger meeting. The World Health Organization published a document[50] on the health hazards of the human environment, prepared by some 90 specialists in 15 countries. The 10-day conference in Stockholm was in effect a double meeting. The formal sessions were attended by 1,250 official delegates from most nations. Delegates consisted of diplomats, econo- mists, and professionals from the health and related fields. In addition to the formal delegates, the meet- ing was attended by about 3,000 interested indi- viduals, some of whom represented professional or conservation organizations, but a great many of whom came on their own initiative because of per- sonal concern. In the course of the sessions these "unofficial" participants developed and held ses- sions of their own. There was worldwide news cov- erage by about 1,500 journalists.

This momentous and unique international con- ference was not without problems. Several impor- tant nations did not attend for political reasons. Per- haps the most difficult problem was a difference of opinion that arose early between the more affluent industrialized nations, who urged a slowing down of development and resource use, and the devel- oping nations, who understandably insisted on their opportunity for economic and industrial progress. Despite such limitations, the outcome was 106 rec-

and territories and 45 major cities, United States, 1969

Food process sanitation	Milk sani- tation	Shellfish sani- tation	Housing hygiene	Vector control	Injury control	Pesticide surveillance	Recreation sanitation	Hazardous products	Drug surveil- lance
23	22	9	15	33	35	3	11	13	15
1[g]	3[g]	2[i]	2[l]	1[g]	4[p]		1[b]		2[g]
			3[n]	1[o]					
26[g]	13[g]	1[g]	5[l]	1[g]	1[p]	4[g]		4[g]	15[q]
1[k]	1[b]					1[i]		1[i]	3[g]
1[i]									3[i,m]
1	14	40	28	17	13	45	41	35	10
	31	6	10	19	15	2	8	2	
	4[g]		1[i]	1[i]					
			2[s]	1[s]	1[d,e]				
	3[g]		6[l]	1[d]	1[t]				
				1[s]					
					15				
	7	39	26	22	13				

ment of Public Works, Public Service, or Sanitation; e, Department of Labor, Labor and Industry, Industrial Relations, or tection Agency; i, State Laboratory or State Chemist; j, Fisheries Department or Commission; k, Department of Conserva- Vector Control Commission; p, Department of Motor Vehicles, Police, or Public Safety; q, Board of Pharmacy; r, Building

ommendations that related to three major decision areas:

1. A Declaration on the Human Environment containing a set of principles designed to guide nations toward a safer environment
2. A resolution calling for the establishment of a United Nations mechanism, including a voluntary Environmental Fund to support international action on global problems
3. A recommendation for an Action Plan to attack global environmental threats through a combination of governments and international organizations

Action on each of these followed promptly. A widely publicized declaration was developed, a Secretariat for the Environment with a Governing Council of 54 members was established within the United Nations, and special financing for the program was arranged. A permanent implementing agency was established with headquarters in Nairobi. In commenting on the conference, Maurice F. Strong of Canada, who served as Secretary-General of the conference and who was overwhelmingly selected as the first Director of the permanent Secretariat for the Environment declared: "We have taken the first steps on a new journey of hope for the future of mankind. The fundamental task of the Stockholm Conference has been to take the political decisions that will enable the community of nations to act together in a manner consistent with the earth's physical interdependence."

REFERENCES

1. U.S. Department of Health, Education, and Welfare: Changing environmental hazards, challenges to community health, Report of the Task Force on Environmental Health of the National Commission on Community Health Services, Washington, D.C., 1967, U.S. Government Printing Office.
2. Description of environmental health, Am. J. Public Health 55:928, June 1965.
3. Environmental determinants of community well-being, Scient. Pub. No. 123, Washington, D.C., 1965,

Pan American Health Organization–World Health Organization.

4. Kates, R.W., and Wohlwill, J.F., editors: Man's response to the physical environment, J. Soc. Issues **22**(4), Oct. 1966.

5. U.S. Department of Health, Education, and Welfare: A strategy for a livable environment, Report of the Task Force on Environmental Health and Related Problems, Washington, D.C., 1967.

6. Stead, F.M.: Levels in environmental health, Am. J. Public Health **50:**312, March 1960.

7. U.S. Public Health Service: Environmental health planning guide, PHS Pub. No. 823, Washington, D.C. 1967.

8. American Public Health Association: Resolution and policy statement: environmental health planning, Am. J. Public Health **67:**89, Jan. 1977.

9. Okun, D.: Drinking water for the future, Am. J. Public Health **66:**639, 1976.

10. A water policy for the American people, Report of the President's Water Resource Policy Commission, Washington, D.C., 1950, U.S. Government Printing Office.

11. Muskie, E.S.: Water pollution control needs for next 6 years, Congressional Record, E6377, July 8, 1970.

12. Hunter, J.S.: Shortcomings and remedies for the water quality improvement programs of the United States, Am. J. Public Health **63:**345, April 1973.

13. Waste management and control, Report to the Federal Council for Science and Technology, Washington, D.C., 1966, National Academy of Sciences–National Research Council.

14. Public health agencies 1980: a report on their expenditures and activities, Washington, D.C., 1981, Association of State and Territorial Health Officials.

15. Wands, R.: Solid waste disposal: a long standing public health problem comes of age, Am. J. Public Health **67:**419, May, 1977.

16. Walker, B., Ellis, E., and Murphy, W.: Food protection has many facets, J. Environ. Health **34:**382, Jan.-Feb., 1972.

17. Dauer, C.C.: Summary of disease outbreaks and a 10 year résumé, Public Health Resp. **76:**915, Oct. 1961.

18. Center for Disease Control: U.S. Department of Health, Education, and Welfare: Foodborne outbreaks, annual summary, DHEW Pub. No. (HSM) 73-8185, Atlanta, 1972.

19. Isaac, P.C.: Air pollution and man's health: in Great Britain, Public Health Rep. **68:**868, Sept. 1953.

20. Larson, G.P.: Air pollution and man's health: in Los Angeles, Public Health Rep. **68:**873, Sept. 1953.

21. Heimann, H.: Status of air pollution health research, 1966, Arch. Environ. Health **14:**488, March 1967.

22. Firket, J.: Sur les causes des accidents survenus dans la vallée de la Meuse, lors des brouillards de décembre 1930, Bull. Acad. R. Med. Belg. **11:**683, 1931.

23. Townsend, J.G.: Investigation of the smog incident in Donora, Pennsylvania, and vicinity, Am. J. Public Health **40:**183, Feb. 1950.

24. Ciocco, A., and Thompson, D.J.: A follow-up of Donora ten years after, Am. J. Public Health **51:**155, Feb. 1961.

25. McCabe, L., and Clayton, G.: Air pollution by hydrogen sulfide in Poza Rica, Mexico, Arch. Ind. Hyg. Occup. Med. **6:**199, Sept. 1952.

26. Scott, J.: Fog and deaths in London, December, 1952, Public Health Rep. **68:**474, Mary 1953.

27. Bugher, J.C.: Health perspectives of our radioactive world, Am. J. Public Health **52:**727, May 1962.

28. Committee on Local Control of Ionizing Radiation of the Conference of Municipal Public Health Engineers: The responsibility of local health agencies in the control of ionizing radiation, Am. J. Public Health **53:**1136, July 1963.

29. Brodsky, A.: Balancing benefit versus risk in the control of consumer items containing radioactive material, Am. J. Public Health **55:**1971, Dec. 1965.

30. American Public Health Association Committee on the Hygiene of Housing; Winslow, C.-E.A., chairman: An appraisal method for measuring the quality of housing. I. Nature and uses of the method, 1945, The Association.

31. Anderson, G.W.: The present epidemiological basis of environmental sanitation, Am. J. Public Health **33:**113, Feb. 1943.

32. Bauer, C.: The provision of good housing, Am. J. Public Health **39:**462, April 1949.

33. Molner, J.G., and Hilbert, M.S.: Responsibilities of public health administrations in the field of housing. In Housing progammes: the role of public health agencies, Geneva, 1964, World Health Organization.

34. Galanter, R.: Land use: public health is the bottom line, Am. J. Public Health **68:**447, May, 1978.

35. Ascher, C.S.: Regulation of housing: hints for health officers, Am. J. Public Health **37:**507, May 1937.

36. Mood, E.W.: Health and housing programs in large cities, U.S.A., 1965, Am. J. Public Health **56:**1540, Sept. 1966.

37. Policy statement on accidents: a public health problem, Am. J. Public Health **51:**122, Jan. 1961.

38. Haddon, W., Suchman, E.A., and Klein, D.L.: Accident research: methods and approaches, New York, 1964, Harper & Row, Publishers, Inc.

39. Iskrant, A.P.: The epidemiological approach to accident causation, Am. J. Public Health **57:**1708, Oct. 1967.

40. U.S. Department of Health, Education, and Welfare, Office of the Assistant Secretary for Program Coordination: Program analysis, selected disease control programs, Washington, D.C., 1966, U.S. Government Printing Office.

41. National Commission on Product Safety, final report, Washington, D.C., 1970, U.S. Government Printing Office.

42. Baker, S.P.: Determinants of injury and opportunities for intervention, Am. J. Epidemiol., **101:**98, Feb. 1975.

43. Dershewitz, R.A., and Williamson, J.W.: Prevention of childhood injuries: a controlled clinical trial, Am. J. Public Health, **67:**1148, Dec. 1977.

44. Hatlen, J.B.: Basic academic preparation for a professional sanitarian, J. Environ. Health **33:**33, July-Aug. 1970.

45. Koren, H.: Environmental technician curriculum guidelines, J. Environ. Health **33:**155, Sept-Oct. 1970.

46. Austin, J.H., McLellon, W.M., and Dyer, J.C.: Training the environmental technician, Am. J. Public Health **60:**2314, Dec. 1970.

47. Hanlon, J.J.: Who manages the environment, J. Environ. Health **32:**409, Jan.-Feb. 1970.

48. E.P.A. at the crossroads: a view from the top emphasizes health, Environ. Health Lett. **17:**2, April 15, 1978.

49. Sargent, F.: Man-environment: problems for public health, Am. J. Public Health **62:**628, May 1972.

50. Health hazards of the human environment, Geneva, 1972, World Health Organization.

PART SIX

Health and human development

In building a public health program, as with so many other things, the best place to start is at the beginning. Life is a continuous spiral with a myriad of interlocking biologic, environmental, and circumstantial factors blending to determine genesis. That event in turn brings to bear a new panoply of factors over which the life that has been brought about has absolutely no control—the characteristics of the bearing mother, her socioeconomic circumstances in the broadest connotations, her habits, mental condition, and state of nutrition. Then when the cord is cut, the still helpless and dependent creature has need for physical and mental care and comfort through a long period of maturation, learning, and development. Childhood can and should be a time of joy and happiness, but biologically it is also a time of preparation for the hopefully fruitful years of adulthood.

Living begins at birth. So, in a sense, does aging. From childhood to adolescence, from young adult to senior citizen, humans change and evolve, shucking off old problems for new ones and reaping the harvest or the bitter fruits of past practices, the environment, and the pool of genes. The middle and last thirds of life are important to those who live them and to public health workers. These phases and transitions are considered in the following chapters on maternal, infant, preschool, school-aged, adolescent, and maturing health problems and opportunities.

CHAPTER 22

Maternal, infant, and preschool health

The utmost reverence is due a child.

Juvenal

A CRITICAL PERIOD

The field of public health is concerned with the well-being of all people, regardless of age, sex, race, or other characteristics. Traditionally, however, there have been two groups to whom particular attention has been given: pregnant women and young children, particularly infants. There are sound reasons for this. Special attention to a pregnant woman brings double health benefits: first, to her as an adult member of society and, second, to the product of her pregnancy. Other reasons are that pregnancy is a period of particular physical stress during which the woman may face unusual risk. Undesirable influences during the prenatal period may jeopardize the health of both the mother and the expected infant. Short of fatalities, these effects may result in health and economic disadvantages for the woman and child and even for the rest of the family if the mother's health is permanently impaired.

Remarkable progress has been made in many parts of the world in protecting the lives of expectant mothers and their infants. In the United States during the last 50 years maternal mortality declined about 99% and infant mortality about 75%. This may be attributed to many factors, of which public health progress is only one. Hospital and medical standards have improved, as have nutrition and the general standard of living. Many new preventive and therapeutic agents and techniques have been introduced. Almost every aspect of public health has had an effect on the health and welfare of expectant mothers, infants, and young children. In undeveloped areas, the institution of an effective program of environmental sanitation involving the purification of water, the sanitation of milk and food, and the promotion of satisfactory facilities for the disposal of human wastes will show its first effects in a reduction in infant morbidity and mortality. Vital statistics are involved in the maternal and child health program in various ways, especially by pinpointing specific problem areas. The public health laboratory is an essential tool, particularly in prenatal management where tests must be performed to detect the presence of venereal diseases, the Rh reaction, inborn metabolic disorders of the fetus, diabetes, tuberculosis, and other problems that increase the risk of pregnancy and to determine appropriate medical management that must be followed. Throughout the entire antenatal, natal, and postnatal period there must be woven a strong thread of health education. The expectant mother must be constantly protected against communicable diseases, particularly those of a viral, streptococcal, and influenzal nature; the use of many hazardous substances, including alcohol and tobacco, must be restricted; and early attempts must be made to protect the newborn child against gonorrheal ophthalmia, whooping cough, diphtheria, measles, and other communicable diseases as well as genetic disorders. It is obvious therefore that the maternal and child health program cannot be considered by itself.

BACKGROUND OF MATERNAL AND CHILD HEALTH PROGRAMS

The development of maternal and child health programs has been discussed in Chapters 2 and

8. Some additional background will be presented here.

The opening of the first milk station in 1893 in New York City to combat the tremendous incidence of summer diarrhea in infants and children of the underprivileged by providing them with safe milk during the summer heat was a significant event. Observance of the benefits that resulted from this meager start led to the establishment of numerous infant welfare societies designed to bring medical and nursing knowledge and care to those in need. In 1908 the New York City Association for Improving the Condition of the Poor, in conjunction with the New York Outdoor Clinic, began to provide prenatal care for expectant mothers in the lower income groups. Simultaneously a Bureau of Child Hygiene was established in the New York City Health Department. These two moves were subsequently duplicated by many other communities throughout the nation. In 1909 a conference on the prevention of infant mortality was held by the American Academy of Medicine. This was followed the same year by the first White House Conference on Children and Youth called by President Theodore Roosevelt. Its purpose was "to discuss what might be done at the federal level to stimulate and help finance state and local health and social welfare programs for children." It resulted in several legislative proposals, one of which was signed into law in 1912 by President Taft to establish the Children's Bureau. Its initial charge was limited—essentially to conduct studies and report—but on this modest base astute leadership was able over the years to develop a broad program of far-reaching significance.

Another development of significance at about the same time was the formation of the American Association for the Study and Prevention of Infant Mortality. This group was composed of pediatricians, infant welfare nurses (who in a sense were the precursors of the present-day public health nurses), social workers, public health officials, and other interested persons. The organization was the beginning of what in 1923 became the American Child Health Association, which provided effective leadership until the time of its disbandment in 1935. The growing interest in child health and welfare commanded national attention that resulted in the passage of the Sheppard-Towner Act. This pro-vided the beginning of a federal grant-in-aid program to encourage and enable states to develop programs in maternal and infant care. The act functioned only from 1922 to 1929, but its goals and principles were subsequently influential in the broad national consideration of maternal and child health problems in the Social Security Act, which was approved in August 1935. The struggle to renew and continue the Sheppard-Towner Act pitted conservative against liberal forces in Congress. The American Medical Association was opposed to the legislation, and a group of pediatricians split off from the AMA to form the American Academy of Pediatrics, a group that has continued to make substantial contributions to the improvement of child welfare programs.

In 1963, recognizing that about 3% of babies born are mentally retarded and that much of this problem is attributable to inadequate maternal and infant care, Congress passed the Maternal and Child Health and Mental Retardation Planning Amendments. This made possible the start of a 5-year, $265 million program to improve maternal and child health services, especially for high-risk prospective mothers who have or are likely to have conditions hazardous to themselves or to their infants during pregnancy. Particular emphasis was placed on those who otherwise would not receive care because of low income or for other reasons beyond their control. The act also provided grants to states to plan comprehensive programs to combat mental retardation.

For health, 1965 was a banner year. The nation, through its Congress and the President, entered into an unprecedented assault on its health problems.[1] More progressive health legislation was passed during that year than at any time previously. The single most significant public health measure passed was the Social Security Amendments Act of 1965 (P.L. 89-97), which modified Title V of the act (the Maternal and Child Health and Crippled Children's Services) and added Title XVIII (Medicare) and Title XIX (Medicaid) to provide payment for health services to the elderly and the poor respectively. The Medicaid program has become the largest governmental program (more than $3 billion by 1978[2]) for the provision of health services to mothers and children. It is not a service delivery program but a federally supported, state-managed vendor payment system that pays for medical services provided to children in families meeting the low-income requirements of the program in that state. If one child is eligible, the mother and other children become eligible as well. The Medicaid act was amended later to require early and periodic screening, diagnosis and treatment (EPSDT) for all low-income children. This latter program was never successfully implemented because of confusion about objectives and methods and the responsibilities of different governmental agencies,[3] but it signaled the interest of Congress in addressing the health needs of virtually all children in the United States and remains as a point of discussion for future expansions of child health programs.

The same Social Security Amendments Act of 1965 extended several provisions, including the Maternity and Infancy Program that resulted from the 1963 legislation, enabling state and local health departments to develop comprehensive health service programs—medical, dental, and psychologic—for preschool and schoolchildren.

Another event of considerable significance to maternal and child health was the passage of the Economic Opportunity Act of 1964 (P.L. 88-452). Through the provision relating to the Head Start program, medical and dental examinations and in some cases treatment and nutritional services were provided to economically disadvantaged preschool children.

P.L. 93-53 amended Title V of the Social Security Act in 1973 by essentially transferring responsibility for the development of maternal and child health programs to the states. The project grants were to be discontinued, and the money was to be allocated to the states as part of a formula grant program. The change was twice postponed but finally implemented on July 1, 1974. Each state was supposed to receive at least as much money as it had received under the two previously separate approaches (project grants and formula grants) and had to develop a "program of projects" and a Maternal and Child Health Services Plan. The program had to include maternity and infant care, family planning services, infant intensive care, health services for children and youth, and dental care. By fiscal year 1980 state health agencies reported spending $604 million on maternal and child health programs and more on other, related services that were not organizationally a part of their maternal and child health programs, such as dental health, immunization programs, nutrition services, and others.[4]

By 1980 the federal appropriation for maternal and child health programs was $394.7 million:

$243.4 for Maternal and Child Health, $102 million for Crippled Children's Services, $31.8 million for research and training, $2.8 million for sudden infant death syndrome programs, $3 million for services for children with hemophilia, and $11.6 million for genetic disease programs. The total rose to $456 million in 1981, but President Reagan and a budget-cutting Congress grouped those separate authorities into one block-grant program for fiscal year 1982 and cut the total to $347.7 million. With inflation running at more than 10% per year, this represented a cut in spending power of more than 30%, and that pattern was continued in the 1983 budget.

There are many other sources of funds for maternal and child health programs. The U.S. Department of Agriculture spent about $630 million for the Supplemental Feeding Program for Women, Infants, and Children (WIC) in 1980 (see Chapter 17); family planning expenditures under Title X of the Public Health Service Act amounted to $159 million; and EPSDT expenditures were $43 million. In all, the state health agencies spent about $1.234 billion for maternal and child health programs in 1980, and about 25% of that money came from the states and local programs.[4] If the WIC program (which was virtually 100% federally funded) is excluded from the calculations, state and local expenditures were about 50% of the total. Although the amounts seem large in absolute terms, Budetti and his colleagues as well as other spokespersons for child health and welfare contend that the amounts are relatively small compared to need.[2] Per capita public expenditures for child health in 1978 were about $82, whereas $218 was spent on adults aged 19 to 64, and $1,280 on those aged 65 or more.

Title V of the Social Security Act was meant to stimulate state programs for maternal and child health, and the substantial level of effort by the states suggests that this objective was attained. About 34% of the $4.3 billion spent for personal health service programs by the states and local health agencies in 1980 was for maternal and child health programs, but 45% of that 34% was spent for the WIC program funded by the Department of Agriculture. George Silver and his colleagues[5] at Yale have concluded that the Title V programs did stimulate the development of administrative systems at the state level but did not increase the amount of state money appropriated for the programs. Most of the required matching funds came from the enumeration of existing services and efforts. By contrast, the Title XIX program (Medicaid) did result in more state money but this was for payments to physicians, hospitals, and other private health service providers. Those groups were the primary lobbyists for such increases in state appropriations. The intended recipients of both Title V and Title XIX services were either left out of the discussions at the state level or ineffective as lobbyists. Individual groups, such as the Parents of Autistic Children or the Parents of Children with Cerebral Palsy, were effective in obtaining state support for specific programs, but the generalized concept of child health has apparently been too general to elicit vigorous and successful support. Public health workers concentrate on Title V programs in their planning, programming, budgeting, and legislative activities, since the state health agency is the single state authority for all Maternal and Child Health programs and almost all Crippled Children's Services Programs. The federal budget for Title V programs, however, is only about 11% of the Medicaid expenditures for children by the single state agency responsible for Title XIX administration, the state welfare agency in most cases.

In 1978, Congress authorized the establishment of a Select Panel for the Promotion of Child Health to "a) formulate specific goals with respect to the promotion of the health status of children and expectant mothers in the United States; and b) develop a comprehensive national plan for achieving these goals and otherwise promoting the health of children . . ." (P.L. 95-626, November 10, 1978). There was considerable concern about the repeated assertions that the United States still experienced an unnecessarily high infant mortality rate in spite of its investments in research and services, and Congress as well as experts in maternal and child health believed that the federal and state agencies responsible for providing or developing services were poorly coordinated and linked. In addition, maternal and child health leaders in the federal government and in the states were dissatisfied with the reduction in status of the remains of the Children's Bureau, which had dropped from bureau status just below a Secretary to office status in the

Bureau of Community Health Services, which reported to the Health Services Administration, which reported in turn to the Office of the Assistant Secretary for Health.

The Select Panel, chaired by Lisbeth Bamberger Schorr, concluded its 2-year effort in December 1980 in a four-volume report to the Secretary[6] that, together with *Maternal and Child Health Practices,*[7] serves as the principal text for students of the subject. The report of the Select Panel verified the concerns of its sponsors and called for stronger, more centralized federal leadership.

The Select Panel found that the health of children had improved considerably during the past 2 decades but that the organizational, administrative, fiscal, and training aspects of the current system of health care had not kept pace with changing needs, technology, and epidemiologic research. They proposed that more attention be given to the prevention of disease and injury through environmental programs, concentration on the relationships between behavior and health, and improved nutrition. The Panel members reached a consensus that three broad classes of services were so essential that unfettered access to them should be guaranteed to all citizens:

- Prenatal, delivery, and postnatal care
- Comprehensive health care for children from birth through age 5
- Family planning services

The Select Panel urged the formation of organized systems of care with group practice arrangements for physicians and other care givers and special support for the expansion of community-owned comprehensive health centers. They differed with the American Academy of Pediatrics and many school officials by urging that the school site be organized as a logical and practical place for a comprehensive health services program. (See Chapter 23 for a discussion of the different opinions on the role of a school health program.)

Predictably, the Select Panel urged that the Children's Bureau be reconstituted as a new Maternal and Child Health Administration within the Public Health Service, and that its reporting channel to the Secretary of the Department of Health and Human Services be shortened from four to three steps or even to two steps. The Select Panel decided not to recommend that Medicaid, EPSDT, or the WIC program be transferred to the new Maternal and Child Health Administration but did recommend that the states be urged to consolidate their functions under the control of a single state agency. This disparity probably resulted from the proximity of the Select Panel to the federal agency program managers, who played a significant role in organizing the work of the Select Panel, and its relative isolation from the organizational relationships of the state agencies.

THE PROBLEMS

Many of the problems that plagued maternal and child health 50 years ago have been stripped away by improvements in the standard of living generally and in health care particularly, leaving a central core of problems that are more difficult to correct. They are related more to education and the distribution of resources than with medical care or specific public health practices.

A substantial proportion of the nation's children move through puberty to adolescence without either the intellectual and emotional ability or the environmental support needed to achieve and maintain an effective family structure. Approximately 1 million teenagers become pregnant each year. Many have abortions. For pregnant girls under the age of 15 there are nearly as many abortions as there are live births: 1,362 abortions per 1,000 live births for white girls and 670 for black girls. In the 15 to 19-year age group, white girls have 690 abortions per 1,000 live births, and black girls have 358.[8] Even though abortion is legal, many pregnant adolescents find it difficult to obtain needed medical care, since Congress has prohibited the use of federal funds for such purposes. Many of the girls do not know about or use effective contraceptive techniques, and most of them do not have ready access to a source of continuing health care.

Alcohol, tobacco, and drug abuse have a pronounced impact on the outcome of pregnancy, reducing the birth weight and increasing the infant mortality rate.[9] Substance abuse is more common in adolescent pregnancies than in those of older women, and it seems likely that adolescent girls are less willing or able to change those practices during pregnancy. Statistically, teenagers are a high-risk group, but studies have shown that the risk is not inherent in the biologic age of the mother (except for those under the age of 14), but rather in her education, behavior, and socioeconomic status.[10]

Other toxic influences in the preconceptual and prepartum periods reside in the environment.[11,12] Many workplaces expose both men and women to chemical and physical hazards that can have an impact on the development of sperm and ova: dry-cleaning establishments, electronics industries, laboratories, chemical plants, and paint manufacturers, to mention a few. The harm is often done in the first few weeks of pregnancy, before the woman knows she is pregnant. Men also are affected and may have damaged sperm or a lower sperm count as a result of toxic exposures. Some plants have attempted to exclude women from areas where such exposures may occur rather than alter the environment. Unless evidence exists to the contrary, it is prudent to assume that if a chemical or other hazard can harm a developing fetus, it can harm spermatozoa as well.

The hazards faced during a pregnancy have changed substantially in the last 50 years. Although the risk of environmental harm has increased, most other factors have improved, including the general state of nutrition and the standard of living. Problems exist in the organization and availability of services. Maternal mortality was 67.3 deaths per 10,000 live births in 1930 but declined to less than 1 by 1978. There is still a pronounced racial difference, the rate for white women being 0.64 per 10,000 live births, whereas the rate for nonwhite women is 2.3. These differences in the rates of maternal deaths by race are reflected in the variations among the states with higher rates occurring in the south. There is no reason to believe that true racial or geographic differences should naturally exist.

Before World War II, most black mothers delivered at home, and nearly half did not have adequate medical care (Table 22-1). Falk and his associates,[13] writing for the Committee on the Costs of Medical Care in 1929, said that 30% or more of the births in the southern states were attended by midwives who were "often ignorant, untrained, dirty and superstitious." The Committee went on to point out that with proper supervision and backup, even the midwives of 50 years ago could provide a valuable service, and the situation has changed dramatically since then. Overall in the nation, by 1979 not only did almost all white births (99%) occur in hospitals but the proportion of black births in hospitals rose from 31.5% in 1943 to 99.2% in 1979, and medically attended black births rose from 55.9% to 96.8%. Recently there has been a slight trend toward home deliveries and deliveries in nonhospital-

Health and human development

TABLE 22-1. Births by race, location, and type of attendant, United States, 1943, 1955, and 1979

		Location		Attendant	
Race and year		Hospital (%)	Elsewhere (%)	Physician (%)	Other (%)
White	1943	77.2	22.8	97.8	2.2
	1955	97.5	2.5	99.2	0.8
	1979	99.0	1.0	97.7	2.3
Nonwhite	1943	31.5	68.5	55.9	44.1
	1955	76.0	24.0	82.8	17.2
	1979	99.2	0.8	96.8	3.2

based birthing centers, partly as a choice based on life-style and partly because of the high cost of delivery in general hospitals. The American College of Obstetricians and Gynecologists has opposed such practices, and official vital statistics reports indicate a higher incidence of complications in out-of-hospital deliveries, including a higher neonatal death rate (deaths occurring in the first 28 days of life), but the figures include both accidental and poorly planned out-of-hospital births as well as planned and attended births. With careful risk assessment (see the section on Approaches to the problems) and a well-trained attendant, the available evidence suggests that the outcomes for home deliveries may be as good as they are in a hospital environment.

Maternal mortality rates are higher in very young mothers and mothers over 35, although the risks are generally very low. The principal causes are still infection, hemorrhage, and toxemias of pregnancy. The striking reductions in maternal mortality that have occurred, particularly during the last 30 years, are because of improved medical care in the prevention and treatment of infection and better management of shock with intravenous fluids and blood. It is not clear whether toxemia is decreasing, but improvements in diet counseling should lead to an improved outcome. For many years small babies were considered to be better than large ones since they were presumed to have a less difficult transit through the birth canal, and physicians sought to keep weight gain below 15 pounds. Nutritionists knew that the restrictive diet practices were causing, not preventing, problems, and as physicians have become more cognizant of the in-

formation, weight gains of 25 pounds have become the norm with much better results.

Whether pregnancy should be treated as a natural process or as a medical problem has become an increasingly important argument. As shown in Table 22-1, efforts to improve the environment in which delivery occurs and the qualifications of the attendants at birth have succeeded dramatically, and the statistics indicate that there has been a parallel improvement in the outcomes. However, in recent years many have advocated the return of the birthing process to a more natural, homelike environment with family involvement. In a study of high technology interventions, the General Accounting Office found that 11.8% of births were induced rather than allowed to begin spontaneously; that 80.8% were carried out with the mother under anesthesia, 25.6% with the use of forceps; and that 13.6% were performed by cesarean section.[14] Electronic monitoring of the fetus is becoming an increasingly common practice, and many believe that this results in still more interventions. A study of 66,049 live births in Arkansas showed that the events were disproportionately distributed by day of the week, with a relatively low number occurring on weekends and holidays.[15] Increasingly, births are being managed as elective medical procedures in a high technology environment that is very costly and, some believe, unnecessarily risky for most of the families involved.

Advocates of "demedicalizing" maternity point out that 70% of all pregnancies are perfectly normal with no known risk factors that might serve to complicate the process. As long as medical backup is promptly accessible, most of these births could occur in a less intense environment with less risk, fewer interventions, and considerably less cost.

Abortion

Most maternal deaths from abortion in earlier years were caused by illegal abortions induced either by unqualified individuals or by women themselves, usually under extremely unsatisfactory and unsanitary conditions. This resulted in its recognition as an important social and public health problem. During the 1960s and early 1970s, an increasing number of nations liberalized their laws with regard to medically induced abortion.[16] Several states in the United States revised their laws to allow induced abortion under medically acceptable circumstances. The Public Health Service established an Abortion Surveillance Program in 1968 in cooperation with state and local health departments, which were encouraged and assisted to develop abortion reporting systems. The purpose was to be able to observe and study changes in fertility as well as maternal morbidity and mortality.

Meanwhile, many professional and other organizations passed strong resolutions endorsing the trend. This long-overdue movement culminated in a landmark decision by the United States Supreme Court in January 1973.* The court did not remove restrictions entirely. For the first 3 months of pregnancy, it said, the decision rests with the woman and her physician—a "right of privacy" in which the state cannot interfere. For the next 6 months states, if they wish, may "regulate the abortion procedures in ways reasonably related to maternal health," such as licensing and regulating the persons and facilities involved. For the last 10 weeks of pregnancy, when the fetus "has the capability of meaningful life outside the mother's womb, states may prohibit abortion except as it may be indicated to preserve the life or health of the mother." The Supreme Court stressed that the ruling did not give a woman the right to abortion on demand, nor could a physician (or presumably a hospital) be required to perform an abortion. The American Public Health Association[17] and the American College of Obstetricians and Gynecologists[18] have published guidelines for abortion services.

Reports from various countries indicate that the risk from induced abortion under proper circumstances, and especially during the first trimester of

*Rowe V. Wade 41 USLW 4213, 1973; Dow V. Bolton 41 USLW 4233, 1973.

TABLE 22-2. Ratios of induced abortions per 1,000 live births by marital status and race of woman, seven-state area, 1978

Race	All women	Married	Unmarried
All races	296.6	97.9	1,177.2
White	259.9	77.0	2,154.4
Black	356.3	185.2	484.3

pregnancy, is extremely low. There were only 16 deaths caused by abortions in the United States in 1978, and several of these were spontaneous rather than planned abortions. In a seven-state survey area, the reported ratio of induced abortions in 1978 was 296.6 per 1,000 live births. The rate for whites is lower than for blacks, but white unmarried women have a rate nearly 4.5 times as great as black unmarried women (Table 22-2).[8]

The complex reasons for these differences by marital status and race are not well understood, but white women generally have better access to elective medical care, making it easier for unmarried white women to obtain abortions. Moreover, white families generally have been less willing to accept an out-of-wedlock pregnancy and have been less successful in providing an effective parenting environment for such children when they are born.

In recent years some groups have succeeded in reinstituting barriers to abortion, particularly for low-income women, by obtaining Congressional interdictions of the use of any federal funds for abortion purposes. This includes counseling by professional staff in a clinic that is only partially funded by federal money. The tactics of committed, single-interest groups are frequently effective, even though the majority of Americans favor broader access to needed abortion services. It is not clear what the effect of restricting access will be on maternal and child health, but it probably will increase the infant mortality rate and the frequency of mental retardation and other severe congenital anomalies.

Infant mortality

As would be expected, the factors involved in the problem of infant mortality and the improvements that have been made closely parallel those described for the mothers of the infants. Although

Health and human development

there is cause for satisfaction in the reduction in infant mortality, much remains to be accomplished. The nation still suffers a loss of about 45,000 infants each year. In 1981 this resulted in an infant mortality of 12.5 per 1,000 live births. Between 1915 and 1949, infant mortality dropped dramatically from 100 to 28 per 1,000 live births. Then the rate of decrease slowed noticeably. During the 16 years from 1965 to 1981, however, the decrease was 50%.

Although infant mortality has been steadily decreasing, as in the case of maternal mortality, internal disparities are to be noted: In 1980 the rate varied from 10.3 in the New England states to 14.2 in the east-south central states.[19] In almost all regions, the rate for black infants was double the rate for white infants. Although both the white and the black infant mortality rates have been declining, the disparity has not diminished appreciably. Again, as in the case of adult women, there is no convincing evidence that the nonwhite infant is intrinsically less viable than infants born to white mothers.

The infant mortality rate can be partitioned into an early neonatal mortality rate (the first 28 days of life), and a postneonatal rate from the twenty-eighth day to the end of the first year. In 1981 the national rates were 8.4 and 4.1 per 1,000 live births respectively. A higher early neonatal death rate suggests inadequate access to delivery services, whereas a higher postneonatal death rate indicates the existence of environmental problems in the home and a lack of access to child care services.

In one sense, infant deaths are most commonly caused by congenital anomalies, respiratory distress, the sudden infant death syndrome, and premature delivery. Underlying all other causes, however, is low birth weight. The dividing line is 2,500 grams, although there is some evidence that low birth weight in black infants may begin at 2,250 grams. The infant mortality rates within each weight-specific group in the United States are better than those of most other countries, and the rates have improved within each weight group over the past 2 decades, but the frequency of low birth weight has not changed. It still occurs in 13% of black births and 6.2% of white births.[20,21] It is more common in women with fewer years of education. It is also more common in women who obtain prenatal care late or not at all during the pregnancy,

and it is more common in unmarried than in married women. These factors (race, education, prenatal care, and marital status) overshadow all other variables in their relationship to low birth weight and therefore to higher infant mortality and morbidity rates. Race is consistently the most powerful determinant, but it appears that that is mediated through the problems of generally lower socioeconomic status and fewer years of education.

The principal effort of public health workers in the United States has been to initiate prenatal care as soon as possible for all women. That effort is reflected in the policies of interested associations and governmental agencies that seek to either provide or pay for prenatal care, particularly for high-risk mothers.[22] Until recently, few people have inquired into the reasons for the relationship, since pregnancy has been considered a medical problem and it is assumed that medical problems respond favorably to a medical intervention. However, it seems unlikely that an early rather than a later visit to a physician can have much influence on the major factors that retard fetal growth, such as alcohol consumption, cigarette smoking, or other environmental or behavioral phenomena, because the management of such problems is not a part of most medical practices. By 1979, 77.1% of all white births occurred in situations in which the mother had begun prenatal care during the first 3 months of her pregnancy. This was true for only 59.4% of black births. Only 57% of white teenagers and 47% of black teenagers began prenatal care during the first 3 months.[23] Within those groups the percent of low-birth-weight infants was more strongly related to the number of years of school completed by the mother than the time at which prenatal care was begun, except for those mothers who obtained no prenatal care at all. This latter group, by definition, included a disproportionate number of women with premature deliveries.

From a medical as well as a public health point of view, early initiation of prenatal care remains the most practical thing that can be done to improve infant health, since the systems as well as the beliefs are in place to support such an effort and there is no wide-spread consensus that increased efforts should be made to alter socioeconomic status and the strength of the educational system, even though such changes would have a greater long-term impact. This may not necessitate the universal provision of medical care, however. Most of the beneficial changes that can be made during the average pregnancy are not the result of medical diagnosis or prescription, but counseling, guidance, and risk assessment that can be more effectively carried out by nurse-midwives and other trained maternity counselors in most instances.

As noted before, the infant mortality rates in the United States within each weight-specific group are very good compared to other countries. This has occurred because of improved care at the time of delivery. Hospitals and physicians have not addressed the problems that underlie low birth weight but have done what they know how to do: intervene effectively in a crisis situation after it has developed. The cost is, of course, very high. In one study, the cost of ensuring that an infant weighing 1,000 grams or less (2.2 pounds) will leave the hospital healthy was $115,356 at 1977 rates.[24] Pneumonia of the newborn used to be a much more important cause of neonatal death but has been reduced by improved nursery management and the use of antibiotics. Some inroads have been made in recent years not only against birth injuries but even against congenital malformations by means of more stringent control of environmental hazards and by examinations of amniotic fluid early in pregnancy followed by abortion if a malformed fetus is discovered.

Survival of the first few days or weeks of life does not mean that the health and life of the infant are no longer subject to risk. Until only a few years ago infectious diseases were common. Now they are of secondary importance, with the exceptions of pneumonia and influenza and gastroenteritis. Even these have been greatly reduced in recent years—the first by better nutrition and antibiotics and the second by improved sanitation, nursery techniques, and chemotherapy. Nevertheless, the large proportion of infant deaths attributable to a variety of respiratory ailments is notable. Numerous recent studies implicate the improper or excessive use of various drugs, pharmaceuticals, and anesthetics, including some used in obstetric practice, as a cause of or contributor to respiratory distress in the newborn. A significant number of infant deaths are caused by accidents and homicides. Accidents represent the second leading cause of infant death after the first month of life is passed. With regard to homicides, attention is called to the discussion of the "battered child syndrome" in Chapter 29. Also surprising is the occurrence of heart disease and malignancies as a cause of some infant deaths. Some success through early diagnosis and surgery

is beginning to be achieved against congenital heart defects.

The infant requires a spectrum of precautions and services to get through the hazardous first year: adequate and sanitary feeding, protection against infections and accidents, supervision preferably by a family pediatrician, home follow-up if necessary by a public health nurse, prompt correction of any defects that may exist, early diagnosis and treatment of any illnesses that may occur, and the provision of a satisfactory emotional environment. Failure to meet these needs invites more serious difficulties later in life.

The preschool child

There are in the United States approximately 16.3 million children under the age of 5, customarily referred to as the preschool period. After that first birthday, the child enters a phase of development that is most favorable from the standpoint of the risks of mortality. Currently the risk of death between the first and the fifth birthday is 0.66 per 1,000. This was not always the case. At the beginning of the century the death rate of this age group was about 20 per 1,000. The preschool period benefited most from many of the greatest triumphs of preventive medicine and public health. The dramatic decreases in deaths, illnesses, and disabilities in this group may be credited chiefly to the prevention of the acute communicable diseases of childhood. This is emphasized by a comparison of the leading causes of death in this age group in 1925 with those in 1978 (Table 22-3). In the earlier year (1925), diarrhea and enteritis accounted for 109.8 deaths per 100,000 children aged 1 to 4. Fifty years later, the rate had dropped to less than 1 per 100,000, primarily because of improved environmental conditions. The overall decline in mortality is striking for almost all causes. It is somewhat surprising to note that the death rate from motor vehicle accidents was less in 1978 than in 1925. Such figures can serve to illustrate a particular point, such as the change in the nature of the phenomena that may place the preschool child in jeopardy, but the observer has to beware of the kinds of groupings that can occur to make a particular item the number one cause. If the category of "accidents (other than motor vehicle)" were subdivided into its various components, the category of "mo-

TABLE 22-3. Mortality in the 1 to 4 age group, United States, 1925 and 1978

Cause of death, 1925	Rate per 100,000 population	Cause of death, 1978	Rate per 100,000 population
Diarrhea and enteritis	109.8	Accidents (other than motor vehicle)	18.2
Accidents (other than motor vehicle)	57.7	Motor vehicle accidents	10.6
Pneumonia	44.7	Congenital anomalies	8.4
Diphtheria	43.0	Malignant neoplasms	4.9
Tuberculosis	28.9	Influenza and pneumonia	2.9
Whooping cough	28.6	Homicide	2.6
Measles	14.4	Heart disease	2.3
Scarlet fever	11.7	Diarrhea and enteritis	0.5
Motor vehicle accidents	11.5	Nephritis	0.2
Heart disease	8.9	Tuberculosis	0.1

Modified from Monthly vital statistics reports, National Center for Health Statistics.

tor vehicle accidents" would rank number one. In addition to ranking, the actual rates merit attention. Although it is shocking to find homicide on the list of the leading causes of death in any age group, the rate (2.5 per 100,000) would not have made the list at all in 1925, when such diseases as diphtheria had death rates in excess of 40 per 100,000.

Of greater significance than the forces of mortality in the preschool years is the fact that although deaths are infrequent, morbidity is high. Thus the National Health Survey indicates an annual frequency rate of acute conditions during the first 6 years of life of 376.2 per 100 children. Similarly, restricted activity days and bed disability days are high during this period of life. Fortunately, not only is the recovery rate for preschool children high but the duration of their illnesses is brief.

The preschool years represent a period of significant nutritional and emotional change for the child as well as of increased effective contacts for the acquirement of communicable diseases and involvement in accidents. From the point of view of the public health approach, therefore, this stage of life is now one to which more attention must be given, not so much for the prevention of death as for the prevention of physical and mental illnesses and trauma that may handicap the future lives of those concerned. Since the individual in this age span is undergoing extremely rapid growth and development, what may often appear at the moment to be inconsequential influences of a nutritional, emotional, dental, or physical nature may have an ultimate cumulative effect far out of proportion to their initial appearance. The need therefore is for programs designed to minimize the daily impact of influences of this nature, programs for nutritional improvement, accident prevention, and continuous health and dental supervision, including techniques for the prevention of dental caries, such as topical application of sodium fluoride. Mental illness is one of the greatest causes of disability in the adult population at the present time. It is during the preschool period that the seeds of much of this are sown. There is an important need, therefore, for the application of sound mental health principles and for the more widespread establishment and use of mental health and child guidance services.

APPROACH TO THE PROBLEM

Since so many factors can affect the well-being of mothers and children, programs related to them must be multifaceted and involve the coordinated efforts of many disciplines, organizations, and agencies. For children, of course, well-informed and concerned parents necessarily must provide the keystone for the arch of proper child care and development. There are many important and sometimes critical roles for the health department.

To meet adequately the many problems in maternal, infant, and child health, the official health agency of a community should carry out a well-conceived and coordinated series of activities, each of which looks forward to the subsequent periods of life. Personal and community services and education are involved.

Arden Miller,[25] speaking before the National Health Forum in 1974, gave a specific prescription in five parts: (1) a national health service for mothers and children to include prenatal care, obstetric and midwifery services, homemaking assistance and mothercraft, postnatal care, family planning services, well-child and developmental checkups, routine immunizations and anticipatory guidance, preschool screening and school health services, including a mandate to treat and correct the defects found and provide care for illnesses of those not able to use private medical care effectively; (2) a public feeding program; (3) national housing reform; (4) community-based family support centers, including day care; and (5) performance standards for state and local health departments as well as for private providers. Miller said that we could afford to do it and that we could not afford not to. In this regard, Lowe,[26] Special Assistant for Child Health Affairs in the Office of the Assistant Secretary for Health, said that in 1975 the United States spent $15.4 billion for health services for 70.5 million children under the age of 19, or about $218 each. According to him, it should have taken only about $200 per child per year, meaning that about $1.3 billion had been wasted through inadequate planning, coordination, and delivery mechanisms.

In Cambridge, Massachusetts, the city operated a separate hospital and health department until 1968, when they were combined in an effort to bring about better coordination of public health programs. The Chairman of the Department of Pediatrics in the hospital (Dr. Philip Porter) became the director of the combined maternal and child health program and moved to both consolidate the administration of the programs and decentralize the delivery system into selected schools in areas that had the greatest child health problems. With the expanded use of nurse practitioners, a comprehensive program has been developed with the resources that were available.[27]

The state health agency is responsible for the overall effort. The Federal Office of Maternal and Child Health has described 14 functional elements in a state-based maternal and child health program:[28]

1. Leadership
2. The assessment of problems, needs, and resources
3. Planning
4. Resource development and allocation
5. Standard setting for providers
6. Quality assurance reviews
7. An information system and data analysis
8. Education for the public and providers
9. Technical assistance for local health departments and community organizations
10. Coordination of multiple programs
11. Evaluation
12. Administration
13. Direct services where needed
14. Research

The health department cannot function alone. In fact, no other part of the health department program requires the cooperation of so many people and agencies in the community. Except in economically disadvantaged areas, much of the direct medical and dental service to mothers, infants, and children will be rendered by private physicians and dentists. Similarly, the health department can never substitute for the health teaching of children in the home and in the classroom under the guidance of intelligent parents and professionally trained teachers. No other phase of the public health program requires so many cooperative contacts with nonofficial health agencies and with the many social agencies that usually exist in the community.

Community health centers, frequently initiated with federal project grant support, and health department clinics provide a substantial proportion of the maternal and child health services in the United States, especially in areas that are otherwise disadvantaged or are medically underserved. No one knows the exact proportion, but as much as 20% of all such health services may now be provided by the public sector in organized settings. Beyond this, the active cooperation and assistance of many lay persons and community groups must be obtained. In addition to using lay advice and support by means of advisory committees, maternal health councils, or similar techniques, many health departments have found it possible to improve and expand their service programs considerably by using volunteer workers both in clinics and in the field.

One further general consideration deals with the necessity to conduct continuous research and surveys to keep the total health program in balance with maternal and child health needs. In areas with good reporting, morbidity and mortality data provide the most obvious source of guidance. The Bureau of the Census and the National Center for Health Statistics and the Bureau of Community Health Services of the Public Health Service are especially good sources of data. In addition, state and community agencies can provide regionally and locally pertinent information.

Generally speaking, the statistical needs for maternal and child health programs can be divided into two categories: vital statistical data and supplemental statistical information that is usually necessary for the proper interpretation of the vital statistics. The following vital statistics relating to maternity and infancy are usually available for any state, county, or large city and are a part of the basic information in planning any health service for mothers and infants:

1. Live births and fetal deaths (number and rate)
   a. Urban, rural
   b. Resident and nonresident
   c. In hospitals, in homes
   d. Attended by physician, not attended by physician
   e. Race, marital status, and age of mother
2. Maternal deaths (number and rate)
   a. Urban, rural
   b. Resident and nonresident
   c. In hospitals, in homes
   d. Attended by physician, not attended by physician
   e. Causes of death
3. Neonatal deaths (infant deaths under 1 month of age) (number and rate)
   a. Urban, rural
   b. Resident and nonresident
   c. In hospitals, in homes
   d. Attended by physician, not attended by physician
   e. Race and age of mother
   f. Causes of death
   g. Age at time of death

This list must be supplemented by information relating to available medical, nursing, and hospital resources; the occupations of women in the childbearing ages; and educational, cultural, and many other socioeconomic factors. In addition, data must be sought with regard to the quality of health care available and the complications of pregnancy and infancy that occur in the geographic area under consideration. There should also be conducted and

available to the health agency periodic analyses of hospital and medical records. This is best done by an acceptable and unbiased peer review procedure.

MATERNAL HEALTH PROGRAM

The natal process divides into several discrete physiologic phases, each of which presents certain problems and needs.

Preconceptional period

An adequate maternal health program should begin long before the child is conceived and even before the expectant mother reaches physiologic maturity. The preconceptional aspects of the program involve a threefold approach of education, health service, and developmental counseling. Much education that may have a direct and significant influence on future parenthood can be accomplished with the high school and even grade school girl and boy. Scientifically correct and socially acceptable facts may be presented to schoolchildren in relation to many phases of social hygiene, including the anatomy and physiology of reproduction, the problem of sexually transmitted diseases, the importance of qualified supervision during pregnancy and infancy, and the responsibilities of parenthood. One of the most important problems in junior and senior high schools is pregnancy and sexual behavior that is unaccompanied by adequate knowledge of reproduction, birth control, and contraception or a thoughtful approach to psychologic development and self-esteem as well as the ethics of responsibility. The tendency has been to focus on educational programs for teenage girls, but many school boards have found themselves faced with stiff parental opposition when the school attempts to teach what the parents have not or cannot. Moreover, it is probably better to conduct such teaching in a coeducational environment since that is a more natural setting. It is important to encourage both boys and girls to understand their responsibility for their sexual behavior, especially when it results in the birth of a child. Faced with parental opposition, some programs have explored techniques for identifying the high-risk girl so that she can be singled out for individual counseling. Health department staffs can work collaboratively with school staffs in settings outside the school, which may ameliorate parental opposition.

Many states have begun to provide genetic counseling services and, by referral, the technique of amniocentesis for high-risk pregnant women (those with a prior history of a congenital anomaly, those with a genetic trait that may jeopardize the outcome, or women over the age of 35, who are more likely to have a baby with Down's syndrome).

Family planning is an essential part of public health programs. In fact, most contraceptive supplies are now distributed through the many public programs. In 1980, 47 state health agencies reported the provision of contraceptive services, 42 reported that they offered services for infertile couples, and 34 provided sterilization services, although it was not specified whether these included both vasectomies and tubal ligations. Nearly 3.4 million people received such services.[4]

Health departments may also be involved in the process whereby sterilization procedures are provided either voluntarily or involuntarily. The techniques of vasectomy and tubal ligation are now quite simple, safe, and relatively inexpensive; and a growing number of men are seeking sterilization as a simpler and safer approach to family planning than the continued use of contraceptive devices by the woman or sterilization of the woman. It is especially important to deal with the consent process in an informed and thoughtful way, and many agencies require a waiting period of a few days to allow the client to think about what is, practially speaking, an irreversible decision. Involuntary sterilizations are now uncommon, but there are some indications for their performance. Careful guidelines need to be developed in any state that still makes provisions for such procedures, and public health personnel should be involved along with those whose expertise is in law or ethics. By 1976, 30.2% of all married couples with a woman aged 15 to 44 were sterile, most of them for purposes of contraception. Another 46.8% used some form of contraception: 46% of those used an oral contraceptive, 14.8% used condoms, 12.5% used an intrauterine device, 6.9% used the rhythm method, 6.2% used vaginal foam, and 6% used a diaphragm.[29] These figures differ from those published by the National Reporting Program for Family Planning Services in 1982,[30] which indicated that 63.7% of the patients in the study group used an oral contraceptive, 7.1% used an intrauterine device, and 7.2% used a diaphragm. These figures, however were for patients in organized clinics only, whereas the earlier figures included patients who obtained family planning services in a private physician's office.

The family planning movement has been significant in many ways in the United States. It was started by Margaret Sanger, who saw it as a political and social action movement to improve the status of women; but the movement quickly became "medicalized" and the term that was applied to it— *family planning*—implied that the purpose was still to raise a family, albeit a planned one.

Family planning programs should include a variety of contraceptive methods; good record keeping, including pertinent medical, social, and reproductive historical information; initial and annual examinations, including breast examinations, abdominal and pelvic examinations, Pap smears, and screening for hypertension; and effective referral for any medical problems detected.

Although services are now widely available, they are still not being used effectively by teenagers. Most girls who use family planning clinic services have had sexual intercourse before they are 16 years old. Many teenagers are contraceptive "failures" who become pregnant either accidentally or deliberately to attain some sense of accomplishment and control in their lives. Services need to be easily accessible for teenagers, and the staff requires special training to cope in a supportive manner with the special problems and demands of these young people. Recent efforts by the federal government to require that clinic personnel inform the parents before providing services, if implemented either by federal requirement or local initiative, may drive many young girls away from one of the few places where they are able to get sound advice.

Programs and services such as those described may be implemented in several ways: through supplementary service in maternal health clinics, through specifically established planned parenthood clinics, and through referral to private physicians. Public health nurses and other trained family planning workers and counselors can provide effective and acceptable services, although a physician is still a desirable participant, at least to conduct the initial physical and annual follow-up examinations as well as initiate prescriptions for oral contraceptives. In practice, all of these functions can be performed by trained nurse practitioners and auxiliary personnel if medical backup is available on referral, but most states have not modified their medical and nursing practice laws to permit such activities.

Women's health groups have formed health centers where much of the indignity of the gynecologic examination has been ameliorated. In addition, some of the groups have published outstanding self-help texts that have contributed significantly to teaching women how to take better care of themselves. *Our Bodies, Ourselves*[31] is a notable example. It is significant that similar activities and publications have not been developed by and for men. The exploited feelings of women, when faced with the masculine medical care system, have led them to develop a strong consumer-oriented focus that promises to be effective in improving self-help and a sense of self-responsibility for both sexes.

One other problem that should concern public health workers is that of rape. Many communities have established rape counseling centers and hot lines. A great deal of attention has been focused on the problems of women who have been raped: the probability that police involvement will involve male officers, the trauma of the emergency room examination—also usually performed by a male physician, the suspicion that a rape victim may have enticed the attack, and, more recently, the difficulty in distinguishing between the overtly violent act of rape as it has been customarily described and the more covert forms of psychologic rape that involve a more subtle but no less serious form of violence to the woman's self-esteem. Health department staff, particularly public health nurses who have had special training or who have special empathy, can and should be involved in helping the victims.

Antepartum and intrapartum period

The antepartum period of pregnancy is most important. The objective is to involve the pregnant woman in an organized system of care as early as possible. In the United States this usually means medical care, although it should include the involvement of a nurse-midwife, access to nutrition counseling, the availability of childbirth and parenting classes for both parents, and an organized approach to special needs such as support and counseling for unmarried women, abortion services if they are not prohibited by law, care for women engaged in industry during pregnancy, and such technical problems as the management of Rh incompatibility.

It is necessary to set up some administrative procedure to locate pregnant women as early in their pregnancies as possible, especially those who may be at high risk either because of age, income, education, physical problems, or a combination of factors. The need for and manner of doing this varies from one community to another. The health department has at its disposal several sources of information. Knowledge of pregnancies may come to the health department staff through their personal observations during their daily rounds, by statements or suggestions from neighbors of expectant mothers, from previous patients, and from school personnel. A highly desirable goal is for the private physicians as well as those in community programs to notify the health department of each new obstetric case. Part of the problem is already solved in that the patient in question is under medical supervision. However, even here the health department may render service through public health nursing supervision and education and with follow-up of women who miss appointments.

A Committee on Perinatal Health was formed by the American Academy of Family Physicians, the American Academy of Pediatrics, the American College of Obstetricians and Gynecologists, and the National Foundation–March of Dimes to develop standards for prenatal and delivery services. The committee recommended a regionalized system of perinatal care and stratified centers into three levels: level I centers are designed to take care of the uncomplicated delivery (even here, however, the backup services and laboratory requirements are extensive); level II centers have a more complete range of maternal and neonatal care services and should be able to handle most of the complicated cases; level III centers are designed to have the full spectrum of services, including neonatologists and other highly skilled personnel. These centers are designed to serve an area with 8,000 to 12,000 deliveries per year, and the committee established a model budget of $2.637 million. (The committee's report[32] has an excellent bibliography, principally dealing with high-risk situations.)

The regionalization of perinatal care has received a great deal of attention by the American College of Obstetricians and Gynecologists and the Robert Wood Johnson Foundation, which has invested heavily in the development and evaluation of such systems. As Ruth Watson Lubic[33] and others have pointed out, however, regionalization of perinatal care serves to strengthen the "medicalization" of the birthing process and to channel people upward toward higher technology care rather than deflecting them from such systems and into appropriate lower technology alternatives.

Some members of the American College of Obstetricians and Gynecologists believed that the report of the Committee on Perinatal Health did not sufficiently deal with rural areas, and they developed a separate report,[34] which is fascinating in its reliance on nonmedical personnel. In fact, the organization of this latter model is very similar to some health care delivery models in underdeveloped countries. The organizational chart starts with the family units at the top rather than at the bottom and recommends the services of a health advocate for each family—a skilled person such as a successful mother—who will serve as a guide for the family. Then comes the primary perinatal health care provider, who does not need to be a physician but may be a public health nurse or, preferably, a nurse-midwife. Below this in the organizational structure come the level I, II, and III centers as described by the original committee. (This second report also contains an excellent bibliography.)

The American Public Health Association has published guidelines and standards in a book titled *Ambulatory Maternal Health Care and Family Planning Services: Policies, Principles, Practices,*[35] which includes chapters on prenatal, postpartum, and interconceptional care; family planning; adolescent pregnancy; health education; nutrition services; social services; the role of the consumer; the human resources needed, as well as facilities, equipment, and supplies; guidelines for evaluation; and an excellent bibliography.

Considerable emphasis has been given in recent years to the family nature of birth. Increasingly fathers are becoming active participants in the delivery, and the concept of "bonding" has become of considerable importance. This is simply assuring virtually immediate contact of the mother and the newborn baby so that eye and skin contact can be made as quickly as possible. Although the nature of the psychologic merits are hotly debated, few would deny that early bonding and a continuing personal relationship can do much to improve the health of both mother and baby in the immediate postpartum period as well as in subsequent growth and development. Family-oriented childbirth is simply another way of saying that it is the family—not the hospital, the doctor, or the nurses—who is having the baby.

One of the most significant developments in recent years in the United States has been a changing attitude toward the use of professionally trained nurse-midwives and out-of-hospital births. The American College of Nurse-Midwives conducted a survey in December 1976 and obtained data from 1,299 respondents. Fifty-one percent of the nurse-midwives were in clinical practice and, of those, 84% managed deliveries, which may have accounted for 1% of all deliveries in the United States in that year.[36]

It is difficult to know how many deliveries are actually performed by someone other than a physician. The figures in Table 22-1 indicate that between 2.3% and 3.2% of births are attended by someone other than a physician, a slight increase since 1975, but many more deliveries were undoubtedly performed by nursing personnel, both untrained and trained. Physicians often "miss" the delivery by arriving too late at the hospital, but still sign the birth certificate, which results in the official tabulation of births by attendant. In recent years, as hospitals and medical staffs have accepted nurse-midwives in the delivery room, they have been less apprehensive about allowing the nurse to sign the official documents. Still less is known about the number of births that are assisted by nursing personnel with no medical supervision at all. In many states, such practices are thought to be illegal, and the people offering such services are necessarily nervous about their visibility. Should a death occur, some county medical societies and prosecuting attorneys might well force prosecution on a charge of manslaughter. The situation is slowly changing as more states amend their practice laws to allow certified nurse-midwives to perform deliveries in out-of-hospital settings.

The Maternity Center Association of New York City established the first school of midwifery in 1932 and the first formally organized out-of-hospital delivery program, the Childbearing Center, in 1974.[37] After several years of effort they were successful in obtaining formal recognition from the city and the state and were recognized as an acceptable provider by Blue Cross shortly thereafter—the first such contract in the nation. By 1981 there were between 125 and 150 such centers in 27 states. The Association was instrumental in establishing the Cooperative Birth Center Network to provide information and technical assistance to interested groups. Model standards for alternative birthing

Health and human development

centers were published by the Network in their newsletter in 1982.[38]

An important part of the standards are the criteria used for risk assessment. Each applicant for an out-of-hospital delivery program needs to be carefully screened for behavioral, environmental, physical, mental, or genetic factors that might increase the probability of an unsuccessful outcome. Individuals with certain risk factors warrant a referral for further evaluation by a specialist before being accepted into the program. In practice, competent nurse-midwives are very thorough in their assessments and insist on client compliance with nutritional and substance-abuse guidelines. Other useful descriptions of the concept are contained in a policy paper adopted by the American Public Health Association in 1979.[39] The review by Bennetts and Lubic[37] includes a study of 1,938 pregnancies in 11 birthing centers, which indicated the safety and reliability of the practice. It has not been possible to develop a controlled, randomized trial, since most physicians would not cooperate in a randomized experiment and most women who choose a birthing center would not accept referral to a hospital unless it were medically necessary.

Hospitals have been quick to adopt the birthing center concept in an effort to satisfy consumer demand. It provides a lower cost labor and delivery area and a more homelike environment for the family. Many hospitals authorize attendance by nurse-midwives in the birthing center. They are able to move quickly to a more traditional, medical environment if that becomes necessary. The hospital-based birthing center is a partial response to the overall problem of high-cost and high-technology obstetric care, but its most important feature may be the evidence that a hospital can respond to consumer pressure and meet community needs, especially when competition is available in the community.

Most states now have one or more requirements related to the screening of the newborn infant for metabolic diseases such as phenylketonuria (PKU) or thyroid problems that if undetected and untreated can lead to cretinism. At least 20 such screening tests can now be performed, but the availability of the technology is not a sufficient reason for doing it.[40] There should be a reasonable probability that affected subjects will benefit from treatment, that affected subjects and their families will be apprised of hazardous situations that should be avoided, or that affected families can be counseled about the risks of recurrence.

Postpartum period

As in the antepartum program, the first essential in the postpartum program is case finding. The location of women who have recently delivered can be accomplished with relative ease where an efficient birth registration program is in effect. In addition to this is the arrangement achieved in some localities whereby hospitals promptly notify the health department of all deliveries. In many instances the health department is notified when the patient is about to return home. Many women and children are now being discharged within 24 hours and routinely within 2 days. In birthing centers the mother is often discharged in 4 to 6 hours if there is no bleeding and within 12 hours in most cases. Notification through the routine birth registration route no longer suffices: some women may be home for a week in a hostile and risk-laden environment before the health department even knows of the birth. It is far better to arrange for someone in the delivery area to notify the health department on the day of birth. Early discharge is advantageous to the family economically, and it facilitates a more rapid reformation of the family, but it reduces the time for contemplation, rest, learning, and the management of special problems such as congenital anomalies and out-of-wedlock births. The immediate postpartum period is often a very effective time to learn about family planning techniques and services, especially for those women who were unaware of such programs.

Unfortunately a great many postpartum public health nursing visits are first made after the mother and her new infant have been home for some weeks. By then much of the potential value is lost. It is when the woman first returns to the confusing cares of her home with the added burden of a new infant that she really needs and appreciates help. It is generally not possible to provide services to every mother and child on their return home, nor is it necessary to do so; but, depending on resources, procedures should be established to make contact with those mothers who may be facing an unusual problem or who are at high risk, such as the adolescent, the socioeconomically disadvantaged mother, the woman over 35 with her first baby, or the mother whose child has a congenital anomaly (often reported on the birth certificate or by the hospital). Contact should also be made in situations of multiple births and families that have had previous problems.

The value of meeting the mother and infant at the doorstep of the home has been demonstrated by several health agencies, and the secret of its accomplishment is one of interagency cooperation and administrative timing. The problem of contacting women and infants after delivery has been greatly complicated during recent years by the frequency of change of address and by the fact that many women come into cities for hospital delivery as a convenience but return to small communities or rural areas after discharge from the hospital.

The health department's postpartum program has two purposes: to provide whatever public health nursing service and education to the mother is indicated in each case and to accomplish a smooth and automatic carry-over to the infant health program. The nurse should instruct the mother in proper postpartum care, in infant care, in the advantages and hygiene of breast-feeding, and in the preparation of infant formulas if they are necessary. The nurse should make certain that the birth of the infant has been registered and that the mother and infant are both under medical supervision. The nurse should also maintain a watchful eye for the development of postpartum complications in the mother and of illness in the infant, and make referrals to appropriate agencies wherever medical, economic, or social problems are found to exist. Finally, the nurse should lay the groundwork for the pediatric supervision of the infant, including all indicated protective treatments from either private physicians or health and well-baby conferences and clinics.

Newborn and infant feeding have attracted particular attention in recent years. Several decades ago, it became fashionable for women to use bottles and later prepackaged formulas to feed their babies. It was thought to be uncivilized to nurse a baby. In recent years mothers and nutritionists have rediscovered the benefits of breast milk: it enhances bonding, provides the baby with a substantial dose of antibodies against infections, maintains natural uterine contractility and recovery, and avoids the problems of allergy to cow's milk. Breast-feeding should be encouraged in every birth unless there are real physical or psychologic problems.[41]

THE INFANT AND PRESCHOOL PROGRAM

With regard to the neonatal program, early case finding is again a prerequisite and may be accomplished by means of (1) a routine check of birth certificates; (2) notification by the attendant at birth (accoucheur), the hospital, or the family itself; or (3) the records of prenatal clinic attendance. Neonatal cases should be classified into priority groups, with premature infants at the top of the list, followed by those known to have been born with physical defects, and those who have become ill or injured during or after birth. Many health departments maintain several portable infant care beds that may be loaned to parents of premature babies who have worked out arrangements with other agencies such as fire or police departments for resuscitation services and for emergency transfer to hospitals. Intensive infant care programs have been developed in most states, including provisions for the transfer of fragile, high-risk, or damaged infants and the development of intensive neonatal care centers with trained neonatologists (a subspecialty of pediatrics) and other trained personnel and technicians as well as special devices and instruments to aid in the care and treatment of these very fragile babies. Specially equipped ambulances with controlled environment systems and trained staff as well as the use of similarly equipped helicopters are becoming more available and are especially useful in rural areas.

Of course, it is better to try to identify the high-risk situation before birth and transport the pregnant women to a level II or III center for the delivery. Intensive infant care services are expensive, as noted earlier, with an average cost per surviving infant exceeding $100,000 in one study.[24] It should be stressed that public health departments ought to concentrate on preventing the need for such heroics and that no community should be encouraged to make such investments in hospitals and personnel before it has adequately developed family planning, prenatal care, and nutrition services as well as public health education programs for prospective mothers, genetic counseling services, and the availability of detection and screening services to find the high-risk cases before or during pregnancy.

The health department has a role to play in helping every child develop to the fullest potential. This involves the availability of guidance, counseling, screening, referral, and treatment services as well as special programs to deal with child abuse, mental health, dental education, immunizations, and nutrition. The majority of children have access to a private physician, either a family practitioner or a pediatrician. Even here, the health department has a role to play in providing screening services and in helping the parents understand what is necessary for the healthy development of their children. In many cases, public agencies or private, nonprofit organizations are the main source of care for young children and their families and the health department should be closely involved in such activities, either as a provider of services or as a coprovider and referral agency.

Well-child clinics have been commonly used by health departments as a means of providing guidance and counseling for parents. The paradox of discontinuing services when the child is sick and referring the family elsewhere has led many health departments to expand their services, so that the well-child clinics have become child care centers, providing comprehensive child health care and educational services. This transition should be encouraged where need can be demonstrated. There are many areas where private practice has adequately covered virtually the whole population; but in areas where that is not the case, health department programs can be made more comprehensive, often in collaboration with local practitioners.

The American Academy of Pediatrics[42,43] has published a fairly extensive guide to the standards that should be maintained in an effective program. The latest edition makes a point of avoiding a rigid prescription for how many visits should be made to a physician at any particular age, stating that such schedules need to be individualized. Nonetheless, they suggest that the child be seen at least five times during the first year and about three times during the second year of life. They suggest about three visits during the preschool years (at the age of 2, 3, and 5 or 6), and then at least four visits during the school years between ages 6 and 18. Not all of the visits need to be to a physician. The academy's report notes that there were at least 50 programs training pediatric nurse practitioners in January 1975 and that 85% of the graduates were working in public programs, whereas only 15% were working in the offices of private practitioners.

Their use in doctors' offices may expand, but it is also possible that independent nursing practices may develop, making access to a well-trained, low-technology health guide much easier for many people.

Immunization programs have been increased in recent years, partly as a result of the interest expressed by Secretary Califano of the Department of Health, Education, and Welfare after his experience with the swine flu program in 1976 and 1977. The percentage of children who were fully immunized against polio, diphtheria, tetanus, pertussis, and measles declined sufficiently that scattered outbreaks of measles began to occur in 1977 and 1978. As a result of an aggressive program by the Centers for Disease Control and state health agencies, the number of doses of vaccine administered increased sharply, boosting coverage to over 90% in most areas of the country. It is still difficult to maintain such protection levels, and a threat of diminished federal support in 1982 made it apparent that the effort can never be neglected.

Almost every state attempts to develop its own recommended schedule for immunizing children, and a great deal of confusion exists both among practitioners and parents. It would be sensible to follow the schedules recommended by the American Academy of Pediatrics in their *Report of the Committee on Infectious Diseases*[44] (known as "the Red Book"), which is published periodically.

The influence of poverty on health has been particularly well described by Kessner and Calk[45] and by Kosa and associates.[46] Health departments have traditionally concentrated a large part of their resources on the children of low-income families, but much more needs to be done. Special nutrition services such as the WIC Program (for women, infants, and children) have been of great value (see Chapter 17). Even in Great Britain, with a National Health Service, it has been found that the poor do not use health services as effectively as the nonpoor or as much as they need to, and special efforts have had to be incorporated into the programs to be sure that services adequately reach those who need them most. As mentioned earlier and as pointed out by Miller, environment, education, housing, and the employment prospects for parents have a powerful impact on health even when access to health services is technically available.

Special programs for the provision of services to handicapped children are a feature of many health departments, although responsibility is often placed with welfare and educational agencies. Most state health agencies provide Crippled Children's Services,[4] but the bulk of the services that are made available to children with developmental disabilities is the responsibility of educational institutions. Federal legislation (P.L. 94-142) requires that educational services for all children be provided in as normative and nonrestrictive an environment as possible and that all other services, including the detection, diagnosis, and correction of defects necessary to make education possible must be provided. Health departments at the state and local level should be involved with departments of education in planning and providing these services, although recent changes in block-grant legislation have removed many of the specific requirements.

The special problems of child abuse also require the attention of health departments, usually in collaboration with other agencies, particularly social service agencies. Many states have made the suspicion of child abuse a reportable event, and every effort is made to provide a supportive, therapeutically oriented program for the child and the parents. The best approach to child abuse is a team approach involving public health nursing, mental health workers, social workers, pediatricians, and a lawyer. A great deal can be done to help these troubled families with such an approach, although an out-of-home placement for the child is sometimes the only solution possible.

THE FUTURE

Whether such a program of projects can become a national and comprehensive set of services, linked together in some coherent way to provide sensible and holistic services for women and children, remains to be seen. The United States has made great progress since the Children's Bureau was established; but whether a truly comprehensive program containing the five elements recommended by Miller[25] can be established is doubtful. The EPSDT program, as discussed earlier, was part of an effort to do just this, but a lack of ability or determination by Congress and the Department of Health, Education, and Welfare to declare explicitly what was intended impeded the development of the program. The managers of the program wrote encouraging words about its possibilities, but others have written about the failures. Foltz[47] particularly describes the legislative and administrative problems that befuddle attempts to create clear policy. This is a continuing problem throughout public health but is par-

ticularly true in maternal and child health where broad, general visions are often defeated by the particularistic notions of groups with special interests and a political process that responds to people who can vote now rather than the needs of those who will shape the future.

REFERENCES

1. Forgotson, E.H.: 1965: the turning point in health law—1966 reflections, Am. J. Public Health **57**:934, June 1967.
2. Budetti, P.P., Butler, J., and McManus, P.: Federal health program reforms: implications for child health care, Milbank Mem. Fund Q. **60**(1):155, Winter 1982.
3. Foltz, A.-M.: Uncertainties of federal child health policies: impact in two states, U.S. Department of Health and Human Services Pub. No. (PHS)78-3190, Washington, D.C., April 1978.
4. National Public Health Program Reporting System: Public health agencies 1980: a report on their expenditures and activities, Washington, D.C., 1981, Association of State and Territorial Health Officials.
5. Silver, G.A., and others: Impact of federal health policies in the states of Connecticut and Vermont, final report of the National Center for Health Services Research, National Technical Information Service Pub. No. PB262-959, Springfield, Va., 1976.
6. The Select Panel for the Promotion of Child Health: Better health for our children: a national strategy, Vols. 1 through 4, U.S. Department of Health and Human Services Pub. No. (PHS)79-55071, Washington, D.C., 1981.
7. Wallace, H.M., Gold, E.M., and Oglesby, A., editors: Maternal and child health practices, ed. 2, New York, 1982, John Wiley & Sons, Inc.
8. National Center for Health Statistics: Induced terminations of pregnancy: reporting states, 1977 and 1978, Monthly Vital Statistics Report (Suppl.) **30**(6), September 28, 1981.
9. Cushner, I.M.: Maternal behavior and perinatal risks: alcohol, smoking, and drugs, Ann. Rev. Public Health, **2**:201, 1981.
10. Merritt, T.A., Laurence, R.A., and Naeye, R.L.: The infants of adolescent mothers, Pediatr. Ann. **9**(3):32, March 1980.
11. Messite, J., and Bond, M.B.: Reproductive toxicology and occupational exposure. In Zenz, C., editor: Developments in occupational medicine, Chicago, 1980, Year Book Medical Publishers, Inc.
12. Dixon, R.L.: Toxic responses of the reproductive system. In Doull, J., Klaassen, C.D., and Amdur, M.O., editors: Casarett and Doull's toxicology: the basic sci-

ence of poisons, ed. 2, New York, 1980, Macmillan Publishing Co., Inc.

13. Falk, I.S., Rorem, C.R., and Ring, M.D.: The cost of medical care, Chicago, 1922, University of Chicago Press.

14. Comptroller General: Evaluating benefits and risks of obstetric practices: more coordinated federal and private efforts needed, General Accounting Office Pub. No. HRD-79-85, Washington, D.C., September 24, 1979.

15. Mangald, W.D.: Neonatal mortality by the day of the week in the 1974-75 Arkansas live birth cohort, Am. J. Public Health **71**(6):601, June 1981.

16. Cook, R.J., and Dickens, B.M.: A decade of international change in abortion law: 1967-1977, Am. J. Public Health **68:**(7):637, July 1978.

17. Recommended program guide for abortion services, Am. J. Public Health **62**(12):1669, December 1972.

18. Guidelines on abortion, Chicago, February 1973, American College of Obstetrics and Gynecology.

19. National Center for Health Statistics: Annual summary of births, deaths, marriages, and divorces: U.S. 1980, Monthly Vital Statistics Report **29**(13), September 17, 1982.

20. Kleinman, J.C. (National Center for Health Statistics): Trends and variations in birth weight, Paper presented at the annual meeting of the American Public Health Association in Los Angeles, November 1981.

21. National Center for Health Statistics: Factors associated with low birth weight, 1976, U.S. Department of Health, Education, and Welfare Pub. No. (PHS)80-1915, Hyattsville, Md., April 1980.

22. Lee, K.S., and others: Neonatal mortality: an analysis of the recent improvement in the United States, Am. J. Public Health, **70**(1):15, January 1980.

23. National Center for Health Statistics: Advance report of final natality statistics, 1979, Monthly Vital Statistics Report (Suppl. 2) **30**(6), September 29, 1981.

24. Pomerance, J.J., and others: Cost of living for infants weighing 1,000 grams or less at birth, Pediatrics **61**:908, June 1978.

25. Miller, C.A.: Health care of children and youth in America, Am. J. Public Health **65**:353, April 1975.

26. Loewe, C.U.: A proposal for new federal leadership in maternal and child health care in the United States, Paper presented at the annual meeting of the Association of State and Territorial Maternal and Child Health and Crippled Children's Services Program Directors, Washington, D.C., March 1977.

27. Porter, P.J.: Realistic outcomes of school health service programs, Health Education Q. **8**(1):81, Spring 1981.

28. Office of Maternal and Child Health: An organized system of child health care in every state: need, potential, mission, A staff paper of the Office of Maternal and Child Health, U.S. Department of Health and Human Services, June 1980.

29. National Center for Health Statistics: Contraceptive utilization in the United States: 1973 and 1976, Advance data no. 36, August 18, 1978.

30. National Center for Health Statistics: Contraceptive use patterns, prior source, and pregnancy history of female family planning patients: United States, 1980, Advance data no. 82, June 16, 1982.

31. Boston Women's Health Book Collective: Our bodies, ourselves: a book by and for women, New York, 1976, Simon & Schuster.

32. Committee on Perinatal Health: Toward improving the outcome of pregnancy, White Plains, N.Y., 1977, National Foundation–March of Dimes.

33. Lubic, R.W.: Evaluation of an out-of-hospital maternity center for low-risk patients. In Aiken, L.H., editor: Health policy and nursing practice, New York, 1981, McGraw-Hill, Inc.

34. Health care for mothers and infants in rural and isolated areas, Chicago, 1978, American College of Obstetricians and Gynecologists.

35. Committee on Maternal Health Care and Family Planning: Ambulatory maternal health care and family planning services: policies, principles, practices, Washington, D.C., 1978, American Public Health Association.

36. Research and Statistics Committee: Nurse-midwifery in the United States: 1976-1977, Washington, D.C., 1978, American College of Nurse-Midwives.

37. Bennetts, A.B., and Lubic, R.W.: The free-standing birth center, Lancet **1:**378, February 13, 1982.

38. Cooperative Birth Center Network: Information for establishing standards or regulations for free-standing birth centers, Perkiomenville, Pa., CBCN News **1**(2-3), Feb.-May, 1982.

39. American Public Health Association: Alternative in maternity care, Am. J. Public Health **70**(3):310, March 1980.

40. Bureau of Community Health Services: Newborn screening for genetic-metabolic disorders: process, principles, and recommendations, U.S. Department of Health, Education, and Welfare Pub. No. (HSA) 77-5207, Rockville, Md., 1977.

41. Jelliffe, D.B., and Jelliffe, E.F.P.: Recent trends in breast feeding, Ann. Rev. Public Health **2:**145, 1981.

42. Committee on Standards of Child Health Care: Standards of child health care, ed. 3, Evanston, Ill., 1977, American Academy of Pediatrics.

43. Committee on School Health: School health: a guide for health professionals, 1981, Evanston, Ill., 1981, American Academy of Pediatrics.

44. Committee on Infectious Diseases: Report of the Committee on Infectious Diseases, ed. 18, Evanston, Ill., 1977, American Academy of Pediatrics.

45. Kessner, D.M., and Calk, C.E.: Contrasts in health status, vol. 2, A strategy for evaluating health services, Washington, D.C., 1973, National Academy of Science.

46. Kosa, J., Antonosky, A., and Zola, I.K.: Poverty and health, Cambridge, Mass., 1969, Harvard University Press.

47. Foltz, A.-M.: The development of ambiguous federal policy: early and periodic screening, diagnosis and treatment (EPSDT), Milbank, Mem. Fund Q. **53:**35, Winter 1975.

CHAPTER 23

School and adolescent health

The excesses of our youth are drafts upon our old age, payable
with interest about thirty years after date.

C. C. Colton

THE SCHOOLCHILD

After the preschool period children enter a world
that involves more extensive contacts, a wider geographic range, an increasing number of personal
and social conflicts, and many varied learning experiences. There are at the present time about 56.1
million children in the age group between 5 and
20 years. The majority are enrolled in primary and
secondary schools. In addition, some in the lowest
age are in kindergarten, and many in the highest
2 or 3 years are enrolled in colleges, universities,
or technical schools.

The situation with regard to mortality and morbidity among schoolchildren is similar to that of
preschool children. The death rates are low, having
dropped from about 4 per 1,000 in 1900 to 0.6 per
1,000 at the present time. This reduction is largely
attributable to the prevention of acute communicable diseases of childhood (Table 23-1). The lowering of the threat of tuberculosis is noteworthy. In
1900 approximately 6,100 children in the age group
5 to 14 died from tuberculosis. In 1978 there were
only seven such deaths. Of further interest is the

reduction in the number of deaths of school-aged
children from cardiorenal diseases, caused largely
by much less hemolytic streptococcal infection.

Death occurs unevenly among different segments of the school-aged population. Rates go up
as age increases. Perhaps more significant are the
sex and race discrepancies, which also become
greater in each successive age group (Table 23-2).
Thus in the age group 15 to 19 years, rates for boys
were 2.5 times higher than rates for girls, largely
because of motor vehicle accidents. Socioeconomic
factors result in a higher death rate among black
children aged 5 to 9.

As in the case of the preschool child, mortality
data provide a poor measure of health problems and
progress for school-aged children. Schoolchildren
constitute a group that although subject to low
death rates, experiences a high incidence of acute
illnesses. This is illustrated by Table 23-3, which
presents the number of acute conditions in each
broad age group. It may be noted that the rates drop
following the childhood and adolescent years. With
reference to types of acute conditions that most

TABLE 23-1. Leading causes of death for children 5 to 14 years of age, United States,
death registration area, 1900 and 1978

1900	Rates per 100,000 population	1978	Rates per 100,000 population
Diphtheria	69.7	Motor vehicle accidents	8.8
Accidents, nonmotor vehicle	38.3	All other accidents	8.4
Pneumonia and influenza	38.2	Congenital malformations	1.8
Tuberculosis	36.2	Homicide	1.3
Diseases of the heart	23.3		

frequently affect the school-aged population, Table 23-4 shows that respiratory illnesses were predominant in 1978.

Many child health problems are difficult to evaluate epidemiologically since they may not become apparent until the child enters school or even later when he or she becomes too large to care for in the home. Behavioral disorders and many developmental disabilities are still kept within the family either out of shame or ignorance. Repeated efforts to measure the prevalence of such problems have resulted in a minimal estimate of "clinical maladjustment" rates of about 11%. These are children who in a group setting have a difficult time adapting to the presence and needs of the others in the group.[1] There are no accurate estimates of the prevalence of psychotic conditions. They are rarely encountered in a form that is recognized as such in children. Research efforts are aimed at detecting the precursors of adult and adolescent mental illness in young children.

Behavioral problems are a major source of con-

cern to both parents and school teachers because they impede the education and development of the child and the other students in the group. In recent years parents, teachers, psychologists, and sociologists have turned their attention to the impact of television on the growth and development of children. It has been a vigorously contested debate, but the consensus is growing that violence on television does increase aggression in children.[2] The exposure is enormous: preschoolers will have spent 6,000 hours watching television by the time they enter first grade; by high school graduation, students usually have watched 15,000 hours of television compared to 11,000 hours spent on formal education; children watch approximately 20,000 food product commercials, "most of them devoted to snack foods, soft drinks, and breakfast cereals."[3]

THE HANDICAPPED SCHOOLCHILD

Of particular concern to the school health program are measures designed to meet the special needs of certain handicapped children. It is estimated that about 2.3 million children under the age of 17 years have one or more chronic disabilities that limit activities. This represents 3.9% of all those in that age group. Among the disabilities or impairments in children under 17 years of age are visual defects (11.3 per 1,000), hearing defects (14.3 per 1,000), speech defects (15.2 per 1,000), and paralysis, complete or partial (2 per 1,000).[5] In addition, of course, are children with other types of physical and mental defects. Most of these children

TABLE 23-2. Death rates per 100,000 by age, race, and sex, United States, 1978, selected age groups

Age group	Nonwhite female	White female	Nonwhite male	White male
5-9	34.4	26.3	51.5	26.3
10-14	28.6	23.7	53.1	41.8
15-19	55.9	55.2	136.1	146.9

From National Center for Health Statistics: Health: United States, 1981, U.S. Department of Health and Human Services, Pub. No. (PHS) 82-1232, Hyattsville, Md., 1981.

TABLE 23-3. Acute conditions by age, United States, 1978

Age group	Acute conditions (in 1000s)	Acute conditions per 100 persons
Under 6	71,354	387.6
6-16	110,815	272.9
17-44	198,942	224.5
45	85,436	129.1
TOTAL	466,547	218.2

From Current estimates from the health interview survey, United States, 1978, DHEW Pub. No. (PHS) 80-1551, Ser. 10, No. 130, Hyattsville, Md. 1979, National Center for Health Statistics.

TABLE 23-4. Acute conditions by type, ages 6-16 years, United States, 1978

Type of condition	Acute conditions per 100 persons	Lost school days per 100 persons
Respiratory	152.8	302.1
Injuries	39.6	42.1
Infectious and parasitic	36.9	75.3
Digestive	13.3	21.1
All other	30.3	40.1

Modified from Current estimates from the health interview survey, United States, 1978, DHEW Pub. No. (PHS)80-1551, Ser. 10, No. 130, Hyattsville, Md., 1979, National Center for Health Statistics.

are educable, and for the majority educational services can be met in conjunction with special care necessitated by physical or mental handicaps.

In the past many localities followed a policy of complete segregation of these children, if not in special institutions, then in separate classes for the blind, hard of hearing, or those with developmental disabilities such as mental retardation or cerebral palsy. Although segregation into such classes can provide specialized care, they have the undesirable result of making the handicapped child feel still more apart and different from other children. This is not conducive to good mental health and development or to complete rehabilitation. Most authorities consider that the best policy is to encourage the handicapped children to intermingle with other children in the same general classrooms and to provide special classes or rest periods if needed for them, depending on their handicap. This policy has a beneficial effect on both the handicapped children and their more fortunate classmates and results in all children considering each other as at least basically the same.

Programs of this nature have been criticized as impractical, time consuming, and expensive. In many instances specially trained teachers are needed. By careful curriculum and administrative planning and by using the specialized personnel partly as consultants and in-service trainers for the general teaching staff, more can be accomplished than by any other approach to the problem.

Federal law (P.L. 94-142. providing for education of the handicapped child) now requires the provision of educational services for the handicapped in as normal an environment as possible and that all ancillary services needed to attain this goal be provided as a condition of receiving any federal money for public or private education.

THE ADOLESCENT

Adolescence begins at puberty (when physical maturation reaches the point at which reproduction is possible) and ends indistinctly sometime after the latter half of the "teen" years. It is a period of physical and cognitive change (the ability to deal with abstraction and the future), psychosocial growth, and the development of a sense of identity and reciprocal relationships.[6] The age of puberty has shifted gradually to earlier years, and a lengthened

period of education and dependency has served to expand the length of adolescence, making it possible for more events to occur during the adolescent years.[7] Although it is a period of impressive growth and change, it has, at least in part, been invented by a culture that segments its population into groups to better market its products and services.

Two circumstances are of considerable importance to the community health program as far as the adolescent student is concerned: throughout this period the individual is preparing for living by learning, and the adolescent of today is the parent and citizen/voter of tomorrow. Both of these factors should have a direct bearing on the success of the public health program in any community. In other words, this receptive, impressionable period should be the most fruitful for the dissemination of health knowledge, the development of healthy life-styles, and the establishment of understanding and support of community health measures. Often it is not.

During this period of life, the stresses of rapid growth become evident and are manifest both in physical and mental changes and in the sexual maturation of the individual. Braceland[8] has provided insight indicating that in addition to the physiologic changes being experienced, as the adolescent tries to find a place in the scheme of things, there is a growing need for intimate peer exchange, friendship, and acceptance as well as for social relationships with the opposite sex. Braceland emphasizes that all of these are important in the development and characterization not only of the adolescent but also of the subsequent adult. If there is nonacceptance of the adolescent's role as an individual and as a male or female, there is apt to develop a defiant loneliness, feelings of rejection, and an unbearable resentment or even hatred of oneself or of one or both parents that may transfer to all members of a particular sex or social group or to society as a whole with disastrous consequences.

Out of this turmoil there may develop a panoply of special medical and social problems. Some are related to genetic factors and some to physiologic changes within the individual, whereas others develop from the search for identity and purpose with concomitant rebellion against a real or apparent restraining society. Not infrequently the causes are interrelated and mutually reinforcing, such as defiance of parents, drinking or drugs, pregnancy, and venereal disease, leading back to greater intergenerational discord.

The death rate for the age group 15 to 19 years

is triple the rate for the immediately preceding age interval. Perhaps more germane would be consideration of the leading causes of death during this period. The picture as shown in Table 23-5 is distressing and illustrates forcefully some of the consequences of the internal and external stress that have been mentioned.

The table shows that of 100,000 white males who reach their fifteenth birthday, 688 will die before the end of their nineteenth year: 326 from motor vehicle accidents, 133 in other accidents, 59 from suicide, and 37 from homicide. Nonwhite males have a slightly higher probability of dying during these 5 years, with homicide as the leading cause of death. The death rate from motor vehicle accidents is half that for white males, probably because of less access to the use of an automobile.

Females are far less likely to die during these same years, with the principal difference attributed to motor vehicle accidents. Nonwhite females are slightly more likely to die than white females. For all four groups, phenomena that are neither "medical" in their etiology nor preventable through a medical care system predominate. Of the 10 leading causes only 10.6% of the deaths among the white male group are caused by "medical" problems such as diseases of the heart or congenital anomalies. Except for motor vehicle accidents, violence is a stronger force of mortality in nonwhite females than in white females, but medical problems are also more important, probably because of the relatively greater difficulty nonwhite people have in obtaining access to medical care. (The category

TABLE 23-5. Ten leading causes of death, rank-ordered by 5-year rate per 100,000, age group 15-19, by sex and race, United States, 1976

Rank	White male	Nonwhite male	White female	Nonwhite female
1	Motor vehicle accidents (326)*	Homicide (215)	Motor vehicle accidents (119)	Homicide (52)
2	All other accidents (133)	Motor vehicle accidents (157)	All other accidents (28)	Motor vehicle accidents (45)
3	Suicide (59)	All other accidents (140)	Malignant neoplasms (22)	All other accidents (31)
4	Homicide (37)	Suicide (42)	Suicide (17)	Malignant neoplasms (19)
5	Malignant neoplasms (37)	Malignant neoplasms (34)	Homicide (15)	Diseases of the heart (17)
6	Diseases of the heart (10)	Diseases of the heart (27)	Congenital anomalies (6)	Suicide (12)
7	Other external causes (10)	Other external causes (16)	Diseases of the heart (5)	Influenza and pneumonia (11)
8	Congenital anomalies (8)	Congenital anomalies (11)	Influenza and pneumonia (5)	Other external causes (8)
9	Influenza and pneumonia (7)	Cerebrovascular diseases (9)	Cerebrovascular diseases (5)	Cerebrovascular diseases (8)
10	Cerebrovascular diseases (5)	Influenza and pneumonia (8)	Other external causes (4)	Complications of pregnancy (6)
TOTAL rate, all causes	688	746	263	284
TOTAL rate, 10 leading causes	632	659	226	209
Percent of 10 leading causes that are medical in nature	10.6%	13.5%	19.0%	26.3%

Modified from Leading causes of death and probabilities of dying, United States, 1975 and 1976, Atlanta, Ga., 1979, U.S. Department of Health, Education, and Welfare, Centers for Disease Control.
*Numbers in parentheses are rates per 100,000.

"Other external causes" includes deaths from injuries in which it cannot be determined whether the event was deliberate or accidental, plus deaths caused by acts of war.)

Although the table reveals striking sex differences, the impact of violence in this age group, and significant racial differences, it also reveals the durability of the group. Another way of stating the results is that more than 99% of children who reach 15 will survive all of these problems and reach their 20s. Although motor vehicle accidents, suicide, and homicide are important problems, indicative of much of the stress of growing up, 99.7% of all children who reach 15 will not die from these phenomena.

Many interested experts point out that society has not provided health services designed to meet the needs of adolescents, but the problem may not be disinterest so much as the habit of thinking that a health problem requires a medical solution. In the Surgeon General's report *Healthy People,* the low priority given to adolescents is in part attributed to such factors as their low mortality rate generally, the difficult problems of consent and confidentiality, and the lack of a recognized medical specialty group.[9] The needs have been medicalized in their descriptions by health experts, and since there are few obvious provider resources available to meet those needs as they have been defined, the needs are said to be unmet. It is true that they are unmet in most communities, but the resources most needed are teachers, counselors, and better educated parents, not physicians, hospitals, and clinics. Such resources may not be well developed because there is not a good source of payment for the services similar to the public and private insurance mechanisms available to support the medical services industry. Health facilities are needed for teens—they are a special group with special health problems, but social and behavioral problems are more important.

Adolescent health problems may be considered to fall into certain categories in relation to origin, severity, and behaviorism, about which parents, physicians, health agencies, schools, and society should be aware. One such category is the extensive group of congenital conditions, some genetic and some acquired. Included are metabolic conditions such as diabetes and certain enzymatic dys-crasias, anatomic conditions such as cardiac and alimentary canal malformations, physiologic conditions such as phenylketonuria (PKU) and certain anemias, psychiatric or neurologic conditions such as Huntington's chorea and schizophrenia, and finally, certain infections that may be acquired congenitally, of which syphilis is a well-known example. In the educational environment some of these merit focused attention in the nature of special classes, referrals, examinations, and other considerations.

In another dimension are the increasingly significant behavioral problems of adolescents that may have serious consequences. Cigarette smoking remains the most significant preventable health problem of both adolescents and adults. The proportion of adolescents who smoked increased steadily until 1974 and then began to decrease, primarily because of nonsmoking by boys. About 34% of all teenagers smoked in 1979, with girls more likely to be smokers than boys.[10] The use of marijuana and other illegal drugs increased rapidly from 1972 to 1977 and then more slowly. By 1979 about 31% of adolescents had tried marijuana. About a quarter of them had only used it once or twice, but an equal number had used it 100 or more times.

Alcohol consumption remains the most significant drug abuse problem among adolescents, as it is among adults. Seventy percent of all adolescents had tried alcohol in 1979. More than one third were current drinkers. The Alcohol, Drug Abuse, and Mental Health Administration estimated that there were 3,300,000 problem drinkers aged 14 to 17, or 19% of the age group.[11] Problem drinking in this age group means an acute problem such as a motor vehicle accident or a fight, not the more common chronic problems associated with adult alcoholics. It is not known whether adolescents who may be labeled as problem drinkers are more likely to become alcoholics than are other adolescents.

The emerging sexuality of the adolescent presents both opportunities and problems. Girls mature earlier than boys. Both develop sex roles based on the models and examples established by their parents, their relationships with their peers, and external influences such as magazines, television, and most importantly, their school experiences. The prevalence of teenaged girls who had experienced sexual intercourse increased during the 1970s so that in 1976, 55% of those who had never been married had had intercourse by the age of 19. The rates were higher for black teenagers than for white. By the age of 15, 38.4% of all black, never-married teenagers had had intercourse, increasing to 83.6% by the age of 19. The rate for white teenagers increases from 13.8% to 48.7%.[12] Despite these high rates of sexual activity, teenagers were relatively abstemious: about half of all the never-married 15- to 19-year-old girls had not had intercourse in the month before the survey.

Thirty-six percent of the teenaged girls make their first visit to a family planning clinic because they suspect that they are pregnant, and another 50% come seeking contraceptive advice and services sometime after they have begun sexual activity. Only 14% came before the first time they had had intercourse.[13] The most frequently stated reasons for not coming to the clinic before beginning to have intercourse were (1) procrastination, (2) fear of parental discovery, and (3) apprehension about what would happen during the clinic visit. Underlying these three reasons is a substantial degree of ignorance about reproduction generally and contraception and contraceptive services specifically. Boys know even less about the subject than girls and appear to believe that it is the girl's responsibility to take care of such matters—a manifestation of the role development process that raises questions about the ability of many parents to provide a useful base for the development of a child's sexuality. About 1 million teenaged girls become pregnant each year and about one half of all of the pregnancies occur in the first 6 months of sexual activity, which makes the reasons for the delay in seeking competent help important.[14]

Except for very young girls (aged 14 or less) the biologic age of the mother does not appear to have an adverse impact on fetal growth and development, but other factors associated with early onset of sexual activity and pregnancy, such as smoking, drinking, or other risk-taking ventures, do have a retardant effect.[15] In addition to the fetal and infant problems associated with teenage pregnancy (see Chapter 22), it can have a devastating impact on the development of the mother as well as the father. Many teenage pregnancies end in abortion and, although this may be a better outcome than motherhood and disrupted schooling in many cases, it is hardly a desirable sequence of events.

Adolescent mental health problems are more noticeable than they usually are in preschool and elementary schoolchildren, in part because they are more pronounced and in part because adolescents make more of a pronouncement about themselves than do younger children. Adolescents are much more likely to need and seek mental health care, but services for them are not well developed. There are few qualified mental health professionals who can work effectively with adolescents. Since adolescents are more capable of making their behavioral problems noticeable as well as more inclined to do so, they are more frequently placed in institutions than are younger children who are more easily managed in the home (managed, but not necessarily treated). There are striking differences in institutionalization rates by race and sex (Table 23-6). The high rates for nonwhite males are the result of a much higher rate of institutionalization in correctional facilities: 618 per 100,000 versus 133 for white males. Subtracting those rates from the totals for males leaves rates of 299 per 100,000 for white males versus 385 for nonwhite males in mental health and developmental disability institutions. It is not known whether these differences represent a significant difference in pathology or simply a different form of societal response to deviant behavior based on the race of the offender. People who come from a dominant community group are more likely to be accorded a sick role, whereas minority group members are more often assigned a criminal label.

As previously discussed, suicide is a distressingly common phenomenon during the adolescent years. It may result from a particular incident, but it usually follows a pattern of vulnerability: unsuccessful adaptations, lack of effective peer relationships, and a sense of repeated failure with no hope for a better

TABLE 23-6. Rate of institutionalization per 100,000 adolescents by race and sex

Type of institution	White males	White females	Nonwhite males	Nonwhite females
Correctional	133		618	
Health	299		385	
TOTAL	432	239	1,003	342

From The President's Commission on Mental Health. In Healthy people: the Surgeon General's report on health promotion and disease prevention, background papers, U.S. Department of Health, Education, and Welfare Pub. No. (PHS) 79-55071A, Washington, D.C., 1979.

future. Warning signs are usually evident and may include expressions of worthlessness, depression, giving away valued possessions, and mention of suicide. Even though most such behavioral patterns do not end in suicide, they are indicators of a potentially serious problem and should be treated accordingly.

It is obvious that all of these behavioral problems confront the educational and public health professions with very difficult and perplexing challenges. A common characteristic of each is that they affect more than one person. Also, they have far-reaching implications for education, medicine, longevity, productivity, and, in some instances, jurisprudence. Another shared characteristic is that all of them require the development of successful motivational approaches for their prevention. In the absence of truly effective prohibitions or restraints, education and propaganda appear to be the only available counterforces. Meanwhile, educational institutions in company with health agencies and the health professions should be alert to the problems and provide appropriate programs and services, such as sex education, special prenatal and postnatal clinics, contraceptive and—if possible—abortion programs, special class schedules for pregnant and postdelivery students, social counseling, and referrals for emotionally disturbed students and those suspected of substance abuse.

SCHOOL AND COMMUNITY HEALTH

Between the fifth or sixth year and early adulthood, children spend a large part of more than half the year in a school environment. During this important formative period, the essential influences for physical and mental health and for education are shared by the home, the community, and the school. If the schools are to meet their responsibilities, it is necessary to formulate and to put into effect sound policies and programs for health protection and promotion during the hours of school experience.

The school is of particular importance for several reasons. In addition to its potential importance with regard to health instruction and the development of desirable habits, it represents a gathering place for a population group that is particularly susceptible to many illnesses and accidents. School health, therefore, must be thought of as one part of the total community health pattern, with its efforts concentrated on the individual during a specific period of existence. School health is actually the common concern of the school, the parent, and the community at all levels of government. The success and effectiveness of the school health program depend in large measure on the common understanding on the part of each of these groups and each individual involved as to (1) the precise scope of its sphere of action, (2) its role in the total community health picture, and (3) the need for consistent cooperation in its implementation. In other words, at its best, the program must be a concerted attempt to put into practice for the school-aged child the thought embraced in the Children's Charter: "Every child has the right to be well-born and to attain the best possible quality of health of which it is capable."[16] All community health personnel need to pool their efforts to realize this obviously desirable goal to the greatest degree possible. This has been emphasized by the American Public Health Association in a position paper on Education for Health in the School Community Setting[17]: "Thus it seems that the school should be regarded as a social unit providing a focal point to which health planning for all other community settings should relate."

THE SCHOOL HEALTH PROGRAM

William Alcott in an "Essay on the Construction of School Houses" suggested the attendance of a physician at school in 1832.[18] Since education is a state and local affair, the patterns of development are varied. There have been three phases in the development of school health programs: (1) a concern about basic protection involving the control of communicable diseases and school sanitation, which has expanded into a more comprehensive service program in some jurisdictions, (2) the development of a national effort to deal with the problems of handicapped children, beginning with the Crippled Children's Services program (see Chapter 22) and expanding into federal legislation to assure an adequate education for all handicapped children in 1975 and (3) the involvement of an expanded variety of health and social service professionals as well as an increased emphasis on the health training of teachers.

There are many good descriptions of school health programs.[18-21] The American Academy of Pediatrics typifies some of the differences of opinion about management and scope.[22] Its official recommendations are that a physician should be the director of the program and that it should rely on the private practitioners in the community for medical care. The physician should determine goals and objectives, establish an organization, advise the board of education about policies and procedures, and supervise all health-related activities, including counseling, nutrition, and accident prevention. As noted earlier, most of the health problems of schoolchildren and adolescents are not medical problems, and most physicians are not especially or uniquely well trained to carry out the suggested tasks.

A school health program includes a systematic concern for the environment of the school; the promotion and protection of the health of the children, including the provision of necessary services; and a comprehensive approach to health education. With this triad in mind, the basic components of the school health program and the activities involved in each of them are presented in Table 23-7. Of necessity, there is a certain amount of overlapping and interrelationship among these. This is desirable, since each part of the program should be designed and used as much as possible to augment other parts. Thus certain aspects of the school environment or health appraisal activities should provide valuable firsthand health instructional material.

TABLE 23-7. Components of the school health program

School environment	Health protection and promotion	Health instruction
Maintenance of a safe sanitary plant	Health appraisal	Planned, direct health teaching
Buildings	Periodic medical examination	Indirect health education
Grounds, playfields	Screening examinations	Assembly programs
Gymnasiums, swimming pools	Dental examination	Exhibits, etc.
Health service unit	Special examinations	Incidental health education
Seating, lighting, ventilation, heating,	Referrals	Integrated health education
sanitation, drinking fountains	Athletes	Correlated health education
Safety and accident prevention	Follow-up procedures	Health units in other subject
Protective equipment	Referrals	courses
Fire drills	Correction of remediable defects	In-service health education
General safety	Care of exceptional children	School personnel
Civilian defense and disaster	Prevention and control of disease	Planning sessions
Safety patrols, traffic safety	Planned emergency care	Workshops
Transportation	Illness	Conferences
Driver education	Injury	Courses
Administrator-teacher-pupil relationships	Health counseling	Parent education
Recreation program	Health of school personnel	Preparation of health curriculum
School luncheon	Cooperation with community	guides
Custodial care	agencies	Use of resources
Healthful school day	Official	Teaching aids
Length	Voluntary	Textbooks, supplementary
Class size	Civic	books, periodicals
Routine	Parent	Community personnel
Grading and marking procedures	Program coordination	Community facilities
Promotions		Museums
Classroom procedures		Libraries
		Health centers
		Cooperation with community
		health education efforts
		Official agencies
		Voluntary agencies

Modified from Hanlon, J.J., and McHose, E.: Design for health: the teacher, the school, and the community, ed. 2, Philadelphia, 1971, Lea & Febiger.

The school environment

In relation to schools, the term *environment* should be interpreted in its broadest sense. It should take cognizance not only of the immediate school premises but also of its surroundings, and not only of its sanitation but also of its location and safety. In other words, it should include consideration of every potential physical, mental, and moral hazard with which the child may come in contact in connection with the school experience. As stated by the National Committee on School Health Policies,[23] "The authority which requires pupils to attend school implies the responsibility to provide an environment as evocative as possible of growth, learning and health."

A discussion of the details of each of the many factors involved in the school environment is beyond the scope of this book. Attention should be directed, however, to the general factors that call for supervision by public health and other authorities. Of primary importance is the location of the school. It should be chosen with an eye to accessibility, salubrity, and adequacy. Proper choice of location will preclude the development of many sanitary problems. Attention should be given to drainage, shade and sunlight, and freedom from industrial wastes, excessive noise, and excessive traffic. Provision should be made for adequate recreational space and for the possibility of future expansion. Although the actual choice of location is not a responsibility of the public health department, the health department should offer its consultative services to whatever agencies are involved.

The health department should play a role in the assurance of the proper construction and maintenance of the school. Conformance with accepted sanitary and safety standards should be assured by frequent inspection by representatives of the public health agency and by consultation with the school authorities. Consideration must be given to ventilation, lighting, heating, and acoustics; to adequacy and location of stairways and exits; to construction materials and methods from the viewpoints of sanitation and safety; and to the adequacy and design of toilet and handwashing facilities. Because of the numbers and characteristics of those involved, the water supplies and sewage disposal facilities serving schools are considered of a public nature. Even if they are part of larger municipal systems, facil-

ities of this type merit particular scrutiny and supervision. In rural and developing suburban areas, the provision and maintenance of satisfactory water and sewage disposal facilities are particularly troublesome and require especially persistent supervision by the health department. In many such areas, the health department should assist in the development of an on-site water fluoridation system (see Chapter 32).

Many schools, even in rural areas, provide lunchrooms and cafeterias that often have rather extensive facilities for the preparation and serving of foods. Such facilities should be under the constant surveillance of the sanitation staff of the health department to prevent their becoming a threat rather than a benefit to the children who use them. In addition, as discussed in Chapters 17 and 18, the staff of the public health agency should work closely with school authorities and staff to make school meals and lunchroom sanitation a practical firsthand learning experience.

Schools that contain gymnasiums, play areas, and swimming pools place an added supervisory responsibility on the health department. Standards of construction and maintenance should be established by the health agency and enforced in cooperation with the school authorities. This becomes particularly important in view of the laudable trend toward making such facilities available to the entire community rather than restricting their use to schoolchildren during school hours. Related to these facilities and to the school as a whole should be adequately equipped and adequately staffed health service rooms for the provision of first aid. This is mentioned further in relation to health protection and promotion.

The most ideally located and constructed school can rapidly deteriorate and become a sanitary menace unless provision is made for its proper maintenance. As implied earlier, many aspects of the physical school plant must be subject to frequent inspection. In addition, the health department staff, as a matter of policy, should annually conduct a complete and detailed survey of the sanitary conditions and facilities of each school, public or private, within its jurisdiction. Often this is best done during the summer months, when some of the other community problems slacken and during which time whatever repairs as may be indicated may be made before the reopening of the schools in the fall. Written reports with recommendations for improvements should be submitted to the school principal and the superintendent of schools. Short-comings should be discussed with them and all possible assistance given to remedy whatever defects are found. Subsequently, follow-up inspections should be made to assure the correction of any undesirable conditions.

Health protection and promotion

Present-day thinking indicates a social responsibility to prepare schoolchildren physically and psychologically as well as intellectually for adulthood. For many individuals this means graduating them in better physical condition than when they entered school. To accomplish this purpose, it is necessary to establish baselines by means of physical examination. At one time it was the custom to attempt to examine every schoolchild every year. Eventually this was realized to be inefficient and pointless. This procedure had two undesirable features: (1) so many children had to be examined each year that they usually received what amounted to a cursory scanning rather than ever getting a truly complete physical examination, and (2) so much attention was given to getting the children examined that it either became an end in itself or else left no time for the follow-up necessary to secure the correction of defects.[24-27]

Accordingly, a more reasonable approach has been developed and is followed by progressive communities. Children should be examined at least three or four times during their school experience: for example, at entrance to grade school, the fourth grade, junior high school, and senior high school. Preferably a parent should be present at the examination of elementary school children for purposes of explanation and education. The examinations must be carefully conducted and complete, regardless of the circumstances under which they are performed. With a reduction in the total amount of time spent on examinations, more funds and personnel time and energy are left available for securing the correction of defects.

The arrangements whereby schoolchildren are examined vary. In some communities salaried school physicians do the work, whereas in others private physicians are employed on an hourly or daily basis. Some communities follow the interesting policy of restricting the school medical work, particularly in relation to periodic examinations, to the younger and newer physicians just entering practice in the community. The philosophy is that all concerned benefit. The schools and health de-partment get the examinations accomplished; the new physicians not yet completely established benefit from the part-time salaries and from the experience and family contacts; and the children are given more thorough examinations because the younger physicians usually relate better to children and devote relatively more time to the examination; whereas more established practitioners are spared the necessity of using their time in routine examinations in which they often are not too interested. Finally, a learning situation is provided in which hopefully the younger physicians experience a satisfactory and helpful relationship with the health department that should bear sound fruits in terms of future professional relations.

Probably the most desirable system in the long run is one in which the health department and the schools educate and prompt parents to the maximum extent possible to take their schoolchildren to their family physician, if they have one, for periodic physical examinations and other protective and promotive services as well as for their illnesses. Furthermore, when the schoolchildren become accustomed to going to their own physicians for such services, the likelihood of continuing to consult a physician after the school years is considerably greater than if children come to expect such services from a full-time school physician.

There has been a general attitude that schools should not become deeply involved in the provision of medical care services and that school health personnel should cope with nonmedical problems and refer medical problems to the child's private physician. In many communitiies this is appropriate and satisfactory, but in many others such care is not available or is too expensive. In many cases, follow-up is difficult because of working parents or ignorance of health and medical care in the family. In areas of the community where services are not available and family income is insufficient, an effort should be made to incorporate comprehensive child health services into the school health program. This has been done successfully in Cambridge, Mass.,[28] as well as other communities. More will be said near the end of this chapter about the organization of child health services.

An important administrative technique that is of value as an adjunct to the periodic physical examination is the screening of pupils by their classroom teachers. The health department may cooperate by providing in-service training for teachers to acquaint them with the signs and symptoms of illness, particularly the communicable diseases. Without attempting to make diagnosticians out of them or to overburden them, the department encourages teachers to survey their pupils briefly each morning, referring any pupils with suspicious indications to the medical personnel available to the school. Comparative tests have demonstrated the ability of teachers of pick out sick or ailing children without reference to the exact cause.

Certain screening tests have been sufficiently validated as to warrant their use in the school setting by trained health professionals or technicians. Vision and hearing screening are particularly important. A substantial number of children enter school with hearing and vision defects that, if uncorrected, will impede the learning experience throughout the school years. Such programs require careful attention to be sure that they are properly carried out and that effective referrals with follow-up are made. Once established, the programs require periodic reevaluation to be sure that they are continuing to function effectively. In many schools, public health nurses have been taught to screen school children for curvature of the spine (scoliosis), which is a simple and inexpensive screening technique.

The discovery of physical and mental defects or illnesses in schoolchildren in itself is of relatively little value. In fact, whatever value it has is contingent on what is done with the information obtained. This means a successful follow-up program from the school and health department to the home, to the private physician or dentist, or to the social agency, whichever is needed for correction of the condition.

Another phase of the school health protection and promotion program deals with the control of communicable diseases. Of primary importance is the degree to which the parents of the community bring their children to school already protected against acute communicable diseases such as diphtheria, whooping cough, measles, and poliomyelitis. Most school systems attempt to secure these protections by mandate. When this approach is followed, some parents tend to delay immunizations until the time of school entrance, which is later than desirable.

On the other hand, a high degree of community and school protection may be obtained by educational methods, and it is foolish for a health department to make lasting enemies for its general program by stubbornly and needlessly insisting, on the basis of law or regulation, on the immunization of every last child. To prevent outbreaks it is necessary to immunize 93% to 95% of the population. If there are a few families who have strong religious convictions against immunization (such as the Christian Scientists), it should still be possible to achieve those levels without insisting on a rigorous application of school entry requirements, especially if the health authorities have maintained a good working relationship with the school authorities. As with other health protection programs, periodic reevaluation of the appropriateness and the implementation of such requirements is necessary. When this does not happen, immunization levels tend to slowly decline until they fall below 83% to 85%, and a new outbreak of measles will occur. Although once accepted as a necessary part of growing up, it has since been recognized that measles is a serious disease and repairing the damage after the immunization levels have declined is expensive for the community and painful for the victims and their families.

A question that inevitably arises in every community is whether schools should be in session during epidemic periods of communicable disease. In general, the public tends to want the schools closed. However, when this is done, greater and more intimate contact between children usually follows, since they tend to play in their neighborhoods and circulate among crowds rather than remain at home. Therefore in communities with well-organized and efficient public health and school health services, epidemics can best be controlled if the schools remain open and engage the children in controlled activities under intelligent and watchful surveillance.

In discussing the subject, the National Committee on School Health Policies suggested that the decision regarding the closing of schools when epidemics occur or threaten may be decided locally by answering the following two questions: (1) Are nurses and medical staffs so adequate and the teaching staff so alert that the inspection, observation, and supervision of students will keep sick students out of school? (2) If schools are closed, will students be kept at home and away from other students, so that the closing of schools will not increase opportunities for contact with possible sources of infection?

As a general policy, when the first question can be answered affirmatively or when the second question is answered negatively, schools should be kept open in the face of an epidemic. This is most often the case in large public schools and in thickly settled communities. Schools should be closed when the first question is answered negatively or the second question affirmatively. In smaller communities with scattered homes, where chances for personal contact are limited, this is frequently the situation. In rural communities where pupils are transported in buses and close contact is unavoidable, it also may be advisable at times to close the schools.

It is easy to lose control of such situations, and a health department may find itself in the middle of a school squabble involving parents, teachers, and the school administration. Some parents cannot accept the possibility that scabies may have been acquired in the home and insist that the school must be the source. Such allegations may fall on fertile soil if there is a difference of opinion about the school health program, and parents may get together to insist that the health department step in and override the school's policies. In one instance, the mothers were upset at what appeared to be a suggestion of a lack of sanitation in the homes and insisted that the schools be closed. It was discovered that the fathers, who were almost all employed at the same manufacturing plant, were on strike, and if the school were closed by the health department, the entire family could take a week's vacation at the height of the spring fishing season. An unwary public health director can be easily ensnared in such situations if there is not an effective means of communication among all three parties.

Health instruction

Schools are primarily places where children go to learn for living. Most people consider health important for successful living. It logically follows therefore that schoolchildren should have presented to them in an understandable and interesting manner a considerable amount of information dealing with the present and future health of themselves and their community. Customarily, "health teaching" is a requisite in most school curricula. However, in a great many instances the job is poorly done. Too often "health classes" turn out to be physical training periods. With equal frequency the material is presented by unqualified and sometimes disinterested persons. On about the same level are the situations where didactically unsuited members of the health department staff or private physicians are asked to give "health talks" to the students. All of these are poor substitutes for what is really needed. Empathy with students is a highly important ingredient for success in this field.

Teaching is a profession in itself. Everyone is not fitted by temperament and training to teach. Certain skills, aptitudes, and training are necessary to accomplish a satisfactory result. Therefore, inasmuch as possible, the teaching of health as well as of arithmetic and geography should be left to the trained classroom teacher who is already well acquainted with the pupils. The health department can be of greatest assistance to this person by offering advice, consultative service, in-service training, and teaching materials and by aiding the teacher in planning the health teaching program. This can best be done by a health educator or health counselor, who may meet with the teachers collectively and individually to discuss goals and problems. Ever-enlarging sources of visual aids are becoming available, and the health department, as one of its justifiable activities, should make them accessible to the schools of the community.

Green and Iverson[29] and McAlister[30] have emphasized the need for rationality and consistency in the school health education effort as a part of the total school health program. The ecology of the school has as much impact on shaping health behavior as the more didactic classroom work. The purpose of health education is to impart knowledge with the expectation that knowledge will shape attitudes that will in turn affect behavior. There has been a great deal of skepticism about the efficacy of school health education efforts. Many programs have been so poorly done as to justify the skepticism, but there is much evidence that a well-designed school health education effort can improve nutrition, reduce risk-taking behavior such as drinking and smoking, and prevent pregnancy. Green and Iverson address the need to develop consistency in the approach to predisposing factors or knowledge about biology and health, enabling factors such as the skills needed to floss teeth or easy accessibility to family planning services in a community clinic, and reinforcing factors that include the environment and the attitude of the teachers and the administrators in the school and the cafeteria. They have reported very good results when schoolchildren are taught how to resist peer pressure. Consistency and rationality are the crucial ingredients: an effective classroom program can be eroded by a poor food service system or the faculty smoking lounge.

Bearing in mind that there are three components to the school health program (the environment, health services, and health education), there are three organizational models: the board of education can operate the entire program; the board of health, or the health department where there is no board of health, can operate the school health program; or they can jointly govern it. If the past history of the community is favorable, the joint governance of the program is preferred. If not, then it is probably better for the board of education to govern the program, even though it will need a good working relationship with the health department to carry out a permissible program of sanitary control. The board of education is legally responsible for the health and safety of the children in school, and if collaboration is not possible it must assume that responsibility directly. In most states the health department has statutory responsibility for many aspects of the school environment and must carry out that responsibility by working with the school officials.

In a combined program, the school staff should have the lead role in developing and implementing the health education program, with the support of the public health department and its staff when indicated. Health professionals should serve in a consulting capacity and only become involved in direct teaching when they are particularly effective or when school personnel cannot handle the assignment. The environmental program must be carried out by school personnel, but health department staff must set the standards and should conduct periodic inspections and provide technical assistance in overcoming problems. Environmental health workers should be involved in the planning of any new school. The service program, which is designed to protect and promote the health of the children, is more appropriately placed under the general supervision of the health department personnel who must plan and carry out their work in close collaboration with the school faculty and staff.

In some large cities, the board of education may have a well-developed school health program including health services, and there is no need to make fundamental changes in organizational responsibility of such programs. In smaller and rural communities, it is more likely that the school system will have to depend on the health department for the school health program. Ownership of the school health program has been both a theoretic as well as a political argument in many communities to the detriment of the program and the health of the children. More recently the argument has centered around who can afford it. As school costs have increased and citizens have resisted increases in school taxes, school boards have often reduced their support for school health service programs, leaving them by default to the local health department, which often has not had the resources to absorb the added work load. Taxpayer support for school systems in general and school health programs especially has become a significant problem, especially as the population ages and the fertility rate declines. In many communities, including some major cities, less than 25% of the households have a member in a public school, which means that the constituency that is needed to support school tax increases has diminished in size.

Many local health departments and school authorities have developed programs of field trips and special health study projects designed to demonstrate to schoolchildren community activities that have an influence on the health and well-being of themselves and their families. When properly planned and carried out, these study programs can have a considerable educational impact. A few health departments have progressed further to the point of allowing high school students to take turns working at simple jobs in the health department offices or even clinics as volunteers or at a nominal temporary salary. This is a doubly worthwhile venture by virtue of its educational effect and because it is also a form of vocational guidance. To be of value, however, a judicious choice of jobs and constant supervision are necessary. Since, if properly planned and conducted, it represents a learning process under supervision, the granting of academic credit for the time spent is considered justified.

Every school and school system should have a health council or committee with representation from all groups concerned with school health. At the top level in the community, where general cooperative community relationships and policies are best developed, membership should include such persons as the superintendent of schools, the local health officer, the president of the Parents and Teachers Association, a representative of the medical and dental societies, and whatever other individuals may be in key positions with relation to the health and well-being of the schoolchild. The relationship of the central school health council to each of the individual school health councils or committees is best determined by experience in each community. In general, it has been recommended that the central council guide and give leadership but leave each individual school health council with considerable authority.

The health council or committee of each school need not follow any particular pattern. In a one-room rural school it might consist only of the teacher, an interested parent, and a public health nurse. In larger schools the numbers of those who may play an active role are many and varied and depend on local circumstances. The essentials are that they be representative of all in the community who are concerned and may be helpful and that they provide a simple, democratic, and orderly means of determining and implementing wise school health policies.

THE FUTURE

There are many good texts on the subject of child[3,31,32] and adolescent[33-36] health and development, but the essential problems are perhaps best expressed by Arden Miller,[37] who has proposed a comprehensive national program of organized health services for mothers and children, and George Silver,[38] who makes the same recommendation. Concern for the health of children, according to Silver, is in third place after concern for the role of the family, even though the family is regrettably the source of the problem in some instances, and concern for protecting the entrepreneurial role of private medical care. Much of what is needed cannot be provided because many people feel that values and behavior are the province of the family, not social institutions, and many services are lacking because of a traditional reliance on private practice. The public organization of school and community health services for children and adolescents is a tattered fabric woven to protect those concerns while still serving the needs of the child. Although many efforts have been very creative and have resulted in well-balanced programs,

the effort to construct such programs without addressing the core problem is tedious, expensive, and inadequate. Reliance on the traditional concepts of private, fee-for-service medical practice supported by sickness insurance cannot produce the sort of social health organization needed. A comprehensive program that includes medical services as one essential component rather than as the controlling component is needed. It is not a likely prospect in the next decade, and the social indicators of literacy, pregnancy, substance abuse, behavioral disorders, and child abuse will continue to reflect the failure to change.

REFERENCES

1. Dohrenwend, B.P., and others: Mental illness in the United States: epidemiological estimates, New York, 1980, Praeger Publishers.
2. Comstock, G.: Influence of mass media on child health and behavior, Health Educ. Q. **8**(1):32, Spring 1981.
3. The Select Panel for the Promotion of Child Health: Better health for our children: a national strategy, vol. 1, U.S. Department of Health and Human Services Pub. No. (PHS)79-55071, Washington, D.C., 1981.
4. National Center for Health Statistics: Current estimates from the health interview survey, United States, 1978, U.S. Department of Health, Education, and Welfare Pub. No. (PHS)80-155, Series 10, No. 130, Hyattsville, Md., 1979.
5. National Center for Health Statistics: Prevalence of selected impairments, U.S. Department of Health and Human Serivces Pub. No. (PHS)81-1562, Series 10, No. 134, Hyattsville, Md., 1981.
6. Daniel, W.A.: Overview of adolescent health problems, South. Med. J. **74**(5):569, May 1981.
7. Doyle, K.K.L., and Cassell, C.: Teenage sexuality: the early adolescent years, Obstet. Gynecol. Annu. **10**:423, 1981.
8. Braceland, F.: The devious paths of loneliness, M.D. **22**(1):11, Jan. 1978.
9. Brown, S.S.: The health needs of adolescents. In Healthy people: the Surgeon General's report on health promotion and disease prevention, background papers, U.S. Department of Health, Education, and Welfare Pub. No. (PHS)79-55071A, Washington, D.C., 1979.
10. The Select Panel for the Promotion of Child Health: Better health for our children: a national strategy, vol. 3, U.S. Department of Health and Human Services Pub. No. (PHS)79-55071, Washington, D.C., 1981.
11. Alcohol, Drug Abuse, and Mental Health Adminis-

tration: The alcohol, drug abuse, and mental health national data book, Rockville, Md., 1980, U.S. Department of Health, Education, and Welfare.

12. Zelnik, M., and Kantrer, J.F.: Sexual and contraceptive experience of young unmarried women in the United States, 1976 and 1971, Fam. Plann. Perspect. **9**(2):55, Mar./April 1977.

13. Zabin, L.S., and Clark, S.D.: Why they delay: a study of teenage family planning clinic patients, Fam. Plann. Perspect. **13**(5):205, Sept./Oct. 1981.

14. Freeman, E.W., and others: Adolescent contraceptive use: comparisons of male and female attitudes and information, Am. J. Public Health **70**(8):790, Aug., 1980.

15. Merritt, T.A., Laurence, R.A., and Naeye, R.L.: The infants of adolescent mothers, Pediatr. Ann. **9**(3):32, Mar. 1980.

16. The White House Conference, New York, 1931, The Century Co.

17. Education for health in the school community setting: position paper of the American Public Health Association, Am. J. Public Health **65**:201, Feb. 1975.

18. Schaller, W.E.: The school health program, ed. 5 Philadelphia, 1981, Saunders College.

19. Mayshark, C., Shaw, D.D., and Best, W.H.: Administration of school health programs: its theory and practice, ed. 2, St. Louis, 1977, C.V. Mosby Co.

20. Cornacchia, H.J., and Staton, W.M.: Health in elementary schools, ed. 5, St. Louis, 1979, The C.V. Mosby Co.

21. American Public Health Association: Health of school-age children (Resolution No. 7905), Am. J. Public Health, **70**(3):304, Mar. 1980.

22. Committee on School Health: School Health: a guide for health professionals, 1981, Evanston, Ill., 1981, American Academy of Pediatrics.

23. Suggested school health policies, ed. 4, Washington, D.C., 1966, National Education Association and American Medical Association.

24. Yankauer, A., and others: A study of periodic school medical examinations, I., Am. J. Public Health **45**:71, Jan. 1955.

25. Yankauer, A., and others: A study of periodic school medical examinations, II., Am. J. Public Health **46**:1553, Dec. 1956.

26. Yankauer, A., and others: A study of periodic school medical examinations, III., Am. J. Public Health **47**:1421, Nov. 1957.

27. Yankauer, A., and others: A study of periodic school medical examinations, IV., Am. J. Public Health **51**:1532, Oct. 1961.

28. Porter, P.J.: Realistic outcomes of school health service programs, Health Educ. Q. **8**(1):81, Spring 1981.

29. Green, L.W., and Iverson, D.C.: School health education, Ann. Rev. Public Health **3**:321, 1982.

30. McAlister, A.L.: Social and environmental influences on health behavior, Health Educ. Q. **8**(1):25, Spring, 1981.

31. Wallace, H.M., Gold, E.M. and Oglesby, A., editors: Maternal and child health practices, ed. 2, New York, 1982, John Whiley & Sons.

32. Fox, J.A.: Primary health care of the young, New York, 1981, McGraw-Hill Book Co.

33. Cole, R.: Children of crisis, col. 1 through 5, Boston, 1964-1977, Atlantic Monthly.

34. Blum, R.W., editor: Adolescent health care: clinical issues, New York, 1982, Academic Press.

35. Shen, J.T.Y., editor: The clinical practice of adolescent medicine, New York, 1980, Appleton-Century-Crofts.

36. Daniel, W.A.: Adolescents in health and disease, St. Louis, 1977, The C.V. Mosby Co.

37. Miller, C.A.: Health care of children and youth in America, Am. J. Public Health **65**:353, April 1975.

38. Silver, G.A.: Redefining school health services: comprehensive child health care as the framework, J. School Health **51**(3):157-162, Mar. 1981.

CHAPTER 24

Aging

Is it with us as clearly shown
By slant and twist, which way
The wind hath blown?

Adelaide Crapsey
On seeing weather-beaten trees

Title VII of the Older Americans Act considers people eligible for nutrition programs at age 60. The Department of Housing and Urban Development makes housing supports available to people who are 62. The Medicare program begins paying hospital bills when people reach age 65. However, biologically, aging starts with conception, and people begin to show some signs of diminished functional capacity by the time they reach 30. From that time on, the prevalence of chronic diseases, the use of medical services, and the degree to which people are dependent on others to carry out what might be considered normal daily activities increases. Is aging a disease or a normal process? It is clear that some people become frail, disabled, or dependent earlier than others, and there are certain characteristics of their lives that have some bearing on the process. Gerontologists have given up trying to define aging and have urged others to abandon the effort. It consumes too much work with no real benefit.

Aging is a process that cannot be reversed. To the extent that its consequences make people excessively dependent on others, much can be done to prevent the dependency or to reduce it. To the extent that dependency is irreversible, its impact on personal security can be mitigated by a spectrum of community supports. The purposes of those community support systems are to maintain maximum possible functional independence, to help restore functions that have been lost, to provide humane care for people who are permanently dependent, and to support the final release from dependency during the dying process with dignity.[1] Those purposes are incidentally a rephrasing of the basic concept of prevention (primary, secondary, and tertiary) to suit the target group.

THE EMERGING PROBLEM

In 1900 there were 2.5 million people aged 65 and over in the United States, representing 4.1% of the total population. By 1980, there were 25.5 million people aged 65 and over, representing 11.3% of the population. Within those summary figures a number of important shifts have been taking place and will continue to emerge over the next 50 years. By then most of the aged will be widowed females living alone.

It is difficult to project population estimates with confidence at this time because a number of surprising changes have been occurring in the last 20 years that have altered mortality expectations dramatically—especially the rapid decline in deaths from cardiovascular disease. This decline has affected the over-65-year age group as well as younger adults. If these changes continue to occur over the next 20 years, their impact on the age distribution of the nation's population will have important consequences. The census bureau has developed high, low, and midrange estimates. Looking at the midrange figures, the over-65 age group will increase from 25.5 million to 55 million by 2040, and the over-75 group (the group that begins to use health and social services in significant amounts) will increase from 9.4 million to 28 million. At that rate of increase, the over-65 group will represent 15.2% of the population.

The age-dependency ratio is derived by dividing the number of people aged 65 and over by the number of people aged 18 to 64. It is a figure sometimes

Health and human development

used to illustrate the extent to which working people will have to support nonworking adults, although it ignores the contributions of many people over 65 and the dependency of many younger people. In 1920 the ratio was 0.08. By 1980 it had increased to 0.18. By 2020 it will increase to somewhere between 0.23 and 0.29.[2]

The biggest increases will be in the over-85 group, which will increase by a factor of four by 2050. This is the group that needs the most assistance with activities of daily living such as toileting, dressing, eating, and bathing. By that time there will be two older women for each older man. Women have higher rates of dependency and activity limitation than men. There are sharp differences in mortality between adult men and women and between whites and nonwhites (Table 24-1). According to 1976 mortality data, during the 5 years from age 40 to 44, 1,749 out of 100,000 white men died— almost one third of them from diseases of the heart. By age 70 to 74, the total increased to 23,653, and nearly half of the deaths were from diseases of the

heart. At both ages, nonwhite men had a considerably worse experience, although by age 70 to 74 both groups had about the same experience with heart disease. The chances that a white woman would die during those 5-year intervals were considerably lower for both age groups—almost half the rates for white men. Nonwhite women were more like white men in their mortality expectations. Most of the sex and race differences in the older age groups were because of diseases of the heart and cerebrovascular disease. Both of these categories have declined as a cause of death during the last 20 years. Although there is no reason to believe that the racial and sexual differences have decreased in importance, sharp reductions in those two categories will clearly have a significant effect on longevity. It does not appear that overall life-span will increase very much but that the mortality curve during the last 40 years of life will become more nearly rectangular, with a sharp fall after age 85. With more and more people living through their seventh and eighth decades of life, the size of the potentially dependent population may increase even more dramatically than has been portrayed.

TABLE 24-1. Chance in 100,000 of dying during the 5-year age interval, by sex and race, 10 leading causes of death,* United States, 1976

	Men				Women			
	Aged 40-44		Aged 70-74		Aged 40-44		Aged 70-74	
Cause of death	White	Nonwhite	White	Nonwhite	White	Nonwhite	White	Nonwhite
Diseases of the heart	542	804	10,266	10,123	126	376	5,269	8,046
Malignant neoplasms	292	490	5,535	6,777	353	466	3,108	3,621
Motor vehicle accidents	128	195	NA	NA	45	57	NA	NA
All other accidents	136	303	284	443	40	68	154	221
Suicide	119	76	NA	NA	58	NA	NA	NA
Homicide	61	486	NA	NA	16	78	NA	NA
Cirrhosis	117	362	260	NA	58	186	102	101
Cerebrovascular disease	58	195	1,963	3,292	58	186	1,471	3,138
Influenza and pneumonia	30	119	591	802	18	57	294	443
Diabetes	21	60	355	581	15	55	384	1,006
Bronchitis, emphysema, and asthma	NA	NA	662	304	NA	NA	141	NA
Other diseases of the arteries	NA	NA	520	360	NA	NA	179	262
Arteriosclerosis	NA	NA	213	277	NA	NA	141	241
Nephritis and nephrosis	NA	NA	NA	277	NA	34	NA	282
All other causes	245	892	3,004	4,426	179	548	1,547	2,756
TOTAL causes	1,749	3,982	23,653	27,662	966	2,111	12,790	20,117

From Center for Disease Control: Leading causes of death and probabilities of dying, United States, 1975 and 1976, Atlanta, Georgia, March 1979, U.S. Department of Health, Education, and Welfare.
*NA indicates some probability of dying, but the cause is not on the top list for that group at that age.

Disability

The elderly have more health problems and use more health services than do young adults. They are not more likely to have acute problems or injuries, but they are more likely to have troublesome and lingering consequences and are more likely to have chronic problems that result in more physician office visits and days of hospital care (Table 24-2).

Chronic conditions become more common with age, and they cause an increasing amount of dependency (Tables 24-3 and 24-4). The increasing prevalence of chronic conditions as people age causes them to use more and more medical care. Those 65 and older, while representing about 11% of the population, use 15% of all physician office visits. Of more importance is the fact that they use about 34% of all short-stay hospital days and 89% of all nursing home beds. All told, they use 29% of all the money spent on medical care.[3] Assuming that some of the changes just described occur, the rapid increase in the older age groups, coupled with

their heavy use of medical services, means that those 65 and over may use 50% or more of all the medical care produced in the United States by the year 2040. This may cause some serious cost problems. It also raises important social and political issues: Will the national government find it necessary to again stimulate an increase in the training of health manpower and the construction of hospital beds, and will younger age groups manifest increasing dissatisfaction with the rising costs and/or increasing scarcity of medical care for themselves and their children? According to Van Nostrand[4] of the National Center for Health Services Research, the elderly have increased their use of short-stay hospitals by 46% since the passage of Medicare in 1965. She combined data such as the above to make some tentative projections: nursing home care will continue to be the most rapidly expanding segment of health care; costs for nursing home care will increase to about $82 billion per year by 1990; and there will be an increase in the shift of the elderly from family care to formal systems of care.

Social problems

There are other dimensions to the aging phenomenon. Family size is decreasing, and the divorce rate is increasing. Although more of the elderly have a living child now than 2 or 3 decades ago, the ability or the willingness of that child to care for an aged parent is decreasing. Houses are physically smaller as building costs rise. Family separations are more likely to result in an aged individual living alone, lost to the children as a functioning member of the family unit. When an elderly

TABLE 24-2. Number of physician visits per person per year by age and sex

Age group	Males	Females
under 17	4.2	4.0
17-24	3.0	5.6
25-44	3.5	5.8
45-64	4.8	5.9
65-74	6.4	6.6
75 and older	6.4	6.6

National Center for Health Statistics: Current estimates from the health interview survey: United States, 1977, U.S. Department of Health, Education, and Welfare Pub. No. (PHS)78-1554, Hyattsville, Md, Sept. 1978.

TABLE 24-3. Percent of population with activity limitation because of chronic conditions

Age group	Males	Females
under 17	4.4	3.5
17-44	9.3	8.4
45-64	25.2	23.0
65 and older	49.1	43.9

National Center for Health Statistics: Health characteristics of persons with chronic activity limitations: United States, 1979, U.S. Department of Health and Human Services Pub. No. 82-1565, Hyattsville, Md., Dec. 1981.

TABLE 24-4. Restricted activity days per year because of chronic conditions by age and sex

Age group	Males	Females
under 17	10.8	11.2
17-44	13.0	16.9
45-64	24.0	27.8
65 and older	38.2	44.5

National Center for Health Statistics: Health characteristics of persons with chronic activity limitations: United States, 1979, U.S. Department of Health and Human Services Pub. No. 82-1565, Hyattsville, Md., Dec. 1981.

parent does live with what remains of the family, there is likely to be greater stress because of space and money problems. The value of a family's earned income has begun to decline in recent years, and more women are finding it necessary to work outside the home both to augment income and to find personal satisfaction. Women have been the traditional care givers for elderly parents, and their removal from the home during the time when elderly parents need increasing amounts of assistance with activities of daily living suggests either that the elderly will be less welcome in the home or will be a source of increased stress within the family. The abuse of fragile, elderly family members is not uncommon, and some think it is becoming more common. On the other hand, an older parent in the home may make it possible for both parents to work and provide valuable support for a child.

Repeated studies of mortality patterns show that elderly people living together are more likely to survive and retain their independence than those living alone. As previously noted, death rates for elderly men are substantially higher than for elderly women. Widowhood has a sex-specific effect, increasing the mortality rate of surviving men, but having no or little apparent effect on the mortality rate for surviving women.[6] The death of a spouse is frequently followed by increased dependency in the survivor and the need for family support. Such needs, having been unexpressed for several decades, often fall suddenly on a family poorly equipped by inclination, income, or space to respond well.

Many other difficulties emerge for the elderly: housing, transportation, housekeeping, and the need for social interaction. The elderly are much less likely to live in their own homes than are the young. From age 65 to 74, 85% of men live in households with their wives or another person. Only 65% of women are living with their husbands or someone else in a household during those years and, by the time they are in the over-75 age group, more than half of all women are either living alone or are living in an institution.[7]

There are a variety of living arrangements possible for the elderly, not all of them satisfactory. About 5% of those over the age of 65 are in nursing homes (about 1.4 million people), but many more are in boarding homes or personal care homes, most of which are not licensed or regulated in any way. Personal care homes are usually homes in which the owner or manager provides some limited forms of assistance with activities of daily living but no direct health services. Boarding homes provide no services at all other than some housekeeping and meals. Although some are very well managed and many are operated on the basis of friendship rather than for proprietary purposes (particularly in rural areas), those in urban areas that cater to the needs of the frail elderly, who are often people who have been "deinstitutionalized" from public mental health or developmental disability facilities, are frequently a source of abuse and mistreatment.

Aloneness is increasing, particularly for women, and its impact on dependency, disability, injury, and death is powerful. The mortality rate is much higher for the elderly who live alone than for those who live with a friend or in a family setting. Depression is one of the more important phenomena affecting the elderly living alone. It is frequently confused with dementia, which is the familiar syndrome of failing memory, disconnected thought patterns, and eccentric behavior so often used to characterize the elderly. Dementia is reversible in up to 20% of cases and is not as common as its diagnosis would suggest, but the label is used casually in the United States where geriatrics is still a relatively rare form of medical practice. Depression is more common and more treatable. Unfortunately, although the elderly are often given psychoactive drugs, they are rarely afforded an adequate psychologic assessment by someone trained in geriatrics.

The health of the elderly

The problem of maintaining the health of the elderly is real and growing. Medical care costs are high and rising rapidly. The formal institutions, mainly nursing homes, that have been developed to solve the problem have not only failed to solve the problem but have exacerbated it by increasing family separations, costs, and patient abuse. Yet it is not all a bleak picture. The elderly are truly healthier than ever before and getting more so. Recent trends in the incidence of cardiovascular diseases suggest that more and more people may emulate Dorian Grey, remaining robust and functional to a ripe old age and then dying suddenly without the interventions of a formal medical or social service structure. Disability is more common in the elderly than in the young but still is uncommon. When asked by an interviewer, 80% of the elderly respond that they are feeling pretty well. Branch and Jette[8] are following a group of elderly participants in the original Framingham heart disease study and find that most do not have any unmet needs arising from a social disability. Of this group, 74% have no unmet housekeeping problems, 79% have no unmet transportation problems, 68% have no unmet needs because of a lack of social interaction, 84% are able to get their meals prepared, and 91% have solved any grocery shopping problems they may have had. When they do have problems stemming from unmet needs, they are most likely to involve housekeeping (3%) or transportation (7%). The Framingham population is mostly white and reasonably well off, but the authors have examined other studies and found results not grossly dissimilar. In summary, most of the elderly are healthy; their needs are met either by themselves, their friends, or their families; and they live in private homes, not nursing homes. The development of community-based service systems, described later, should increase wellness even more, and preventive efforts can decrease dependency. Nonetheless, the small proportion of the elderly that is dependent and disabled is a small proportion of a very large and rapidly growing group, which means that that small proportion of partially dependent people includes many people—millions of people—whose needs are often great, and the costs of meeting those needs are high and growing higher. Considering all of the disabled and dependent people in society, regardless of the cause of their disability or dependency, and the fragmented, complex, and costly nature of the formal service structures we have erected to deal with the problems, dependency generally and aging particularly, are the biggest challenges to be faced by public health in the decades ahead.

THE LONG-TERM CARE SYSTEM

A system is an organization of two or more people or parts engaged in the pursuit of a common goal. In that sense, there is no long-term care system: the parts are rarely organized and the people, or parts, have different goals. In a somewhat looser sense of the word, however, the parts define a system that (1) is largely proprietary, (2) is institutionally based, (3) is built on welfare concepts rather than entitlements, (4) is fueled by a fee-for-service approach, (5) treats aging as a health problem rather than a social problem, (6) is not generally attractive to most well-trained professional health

workers, and (7) is "closed-ended," that is, one rarely leaves the system alive.[9] That may be an optimistic portrait. The U.S. Senate Special Committee on Aging said that "the elderly and their offspring suffer severe emotional damage because of the dread and despair associated with nursing home care in the United States today . . . the actions of Congress and of the States, as expressed through the Medicare and Medicaid programs, have, in many ways, intensified old problems and have created new ones. . . ."[10] For an even more graphic portrayal of the problem, the reader may wish to read *Tender Loving Greed,* which describes an industry driven by profit motives and fueled by a government or series of governments that has taken on the problem and made it worse.[11]

Slightly less than 5% of the population aged 65 and over live in a formal institution such as a nursing home. Most of the elderly and the majority of the disabled elderly were still cared for in a family environment in the 1970s. This situation deteriorates with age. Of men aged 65 to 74, 15% live alone or in an institution. About 26% of those over the age of 75 live alone or in institutions. For women, the situation is even worse: more than half live alone or in institutions after the age of 75.[7] Of all men over the age of 65, 14.7% were living alone in 1980, and 32% of women over the age of 65 were living alone.[12]

Institutionalization

No matter what government tries to do, the institutional response gets worse. Faced with pressure to provide more nursing home beds for the disabled elderly, Congress included coverage for such care in both Medicaid and Medicare. The response was rapid. The available beds were filled quickly and more were built as entrepreneurs found the new program would assure quick profits, principally through manipulations of real estate and taxes rather than through services. In 1960 there were 388,000 people aged 65 and over living in nursing homes, or about 2.3% of that age group. By 1970 the number had more than doubled to 796,000. By 1980 it had increased to nearly 1.4 million. As more and more elderly people went into the new beds, Congress attempted to protect them and the budget by establishing standards for admission and for the care services that had to be provided. Although the industry objected, it simply added the services, often in an inadequate fashion, and increased its charges. The costs continued to increase, and the regulatory pressures became worse. Regulations defined door widths, floor coverings, hours of nursing care per patient, safety requirements, and record-keeping procedures, but none of this has been shown to be related to the quality of the care provided.[13]

Nearly 60% of the costs of the nursing home industry are paid for by public funds, with Medicaid absorbing 90% of that public share and Medicare paying about half of the rest. Medicare services and conditions are defined nationally, and use has been controlled by very tight admission and length of stay criteria. The Medicaid program is administered by the states, which pay one quarter to one half of the cost of the program. The pressure of families with no place to put the elderly and of the builders who are quick to show legislators how to provide the care and pay only 25 to 50 cents on the dollar resulted in support at the state level for extensive Medicaid coverage and an expansion of the bed supply. Historically, counties provided sheltered housing for the dependent elderly in what were often known as county poor farms. County commissioners are now anxious to support the building plans of the investors, especially since it means shifting the costs from the county's weak tax base to the state and federally funded Medicaid program. The cost involved in this shift of the elderly from homes, poor farms, and other boarding home environments into nursing homes has increased substantially, but the cost has shifted away from the community, which had customarily paid the bill. Many communities rehabilitated their "old folks' home" to meet Medicaid standards. Although the cost of rehabilitation may be substantial, much of the increased operating cost could then be received as revenue from the state Medicaid program. Whether the elderly got better care is unknown, but it certainly cost more.

For private-paying patients, the process often wipes out the family estate, transferring what used to be an inheritance within the family to the nursing home industry. Once the personal holdings of the elderly have been sufficiently depleted to make them indigent, they become eligible for the Medicaid program, and the cost is shifted to the public purse. Many elderly people shift title to their homes and other assets to their children, making the elderly parents eligible for tax-supported nursing home care. The black and rural elderly are less likely to "benefit" from these changes than are the white and urban elderly. This does not appear to be a direct result of discrimination, but rather a locational phenomenon: investors put nursing homes where they can get patients, preferably those who can pay their own bills because they pay higher rates than does the Medicaid program. That means that the nursing homes are built in more urban and affluent environments.

Nursing homes are not the only institutions used to house the frail or dependent elderly. Some nursing homes are called skilled nursing facilities (SNFs, called "sniffs" by the bureaucrats.) They generally require the highest level of nursing care. Intermediate care facilities (ICFs) were invented to provide care at a lower cost by decreasing the amount and type of care needed, but intermediate care facilities are still health related. Generally the Medicare program will only pay for skilled nursing facility services, since Medicare has a decidedly medical orientation. In many states the Medicaid program will pay for care in both skilled nursing facilities and intermediate care facilities. Personal care homes move away from the medical aspects of aging and provide basic social supports. This may include routine body care, such as grooming, help with the toilet, and washing. Personal care homes cannot participate in either the Medicaid or the Medicare programs. They are often supported by Title XX funds (Title XX of the Social Security Act, which provides for social services designed to keep people out of institutions) or by payment from a cash grant received by the resident who may qualify for old age assistance or aid to the totally disabled. Boarding homes may provide meal serice and some housekeeping, but no personal care. There are no government programs specifically designed to help with the cost of boarding home care. In recent years "congregate" care and "group homes" have become increasingly popular. These are usually organized for a specific group, such as the developmentally disabled, alcoholics, or occasionally the aged. In a sense these are cooperative housing arrangements, often supported by community groups with a genuine social welfare motivation. Arrangements are usually made with community-based service organizations for home health services, meal services, transportation assistance, and occupational and physical therapy, which are easier to arrange and pay for on a group basis.

As previously discussed, most nursing homes are privately owned, although government funds are used in several ways to pay for them. In many states it is possible for a private organization to float a bond issue through a local government as an effort to develop the industrial or commercial base of the community. These bonds produce tax-free income for the bond owners and thus represent a government subsidy for construction. As also noted, most of the operating costs are paid for through public funds. There is no good count of personal care homes or the "beds" available in them or of congregate housing arrangements, since these are usually not licensed. Lacking a statutory reimbursement program such as Medicare or Medicaid, they are less directly involved in governmental processes; hence they are not as well counted. Some official counts by the national government put the number of personal care home and similar beds at about 12,000, but workers in licensure programs are aware of numerous private arrangements that have been made to provide some housing and support for a dependent unrelated person. It seems likely that the total number of such arrangements equals or exceeds the number of formally counted and regulated beds.

The cost of institutional care varies widely, depending on the location and the level of care available. Since most of the bills are paid by Medicaid, rates are generally set to reflect what can be negotiated with the state program, which means that they are different in each state. They may range from as low as $25 per day to $80 per day or more, depending on private pay status and ability to pay. At an average price of $60 per day, nursing home care can cost about $1800 each month. The national cost, at that rate, would be $30.2 billion per year.

Nursing homes often solve problems of behavior or nonconformity by routinely using tranquilizers in large doses. The sexes are often segregated, and late-night visits are discouraged because they appear to be disorderly or disturbing, at least to the staff. These shortcomings make nursing homes and similar facilities the kinds of institutions that dehumanize people. Any unusual behavior is treated by the formation of additional rules or policies rather than accepted as part of the heterogeneity of the community within the nursing home. Policies ac-cumulate over time until virtually all aspects of human conduct are regulated by the institution rather than by the individual. The results are apparent to any visitor of most nursing homes. However, there are exceptions. It cannot be proved that the exceptions are those homes that are run by nonprofit organizations or by religious groups, but it seems that way to any collector of personal impressions and anecdotes. Unfortunately, efforts to measure the quality of care have been very unsatisfactory. Whenever objective criteria are applied to such assessments, either for research or regulatory purposes, the difficulty in defining "quality" becomes apparent. Social workers, nurses, physicians, administrators, and family members all have different impressions of quality care, and the client is usually least able to express his or her preference, which should be the most important one.

Deinstitutionalization

"Deinstitutionalizing" people has become very popular in the United States during the last 3 decades. Major national efforts have been launched to deinstitutionalize the mentally ill, the developmentally disabled, and now the elderly. The motivations are not always related to the benefits to the individual from living outside an institution: many government officials think that it will save money. The original efforts to deinstitutionalize tuberculosis patients were based on improvements in drug therapy and the demonstrated ability to do a better job with outpatients than with inpatients. Tuberculosis hospitals were designed to keep infectious people away from healthy people and were managed somewhat like prisons. It became important for the patients, who often felt well, to outwit the medical and nursing staff who were trying to control their lives, sometimes by taking unauthorized leave or by not taking medications. In addition to creating social problems, the disease was not controlled. A different kind of medical and nursing team found it easier and more effective to form a partnership with the patients and treat them in the community once the initial assessment had been completed and treatment had begun. To convince legislators, who often had a vested interest in the large tuberculosis hospitals that employed many people, the health staff calculated how much cheaper it would be to treat someone as an outpatient. Of course, as the census in the hospital declined, the cost per day for the remaining patients increased, but overall the program change did save money as well as improve care.

The same approach was tried in mental health. Pinel did it in France in the 1790s. It began in the United States in the 1950s as a result of President Kennedy's interest in the development of community service programs. Having learned from the tuberculosis battle, experts touted the low cost of outpatient or community-based care in contrast with institutional care, and several studies seemed to substantiate this. Two problems exist in such comparisons, however: most studies were unable to assess the change in the functional level of the person being deinstitutionalized, and none of the studies was really able to capture all of the public costs incurred on behalf of the deinstitutionalized individual. As will be discussed later, these same problems jeopardize cost-benefit studies of community-based care for the elderly. Often the communities into which most dependent people are deinstitutionalized are not integrated communities with all of the necessary health and social service supports well coordinated in an efficient manner. Even though nursing home environments are often shabby, sometimes brutal, and usually demeaning, they are at least open and available for public inspectors, and they do fix responsibility for the safety of the resident on the institution. This is not the case in the more fractured living arrangements often available in community settings.

Since nursing homes have created such a bad impression and since collectively they cost so much, national, state, and community officials and leaders have tried to develop alternatives. Several studies have indicated that many of the people in nursing homes would not need to be there if other kinds of services were available in the community. Estimates of unnecessary use of nursing homes vary a great deal, depending on the bias of the investigator, but an overuse of about 30% is commonly described. At the same time, other investigators have found at least as many if not more people living in the community, often in very poor environments, who do need nursing home care. Similar to other types of health care, the total may be about right, but decisions about use or nonuse are not made by what an investigator could call

rational means in about 30% of the cases. The problem is one of misuse rather than overuse. The General Accounting Office found that in Cleveland about 12% of the population over age 65 was living in the community with conditions similar to those of 5% of the population living in nursing homes. The principal difference was that those living in the community were married.[14-16]

Case management

Most of the efforts to develop more rational service delivery arrangements involve case management. Simply put, this involves fixing responsibility on one individual for securing needed services for a client. The case manager usually is a member of an organization skilled in assembling the services needed for the particular client group. The principal advantage of case management is that it starts from an assessment of the client's needs and attempts to weave a cloth of services that will fit the client without suffocating him or her. Theoretically, this avoids trying to reshape the client to fit the needs and services of the institution.

To study the needs of a community, standardized assessment forms are used. In the General Accounting Office's Cleveland study mentioned earlier, the Older Americans' Resources and Services Information System (OARS), developed by Duke University, was used to study community needs. OARS is used to develop a baseline of well-being, cataloging social and economic resources, mental and physical health status, and capacity for self-care. OARS has been successfully used in before-and-after comparisons to test the efficacy of specific interventions.[17] The Capacity for Self Care Index is derived by ascertaining if the subject can (1) go out-of-doors, (2) walk up and down stairs, (3) get about the house, (4) wash and bathe, (5) dress and put on shoes, and (6) cut toenails. (If the last item seems foolish, imagine an elderly person with arthritis trying to do it.) Scores range from 0 to 7, with 7 indicating the greatest level of incapacity.[18] There are other survey techniques, such as Activities of Daily Living,[19] but all are aimed at testing physical capability, social strength, and mental status in an effort to understand something about the three areas most likely to be related to dependency: disability, aloneness, and income. These are the three areas that require community services such as home nursing and therapy, homemaker services, appliances such as canes and wheel chairs, companionship and social interaction systems, and income support either through Social Security or through supplemental cash grants, which usually are supplied by the states through what is known as Supplemental Security Income.

Case managers (1) accept referrals, (2) assess the client's needs, often with other specialists, (3) recommend services, (4) connect the client with the needed service, and (5) periodically reexamine the clients to be sure that their needs are being met. Case managers use mental health services, nursing homes, optometrists, physicians, hearing aid dealers, home health agencies, homemakers and chore workers, day care centers, hospitals, and meal services such as Meals on Wheels or senior citizen food programs supported by local agencies for the aging. Their goal is assumed to be to keep the client out of an institution, but sometimes an institution may be the most appropriate setting for the services needed by a client.

Although most experts agree on the need for case management, there is dispute as to whether the agencies should be brokers or service providers. The tendency is to follow the broker model, with the creation of a new agency for case management that arranges or brokers services on behalf of the client, using existing agencies. There are several advantages to this approach: it involves little disruption in the existing pattern of doing things, it allows the case manager the freedom to arrange the most suitable services rather than to try to shape the client's needs to the agencies' array of services, and it should leave the case manager in a better position to serve as an advocate for better care and needed services in the community.[20] The Health Care Financing Administration (part of the U.S. Department of Health and Human Services) seems to favor the brokering type of case management agency in its research and demonstration programs, but this may be because it is reluctant to establish any more large provider organizations, given its difficulties in trying to make sense out of the nursing home industry. Others have advocated a more consolidated or centralized approach, with the case management agency actually providing most of the services needed either directly or through contractual arrangements. This has the advantage of assuring the availability of the recommended service and fixing responsibility for the nature of the care package developed for the client. However, it has the theoretic disadvantage of allowing the agency to continue to use up the service slots it has rather than develop new and possibly more needed ser-

vices. The Social Health Maintenance Organization is the ultimate in centralized case management organizations, depending on a prepaid capitation fee to provide all necessary services for enrolled clients. A major new project is underway under the aegis of the University Health Policy Center at Brandeis University to test the feasibility of social health maintanence organizations. Its goals are to maintain more frail elderly people at home, to not cost any more than existing service systems, to provide better case management than other centralized or brokering agencies, and to attract third-party payors to support the program.

Hospitals, home care agencies, or personal care agencies could manage a consolidated social health maintenance organization, but the development of a new agency that builds its service package through coalitions and contracts would appear to be more desirable to avoid the service biases of the existing agencies. However case management agencies are developed, they must always depend on the assessment of the case manager, which raises questions about the training and orientation of the workers. Nurses are likely to see problems and service needs differently than social workers. If, as most people believe, the problems of aging are more social problems than health problems, it would seem logical to use social workers as case managers, but some have argued that nurses do a better job. The professional discipline is less likely to be as important as the experience and training of the worker. Both disciplines are clearly needed.

Partial day care services and home services are often described as useful alternatives to institutional care. Partial day care services provide either daytime or night-time shelter and a social environment. Day care can provide for needed social interaction, nutrition support, and nursing and physical therapy services in a convenient location. This may be particularly effective for a family that can provide evening support but needs to be at work during the day. Home services may consist of housekeeping assistance, skilled nursing care, physical therapy, speech therapy, or the assistance of a nutritionist. Home health agencies are principally nursing agencies, but to be accredited by Medicare for reimbursement purposes, at least one other skilled service must be available. This requirement plus time-consuming and costly travel requirements have made home care difficult to establish in rural areas. Homemakers and chore services are often paid for by social service agencies with Title XX funds. They provide help with shopping, cleaning, cooking, and other housekeeping needs.

This array of service possibilities would seem to offer many opportunities for better and more appropriate care at a lower cost than is possible through nursing homes, but the evidence, although enthusiastic, does not support the claim. Weissert and associates[21] conducted a controlled experiment using day care and homemaker services for Medicare beneficiaries and found that the costs were considerably higher (60% to 70%) for those maintained at home. Clients did not use the noninstitutional services in the numbers expected, which meant that operating costs per client were higher than anticipated, and they seemed to use the services as supplemental rather than replacement services. They tended to use fewer nursing home and hospital days of care per year, but this was more than offset by the cost of the alternative service programs. Many other studies have enthusiastically reported substantial savings, but they all leave out several public costs, such as subsidized housing, meals, and Supplemental Security Income payments. A review of several state experimental programs by the Intergovernmental Health Policy Project indicates the nature of the savings claimed by the program sponsors, but points out the omissions from the calculations of cost in the community-based systems and concludes that "there is still no available evidence that the provision of community-based services will reduce costs."[22] That is a reasonable assessment of the work done to date, but it leaves out of the equation that the people maintained at home in a well-managed system are functionally better than their institutionalized counterparts in all three dimensions: physical, mental, and social. The question remains, how much is it worth to the taxpayer? Present research is aimed at refining the mix of available services and better identification of those individuals who are most likely to benefit from a well-managed, community-based system and who would otherwise incur significant costs. The Intergovernmental Health Policy Project Review provides a good description of 12 ongoing state projects. In addition, 12 states have received special "channeling" grants from the Health Care Financing Administration to further develop case management systems to better "channel" dependent elderly clients into appropriate service systems. The Robert Wood Johnson Foundation has provided grants to 8 states to foster more effective cooperation between voluntary service provider organizations and public agencies. Fourteen states have developmental grants from the national government. The area is not devoid of experimentation, but there are no quick answers to such complex problems.

PUBLIC HEALTH AND AGING

Aging is not really a health problem. It is a physiologic inevitability that increases the probability of health problems, which may have important social consequences. There are no specific programs for aging that can be established in a public health agency, although public health can contribute a great deal to ameliorating the disability and dependency of aging.

Aging itself cannot be prevented, but some of the health problems associated with aging can be. Heart disease is the biggest health problem of aging. The known risk factors are high blood cholesterol levels, hypertension, smoking, and lack of exercise. Although most of these risk factors fade with age, since age itself appears to become the predominant risk factor, hypertension remains a valid indicator of vulnerability, and it can be controlled. Primary prevention is not yet possible, but early detection and effective management can do much to reduce the consequences of hypertension: renal disease, cerebrovascular disease, and heart failure. It was once thought that blood pressure rose naturally with age, but it is now apparent that high blood pressure is as significant in the aged as it is in the young and that it can be controlled. The death rate from cardiovascular disease has decreased by over 20% in the last 2 decades, and this decrease has occurred in the age group over 65 just as it has in the younger age groups.[23] There are many other risk factors associated with the dependency and disability of aging: inappropriate retirement, aloneness, social activity, heredity, sex differences, race, education, and socioeconomic status. The last three are connected to some extent. The well-established relationship of poverty and lack of education with poor health is very evident in the aged. Some of the risk factors cannot be changed, but their effects can be modified.

Many of the health problems common in the aged

such as arthritis, cancer, vision problems, and hearing problems can only be dealt with through secondary and tertiary prevention techniques once the process has begun, which highlights the need for stronger prevention efforts in the young. There are many approaches to health maintenance such as the *Canadian Periodic Health Examination Report*,[24] *Prospective Medicine and Health Hazard Appraisal* by Robbins,[25] *Preventive Medical Services in National Health Insurance* by Breslow,[26] and *Proposed Preventive Benefits to be Covered on a First Dollar Basis under National Health Insurance* developed by the American Public Health Association.[27] All of these proposals focus on periodic health and social needs assessments, tailored to the known risks and disability patterns evinced by sex and age-specific groups as ascertained through epidemiologic analysis (see Chapter 18). In older age groups, they recommend health assessment every 1 or 2 years and pay particular attention to cancer, heart disease, vision, hearing, housing, nutrition, and socialization.

Many public health agencies have established chronic disease screening programs for such problems as diabetes, glaucoma, and cancer. Most screening programs, either single purpose or multiphasic, have not been effective either in preventing disease or in saving money. The reasons are described in Chapter 16. Generally speaking, they tend to attract those at lowest risk and too often are unable to assure continuity of care for those identified as having a problem. Screening that is not done by an agency with a continuing responsibility for the well-being of the client fails to protect either the client or the public purse.

Some public health agencies operate service programs that provide direct treatment and maintenance services for adults such as general outpatient clinics or special-purpose programs for the maintenance of blood pressure control. Health departments also operate home health agencies, although it is administratively difficult to separate public health nursing, which is not generally reimbursable by Medicare or other third-party insurance programs, from home health nursing with its special certification requirements. The latter programs are usually operated by independent agencies, voluntary or proprietary, but they need close working relationships with public health nursing (see Chapter 30). Public health agencies also have an important role to play in monitoring the long-term care system. In addition to such traditional functions as

inspection and licensure of food-serving establishments (this includes the kitchens in nursing homes and in senior citizen centers), laboratory performance testing, and supervision of inhome health programs, most state health departments and many local health departments have a role in the licensing and certification of nursing homes. State programs to license nursing homes date from the 1950s and the Social Security amendments, which required such regulation if a state wished to participate in the old-age assistance program. Licensure is a state function that can deny an organization the privilege of operating a nursing home if it cannot meet reasonable state standards for services, equipment, safety, and patient care. Certification is a national program that determines whether or not a nursing home can participate in the Medicare program. It is a responsibility of the Health Care Financing Administration but is administered with federal support through state agencies, which carry out the work under contract. The standards for licensing and certification are often different and sometimes result in two different units, sometimes within the same state agency, conducting two separate inspection programs. They should be combined.

In some states, licensing has been delegated to selected local health departments if they have the capability to carry out the program. The nursing home licensure programs have been controversial from their beginning. They are not generally thought to have been particularly effective in improving care or preventing abuse and have been criticized for their failure to serve as effective advocates for better services for the elderly. The programs are fraught with difficulty since it is hard to bring about corrective action except through tedious and time-consuming negotiation and court action. The final weapon is closure and removal of the patients, but this is rarely an effective option, since there is usually no place else for the patients to go. A few states have experimented with legislation that empowers the state health agency to assume direct operating control of nursing homes whose deficiencies cannot otherwise be corrected. These actions have resulted in corrections, but they leave the state with the problem of continued management or some other acceptable disposition of the facility.

The regulatory programs raise a number of policy questions. The Medicare and Medicaid programs have supported and fostered the entrepreneurial approach to nursing home care. Market forces have not been effective in improving services, controlling costs, or preventing client abuse. Most often clients do not pay for the service directly, have few if any alternatives, and too often are not able to advocate or intervene effectively on their own behalf. Since most of the bills are paid through public programs, the only recourse has been regulation. With each attempt by the paying agencies to control costs, the provider organizations have attempted to reduce services or find other ways to increase their profit margin. This has caused the licensing agency to increase its demands on the provider organization, and the battle is joined. Typically, private interests prevail in what is a public market, and the paying and regulating agencies are forced to command behavior that is contrary to the best interests of the provider organizations. The process and the results have left no one happy: the clients, the families of clients, the regulators, the payors, the providers, or the legislators. The problem has arisen as a result of a policy decision to purchase what appears to be a public service in a private market and then regulate the transactions. The regulatory process could be reduced or eliminated if the service became a direct public function through publicly owned nursing homes. Local or state governments could build their own facilities and either operate them directly with a citizens' board as a watch-dog agency, or negotiate multiyear service contracts with proprietary or nonprofit operating agencies. This would at least remove the real-estate transactions from the complex equations of profit and cost, but such proposals would clearly face strong political opposition. The paying agencies could rent the space for a year at a time and allocate that space directly rather than leave it to the client to make the purchase transaction. Since demand for nursing home beds seems to be greater than the supply, "freedom of choice" options are not operative for the clients, although they are for the operators. If the public agency controlled the use of the space, it might be possible to work out more effective admissions. As it is the operators have an incentive to restrain the admission of those people who need the most care in favor of those who need the least, thereby exacerbating the misuse patterns. Clearly

the present approach has not worked effectively for anyone except the entrepreneurs. At this time it seems unlikely that the national government can overcome the political opposition of the industry to change. Much could be learned by encouraging more state-level experimentation with organizational design and incentive systems, but the present trend is to further centralize control in Washington. This is an instance where decentralization could produce a richer variety of alternatives at an acceptable cost, both in terms of money spent and in terms of patient care.

THE FUTURE

As noted at the outset, the problem is large and growing larger. The elderly are increasing in absolute numbers and as a proportion of the total population. The elderly need more health and social services than the young, and our policy is to make the services available. Those over the age of 75 use more services than those between 65 and 74, and those over the age of 85 use the most. The high-use groups, "the elderly old" are increasing even more rapidly than "the young old." As the cost of health services continues to increase, a segment of the population that uses much of the service and is increasing in size presents serious problems to service organizations, to policy makers and to society as a whole. Past efforts will not suffice in the future.

The Federal Council on Aging has 13 themes that should serve well as a guide through the future:[28]

1. Long-term care should be defined in terms of the person, not the program.
2. Long-term care should be based on an assessment of the disability, not a medical diagnosis.
3. Physical and mental health concepts must be integrated.
4. Long-term care is not just a problem for the elderly.
5. Disability is a social problem, not a medical problem.
6. Agencies should try to use natural supports and not supplant them in favor of professional workers.
7. Programs should strive to maintain volunteerism.
8. Some of the fundamental actions have to be carried out at the community level: (a) the administration of a simplified eligibility process, (b) client assessment, and (c) case management.
9. Program management should be locally based.
10. The fiscal resources available in all related federal programs (Titles XVI, XVIII, XIX and XX of the Social Security Act and Title III of the Older Americans Act) should be used creatively and together,

rather than separately by state agencies in support of local programs.

11. Quality control may be elusive, but has to be pursued.
12. The responsibilities of the three different levels of government have to be sorted out.
13. Who is supposed to pay and how is a question that requires an answer.

It is clear that formally organized and highly structured programs, developed to follow federal reimbursement quidelines, cannot provide an acceptable and affordable answer to the problem of aging in America. For the elderly as well as other groups with disabilities that make them dependent in some respects, support for and insistence on the use of more natural community supports is essential. Public health agencies are highly organized and authoritarian by nature. It comes with the training: nurses, physicians, and sanitarians. If they are to play a constructive role in ameliorating the dependency that all too often and unnecessarily accompanies aging, they must learn to play a more collaborative and resourceful role, encouraging the creativity of families and community groups rather than displacing them or attempting to regulate their conduct. Next to poverty and education, dependency will continue to be the biggest problem for public health in the decades ahead.

REFERENCES

1. Callahan, J.J., and Wallack, S.S.: Major reforms in long-term care. In Callahan, J.J., and Wallack, S.S., editors: Reforming the long-term care system: financial and organizational options, Lexington, Mass., 1981, D.C. Heath & Co.
2. Siegel, J.S.: Recent and prospective demographic trends for the elderly population and some implications for health care. In Haynes, S.G., and Feinlein, M., editors: Epidemiology of aging, NIH Pub. No. 80-969, July 1980, U.S. Department of Health and Human Services.
3. Kovar, M.G.: Morbidity and health care utilization. In Haynes, S.G., and Feinleib, M., editors: Epidemiology of aging, NIH Pub. No. 80-969, July 1980, U.S. Department of Health and Human Services.
4. Van Nostrand, J.: Defining need. Paper presented at the Annual Meeting of the American Public Health Association, Los Angeles, November 1981.
5. Hickey, T., and Douglass, R.L.: Mistreatment of the elderly in the domestic setting: an exploratory study, Am. J. Public Health 71(5):500, May 1981.
6. Helsing, K.J., Szklo, M., and Comstock, G.W.: Factors associated with mortality after widowhood, Am. J. Public Health 71(8):802, Aug. 1981.
7. U.S. Bureau of the Census: Current population re-

ports, special studies, Series P-23, No. 59, May 1976, U.S. Department of Commerce.
8. Branch, L.G., and Jette, A.M.: The Framingham disability study. I. Social disability among the aging, Am. J. Public Health 71(11): 1202, Nov. 1981.
9. Kane, R.L., and Kane, R.A.: Directions for reallocating health resources: some next steps. In Morris, editor: Allocating health resources for the aged and disabled, Lexington, Mass., 1981, D.C. Heath & Co.
10. U.S. Senate Special Committee on Aging: Nursing home care in the United States: failure in public policy, Washington, D.C., 1974, U.S. Government Printing Office.
11. Mendelson, M.A.: Tender loving greed, New York, 1974, Alfred A. Knopf, Inc.
12. U.S. Bureau of the Census: Statistical abstracts of the United States, 1981, Washington, D.C., 1981, U.S. Department of Commerce.
13. Beatrice, D.F.: Licensing and certification in nursing homes: assuring quality care? In Altman, S.H., and Sapolsky H.M., editors: Federal health programs: problems and prospects, Lexington, Mass., 1981, D.C. Heath & Co.
14. General Accounting Office: Report of the Comptroller General to the Congress. I. The well being of older people in Cleveland, Ohio, April 19, 1977, Washington, D.C.
15. General Accounting Office: Report of the Comptroller General to the Congress. II. Home health, December 30, 1977, Washington, D.C.
16. General Accounting Office: Report of the Comptroller General to the Congress. III. Conditions of older people, Sept. 20, 1979, Washington, D.C.
17. Fillenbaum, G.G., and Smyer, M.A.: The development, validity, and reliability of the OARS multidimensional functional assessment questionnaire, J. Gerontology, 36(4):428, 1981.
18. Shanas, E.: Self-assessment of physical function: white and black elderly in the United States. In Haynes, S.G., and Feinleib, M., editors: Epidemiology of aging, NIH Pub. No. 80-969, July 1980, U.S. Department of Health and Human Services.
19. Katz, S., and others: Progress in the development of the index of ADL, Gerontologist 10:20, 1970.
20. Kodner, D.L., and Feldman, E.S.: The service coordination/delivery dichotomy: a critical issue to address in reforming the long-term care system. Paper presented at annual meeting of the American Public Health Association, Los Angeles, Nov. 1981.
21. Weissert, W.G., Wan, T.T.H., and Livieratos, B.B.: Effects and costs of day care and homemaker services for the chronically ill: a randomized experiment, U.S. Department of Health, Education, and Welfare Pub. No. (PHS)79-3258, Feb. 1980.
22. Toff, G.E.: Alternatives to institutional care for the

elderly: an analysis of state initiatives, Washington, D.C., 1981, Intergovernmental Health Policy Project.

23. Kannel, W.B.: Cardiovascular risk factors in the aged: the Framingham study. In Haynes, S.G., and Feinleib, M., editors: Epidemiology of aging, NIH Pub. No. 80-969, July 1980, U.S. Department of Health and Human Services.

24. Periodic health examinations: Report of a task force to the Conference of Deputy Ministers of Health, Health and Welfare, Canada, Hull, Quebec, 1980, Canadian Government Printing Center.

25. Robbins, L.C., editor: Prospective medicine and health hazard appraisal, Indianapolis, Ind. 1974, Methodist Hospital Press.

26. Breslow, L.: Preventive medical service in National Health Insurance. Paper prepared for the Office of Management and Budget on behalf of the Association of Schools of Public Health and the Association of Teachers of Preventive Medicine, 1973. In Preventive medicine U.S.A.: task force reports sponsored by the John E. Fogarty International Center for Advanced Study in the Health Sciences, National Institutes of Health, and the American College of Preventive Medicine, New York, 1976, Prodist.

27. American Public Health Association: Proposed preventive benefits to be covered on a first dollar basis under national health insurance, American Public Health Association, 1974. In Preventive medicine U.S.A.: task force reports sponsored by the John E. Fogarty International Center for Advanced Study in the Health Sciences, National Institutes of Health, and the American College of Preventive Medicine, New York, 1976, Prodist.

28. Fahey, C.: Some political, economic, and social considerations. In Morris, R., editor: Allocating health resources for the aged and disabled, Lexington, Mass. 1981, D.C. Heath & Co.

PART SEVEN

Health and behavior disorders

Despite Juvenal's well-known and widely quoted aphorism, *Mens sana in corpore sano*,[1] far too many people, including a substantial proportion of health workers, tend to think of health and illness only in relation to the physical body. This is thrice in error! It errs first in that it ignores the complex of mental and behavioral disorders that afflict a large proportion of people, second in that it ignores the various mental and behavioral conditions that may have their genesis in physical illnesses, and third in that it ignores the fact that few, if any, physical illnesses or injuries are without a mental or behavioral component or consequence.

Much of the problem relates to difficulty of definition. The case has been stated particularly well by Lipscomb[2]:

The attempts to study mental illness, delinquency, alcoholism and drug use have demanded that epidemiologists ruefully accept that they can no longer classify the occurrences of these events by single precise labels—"the alcoholic," "the delinquent." They have had to consider the events under study—drinking, drug use, delinquent behavior—in the ecological context in which an indexed individual lives, a context which inevitably changes over time as the person himself changes.

This is especially evident among those who find themselves, by no personal choice, in socioeconomically disadvantaged circumstances, epitomized by the slum or ghetto, that constitute a complex morass of human problems. The choices open to such marginal persons in their attempts to cope with the intolerable externalities that confront them have been summarized as follows:[3]:

1. He may adopt a delinquent or criminal pattern.
2. He may become a drug addict and consequently a criminal.
3. He may passively accept his lot in life or divorce himself from it as the latent schizophrenics do.
4. He may reject the Horatio Alger myth that appears as the primary ingredient which predisposes him to the above solutions, and he may instead struggle for change in the external intolerable conditions. In so doing, the individual would change himself and the whole world around him.

It is essentially within this conceptual framework that the next group of chapters are presented.

REFERENCES

1. Juvenal: Satires X.
2. Lipscomb, W.R.: An epidemiology of drug use-abuse, Am. J. Public Health **61:**1794, Sept. 1971.
3. Abrams, A., Gagnon, J.H., and Levin, J.J.: Psychosocial aspects of addiction, Am. J. Public Health **58:**2142, Nov. 1968.

CHAPTER 25

Mental health and illness

If a patient is poor he is committed to a public hospital as "psychotic"; if he can afford the luxury of a private sanitarium, he is put there with the diagnosis of "neurasthenia"; if he is wealthy enough to be isolated in his own home under constant watch of nurses and physicians he is simply an indisposed "eccentric."

Pierre Marie Felix Janet (1859-1947)
La Force et la Faiblesse psychologiques

THE PROBLEM WITHIN

The field of mental and emotional health and illness is one of the frontiers of public health that has undergone expanding exploration and action during recent decades.[1] The considerable attention to the subject by the communications media has resulted in an increased awareness of the real or potential relationship between mental illness and crime, violence, juvenile delinquency, prostitution, alcoholism, addictions, accidents, suicides, familial discord, occupational inadequacies, and a host of other social and physical phenomena. These are now recognized as components of what the Committee on Mental Health of the American Public Health Association has referred to as the "Social Breakdown Syndrome."[2] Similarly, the public as well as the medical and health professions have become conscious of the increasing mental stresses of urban and especially of industrialized life.[3-6] Furthermore, the many people in need of professional and institutional care and the great cost of providing it have become matters of common knowledge and concern.

As with many other social problems, initial study and experimentation in this field derived chiefly from the interest of a few individuals and private or voluntary groups or agencies. Until relatively recent historical time, mentally ill persons were incarcerated without treatment in filthy jails and similar institutions, often with criminals and diseased persons; exhibited as curiosities or sources of amusement; and restrained for long periods in chains and straightjackets, cruelly beaten, and rendered stuporous by drugs. Some were even burned at the stake on the assumption that they were witches or possessed by evil spirits. Their most courageous champion was Philippe Pinel in France, who in the 1790s agitated for reforms for their more humane treatment. His efforts to remove their chains, to have them considered victims of illness, and to transfer them from prisons to hospitals were pursued in the face of strenuous opposition and ridicule not only from the public but also from his fellow physicians. About 50 years later a similar movement was begun in the United States by Dorothea Dix. During the late nineteenth century, the foundations of the related fields of psychology and psychiatry were laid, leading to consideration of possible preventive and promotive approaches to the problem.

The mental health movement may be said to have begun in 1908 with the publication of Clifford W. Beers' book *A Mind That Found Itself.*[7] It presented in dramatic and effective manner his experiences as a patient in several institutions for the mentally ill. The narrative ended with a plea for drastic reform and public education in mental health. Prompt encouragement and support enabled Beers to establish the first organization of its type, the Connecticut Society for Mental Hygiene. Its purpose was to combat the widespread ignorance about mental illnesses and their causes. One year later, in 1909, the National Committee for Mental Hygiene was organized. Rapid growth occurred during the ensuing two decades, evidenced by the organization of mental hygiene societies in 19 states

449

and 16 nations. In 1922 the International Congress for Mental Hygiene came into being, and in 1930 it called the first International Mental Hygiene Congress in Washington, D.C.

Meanwhile, a few local and state governmental units, including some health departments, began mental health activities. Usually they were exploratory and experimental and often integrated with some other activities rather than identified separately. A great stimulus came in 1946, when the National Mental Health Act was passed by Congress. It authorized $7.5 million for the construction and equipment of hospital and research facilities by the Public Health Service as a center for research and training in mental problems. Ten million dollars were provided for grants to states to expand their facilities, and an additional $1 million for demonstrations and the employment of personnel. In 1948 these activities were reorganized to form the National Institute of Mental Health (now part of the Alcoholism, Drug Abuse, and Mental Health Administration). This and subsequent legislation made possible much of the expansion of thought and action that since has occurred at all levels of government in the United States.

NATURE AND EXTENT OF THE PROBLEM

In terms of incidence and prevalence, as well as of social and economic consequences, mental illness is one of the most compelling public health problems. So pervasive are its facets into all aspects of community health that Jensen,[8] a sociologist, long ago exclaimed: "If it isn't mental health, it isn't public health." Indeed, it is difficult to think of any aspect of public health work that does not have a mental or psychologic component. Mental illness, like cancer, is not a clear, discrete entity. Rather, it includes a variety of conditions that limit or destroy the individual's effectiveness. By now much concerning the nature, cause and treatment of mental illness has been clarified and classified on an organic basis. A veritable explosion of research is shedding more light on the remaining hidden areas.[9,10] Evidence has been accumulating to indicate that somatic and psychic functions are so closely related that they operate in health and illness as parts of an entity. As a result, the integration of psychiatry with general medicine is considered to be the most significant trend in modern psychiatry. This is evidenced by the increasing movement of psychiatrists and other mental health personnel out of their hospitals, clinics, and consulting rooms and into close relationships with other physicians and groups in the community.[11] Concurrently, there has been increased attention to family and group dynamics.

It is difficult to determine the number of individuals affected by psychiatric or handicapping psychologic or behavioral disorders at any given moment or on an annual or lifetime basis. Too many variables are involved: concepts of mental illness by the public, by those affected, and by health and social personnel; the distribution of psychiatric, psychologic, and related personnel; the availability of inpatient and outpatient facilities; economics; the availability and use of psychotropic drugs; and variations in the frequency of relapses or repeated episodes. The President's Commission on Mental Health[12] indicates that 20 to 30 million people in the United States at any one time need some form of psychiatric attention, ranging from counseling to long-term treatment. The significance of the figures is confused by inclusion of a wide variety of conditions: alcoholism, drug abuse, delinquency, child abuse, and the like. Somewhat more useful, but still subject to many of the variables mentioned, are the average daily census in state and county mental hospitals (145,616 in 1979) and the number of patient-case-episodes in mental health facilities.[13] These are shown in Table 25-1.

Coleman and Patrick[11] found that of patients who visited the Greater New Haven (Conn.) Community Health Center Plan facilities, 15.7% presented emotional problems. This, they noted, was consistent with the 14% in general medical practices in England, Australia, and Austria. It is notable that 72% of the New Haven patients were treated by primary care clinicians alone; the remaining 28% were treated by associated mental health clinicians. It is estimated that of the 20 million patients who go to general hospitals in the United States for physical ailments each year, about 6 million have illnesses caused by emotional disturbances. There is evidence that at any given time about 1 out of every 10 persons in the country has some form of mental or emotional disorder that needs treatment.

Among the many factors that contribute to the increase in mental patients are increased stresses of urbanization and industrialization, extended longevity, increased population and crowding, improved and more acceptable diagnosis, and increased facilities for diagnosis and care. Recently, the National Institute of Mental Health established an Epidemiological Catchment Area Program, the goals of which are to provide more dependable estimates of the incidence and prevalence of mental disorders, to search for etiologic clues and to aid in planning mental health care services and programs. Its methods are fivefold—emphasis on specific diagnosis, integration of community surveys with institutional surveys, collection of prevalence as well as incidence data, systematic linkage of service use data with other epidemiologic variables, and multisite comparative-collaborative efforts. Although none of these are new, it is hoped that their combination will produce new knowledge concerning the extent of the mental health problem.[14]

With reference to the components of the mental health problem, schizophrenia is the most common reason for hospitalization, accounting for 45.6% of the total. The frequencies of other important conditions are mental diseases of the senium, 12.2%; manic depression, 7.6%; syphilitic psychosis, 6.7%; and psychosis with mental deficiency, 6%. Alcoholic and involutional psychoses each account for about 3% of those hospitalized.

The incidence of mental illness depends on many factors. Type of condition in relation to age is especially important. Most mental illnesses have their origins in early childhood but do not become manifest until the developmental or productive years of life. Despite this, schizophrenia is being diagnosed in children with increasing frequency. In general, however, in terms of age at first hospitalization for mental illness, about one half are between 35 and 64 years, about one fourth are between 15 and 34 years, and about one fourth are over 65 years, whereas only about 1% are under 15 years of age. It is interesting that one of the reasons given by Gibson[4] for the increased need for psychiatric help is increased longevity. One's tendency to psychiatric breakdown increases with age, depression being more common in the middle aged and elderly, and pathologic intellectual deterioration occurring most often in the older age groups. Also, as described by Silverman,[15] personal and nutritional neglect as well as more dramatic phenomena such as suicide are common manifestations of depression in the elderly.

As to type of illness, mental deficiency, epilepsy, personality disorders, and schizophrenia usually appear early in life; alcoholic and manic-depressive psychoses are centered in the middle, productive years of life; whereas involutional and senile psychoses occur during the later years. Mental illness seems to be more frequent among women than among men. About 50% more women than men enter hospitals because of schizophrenia and manic-depression. The incidence of psychoneuroses appears to be about twice as common in women as in men, whereas involutional psychoses are three times as high. On the other hand, personality disorders are twice as frequent and alcoholic psychoses are about four or five times as frequent in

TABLE 25-1. Patient care episodes in mental health facilities, 1955-1975

Facility	1955	1965	1978
Inpatient—total	1,296,352	1,565,525	1,816,613
State and county mental hospitals	818,832	804,926	574,226
Private mental hospitals	123,231	125,428	184,189
General hospital psychiatric services	265,934	519,328	571,725
Veterans Administration hospital psychiatric services	88,355	115,843	217,507
Federally assisted community mental health centers	—	—	268,966
Outpatient—total	379,000	1,071,000	4,576,366
Federally assisted community mental health centers	—	—	1,741,729
Other	379,000	1,071,000	2,834,637
TOTAL, ALL FACILITIES	1,675,352	2,636,525	6,392,979

Modified from The world almanac and book of facts, 1982 edition, New York, 1981, Newspaper Enterprise Association, Inc.

men as in women. There is no significant difference between the sexes in the incidence of mental deficiency or of senile psychoses.

These differences by type and age are especially significant in relation to the chances for recovery and play a determining role in the enormous hospital bed requirements and treatment costs for mental illness. This is summarized in Table 25-2, which presents various mental conditions in the order of their general ultimate importance, considering numbers of persons affected, duration of illness, length of hospitalization necessary, and chances of recovery.

Some interesting socioeconomic variations may be noted in the incidence of mental illness. Thus neuroses are twice as common as the more severe psychoses among the wealthy, professional, and top managerial groups; the opposite is true among semiskilled and unskilled laborers. Another way of looking at this is that neuroses are twice as common in the more advantaged socioeconomic groups, whereas severe psychoses occur about twice as frequently in the less advantaged socioeconomic groups of the population. Part of these discrepancies may result from a greater awareness of and economic ability to seek medical attention for neuroses by the more educated and affluent. Similarly, many in the less advantaged socioeconomic group may not consider neurosis as an illness in relation to other problems.[16] On the other hand, some of the causes of the more severe psychoses are more prevalent in the environments and family milieus of the socioeconomically deprived. Gibson[4] notes that the higher one is on the socioeconomic scale, the less the chance one has of developing a psychologic illness, except manic-depressive psychosis.

At present the most dramatic and effective role in mental health is being played by pharmacologic research.[9,10,17] The discovery of ataractics, or tranquilizers, has revolutionized both inpatient and outpatient care. Many who previously would have been institutionalized now are not, and the length of institutional stay for those who have been hospitalized has been shortened significantly. Indeed, the very atmosphere of mental institutions has changed dramatically because of drug therapy. In 1949 an Australian group discovered that lithium salts were effective in abating manic states. Since then investigators in Europe showed that lithium salts were useful as a sort of prophylaxis against the extreme swings of mood in manic-depressive patients.[18] The first psychotropic drug to be successfully used against schizophrenia was the neuroleptic chlorpromazine hydrochloride in 1952. It increased the recovery rate from severe schizophrenia from 20% to about 60%. Frequently, however, long-term maintenance therapy is necessary to prevent relapse. The year 1954 was the turning point in the treatment of manic depression. Investigators of a new antituberculosis drug, iproniazid, noted a remarkable improvement in disposition and behavior

TABLE 25-2. Hospitalization for mental illness by age, sex and chance of recovery

Condition	Usual age at first admission	First admissions (%)			Hospitalized mental patients (%)	Chances of recovery
		Men	Women	Both		
Schizophrenia	16-35	18.6	26.8	22.6	45.6	Poor after age 50; long hospitalization
Manic-depressive psychosis	35-50	3.1	5.3	4.2	7.6	Poor; long hospitalization
Psychosis with mental deficiency	15-44	2.7	1.8	2.3	6.0	Poor; long hospitalization
Alcoholic psychosis	25-54	21.8	5.2	13.7	3.0	Fair; short hospitalization
Involutional psychosis	48-58	3.0	8.3	5.6	3.0	Poor; die soon; short hospitalization
Senile psychosis	Over 60	21.1	20.5	20.8	12.2	Poor; die soon; short hospitalization
Personality disorders (nonalcoholic)	15-34	7.2	3.9	5.6	4.0	Fair; short hospitalization
Psychoneurotic	25-44	6.3	12.4	9.3	6.0	Fair; short hospitalization
Other disorders, each of low incidence	All ages	16.2	15.8	15.9	12.6	Generally poor; long hospitalization

of the dispirited far-advanced invalids who received the drug. Until then, electroconvulsive shock was the only effective treatment for severely depressed patients. This provoked a wave of research that led to the development in 1957 of imipramine, phenelzine, and other neuroleptics that are inhibitors of the monoamine oxidase (MAO) enzyme system, which among other things is somehow involved in the development and maintenance of depressive states.[19]

The effects of these remarkable discoveries were not long in coming. As early as 1955, the number of patients discharged from institutions increased sharply, and the number of people institutionalized declined. In 1955 over 77% of the 1.7 million patient treatment episodes in mental health facilities involved inpatients, as compared with only about 28% of the 6.4 million patient care episodes in 1978. During the quarter century, the resident population of state mental hospitals dropped from 559,000 in 1955 to 146,000 in 1979, and the average length of stay has been approximately halved. The economic as well as humane implications of this change are tremendous. Research does pay!

The limitations of data restricted to hospitalization are obvious. Many individuals receive some psychiatric guidance through public and private medical facilities other than hospitals, but the amount is unknown. Many more are in need of varying degrees of assistance for relatively minor personality adjustment and psychiatric problems but never receive it. In many ways the latter represents perhaps the greatest social and economic aspect of the total problem. In 1970 it was estimated that the overall annual cost of mental illness in the United States was about $21 billion, of which about 43% was borne by those other than the mentally ill or their families. The average annual cost was about $5,400 per patient. Almost $2 billion of the total represented the cost of care and maintenance in public mental hospitals. The annual cost to the Veterans Administration was $1.25 billion. In addition to figures such as the above is the cost of care rendered in community mental health centers and by private psychiatrists. The value of the extensive mental health counseling by other private physicians, public health nurses, family counselors, social workers, clergymen, and others is, of course, unknown.[20] The economic and patient-load changes since 1970 would of course multiply these costs several times.

The possibility of insuring against the costs of mental illness has been raised by many. Although several health insurance organizations and plans that operate their own facilities have psychiatrists on their staffs and some provide mental health clinics, only rarely do they include the costs of psychiatric treatment among their benefits. The few that have attempted to do so have encountered substantial difficulties. Included are the rapid attitudinal and age changes in the population; high costs in a setting where all types of health insurance plans are finding their costs expanding; difficulty in defining and determining mental health care costs, particularly when care over a long period in a hospital or physician's office is required; the question of how mental hospitals and mental health centers should be financed and the respective roles of patient, private insurance, and government in financing mental care; and a rather complete lack of information as to what the use of psychiatric services would be if they were available on an insured basis. Nevertheless, some progress has occurred. An increasing number of state Blue Cross and Blue Shield plans have included provision for payment of certain psychiatric services. The 1967 amendments to the Social Security Act expanded significantly the benefits under Medicare and Medicaid for the mentally ill.[21] Beyond this, the movement toward the development of comprehensive Health Maintenance Organizations implies an increase in community mental health resources. Of special significance was a contract negotiated in 1964 between the United Auto Workers and the automobile and agricultural implement industries under which about 2.5 million workers and their families received coverage for psychiatric care.[22]

In the larger sense, intensified interest in the need for a national health insurance system has provoked increased consideration of the inclusion of benefits for mental health care.[11] If this is to eventuate and develop successfully, certain entrenched ideas must be changed. Fundamental is a charge made by Senator Javits of New York in an address to the American Association of Psychiatric Services for Children in 1977. He pointed out that "the inability of mental health professionals to agree on a common concept of mental illness and to elucidate the roles and responsibilities of each discipline was hindering their coverage in projected national health insurance legislation.[23] In addition,

Mechanic,[24] in reviewing existing insurance coverage for mental health benefits, has noted that such benefits provide incentives for hospital care rather than community care and reinforce the medical approach to what are essentially psychologic disabilities. Moreover, he states, the benefits favor the affluent as compared with the disadvantaged and make little provision for the integration of the chronic mental patient into the community. He urges that if mental health benefits are to be included in a national health insurance plan, care must be taken to avoid reinforcing these patterns.

DEFINITION AND GOAL OF MENTAL HEALTH

Mental health represents a broad field that is difficult to define. Caplan and Caplan[25] described it simply and practically as "the potential of a person to solve his problems in a reality based way within the framework of his traditions and culture." Potentially there are few if any areas of public health with which it is unrelated and to which it cannot make a contribution. The increased provision of facilities and the improvement of techniques for treatment of the mentally ill are not of course the complete or ultimate goals. Rather, the primary concerns include improved and increased detection of psychiatric and prepsychiatric conditions that may result in personal and social handicaps, the study of their causes, and the initiation of efforts to eliminate as far as possible the factors that bring them about. The goal must be a more satisfying and effective life, free of adverse mental deterrents for more people or, to state it even more simply, the development of emotionally mature people.

Lemkau,[26] in his excellent discussion of the field of mental health, has outlined its goals and indicated that desirable program content should be two dimensional. He points out that the vertical or categoric dimension, consisting of early diagnosis and treatment of existing mental ills, as in the case of tuberculosis control, meets several needs: (1) the prevention of the development of more serious and handicapping illness, (2) the removal of sources of stress from family and social environments, and (3) the making available of the services of specialist personnel to the broader horizontal aims of the mental health program. He visualizes the horizontal goals of mental health in terms of the work of

every member of the health agency being influenced by mental health principles.

MENTAL HEALTH PROGRAMS

Differences of opinion still exist concerning what a mental health program should include or who should administer it. However, a consideration of its components is pertinent. The establishment in 1948 of the National Institute of Mental Health provided national leadership of high quality to developments throughout the United States. Among many other accomplishments, it made state and local public health and other types of personnel aware of mental health so that it was integrated into various parts of their programs and activities. Private enterprise was also affected. By now, all states and most localities of significant size have ongoing programs and services under various types of leadership—public health departments, mental health departments, community mental health boards, and in some local instances voluntary agencies. Functions variously include the maintenance of lists or rosters of mental health facilities; the gathering of reports or data on mental health needs and problems; the development of and assistance to state and local, lay and professional educational programs; the direct operation of mental health clinics, inpatient facilities, and day care centers; the promulgation of rules and regulations relating to mental health and the administration of certain aspects of some of them; financial assistance to local agencies; promotional, supervisory, and consultative services to local official and voluntary agencies; and special surveys and research.

In 1963 another milestone occurred—the Mental Retardation Facilities and Community Mental Health Centers Construction Act, which defined a community mental health center as "a facility providing services for the prevention or diagnosis of mental illness, or care and treatment of mentally ill patients, or rehabilitation of such persons. . . ." Its purpose was to assist all levels of government to deal more vigorously with the problems of mental illness and mental retardation. In addition to providing more funds for research, it also authorized grants to states for the construction of additional community mental health centers, the extension of community mental health preventive and promotive programs, and the initial staffing of these facilities and programs. The purpose of the act was extended and strengthened in 1965 by an amendment that provided additional support for community-based programs for the care of the mentally ill and encouraged general hospitals to become major community psychiatric resources.

Since the passage of the Community Mental Health Center Act in 1963 (amended in 1975), significant changes in the philosophy and nature of mental health services have occurred in the United States. By the end of 1974, many community mental health boards with broadly representative memberships had been formed and more than 590 centers established, in addition to over 2,000 psychiatric outpatient clinics. Among other influences, these services have provided physical resources for a more complete use of the new psychotropic drugs, which has resulted in the dramatic shift from state mental hospital inpatient care to community outpatient care.

A necessary accompaniment has been attention to mental health personnel needs. Again, leadership and funds have come essentially from the National Institute of Mental Health, which has provided grants to professional educational institutions to increase the numbers of psychiatrists, psychologists, social workers, nurses, and others. It is estimated that there are now about 28,000 psychiatrists, 10,000 clinical psychologists, 3,500 psychologic counselors, and 31,000 social workers in psychiatric hospitals or outpatient mental health facilities.[24] The number of nurses engaged to some extent in mental health activities in institutions or in the community is impossible to estimate. Without question, their numbers are great.

Despite these considerable gains, as DuVal and Venable[27] have indicated, the greatest hindrances to the development of truly efficient and effective community mental health services have been the lack of coordination and cooperation among the agencies on the several levels of government, on the one hand, and between public or community health advocates and mental health advocates, on the other. With reference to the former, significant progress has been achieved in recent years. Thus the states have been provided with federal stimulus and assistance to enact legislation for the establishment of community mental health services boards and the provision to them of state matching funds for the extension and coordination of mental health activities. Improvement of the second hindrance, however, is still needed. It is true that throughout its history the field of public health generally gave less than adequate attention and leadership to various aspects of mental health and re-

lated fields. This, plus the fact that psychiatry developed a mind-body distinction and a one-to-one concept, led the American Psychiatric Association in the early 1960s to adopt an official position that community mental health services should be organized as separate departments of mental health. As a consequence, there has developed an undesirable situation in which responsibility is divided among departments of public health, mental health, and welfare, or institutions, as well as in some instances, special boards or commissions. Understandably this has resulted in considerable anguish among many public health workers and governmental managers who fear possible program inefficiency and public confusion. Unfortunately, to date truly effective methods of coordination and cooperation have appeared unreasonably difficult to achieve.

It is interesting to note that by 1967 the Conference on Education in Psychiatry of the American Psychiatric Association regarded the mind-body distinction and the one-to-one approach anachronistic and strongly endorsed training and practice to be comprehensive in the total-person sense and in the form of group and community action. Meanwhile, as DuVal and Venable[27] have noted, both the fields of public health and mental health are in active ferment: "In some states each . . . appears to be moving in a different path and often in a different direction, as both search for new methods of approaching the same problems." Still holding the beliefs that the mind and body are irrevocably related parts of the whole, they urge the development not of a single organizational model but of a variety of bilaterally endorsed and supported accommodations based on the customs, mores, relationships, responsibilities, and authorities of the different governmental jurisdictions. It must be realized by all that solutions to the exceedingly complex problems of mental health, especially as they impinge on or are affected by physical health, society, and the environment, cannot be found within any single group or profession. This was emphasized early by Felix and Kramer[28]: "Because of the complexity of the problem, effective research on the community aspects of mental illness must be interdisciplinary, combining the skills and knowledge of the psychiatrist, psychologist, social scientist, public health physician and nurse, psychiatric social worker, epidemiologists, and statistician." This was also clearly indicated years ago in the 1948 report of the National Health Assembly,[29] which stated, "Clergymen, teachers, lawyers, social workers, nurses, recreation and group workers, law enforcement officers, public health personnel, representatives of management and labor, and many others are constantly presented with opportunities for recognizing emotional problems." Important omission by each of these listings, and perhaps the key groups toward which the efforts of all of the others should be primarily aimed, are family physicians and parents. These important concepts have been clearly illustrated by Blain and Robinson[30] as shown in Fig. 25-1.

As has been implied, the relationship between the staffs of mental health centers or programs and the personnel of official public health agencies sometimes presents an administrative problem. It involves especially the relationship between social workers and public health nursing staffs. The obvious goal is for public health nurses and mental health social workers to regard each other as sources of referral and as resources for consultation, advice, and in-service education. This can best be accomplished through joint planning, joint conferences, and joint in-service training. Perhaps the key consideration to be kept in mind by nursing staffs is that social work, especially as it relates to the mentally disturbed, is a specialized field. In turn, the limited numbers of psychiatrically trained social workers must recognize that they are physically incapable of making all the contacts and of meeting all the needs and that public health nurses have wide and well-established contacts and entrée throughout the community. Beyond this, all concerned, including the health officer and the director of the mental health center, should bear in mind that the promotion and maintenance of smooth and fruitful interpersonnel and interprofessional relationships is in itself a manifestation of sound mental

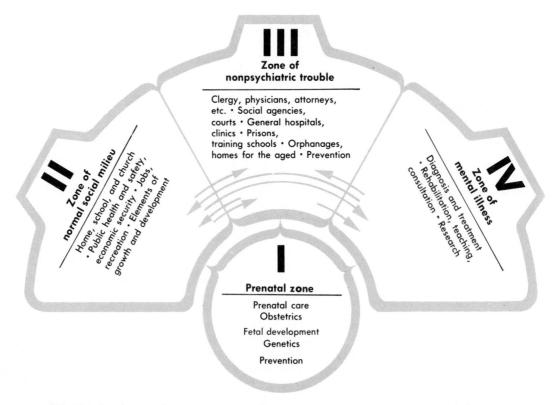

FIG. 25-1. Population and service zones in relation to mental health and illness. (Modified from Blain, D., and Robinson, R.L.: N.Y. J. Med. **57**:257, Jan. 15, 1957.)

health and in turn is a prerequisite to the planning, development, and implementation of an effective community mental health program. An effective and equitable merger of these two intimately related areas of social action appears to offer the most logical solution to many of the basic problems of each.

ROLE OF THE HEALTH DEPARTMENT

At an Institute on Mental Health in Public Health held in the University of California at Berkeley in 1948,[31] it was agreed that one of the most important problems for health departments at that time was to clarify their responsibilities in their communities with respect to mental health in order that citizens and other agencies might know what to expect. It was thought that unless effective organization took place among the various agencies concerned with the problem and unless each understood its specific role and the roles of the others, confusion would result. This was also indicated in the report of the Joint Commission on Mental Illness and Health[32] not only with reference to public health but also in relation to most other types of agencies. Unfortunately some health departments have yet to clarify their positions and roles, and confusion still exists.

Actually, the roots of this problem go back much further. The problem is well illustrated by a provocative statement made by Kelley[33] in 1921 at the annual meeting of the American Public Health Association.

We can scarcely speak of relinquishing . . . mental hygiene, to anybody, never having claimed it. This is the first occasion, I think, when this subject has had a place upon the program of this Conference. I believe there now exists in but one state, provincial, county or municipal health department on this continent an officially organized or recognized division of mental hygiene; yet it is apparent upon the most cursory reflection that mental hygiene is for all future time bound to be recognized as one of the greatest, if not the greatest branch of hygiene. The fact that it is largely rooted in the emotional and psychic life has long blinded us to the fact that this is not only a subject of basic importance to the public health administrator in itself, but in many phases of what is usually considered purely physical hygiene, a satisfactory standard of achievement can never be reached without taking into account the relationship of the emotional and mental life.

Aronson[34] has proposed that the health officer, in attempting to face the challenge of the mental health problem, should turn to well-established patterns used so successfully in the control of communicable disease. First, the health officer looks for broad, well-documented epidemiologic patterns. Second, he or she searches for elements in existing programs that most nearly meet the needs of those patterns. Finally, he or she explores ways to use existing personnel in the new areas of activity. Aronson emphasizes the opportunity for the health officer "to act as a catalyst—to be the voice of the community, in calling for the coordination of the variety of services and efforts being made by a number of agencies, in pointing out imbalance and gaps in available services, and in securing the widest community support for a broad spectrum of mental health services consistent with recognized scientific evidence and readily available to all who need them."

Others[1,35,36] have suggested health department activities to orient and train their own staffs and personnel of other community agencies in mental health and illness, to provide diagnostic and referral services as well as community follow-up after discharge of patients from psychiatric hospitals, to operate community mental health clinics and day care centers for mentally retarded children, to cooperate with industrial mental health programs, and to educate the public in mental health. In addition, attention is directed to the important psychologic and psychiatric implications of children institutionalized for any reason, as well as persons affected by geriatric problems, alcoholism, suicidal impulses, marital and other family discord, crime and delinquency, and accident proneness. And then there is the myriad of the lonely who Braceland[37] has discussed as a masss of psychologically and socially neglected people. Some of these problems are discussed in detail in subsequent chapters.

To assist public health agencies in defining and developing their role, the American Public Health Association has developed a useful handbook on mental disorders and their control.[38] In addition, attention is directed to a highly provocative series of presentations on the potentials for mental health involvement by the various components of traditional health agencies.[39]

FUTURE OF COMMUNITY MENTAL HEALTH

With the ever-increasing complexity of American society, the accelerating pace of living, and the concentrations of people, it is probable that mental and emotional problems will increase in the years ahead. Offsetting this is the increase in understanding of human behavior and the continuing advances in psychopharmacology. For the immediate future, certainly more community-based facilities are needed. In 1964 Felix[40] envisioned very broad, comprehensive multiservice centers designed to provide preventive services, early diagnosis, and treatment of mental illness on both an inpatient and outpatient basis, and to serve as a locus for the aftercare of discharged hospital patients. He itemized the spectrum of services to include the following:

A general diagnostic and evaluation service (precare)
An acute inpatient service and an outpatient service
A day-care service and a night-care service
An emergency service available around the clock
Rehabilitation services
Consultation services
Public information and education services
Supervision of foster homes
Research and training

By means of these, he believed true continuity of mental and emotional care would become possible to the enormous advantage of the patient and of the community of which the patient is a member. Many such comprehensive community mental health facilities have since developed.[41,42] Thus aid for stressful mental problems is being brought ever closer to the people and the sources of their problems. The importance of the establishment and operation of 24-hour emergency mental health facilities deserves particular emphasis.[43] Although it appears in Felix's list, actually it relates to many of the other needs in the list. In view of the nature of the problem, its importance is self-evident.

In his perceptive work on the social organization of health, Dreitzel[44] states:

The creation of mental hospitals was a great achievement for the nineteenth century. For the first time mentally disturbed persons were ascribed the role of the sick and treated accordingly. However, these hospitals, in which most psychotics are still kept, are . . . "total hospitals" with an internal power structure and the norms of a community of prisoners. Though once a humane alternative to almshouses and jails, they serve today as asylums for the socially unwanted, radically isolating the patient from his family, neighborhood, and work. They thus more

often than not function as a self-fulfilling prophecy, producing in the patient the illness that originally served as a pretext to run him in, rather than providing help for his life problems.

Among the rewards of biochemical and humanistic approaches to mental illness and the development of community mental health centers during recent years has been the opportunity for increasing numbers of patients to avoid or escape from the confines of the artificial and generally unhelpful closed institutional environments of the not-so-distant past back to the more normal environment whence they came and wherein may be some true hope and opportunity of social reentry.

REFERENCES

1. Lieberman, E.J., editor: Mental health: the public health challenge, Washington, D.C., 1975, American Public Health Association.
2. Gruenberg, E.M., and others: Social breakdown syndrome: environmental and host factors associated with chronicity, Am. J. Public Health 62:91, Jan. 1972.
3. Society, stress, and disease, Report of symposia, WHO Chron. 25:168, April 1971.
4. Gibson, A.C.: Stress disorders of modern life, R. Soc. Health J. 91:172, April 1971.
5. Segal, J.: Forces that shape the lives of our young, Public Health Rep. 94:399, Sept.-Oct. 1979.
6. Schweitzer, L., and Wen-Huey, S.: Population density and the rate of mental illness, Am. J. Public Health 67:1165, Dec. 1977.
7. Beers, C.W.: A mind that found itself, New York, 1948, Doubleday & Co., Inc.
8. Jensen, H.E.: Mental health: a local public health responsibility, Ment. Hyg. 37:530, Oct. 1953.
9. Segal, J., editor: Research in the service of mental health, Department of Health, Education, and Welfare Pub. No. (ADM) 75-236, Rockville, Md., 1975, National Institute of Mental Health.
10. Keith, S.J., editor: Schizophrenia, 1980: special report, Department of Health and Human Services Pub. No. (ADM)81-1064, Rockville, Md., 1981, National Institute of Mental Health.
11. Coleman, J.V., and Patrick, D.L.: Psychiatry and general health care, Am. J. Public Health 68:451, May 1978.
12. President's Commission on Mental Health: Preliminary report, Washington, D.C., Sept. 1, 1977, The White House.
13. The world almanac and book of facts, 1982 edition, New York, 1981, Newspaper Enterprise Association, Inc.
14. Eaton, W.W., and others: The epidemiological catchment area program of the National Institute of Health, Public Health Rep. 96:319, July-Aug. 1981.

15. Silverman, C.: The epidemiology of depression, Baltimore, 1968, The Johns Hopkins University Press.

16. King, S.H.: Perceptions of illness and medical practice, New York, 1962, Russell Sage Foundation.

17. Psychotropic drugs and mental illness, WHO Chron. **30**:420, Oct. 1976.

18. Gattozzi, A.A.: The psychology and biochemistry of depression. In Yolles, S.F., editor: Mental health program reports II, Public Health Service Pub. No. 1743, Rockville, Md., 1968, National Institute of Mental Health.

19. Gattozzi, A.A.: Norepinephrine II: its possible role in depression and mania. In Yolles, S.F., editor: Mental health program reports III, Public Health Service Pub. No. 1876, Rockville, Md., 1969, National Institute of Mental Health.

20. What are the facts about mental illness in the United States? New York, 1971, National Health Education Commission.

21. National Institute of Mental Health: Mental health benefits of Medicare and Medicaid, PHS Pub. No. 1505, Rockville, Md., 1969.

22. Editorial: Insurance coverage for psychiatric care, Public Health Rep. **80**:1118, Dec. 1965.

23. Gorman, M.: Mental health insurance: problems and prognosis, Am. J. Public Health **68**:445, May 1978.

24. Mechanic, D.: Considerations in the design of mental health benefits under national health insurance, Am. J. Public Health **68**:482, May 1978.

25. Caplan, G., and Caplan, R.: Development of community psychiatry concepts in the U.S. In Freedman, A., and Kaplan, H., editors: Comprehensive textbook of psychiatry, Baltimore, 1967, The Williams & Wilkins Co.

26. Lemkau, P.V.: Mental hygiene and public health, New York, 1955, McGraw-Hill Book Co.

27. DuVal, A.M., nd Venable, J.H.: Mental health and public health—organization of state services, Am. J. Public Health **57**:878, May 1967.

28. Felix, R.H., and Kramer, M.: Research in epidemiology of mental illness, Public Health Rep. **67**:160, Feb. 1952.

29. America's health—a report to the nation by the National Health Assembly, New York, 1948, Harper & Row, Publishers, Inc.

30. Blain, D., and Robinson, R.L.: Personnel shortages in psychiatric services, a shift of emphasis, N.Y. J. Med. **57**:257, Jan. 15, 1957.

31. Ginsberg, E.L.: Public health is people, New York, 1950, Commonwealth Fund.

32. Action for mental health; report of Joint Committee on Mental Illness and Health, New York, 1961, Basic Books, Inc.

33. Kelley, E.R.: Two twilight zones in health administration, Am. J. Public Health, **12**:563, July 1922.

34. Aronson, J.B.: Mental health and the local health department, Am. J. Public Health **51**:89, Jan. 1961.

35. Sparer, P.J.: Mental hygiene in a modern health department program, Am. J. Public Health **51**:892, June 1961.

36. Turner, W.E., Smith, D.C., and Medley, P.: Integration of mental health into public health programs—advantages and disadvantages, Am. J. Public Health **57**:1322, Aug. 1967.

37. Braceland, F.J.: The devious paths of loneliness, M.D., p. 11, Jan. 1978.

38. Mental disorders: a guide to control methods, New York, 1962, American Public Health Association.

39. Goldston, S.E., editor: Mental health considerations in public health: a guide for training and practice, PHS Pub. No. 1898, Rockville, Md., 1969, National Institute of Mental Health.

40. Felix, R.H.: A model for comprehensive mental health centers, Am. J. Public Health **54**:1964, Dec. 1964.

41. National Institute of Mental Health: The comprehensive community mental health center, PHS Pub. No. 2136, Rockville, Md., 1970.

42. Feldman, S., and Goldstein, H.H.: Community mental health centers in the United States: an overview, Int. J. Nurs. Stud. **8**:247, Aug. 1971.

43. Resnik, H.L.P., and Ruben, H.L., editors: Emergency psychiatric care, Bowie, Md., 1974, Charles Press Publishers.

44. Dreitzel, H.P.: The social organization of health, New York, 1971, Macmillan, Inc.

CHAPTER 26

Alcoholism

Every inordinate cup is unblessed and the ingredient is a devil.

Othello II. 3

FRIEND OR FOE

In addition to the communicable and organic disorders to which we are subject and which we often share with other creatures, another group of conditions exists that is peculiarly our own invention. These are behavioral disorders that involve the unreasoned compulsive consumption of certain chemical substances, some natural and some man-made, to our ultimate physical, psychic, and social detriment. It is interesting that all of these substances have numerous beneficial uses and effects when used properly and judiciously and generally adversely affect only a minor proportion of those who use them. Most prominent among these is alcohol, a substance of ancient development and widespread consumption.

Alcohol has played a fascinating role in the history of mankind. The production of alcoholic beverages appears to have been one of our earliest discoveries. Undoubtedly, it was recognized early that among those who consumed it were some who developed an uncontrollable craving for continued use regardless of the consequences. Thus the drunkard is mentioned in the Old Testament. Through time, society typically frowned on the undesirable results of the abuse of alcohol but was at a loss to understand them. Generally they were attributed to innate depravity, an inherited weakness, or the loss of the soul. Such attitudes have continued to the present time. Only recently have more enlightened attitudes developed, based on clearer understanding of the function of the mind, its relationship to the body, and the effects of pressures of society.

Alcohol is used in many different situations and

For excellent overviews of the subject, see references 1 to 4.

for many purposes—in religious ceremonies, as a food, as a relaxant, as a customary base for many social affairs—by many different kinds of people—men and women, young and old, and well-adjusted and emotionally disturbed. Its effects vary in type and extent—an improved appetite, a warm glow of well-being and conviviality, a blackout, or personality deterioration.

Alcohol has a long history of use in medicine and at one time was one of the most commonly prescribed drugs. Often it has been used as an anesthetic. Although some of the supposed health values ascribed to it have been disproved, certain others have been scientifically confirmed. For example, certain alcoholic beverages are now used in the diets of diabetic patients, since alcohol, unlike sugar, does not require insulin for metabolism. It is also used as an aid in the treatment of arthritis, certain digestive diseases, hypertension and coronary disease, and as a tranquilizer or sedative for convalescent and geriatric patients.[5]

The use and effects of alcohol may be regarded in terms of a gradient, with all persons being distributed along a scale of consumption with a concurrent scale of response. Ordinarily the less the intake, the less will be the response, whereas the more the intake, the greater will be the response, its consequences, and the probability of the person becoming an alcoholic. However, the situation is not so simple. Some individuals may actually consume, even on a consistent basis, a considerable amount of alcohol yet never become alcoholics. There are others whose intake may be significantly less or occasional yet may be problem drinkers. The reason for drinking and for continuing to drink has much to do with the making of an alcoholic. Similarly, the attitude toward other aspects of life and the world has much to do with deciding whether or not a person becomes an alcoholic. Still another deciding factor is the relative ease or difficulty of reduction or elimination of the consumption of alcohol.

DEFINITION

The foregoing points up factors that make alcoholism difficult to define. Nevertheless, the more the problem is studied, the more it becomes apparent that certain types of persons, especially under certain circumstances, tend to become alcoholics, whereas others do not. The alcoholic has been defined by some as an individual under emotional pressure who drinks to get away from feeling a certain way but eventually is drinking because of the drinking. This is a practical definition in its emphasis on the initial psychosocial trigger followed by the eventual psychophysiologic entanglement.

From an epidemiologic viewpoint, alcoholism may be defined as an acquired chronic progressive disease involving the compulsive intake of excessive amounts of alcohol and leading in its more advanced stages to certain psychologic, social, and physical deteriorating sequelae. It affects predominantly men to the ratio of 3 or more to 1, although the gap is closing.[6,7] Alcoholism is particularly common in certain occupations, such as those involving nonroutine, pressure, decision making, and transiency. It is significantly greater in urban areas and is more frequently found in certain nationalities, especially Scandinavian, Nordic, Celtic, and Polish, in contrast to its infrequency among Italians, Greeks, and Jews.

EXTENT OF THE PROBLEM

The magnitude of the problem is difficult to determine because so many cases never come to social or medical attention and because of the number of individuals at any time who are on the borderline between problem drinking and chronic alcoholism. A 1964-1965 survey[8] by the Rutgers Center of Alcohol Studies found that 12% of a national sample of adults were heavy drinkers—one fifth of the adult men and one twentieth of the adult women. Similar incidences were reported by Mulford[9] and Gallup.[10]

Of special concern in this and several other countries is the current increase in the use of alcohol among young people. In a 1974 study in the United States, for example, more than a fourth of male students 12 to 13 years old and two thirds of those 18 to 20 years old were classified as moderate to heavy drinkers on the basis of one drink a week, two drinks three times a month, or five drinks once a month. Among female students the incidence was 20% for those 12 to 13 years to 50% after age 17 years.[11]

To complicate the picture further, alcoholism is not a disease primarily of the ignorant or of unskilled labor. To the contrary, about 80% of adult alcoholics are regularly employed up to the point of disability, and three fourths of them belong to the executive class in large and small businesses or are professionals, salespeople, or skilled laborers.

Some further insight on alcoholism is provided from studies by Cisin and Cahalan,[8,12] who distinguished between the characteristics of those who drink at least once a year and those who fall into the category of "heavy drinkers." Their findings are summarized in Table 26-1.

As they note, their survey produced some unexpected findings and confirmed others:

1. It showed that drinking is (at least statistically) normal behavior, and that both abstinence and heavy drinking are statistically atypical.
2. Whether a person drinks at all is primarily related to sociological and cultural variables rather than to psychological variables. This is obvious from the great difference in the proportion of drinkers by sex, age, social status, region, urbanization and religion.
3. However, certain personality measures helped to account for some of the "heavy" drinking—particularly alienation from society, neurotic tendencies, and psychological involvement with alcohol or "escape" drinking.
4. There appears to be a high turnover in the drinker or nondrinker status of many individuals, in addition to the general tendency for older persons to drop out of the drinking and heavy-drinking classes.

The implications of this with regard to social, economic, and professional productivity and morale are obvious. The reality of the problem becomes evident from several business and industrial surveys,[13] which indicate that the average company can expect about 3% of all its employees to be alcoholics in need of special attention. Little wonder that alcoholism is now included among the seven categories of diseases that cause outstanding numbers of deaths and disabilities and that represent major unsolved public health problems. The others are cardiovascular disease, mental illness, crippling

TABLE 26-1. Comparison of groups most likely to be drinkers and heavier drinking groups

Groups in total population with highest rates of drinking at least once a year (total sample, 68%)	Among those who drink, groups with highest rates of "heavy drinking"* (total among drinkers, 18%)
Men 30-34, 88% women 35-39, 73%	Men 40-49, 40%
Men of highest social status, 88%	Men of lowest social status, 33%
Professional people, 81%; semiprofessional or technical, 78%; sales workers, 79%; managers or officials, 75%	Operatives, 24%; service workers, 23%
College graduates, 82%	Men who completed high school but not college, 32%
Single men, 83%	Single men, 26%; divorced or separated men, 21%
Residents of suburban cities of 50,000 to 1 million, 87%	Residents of central cities over 50,000, 22%
Those whose fathers were foreign-born, 80%; especially of Italian origin, 92%	Those whose fathers were Latin-American/Caribbean, 30%; Italian, 22%; British, 21% (Irish, when adjusted for age levels, 33%)
Jews, 92%; Episcopalians, 91%	Protestants of no established denomination, 29%; Catholics, 23%; those without affiliation, 25%

Data from the National Survey, conducted 1964-1965 by the Social Research Group, a national probability sample of 2,746 persons.
*For definitions of "heavy drinkers," see Cahalan and associates.[8] Most "heavy drinkers" drank nearly every day with five or more drinks per occasion at least once in a while, or about once weekly with usually five or more drinks per occasion.

and handicapping conditions, cancer, dental disease, and diabetes. It should be noted, incidentally, that all of these, including alcoholism, are conditions about which something is known and about which something can be done.

COST OF ALCOHOLISM

Although it is obviously impossible to determine, the cost of alcoholism to society must be great. Many factors contribute to the cost, which The National Institute on Alcohol Abuse and Alcoholism estimates at $15 billion annually in the United States. Absenteeism, high spoilage rates, decreased productivity while on the job because of lowered ability and apparent avoidance of work situations that involve hazard or that are likely to indicate the worker's condition, personnel turnover, and lowered morale of the alcoholic and those working with this person account for some of these costs. Added to them is the expense to society of many resources for grappling with various aspects of the problem, for example, police, courts, jails, religious organizations, hospitals and medical care, various social and charitable agencies, departments of welfare, domestic relations organizations, visiting nurse agencies, and industrial presonnel guidance offices. Less tangible is the ultimate cost of detri-

mental effects on family members and friends, for example, on children at school and on other adults at work—either those in the home or colleagues at the alcoholic's place of employment. Still another social loss caused by alcoholism is the amount of crime and prostitution that is related to it as either or both cause and effect. The amount is indeterminate but, on the basis of observations by many, would appear to be significant.

The relationship of alcoholism to accidents is interesting. Some notable surveys carried out by the Yale University School of Alcohol Studies in 1943[14] indicated that the estimated 1.37 million alcoholics employed in industry at that time accounted for 1,500 fatal accidents at work and 2,850 fatal accidents at home, in public places, and in traffic, or for a total of 4,350 fatalities. This was a fatal accident rate of 321 per 100,000 men, or more than twice that of nonalcoholic workers in the same occupations. Subsequent studies,[15] however, have indicated that whereas alcoholics lose more work time than nonalcoholics, they do not appear to suffer a higher rate of occupational accidents. This substantiates earlier studies by Trice,[16] who hypothesized that the alcoholic while actually on the job tends to be overcautious, concentrates more on what he is doing in a deliberate attempt to avoid accidents, is subject to fewer of other types of distractions, develops a well-planned work routine, is sometimes "covered up" by his fellow workers, and if actually in an alcoholic or hangover state, tends to be absent rather than risk discovery or a work accident. The only work relationships in which Trice found alcoholics to indulge their addiction and to have work-related accidents were (1) as participants in fellow-worker drinking groups after working hours and (2) on jobs that require geographic mobility, hence separation from protecting or inhibiting influences coupled with greater accessibility to alcohol.

Alcohol-related accidents away from work present a different picture from the nonmobile work situation. This is best illustrated by the relationship between automobile accidents and alcohol consumption, which has been the subject of many studies. Problem drinkers have about twice as many accidents per mile of driving as the nondrinking population. As little as 0.03% of alcohol in the blood reduces driving skill,[17] and the probability of accidents increases consistently with an increase of alcohol in the blood. The risk with a blood alcohol level at 0.1% has been found to be twice that at 0.05%, whereas an increase in the blood level to 0.15% multiplies the risk tenfold.[18] With this in mind, the percentage of automotive accident fatalities involving persons with significant blood alcohol levels is illuminating. Numerous studies in many places have shown that about 50% of automobile-related fatalities involve significant blood alcohol levels in either or both drivers and pedestrians, if the latter are involved.

It is somewhat more difficult to relate alcohol to home accident fatalities. However, in view of Jellinek's study,[14] in which the total fatal accident rate in alcoholic workers was twice that of nondrinkers, and Trice's study,[16] in which this accident rate was not found to be caused by on-the-job accidents, and because in the United States home accidents (fatal and nonfatal combined) are about twice as frequent as work accidents and at least four times as frequent as vehicular accidents, it would seem reasonably certain that a close relationship exists between drinking and the probability of home accidents. To paraphrase the slogan "If you drink, don't drive," one might say, "If you drink, don't climb a ladder."

In view of its disinhibitory effects, the relationship of alcoholism to internally and externally expressed violence is significant. It is commonly associated with child abuse[19] and with spouse abuse.[20] Numerous studies[21,22] of criminal homicide have shown that 50% or more of the offenders had been drinking before committing murder. With reference to self-destruction, it has been noted that about one half of successful suicide victims have been drinking immediately before their self-destructive act.[23] Furthermore, by means of the technique of "psychologic autopsy," an extremely high proportion of successful suicides were found to have been chronic alcoholics.[24]

EFFECTS OF ALCOHOL

The Alcoholism Subcommittee of the Expert Committee on Mental Health of the World Health Organization has concluded that although alcohol must be regarded as a drug, it can be classified neither as an addiction-producing drug nor as a habit-forming drug but must be placed in a category of its own, intermediate between these two groups. After ingestion, alcohol is rapidly absorbed directly from the stomach and upper intestine into the bloodstream. It is detectable in the blood within 5 minutes after ingestion and by this medium is distributed throughout the body. The average adult body can oxidize about 10 ml of alcohol per hour, releasing energy and carbon dioxide and water. Any that is not oxidized is excreted in the urine and through the lungs. Thus ingestion of excessive amounts gives rise to a buildup in the bloodstream and in the tissues, awaiting either oxidation or excretion. Blood concentrations of 0.2% usually result in mild to moderate intoxication, whereas more than 0.3% causes significant effects. Blood concentrations between 0.5% and 0.8% result in death. Repeated and extensive use of alcohol tends to result in increased tolerance.

Alcohol affects all parts of the body, especially the central nervous tissue. Contrary to common belief, it acts not as a stimulant but as a depressant. In so doing it inhibits the controls of behavior in the cerebral cortex. The pulse increases and vasodilation occurs, especially in the skin, and results in decreased body temperature because of heat loss. Because of this, again contrary to common thought, the use of alcohol to warm the body is not physiologically sound. Vision and sense of balance are impaired relatively early. In more advanced states of intoxication, the centers in the brain that regulate breathing, cardiac function, and body heat are depressed. As with so many things, the moderate consumption of alcohol actually appears to have little or no effect on longevity. There is good evidence, however, that heavy drinking does shorten life in various ways. Some estimates indicate that the life expectancy of alcoholics is about 10 to 12 years less than the average for all people.

Much of the ill effect of excessive consumption of alcohol is because of malnutrition. The alcoholic typically eats inadequately because of the dulling of the appetite and general disinterest in food and because calories for energy are obtained from alcohol. Since the latter are so readily available, what food is eaten often is stored unused in the body. Hence many alcoholics, especially in the earlier stages, may become overweight. Most important among the nutritional deficiencies that occur are those involving vitamin B complex. This may result in polyneuritis, so-called beer heart, with cardiac weakening and enlargement with attending edema, pellagra, and the typical skin and ocular manifestations of riboflavin deficiency. Fatty degeneration of the liver may result, probably from a combination of vitamin B deficiency and direct toxic effects of alcohol on the liver cells. Because of lowered mineral intake, anemia is frequent. Among the more dramatic effects are those relating to the psyche, such as delirium tremens, Korsakoff's psychosis, and personality changes caused by alcoholic degeneration of cortical tissue. In connection with the latter, the advanced alcoholic tends to become socially unstable, careless about appearance or actions, suspicious, irritable, belligerent and quick to take offense, crafty, overemotional, and frequently brutal and callous toward others, especially loved ones. Much of the latter, of course, is attributable to the severe guilt complex that is typically developed.[25]

TYPES OF ALCOHOLICS

It is important to consider first of all how alcoholics differ from the much larger number of persons who drink but are not alcoholics. As Bacon[26] has indicated, there are many reasons for drinking, such as to fulfill a religious ritual, to be polite, to have a good time, to make friends, to experiment, to show off, to get warm or cool, to quench thirst, to go on a spree, or to flavor food. He states, however:

None of these is the purpose of the alcoholic, although he might claim any or all to satisfy some questioner. The alcoholic drinks because he has to if he is to go on living. He drinks compulsively; that is, a power greater than rational planning brings him to drinking and to excessive drinking. . . . Most alcoholics hate liquor, hate drinking, hate the taste, hate the results, hate themselves for succumbing, but they can't stop. Their drinking is as compulsive as the stealing by a kleptomaniac or the continued hand washing of a person with a neurosis about cleanliness. . . . It is useful to think of their drinking behavior as a symptom of some inner maladjustment which they do not understand and cannot control. The drinking may be the outward, obvious accompaniment of this more basic hidden factor.

Many psychiatrists have pointed out that if the alcoholic did not drink, he or she would consciously or subconsciously seek some other outlet for unresolved conflicts and tensions. In addition, there is some evidence that certain physical causes for alcohlism exist. Some investigators believe that the problem drinker may have some abnormal psychologic and physiologic reaction to alcohol that others do not have.[27]

Frank alcoholics are intensely introspective and disinterested in anything except themselves and their problem. They have few if any diversional interests, such as hobbies, entertainment, or social activities. A large proportion of alcoholics are socially unattached to family or social groups, both of which tend to be regarded as secondary to the drinking pattern and to drinking "buddies." This introspection and social isolation presents particular difficulty to persons, programs, or agencies that may try to relate meaningfully to alcoholics to assist them. Sometimes part of the difficulty derives from the sense of failure and guilt that the alcoholic commonly feels and that may even result in a willful rejection of attempts to help. Alcoholics may reject help on the basis that they deserve to be miserable because of their real or imagined failings and because of the compulsive drinking pattern itself, which they developed in relation to their conflicts and failings.

Generally speaking, there are two main types of problem drinkers. The first or primary type is the individual who was maladjusted to begin with. That is, before embarking on compulsive drinking, this person probably was referred to as a neurotic who was subject to a sense of constitutional psychoneurotic inferiority. Usually the personality was developed improperly from early childhood with gradual realization of vague and constant feelings of anxiety, apprehension, inadequacy, or inferiority. Often the person feels defeated before even beginning and fears failure in school, in courtship, in work, and in society and, if at all possible, wants to avoid such situations. Occasionally such a person finds that indulgence in alcohol brings a sense of release and gives some degree of confidence and apparent success. Perhaps more than anything it enables the individual to forget temporarily the feeling of inadequacy and self-dissatisfaction. What is more logical than to repeat the experience? The problem is compounded, however, when the effects of alcohol wear off. There are unpleasant memories or, worse, uncertainties about behavior while under the influence of alcohol, providing additional feelings of anxiety and guilt. This leads to the additional use of alcohol, often the morning after, to overcome the postalcoholic sense of guilt, and a vicious circle is established.

The second type of compulsive drinker begins as an apparently well-adjusted person who is not neurotic; the personality has not been improperly developed; and, in fact, the person appears to get along well in the family, at work, and with the group. If anything, he or she may tend to be an extrovert, becoming involved in situations and with groups, either socially or professionally, that lead to considerable drinking. The person participates with enthusiasm but is not yet an alcoholic. Such an individual is being self-indulgent without having any particular feeling of compulsion. However, the continued use of more alcohol gradually lowers the senses of discrimination and responsibility. The person becomes less efficient, becomes careless, and begins to put things off or to let things slide to meet the preferred social demands. Almost imperceptibly at first, relationships and behavior at home, on the job, and in society begin to deteriorate. This becomes noticeable to the drinker, who because of fear or worry drinks more. Meanwhile, the family, friends, and employer also begin to notice and, although usually indulgent or tolerant at first, soon become impatient. There occurs a mutual loss of regard, and blunt words are exchanged. Because of arguments at home or perhaps a demotion or loss of a job, the individual begins to believe that everyone is down on him and with increasing self-pity

blames it all on the misunderstanding and intolerance of others or on just plain bad luck. The only thing that provides escape or supports the ego is the very thing that began the process—alcohol. Hence again a vicious circle is begun. As time goes by and the situation becomes worse, this second type of compulsive drinker appears on the surface more and more like the primary type of alcoholic. However, because the alcoholism is not superimposed on a basic feeling of inferiority, the chances of recovery and rehabilitation are decidedly better. Fortunately from society's viewpoint the larger proportion of alcoholics appear to fall into this category.

Brenner[28] has found that economic conditions appear to divide people into two divergent categories with relation to alcohol use. One group uses alcohol under conditions of economic prosperity and stability. Their preference appears to be wine and beer. The other group, which is in the minority, resorts to distilled spirits during periods of economic difficulty. Some of these become intoxicated, leading to involvement with the criminal justice or mental health systems. Some others of the second group become long-term alcoholics who develop liver damage and resultant lowered life expectancy. The implication of these observations is that the consumption and abuse of distilled spirits is often stress related, whereas the use of beer and wine is not.

FETAL ALCOHOL SYNDROME

Alcohol-induced impairment of the growth and development of infants was first documented by Dr. William B. Carpenter of the University of London in 1849. Within 2 years it had been reprinted by the Massachusetts Temperance Society.[29] The problem was then essentially ignored until the studies of several French pediatricians during the late 1950s and 1960s. In 1968 some of them reported 127 cases of infants with peculiar facies, considerable retardation in height and weight, and a high incidence of various malformations and psychomotor disturbances. Alcoholic mothers were noted as the common factor. Numerous studies[30,31] since then have confirmed the condition and pointed to its frequent occurrence in this and other countries. Among infants of women with severe chronic alcoholism, there is experienced a 17% perinatal mortality, and 44% of those who survive are mentally deficient. The intelligence quotient of affected children averages 35 to 40 points below normal.[32] The syndrome consists of behavioral, craniofacial, limb, and neurologic anomalies and, in nearly 50% of reported cases, cardiac-septal defects, genital abnormalities, and hemangiomas. Primary anomalies of the head and face include microcephaly, fissures of the eyelids, midfacial defects, and a flattened, elongated vertical groove in the upper lip. Malformations of the hands include abnormal palmar creases and joined, deviated, or permanently flexed fingers and toes.[33,34]

The risk and extent of abnormalities increase with increased maternal intake of alcohol. High blood alcohol levels, as well as frequency of drinking, are important. Physicians and other health advisors should discuss drinking habits with women of childbearing age and inform them of the risks involved. Although totally safe levels of drinking have not been determined, a risk is apparently established with ingestion of the equivalent of 3 oz. of absolute alcohol, or about 6 drinks per day. The risk for lesser amounts is uncertain, but caution is advised.[35] "Binge" drinking should definitely be avoided by pregnant women, and women with chronic and severe drinking problems should be discouraged from becoming pregnant until their alcoholism is brought under control. Because of the uncertainty, it is now recommended that no alcohol be consumed by pregnant women. A still open question is the possibility of an undesirable preconceptional effect of significant alcohol consumption on spermatazoa.

WHAT CAN BE DONE

Until recently and even now in many places, the approach to the alcoholic has been to tolerate the person if possible; "dry the person out" periodically, either in jail, in a public hospital, or in a private sanatorium; or if the condition were beyond recovery, to provide the person with some type of refuge in skid row or elsewhere in which the alcoholic could subsist on handouts from friends, strangers, missions, or other charitable organizations during the intervals between employment at usually undesirable types of work. With the relatively recent acceptance of the condition as a disease and on the basis of an increasing amount of social, medical, and psychiatric study and research, a growing number of programs are being established with increasingly fruitful results. Much is still on the basis of trial and demonstration.[36]

It is interesting that the real impetus arose from within the group affected. This took the form of the organization in 1935 of Alcoholics Anonymous (A.A.). This group considers itself "a fellowship of men and women who share their experience, strength, and hope with each other that they may solve their common problem and help others to recover from alcoholism." It states that "the only requirement for membership is an honest desire to stop drinking," and that it is "not allied with any sect, denomination, politics, organization, or institution; does not wish to engage in any controversy, neither endorses nor opposes any causes." The primary purpose of its members "is to stay sober and to help other alcoholics to achieve sobriety." Since its foundation, A.A. has helped more than 500,000 men and women in the United States, Canada, and many other countries. These people constitute the core of the membership and the nucleus to which others in need of help may relate. There are now many thousands of groups in communities thoughout the world, including those in hospitals and in prisons.

The organization operates on a few simple but sound and effective premises. Participation must be voluntary—there can be no checking up or compulsion. An alcoholic can never indulge in controlled drinking; either the drinking will become progressively worse or the alcoholic must abstain completely from alcohol and develop a new pattern of constructive living. Belief and faith in God is a fundamental source of strength in the attempt toward recovery. A recovered alcoholic can best understand the problems and motivations of the alcoholic and is therefore in the best position to be of assistance. Group meetings for group therapy and open discussion of problems are valuable in obtaining an understanding of the underlying causes of one's alcoholism. Individual anonymous assistance in the form of moral support is instantly available by visit or phone at all times. The process of trying to help other alcoholics in itself is an important aid to staying sober oneself. Members do not swear off alcohol for life or for any other period in the future—they merely concentrate on the 24 hours of today. Contributions toward recovery and rehabilitation by other groups, such as the medical profession and social agencies, are recognized, and members are referred freely as indicated.

In a similar vein have been the efforts of the Salvation Army and various "Gospel Mission" programs. Although they tend to be underrated by many, including health professionals, it must be recognized that in the face of a social and professional vacuum over many years they have provided for a number of important basic needs: psychologic encouragement, shelter, and nutrition.

Meanwhile an increasing knowledge about the psychologic and physiologic causes and effects of alcoholism has been accumulated. One result has been the development of three schools of thought with regard to explaining and handling the problem: the social, the psychiatric, and the medical or physiologic schools of thought. Increasingly it is recognized that rather than conflicting, the three are complementary—each approach contributing to the solution of the problem. Not until recently have attempts been made to apply knowledge as it became available. In 1944 the Laboratory of Applied Physiology at Yale University established two public clinics in Connecticut—one at New Haven and the other at Hartford—to attract and guide alcoholics and to bring to bear the various resources and approaches to their treatment. Soon after, schools of alcohol studies were established, first at Yale then at Rutgers University. A journal, *The Quarterly Journal of Studies on Alcohol,* devoted exclusively to the subject was begun. The success of the Yale clinics led to the establishment in 1949 of a pilot program by the Western Electric Corporation, which now estimates that about 70% of its recognized alcoholics are rehabilitated. Since 1949, the number of companies with planned programs for the recognition and treatment of alcoholics has rapidly increased. For companies without programs, assistance in the form of consultation and information has been made available through the numerous local committees of the National Council on Alcoholism.

ALCOHOLISM PROGRAMS

Until 1945, no state had a program specifically for alcoholism. In that year, largely as a result of the success of the Yale clinics, Connecticut began the first state program under an independent commission. Since then, most states have established programs. There is no consistency with reference to their organizational location. In general, they are distributed about equally among state health departments, state mental health agencies, and independent commissions. The programs carried on are various combinations of educational, research, and treatment activities.

Until recently, federal interest in alcoholism has been minimal, In 1966, however, President Lyndon Johnson dealt with alcoholism explicitly for the first time in U.S. history in his health message to the Congress. New legislation was passed, and a National Advisory Committee on Alcoholism was apppointed. In addition, a National Center for Prevention and Control of Alcoholism was established within the National Institute of Mental Health to provide consultation and grants for education, research, and demonstrations to states and through them to localities and institutions. One of the most significant activities has been to stimulate the formation of state mental health planning agencies and community mental health boards. As a result, a significant and increasing number of competent community mental health programs with well-grounded alcoholism components have been established. These activities were strengthened further by the passage on December 31, 1970, of the Comprehensive Alcoholism Prevention Treatment and Rehabilitation Act (P.L. 91-616), which in addition to making possible more grants and contracts in this field, also created a National Advisory Council on Alcoholism. More recently, several program areas have been combined into the Alcohol, Drug Abuse, and Mental Health Administration of the Public Health Service.

Too often, local programs have tended to be parochial and limited to treatment of cases brought to public attention. There is a trend, however, toward broadening the base of approach by more effectively and extensively using resources of all pertinent fields, professions, and agencies. Among the resources, services, and activities that should be included if possible are the following[2]:

For alcoholics
Information and referral
Intensive care facilities
Extended care facilities
Physicians
Outpatient clinic services
Halfway houses
Day-care facilities
Custodial care facilities
Pastoral counselors
Social agencies

Psychiatrists
Vocational rehabilitation
Industrial health services
Surveys
Case finding
Follow-up
Evaluation
For family members
Information
Consultation
Social assistance
Group analysis
For providers of services
Information and referral
Consultation
Coordination
Training programs
Resource materials
Evaluation and standards
Reports
Morbidity and mortality data
Demographic and social data
Follow-up
For prevention
Information and referral
Consultation
Resource materials
Educational activities
Surveys and reports
Teacher training programs
Social agencies
Research (especially etiologic)
Coordination
For opinion molders
Informational services
Surveys and reports
Coordination
Consultation
Evaluation and standards
Resource materials

The problem is so vast and complex, with multiple causes, different types of cases, and numerous agencies of potential value, that no standard program is possible or even desirable at this time. A quarter century ago, Vogel[37] emphasized:

Treatment of the alcoholic is not the sole province of the psychiatrist, internist, sociologist, minister, or any scientific or lay discipline. Recognition of this is fundamental. . . . A total push is necessary and mobilization of all methods and facilities is necessary to improve results and make help available to more alcoholics. The nonspecificity of present-day treatment should not result in therapeutic nihilism, which is often used by physicians and others as

rationalization to avoid this important problem. There are definitely ways to treat the alcoholic.

Such a multidisciplinary approach, illustrated by a well-planned program developed on a systems basis by the South Central Mental Health Region of North Carolina,[38] is shown in Fig. 26-1.

Bascially there is no reason why the approach to the problem of alcoholism should not follow the well-established principles of epidemiology and program planning that have been so successful in many others areas. This should include the gathering of data by survey, reporting, or other means to determine the extent of the problem. The data should be analyzed to pinpoint problem areas and problem groups, existing or incipient, and to determine places and circumstances in which alcoholism is or tends to become a problem. Early case finding should be carried out by enlisting the participation of public health and visiting nurses, police, clergy, institutional staff, and many others.

Since about one half of problem drinkers are in the preaddict stage, special effort should be made to reach them as early as possible for attempts at prevention of progression. Another 30% of problem drinkers are in the early acute addict stage. This group probably represents the combination of the most accessible and potentially most susceptible to rehabilitation. Treatment centers, providing a spectrum of therapies using the services of A.A., internists, psychiatrists, sociologists, and others, should be available especially for those in the early acute stage. Provision should be made for individual counseling, group therapy, medical treatment as required, and hospital referral if indicated. Increasing use has been made of the drug disulfiram (Antabuse), which taken orally produces no effect unless alcohol is subsequently used. In such an event, acetaldehyde is formed and causes severe nausea, vomiting, increased pulse rate, and decreased blood pressure. This should be prescribed and used only under medical guidance and, if at all possible, should be combined with psychotherapy.

Concurrent with treatment, steps should be initiated for the other aspects of rehabilitation, that is, social, familial, religious, economic, and the like. In the process, the patient's family, especially the spouse, should not be overlooked. The importance of the spouse has been emphasized by Lewis,[39] as follows:

When the wife of an alcoholic remarries, she very often remarries an alcoholic. We often see reciprocal relationships between the alcoholic and his spouse, and as an

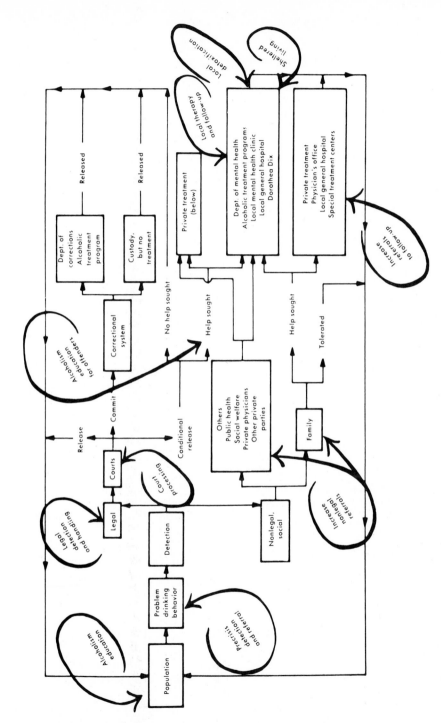

FIG. 26-1. Points of intervention in the public-private system for dealing with problem drinkers. (From the Regional Alcoholism Systems Project, Raleigh, N.C., 1971, South-Central Mental Health Region.)

alcoholic improves the adjustment of the spouse deteriorates. Strange as it may seem, the spouse is often ambivalent about her alcoholic husband's recovery; she frequently derives neurotic satisfaction, which may be unconscious, from his alcoholic binges. The inadequacy of her husband makes her feel needed and more adequate. . . . Wives often resent their alcoholic husband's therapists whom they see as threatening their control of their husbands. A part of this psychological mechanism between husband and wife is the nagging and the pressure which the wife puts on her alcoholic husband, making him feel more inadequate and thus less likely to stop drinking.

Many male alcoholics do tend to exhibit some degree of an Oedipus complex, and not infrequently their wives play the role of the long-suffering but protective mother figure. Literature on female alcoholics, on the other hand, indicates that they have strong emotional conflicts about their womanliness; they have been described[40] as having "a fragile sense of feminine adequacy"; and when confronted with self-doubts, they turn to alcohol in an attempt to gain artificial feelings of womanliness. Steinglass and Weiner,[41] however, have raised the interesting question of "whether the marital structure is the result of the preexisting needs of each partner or the result of stress placed upon the marriage by the introduction of drinking behavior essentially after the fact." To the extent that this may be true, the emphasis perhaps should be not so much on the alcoholic per se as on the quality and form of the marriage.

Suggestions made for meeting this situation are to align oneself with the spouse's positive motivations, to urge the spouse to join Alanon, a group of spouses of A.A. members, or if possible to get the spouse to accept some psychiatric consultation to better understand the other partner's problem and the spouse's own relationship to it.

PREVENTION

The development of most cases of alcoholism is so insidious and the causative factors so complex and often buried in the individual's past that prevention is difficult. Experience has shown that prohibition of alcoholic beverages by law is impractical. Even if it could be achieved, the maladjustments and inferiorities that give rise to alcoholism in the presence of alcohol would still be there. In a utopian world the elimination of these underlying factors might be anticipated, but under existing conditions this is too much to hope for.

Nevertheless, increasing attention to mental health, the greater equalization of social and economic opportunity, and more understanding parents may make some inroads. In the practical sense, however, it would appear that the best chance for prevention still lies along the path of education. This should have as its goal a willingness and ability to discuss, study, and deal with alcoholism and its precursors frankly, dispassionately, and intelligently toward the end of combatting the development of the precursors and of seeking patterns of behavior other than hiding behind the screen of an alcoholic haze. Unfortunately, often this approach is not followed.[42,43] Furthermore, it is pointless for an uninformed teacher to utter prohibitory preachments to students about drinking when they know that they themselves, their own families and friends, and society in general partake of alcoholic beverages to some extent. Far better for an informed teacher to present the realities of living and on that basis to discuss its risks and why and how they may be avoided.

Earlier it is stated that one of the most important needs is to recognize alcoholism for what it really is—a disease. Paradoxically, this is still lacking to a considerable degree in the medical profession.[44] Surprisingly few schools of medicine teach to any consequential extent about alcoholism. Many physicians and, indeed, many public health workers still regard alcoholics as socially undesirable misfits who refuse to pull themselves together. If physicians and public health workers cannot face the problem honestly and properly, how can anyone else?

A few recent events serve to emphasize the point. Only within the past few years have some hospitals begun to take alcoholics on their general wards. Only within the past few years have hospitalization insurance organizations begun to pay for hospitalization because of alcoholism. Even now, only about one half of such organizations do so and benefits vary widely despite the fact that in 1958 the House of Delegates of the American Medical Association unanimously passed a resolution stating that alcoholism is a disease that should be treated by a physician in a hospital when necessary. Its Committee on Alcoholism prepared a manual on alcoholism,[45] which was distributed to all physicians. Also it urged the development of uniform legislation dealing with alcoholism based on scientific fact. This has since been done by the National Conference of Commissioners on Uniform State Laws.[46] The American Medical Association also urges hospitalization insurance organizations to allow hospital benefits for alcoholism; and most important, with its Committee on Professional Education, the Association works toward the much-needed improvement in the teaching of alcoholism as a disease in the nation's medical schools. It is encouraging to note that most schools of public health as well as many schools of nursing and social work have followed suit. In the meantime other organizations, such as the Toronto Addiction Foundation and the U.S. Naval Medical Centers at San Diego and Long Beach, California, have moved successfully into the field of nonmedical treatment of the alcoholic. Obviously, an enlightened and progressive viewpoint by all health-related professionals is crucial to the amelioration of this severe health and social problem.

REFERENCES

1. Alcoholism in the United States, Ann. Am. Acad. Polit. Soc. Sci. **315**:1 (entire issue), Jan. 1958.
2. Cross, J.N.: Guide to the community control of alcoholism, New York, 1968, American Public Health Association.
3. National Institute of Mental Health: Alcohol and alcoholism, PHS Pub. No. 1640, Washington, D.C., 1970.
4. First special report to the U.S. Congress on alcohol and health, DHEW Pub. No. (HSM) 72-9099, Rockville, Md., 1972.
5. Leake, C.D., and Silverman, M.: Alcoholic beverages in clinical medicine, Chicago, 1966, Year Book Medical Publishers, Inc.
6. Zabolai-Csekme, E.: Alcohol and women, World Health, Aug. 1981.
7. Gomberg, E.S.: Female alcoholic. In Tarter, R.E., and Sugerman, A.A., editors: Alcoholism, Reading, Mass., 1976, Addison-Wesley Publishing Co., Inc.
8. Cahalan, D., Cisin, I.H., and Crossley, D.: American drinking practices, Monograph No. 6, New Brunswick, N.J., 1969, Rutgers Center of Alcohol Studies.
9. Mulford, H.A.: Drinking and deviate drinking, U.S.A., 1963, Q. J. Stud. Alcohol **25**:634, 1964.
10. Gallup, G.: Political index; political, social, and economic trends, Princeton, N.J., 1966, American Institute of Public Opinion.
11. Health, United States, 1976-1977, DHEW Pub. No. (HRA) 77-1232, Washington, D.C., 1977, U.S. Government Printing Office.
12. Cisin, I.H., and Cahalan, D.: Some correlates of American drinking practices. In Mello, N.K., and Mendelsohn, J.H., editors: Recent advances in studies of alcoholism. DHEW Pub. No. (HSM) 71-9045, Rockville, Md., 1971, National Institute of Mental Health.
13. Presnall, L.F.: Quoted in Business Week, Sept. 21, 1963.
14. Jellinek, E.M.: Phases in the drinking history of alcoholics, Q. J. Stud. Alcohol **7**:1, 1946.
15. "Observer," and Maxwell, M.A.: A study of absenteeism, accidents, and sickness payments in problem drinkers in one industry. Q. J. Stud. Alcohol **20**:302, 1959.
16. Trice, H.M.: Work accidents and the problem drinker, I.L.R. Research, New York State School of Industrial and Labor Relations, Cornell University **3**:2, March 1957.
17. Loomis, T.A., and West, T.C.: The influence of alcohol on automobile driving ability, Q. J. Stud. Alcohol **19**:30, 1958.
18. McFarland, R.A.: The role of preventive medicine in highway accidents, Am. J. Public Health **47**:288, March 1957.
19. Runyan, D.K., and others: Determinants of foster care placement for the maltreated child, Am. J. Public Health **71**:706, July 1981.
20. Gayford, J.J.: Research on battered wives, J. Royal Soc. Health **95**(6):288, 1975.
21. MacDonald, J.M.: The murderer and his victim, Springfield, Ill., 1961, Charles C Thomas, Publisher.
22. Guttmacher, M.: The normal and sociopathic murderer. In Wolfgang, M., editor: Studies in homicide, New York, 1967, Harper & Row Publishers, Inc.
23. Tabachnick, N., and others: Comparative psychiatric study of accidents and suicidal deaths, Arch. Gen. Psychiatry **14**:60, Jan. 1966.
24. Weisman, A.D., and Kastenbaum, R.: The psychological autopsy: a study of the terminal phase of life, New York, 1968, Columbia University Press.
25. Mello, N.K., and Mendelson, J.H., editors: Recent advances in studies of alcoholism; an interdisciplinary symposium, DHEW Pub. No. (HSM) 71-9045, Rockville, Md., 1971, National Institute of Mental Health.
26. Bacon, S.D.: Alcoholism, nature of the problem, Federal Probation, vol. 11, No. 1, 1947.
27. Zimering, S., and Calhoun, J.F.: Is there an alcoholic personality? J. Drug Educ. **6**(2):97, 1976.
28. Brenner, M.H.: Trends in alcohol consumption and associated illnesses: some effects of economic changes, Am. J. Public Health **26**:1979, Dec. 1975.
29. Mendelson, J.H.: The fetal alcohol syndrome, Portland, Ore., 1979, Raleigh Hills Foundation.
30. Ulleland, C.W.: The offspring of alcoholic mothers, Ann. N.Y. Acad. Sci. **197**:167, May 25, 1972.

31. Jones, K.L., and Smith, D.W.: Recognition of the fetal alcohol syndrome in early infancy, Lancet **2:**999, Nov. 3, 1973.

32. Jones, K.L., and others: Outcome in offspring of chronic alcoholic women, Lancet **1:**1076, June 1, 1974.

33. Hanson, J.W., Jones, K.L., and Smith, D.W.: Fetal alcohol syndrome, J.A.M.A. **235:**1458, April 5, 1976.

34. Ouellette, E.M., and others: Adverse effects on offspring of maternal alcohol abuse during pregnancy. N. Engl. J. Med. **297:**528, Sept. 8, 1977.

35. Little, R.E.: Moderate alcohol use during pregnancy and decreased infant birth weight. Am. J. Public Health **67:**1154, Dec. 1977.

36. Roman, P., and Trice, H.: Strategies of preventive psychiatry and social reality: the case of alcoholism. In Roman, P., and others, editors: Sociological perspective on community mental health, Rockville, Md., 1974, National Institute on Alcohol Abuse and Alcoholism.

37. Vogel, S.: Psychiatric treatment of alcoholism, Ann. Am. Acad. Pol. Soc. Sci. **315:**99, Jan. 1958.

38. Holder, H.D., and Hallan, J.: Systems approach to planning alcoholism programs in North Carolina, Am. J. Public Health **62:**1415, Oct. 1972.

39. Lewis, J.A.: Alcoholism, Am. J. Nurs. **56:**433, April 1956.

40. Wilsnack, S.C.: Impact of sex roles and women's alcohol use and abuse. In Greenblatt, M., and Schuckit, M.A., editors: Alcoholism problems in women and children, New York, 1976, Grune & Stratton, Inc.

41. Steinglass, P., and Weiner, S.: Familial interactions and determinants of drinking behavior. In Mello, N.K., and Mendelson, J.H., editors: Recent advances in studies of alcoholism, DHEW Pub. No. (HSM) 71-9045, Rockville, Md., 1971, National Institute of Mental Health.

42. Finn, P.: The role of attitudes in public school alcohol education, J. Alcohol Drug Educ. **20**(3):23, Spring 1975.

43. Milgram, G.: A historical review of alcohol education research and comments, J. Alcohol Drug Educ. **21**(2):1, Winter 1976.

44. Symposium article: Alcoholics face a "therapy gap," Am. Med. News **15:**8, Feb. 7, 1972.

45. Committee on Alcoholism of Council on Mental Health: Manual on alcoholism, Chicago, 1958, American Medical Association.

46. National Institute of Mental Health: Uniform Alcoholism and Intoxication Treatment Act. In Alcohol and health, DHEW Pub. No. (HSM) 72-9099, Rockville, Md., 1972.

CHAPTER 27

Substance abuse

Not poppy, nor mandragora,
Nor all the drowsy syrups of the world
Shall ever medicine thee to that sweet sleep
Which thou ow'dst yesterday.

Othello III. 3

WHAT ARE DRUGS?

Next to alcohol in prominence and historical discovery are the narcotizing alkaloids. More recently have been added certain substances that have been developed synthetically, usually for therapeutic purposes, such as the barbiturates and related drugs, amphetamines, and, to some extent, certain of the so-called tranquilizers, euphoriants, and ataractics.[1] To these may also be added the psychedelic or psychotomimetic drugs, natural and synthesized, of which mescaline, psilocybin, and lysergic acid diethylamide (LSD-25) are the best known.

Alkaloid-bearing plants were probably discovered very early. Because of the physiologic effects they produced, they soon became important adjuncts to social intercourse, religion, and politics and have played an important part in the literature of all cultures. Through the ages there has been much speculation about them, especially about certain of the psychic effects they produce. They seemed to release the usually pent-up spirit from the tangible body and allow it to wander freely. Sometimes these substances seemed to bring about the phenomenon of second sight. Some mystical results, coupled with the unusual appearance and behavior of the person affected, inevitably led to great wonder and awe, especially on the part of primitive peoples. From the beginning, therefore, although these substances appeared to be similar to other materials ingested such as food and drink, they were nevertheless considered different and special. Indeed, in many instances they were treated as sacred, to be prepared only by certain persons, and to be used only at certain times, such as festivities, religious events, or in instances of individual or group catastrophe.

As with alcoholism, the more severe types of drug abuse confront society with conditions that on the surface are somewhat misleading. Thus the alcoholic is often regarded as a weakling, lacking in self-control and self-respect. Similarly, the narcotic addict usually has been and still is considered depraved and a criminal. This has changed somewhat during recent years with the advent of the so-called drug culture, characterized by peer envy, approval, and imitation.[2] This phenomenon has affected the affluent, educated, and adult components of American and other societies as well as the young and the socioeconomically disadvantaged.

DEFINITION

The World Health Organization's Expert Committee on Addiction-Producing Drugs[3] considered it important to distinguish between drug habituation and drug addiction. It defined *drug habituation* as "a condition resulting from the repeated consumption of a drug," and listed its characteristics as (1) a desire (but not a compulsion) to continue taking the drug for the sense of improved well-being it engenders, (2) little or no tendency to increase the doses, (3) some degree of psychic dependence on the effect of the drug but absence of physical dependence hence of withdrawal or abstinence symptoms, and (4) detrimental effects, if any, primarily on the individual. The majority of affinities to synthetic drugs fall in this category.

On the other hand, the committee defined *drug addition* as "a state of periodic or chronic intoxication produced by the repeated consumption of a drug (natural or synthetic)," and listed its characteristics as (1) an overpowering desire or need (compulsion) to continue taking the drug and to obtain it by any means, (2) a tendency to develop tolerance or decreased effect hence a tendency to increase the dose, (3) a psychic (psychologic) and usually a physical dependence on the effects of the drug, and (4) detrimental effects not only on the individual but also on society. The narcotizing alkaloids and certain synthetic drugs are included. It should be pointed out that the World Health Organization considers alcohol as intermediate between the addiction-producing and the habit-forming drugs. It points out that alcoholism and drug addiction have certain similarities but also certain important differences. Thus the severe symptoms that occur on withdrawal of alcohol can be more dangerous to the individual than those that occur when morphine, for example, is withheld. On the other hand, it takes much longer to develop tolerance to and dependence on alcohol than is the case with narcotics. Also, treatment of alcoholism is much more successful than is treatment of narcotic addiction.[4]

REASONS FOR DRUG USE

The use and misuse of drugs, especially alkaloids, is not new. No culture is without a substance to chew, swallow, inhale, or smoke to transform feelings about reality. Some have been used for many centuries without legal or social restrictions, and on several occasions international strife has resulted from attempts to curtail their open sale and use. It is also interesting to note that in the past, stronger sanctions existed against certain substances that are now accepted than against some substances that are now considered dangerous. Thus in the seventeenth century in various parts of Europe and western Asia the use of tobacco invited flogging, slitting of the lips, life imprisonment, and in some instances even the death penalty. It is notable that none of these severe punishments stopped the use of tobacco. Even tea and coffee were regarded as evil and dangerous. Lewis,[5] a professor emeritus of psychiatry at the University of London, described the attitude that existed in many places as recently as the beginning of the twentieth century.

The results of excessive coffee are painted in alarming colours: "The sufferer is tremulous and loses his self-command; he is subject to fits of agitation and depression. He has a haggard appearance.... As with other such agents, a renewed dose of the poison gives a temporary relief, but at the cost of future misery." Tea is no better: "tea has appeared to us to be especially efficient in producing nightmares with hallucinations which may be alarming in their intensity. Another peculiar quality of tea is to produce a strange and extreme degree of physical depression. An hour or two after breakfast at which tea has been taken a grievous sinking may seize upon a sufferer, so that to speak is an effort. The speech may become weak and vague. By miseries such as these, the best years of life may be spoilt."

The writers quoted were eminent in their days, one a regius professor at Cambridge, another a leading British pharmacologist. Their attitude toward the use of opium presents an interesting contrast, one not at all uncommon in America as well as in Britain and the European continent at that time. They wrote:

Opium is used, rightly or wrongly, in many oriental countries, not as an idle or vicious indulgence, but as a reasonable aid in the work of life. A patient of one of us took a grain of opium in a pill every morning and every evening for the last fifteen years of a long, laborious and distinguished career. A man of great force of character, concerned in affairs of weight and of national importance and of stainless character, he persisted in this habit as being one which gave him no conscious gratification or diversion, but which toned and strengthened him for his deliberations and engagements.

Somewhat similar is the age-old practice of chewing coca leaves by the Indians of the Andes. It is estimated that 6 million, or 2 out of every 5, persons of all ages in that area indulge in this habit. There is some slight stimulating and sometimes a mild hallucinatory effect, but essentially the slow, sustained release of a small amount of cocaine makes possible a tolerance of a depressing existence and an ability to perform otherwise exhausting work at physiologically antagonistic altitudes and temperatures. Indeed, when its common use in the Andes became known, laudatory articles appeared in several leading medical journals both in England and America recommending its use for everything from tuberculosis to impotence.[6]

Without at all intending to minimize the great significance of the problem, it must be recognized that not all drug users are necessarily addicts any more than all people who drink alcohol are alcoholics. It is important to recognize further that there is nothing new about drug use, even common drug use. Addiction, predominantly to opiates and morphine, became prevalent among Civil War veterans who had been administered large amounts of these narcotics in relation to their severe battle wounds and amputations. In fact, morphine addiction was referred to as "the army disease." Ironically, both cocaine and heroin, which were considered to be nonaddictive, were deliberately introduced later as substitutes for morphine.[7]

It is well to realize that it was not until the second decade of this century that serious steps began to be taken against the free and common use even of narcotics. As Brotman and Freedman[8] have pointed out, it is estimated, for example, that in 1910 in the United States narcotics, predominantly opium and cocaine, were used by 1% to 4% of the population, predominantly men, among whom the incidence of use was therefore about 10%. These materials could be openly purchased over the counter with no restrictions in grocery stores and pharmacies. It should also be remembered that into the 1920s many cough syrups, products for soothing babies, headache remedies, and "tonics" for female ailments as well as several popular drinks contained narcotic substances, sometimes in significant amounts.

There are actually many and sometimes complex reasons for drug use and abuse. Addiction that results from medication to relieve severe pain has been mentioned. In this connection it has been pointed out that whereas the pain that led to addiction in the last century was usually physical, today it is mainly psychic. Most of today's addicted persons appear to have discovered that drugs relieve their anxieties, tensions, feelings of inadequacy, and other emotional conditions with which they cannot cope in a normal way. Peculiarly, although it was logically anticipated that a generally improved standard of living and a reduction of poverty would eliminate escape phenomena such as drug abuse and addictions, the opposite seems to have occurred. Under circumstances in which changes are rapid and the beliefs, customs, and values of yesterday are attacked and eroded, affluence allows the time and funds to support drug excesses. When it is no longer necessary to work as much for the necessities of life, some people develop problems of leisure. If one has no viable goals and no motivation or drive to create, to study, or to help others, or is denied the opportunity to do so, one may become

bored or alienated and vulnerable to the temptation of using artificial substitutes.

Some of the factors involved in the recent increase in drug use are as follows[9]:

1. The widespread belief that "medicine" can magically solve problems
2. The easy access to drugs of various sorts in an affluent society and the profit reaped in supplying them
3. Enjoyment of the euphoria or excitement induced by drugs
4. "Peer pressure" which leads an individual, especially a young one, to conform to current styles in dress, behavior, entertainment, and drugs
5. A search for sharpened perception and heightened creativity which some persons believe they obtain from mind-altering drugs
6. The use of drugs, especially marihuana and cocaine, in a social context, with a role similar to that of alcohol
7. The numbers of young people who are dissatisfied or disillusioned, or who have lost faith in the prevailing social system
8. The tendency of persons with psychological problems to seek easy solutions with chemicals
9. The statements of proselytizers who proclaim the "goodness" of drugs
10. A lack of alternatives which appear meaningful to "counter culture"

CLASSIFICATION OF DRUG ABUSERS

Yost[10] has classified drug addicts into the following three groups, to which a fourth may be added:

1. Emotionally well-adjusted individuals who take addicting drugs on medical advice for treatment of pain, sleeplessness, and the like. After protracted use they find they cannot get along without them. This type constitutes only 5 in 1,000 of those hospitalized at the Public Health Service Hospitals at Lexington, Ky., and Fort Worth, Tex.

2. Neurotics who turn to drugs because drugs make them forget their feelings of inadequacy, fear, and the like, making them feel better and more normal, either physically or mentally or both. These constitute the largest group of drug abusers.

3. Psychopaths who take drugs in a deliberate search for thrills and "kicks." This is probably the smallest group numerically.

4. Otherwise relatively normal individuals, usually adolescents, who try narcotics to maintain face

with the group. This would appear to be a variable group, its numbers depending considerably on variations and fluctuations in group behavior and fads and on the extent of law enforcement and availability of supplies.

Yost applies the apt phrases of "addiction prone" to the second and third categories (neurotics and psychopaths) and "accidental addicts" to the first group. As might be expected and in line with the experience with alcohol, the first and fourth categories of addicts present the least important and least difficult part of the problem and are much more susceptible to rehabilitation because undesirable underlying personality and social problems are generally absent. The second and third categories, neurotics and psychopaths, present the core of the problem of addiction in terms of numbers and presence of personality insufficiencies, hence difficulty of cure.

With regard to the type of person who is apt to become an addict, a study in 1951 of 260 boys and girls admitted to Bellevue Hospital in New York City is illuminating. It was concluded that there was a striking uniformity in personalities and backgrounds of the boys. The subjects were all nonaggressive and used passive techniques that gave a superficial appearance of ease and poise. Their interpersonal relationships were weak and superficial, with the notable exception of their relationships with their mothers. They had many acquaintances but few friends, but their relationships with their mothers were extremely close. Often they were their mother's favorite. Many had chosen definitely domestic types of occupations such as cooking or tailoring.

In more recent years there appears to have developed a reversal of this essentially complacent and introverted prototype. The usual and normal level of conflict between adolescents and adults has risen to a high pitch as standards and established social institutions have been increasingly challenged and attacked by the young. It would appear that one manifestation of this has been the use of drugs as familial and social defiance.[11] This is illustrated by the typical new user in Washington, D.C., described by Dupont[12] as "a 17 year old unmarried, unemployed, black male with a criminal record at the time of onset of heroin use." This picture, he says, has been fairly constant all across the United States, the only variation being the racial composition of the user population in different regions.

This fact suggests that drugs are now typically used as a way to cope with psychologic stresses that did not exist a few decades ago. Thus among the factors that are commonly observed in individual drug dependency are underachievement, loneliness, mistrust and fear of closeness, identity problems, social conflicts, the dependence-versus-independence struggle, rebellion, aggressive feelings, and self-destructive tendencies.[13] In other words, the addicted individual often may begin to use drugs not as an escape as much as from frustrated yearnings to be accepted by a society that appears to have rejected him. This is particularly true of young addicts in socioeconomically deprived localities. Substantiating this is an analysis[14,15] in Portland, Ore., of an array of social factors in relation to adolescent drug use. Significant positive association was identified with regard to broken families, low income, adult crime, substandard housing, low valuation of owner-occupied dwelling, and extent of rented occupancy. Obviously most of these are interrelated as well as related to other problems or indices of low socioeconomic status. Significantly, surveys of high school students indicate that they make a sharp distinction between marijuana and more serious drugs. Over two thirds strongly disapprove the regular use of the more serious drugs, but the same proportion approve or are neutral about the use of marijuana. This is also indicated by a study of self-reported use of various drugs during and immediately after high school (Table 27-1).[16]

Table 27-2 presents in condensed form some of the characteristics and effects of various narcotics and drugs that are considered later in this chapter. Alcohol is included for comparison and because it is actually a drug.

NARCOTIC ADDICTION
Extent and cost of the problem

It is very difficult or impossible to determine the extent of narcotic addiction. One must bear in mind the variations through time and place of definition, drug types and concentrations, willingness and methods of reporting, length of time of usage, treatment acceptance and success, and many other factors. For example, current estimates of the prevalence of heroin addiction in the United States range from about 150,000 to over 500,000. Much depends on the biases of those who do the surveying or calculation. The higher figures are estimates based on limited or biased surveys, extrapolations from overdose deaths or numbers of arrests, or on amounts of narcotics known or thought to have entered the country. This, of course, ignores the facts that many individuals use narcotics only once, a few times, or sporadically, that some who use them more often are not necessarily addicted, and that some persons who may be classified as addicts still continue as useful, productive members of society.

As an example of the undependability of data in this field, whereas the federal Bureau of Narcotics and Dangerous Drugs in the late 1960s counted 32,000 "known" narcotic addicts in the state of New York, the New York State Narcotic Control Commission reported about 60,000 addicts, essentially the same figure given by the federal agency for the nation as a whole. Furthermore, a careful survey at about the same time by the New York City Addiction Service Agency concluded that there were about 100,000 narcotic addicts *in New York City alone*. One reasonably firm figure is the 1,259 narcotic-related deaths that occurred in New York City during 1971. This represented an increase from 311 such deaths in 1961 and constituted the leading cause of death in persons between 15 and 35 years of age in that city. A recent report of the

United Nations Fund for Drug Abuse Control estimates about 620,000 active heroin addicts in the United States, about one half of whom live in New York state.

It is impossible to make even a crude guess as to what drug addiction costs society. Included should be the loss or decrease of production by those afflicted; the costs of hospitals, enforcement agencies, and prisons; losses from crime stimulated by the search for money with which to purchase drugs; the costs of accidents and illnesses connected with the use of drugs; and the cost of the drugs themselves.

Most opium, which is the raw source of heroin, morphine, and codeine, is grown in Asia and the Middle East. Large amounts are sold illicitly each year. North America, and especially the United States, is the principal consumer of both the legitimate (morphine) and illegitimate (heroin) refined products. It is estimated that less than one tenth of the amount destined for the United States is seized each year by all enforcement agencies.

The Permanent Central Narcotics Board of the United Nations Economic and Social Council has pointed out that raw opium sells for $30 to $40 per kilogram in areas where there is little control and about 10 times that where there is risk of discovery. Hence the value of the 1,500 or more tons of illicit

TABLE 27-1. Self-reported usage rates during high school years and the year following: results of a national longitudinal study

Drug	During high school		Year after high school	
	Any use (%)	Weekly use (%)	Any use (%)	Weekly use (%)
Marijuana or hashish	21	6	34	10
Hallucinogens	7	1	11	1
Amphetamines	10	2	14	2
Barbiturates	6	1	9	1
Heroin	2	1	2	1
Alcoholic beverages	81	33	89	44
Cigarettes*	66	36	68	41

*Daily cigarette use.

TABLE 27-2. Characteristics of narcotics and drugs

	Slang names	Description
Alcohol (sedative)	Booze, liquor, cocktail, nightcap, moonshine, white lightning, mountain dew, firewater	Liquid, made through natural process by the fermentation of sugars and starches
Amphetamines, or uppers (stimulant)	Bennies, dexies, hearts, speed, pep pills, wake-ups, uppers, copilots, meth	Capsules or pills in a variety of shapes and colors; bitter taste, odorless
Barbiturates, or downers (depressant)	Peanuts, barbs, goof balls, red devils, yellow jackets, rainbows, blue devils, spacers, downers	Capsules or pills in a variety of shapes and colors; bitter taste, odorless
Cocaine (anesthetic)	Snow, dust, flake, stardust, girl, Corine, Cecil, C, coke	White, flaky powder, bitter, odorless; numbs lips and tongue
Codeine (mild depressant)	C, poppys, school boy	Liquid, ingredient in cough medicine
Hallucinogens (includes LSD, STP, DMT, psilocybin, PCP, etc.)	Acid, cubes, sugar, pearly gates, heavenly blue, royal blue, DOM, serenity, tranquillity, peace, angel dust	White crystalline powder or a tasteless, odorless, colorless liquid that can be placed on any type of tablet, capsule, or transporting agent
Heroin (analgesic-depressant; narcotic made from morphine)	Horse, H, smack, white stuff, joy powder, junk, dope, goods, hard stuff, heavy stuff	White (or possibly brown) powder, packed in paper bundles or balloons; bitter taste, vinegar-like odor
Marijuana (*Cannabis sativa;* hallucinogen, stimulant)	Pot, grass, weed, hashish, joint, stick, reefer, roach, Mary Jane, rope, ashes, jive, hay, loco, sweet Lucy, gaga, griefo, bhang	Greenish-brown plant material, coarsely ground, powdered leaf; weedy, burned-rope odor
Mescaline (hallucinogenic drug from peyote cactus)	Peyote, mescal, mesc, buttons	Powder made from cactus plant top; bitter, odorless
Morphine (analgesic narcotic)	Junk, morpho, morphie, Miss Emma, white stuff, hard stuff, dope, goods, stuff, Big M	Bitter white powder or tablets
Solvents (includes glue, paint thinner, gasoline, etc.; volatile chemicals)	Sniffing	Any volatile substance whose fumes are capable of producing an intoxicating effect, such as glue, paint thinner, gasoline, lighter fluid, air fresheners

Effects	How used	Medical use
Slurred speech, incoordination, confusion, tremors, drowsiness, agitation, nausea, respiratory depression; continued use can damage the liver and enlarge and weaken the heart	Orally	For mild sedation and appetite stimulation
Excitability, rapid and unclear speech, restlessness, tremors, insomnia, sweating, dry mouth, bad breath, itchy nose, dilated pupils; continued use results in increased pulse and blood pressure, hallucinations, psychoses	Usually orally or by injection (speed)	For weight reduction, mild depression, narcolepsy
Similar to alcohol intoxication: drowsiness, confusion, incoordination, tremors; continued use results in depressed pulse and blood pressure, possible convulsions	Orally or by injection	For sedation and sleep, analgesic for minor pain; sometimes used as anesthetic for minor surgery
Excitability, talkativeness, headache, nausea; continued use results in increased blood pressure and pulse rate, possible hallucinations and violent or dangerous behavior	Usually sniffed or injected	Has been used (very rarely now) for local anesthesia in oral-nasal surgery
Drowsiness, pinpoint pupils, stupor, sometimes nausea develops; continued use develops a tolerance to drug	Orally	To relieve pain, coughing
Trance, anxiety, confusion, tremors, euphoria, depression, dilated pupils, increased pulse rate and blood pressure; continued use may result in psychoses, possible chromosomal breakdown and organic brain damage	Orally, dissolved on sugar cubes, tablets, stamps, etc., and swallowed or licked; can be injected for faster high; DMT is often smoked in pipe or cigarette	None, LDS has been used for psychiatric experimentation
Relaxation, drowsiness, confusion, euphoria, slurred speech, flushing of skin or face, nausea, constricted pupils, respiratory depression; continued use results in scars or abscesses at injection points	Dissolved in water and injected, called skin popping or mainlining; sometimes sniffed	None in the United States
Euphoria, dizziness, excitability, hallucinations, increased appetite, dryness of mouth, increased pulse and blood pressure, nausea	Usually made into cigarettes (joints) and smoked; sometimes sniffed or swallowed (baked in cookies)	None
Resembles LSD effects: distortion of senses, anxiety, confusion, tremors, euphoria, depression, dilated pupils, increased pulse rate, psychoses, and possible hallucinations	Orally, powder form in capsule	None
Lethargy, drowsiness, confusion, euphoria, slurred speech, flushing of skin, nausea, constricted pupils, respiratory depression; continued use results in scars or abscesses at injection points	Dissolved in water and injected, or sometimes used orally	For relief of pain
Similar to alcohol intoxication: slurred speech, blurred vision, incoordination; ringing in ears, nausea, and vomiting; continued use results in psychoses, hallucinations, liver and blood damage, respiratory depression	Inhaled; fumes from the glue tubes are inhaled by the user after the glue has been squirted into a sack or paper bag	None

raw opium is between $40 and $400 million. But when processed into heroin, it brings thousands of dollars per ounce. Another way of emphasizing the profit, or markup, is that the true cost of 1 kilogram (2.2 pounds) of heroin is about the same as 1 kilogram of potatoes. When it ultimately reaches the street, where it is sold, it is worth more than $50,000. This, of course, is why traffic in illicit narcotics has attracted the criminal classes in various countries and why dealers in illicit drugs so frequently encourage free trials to get additional sure customers "on the hook." Once an addict is hooked, it has been estimated that the average cost of supporting the habit is more than $200 per day. One hard drug addict is worth thousands of dollars per year to a "pusher." Where does the confirmed addict obtain the necessary funds, especially if addiction affects the ability to work? Essentially the source of funds is illegal—theft, prostitution, or pandering. About one half of all street crime in the United States is attributed to addicts, and the Drug Abuse Council[17] has estimated that heroin addicts in the United States steal from $1 to $2 billion annually.

Effects of narcotics

Each narcotic produces certain characteristic effects. Generally speaking, they all cause general stimulation, euphoria, and contentment, with release from pain or concerns that arise from worries, neuroses, and conflicts. Various sensory manifestations occur, such as a tingling of the skin, hallucinations, and feelings of ecstasy. All these pleasures, of course, are of temporary and short duration, for which the addict pays a high price in continued and progressive misery. Contrary to popular opinion, although these substances act generally as stimulants, they depress certain functions, notably the sexual drive. Continued use produces a considerable loss of appetite, resulting in weight loss and nutritional disorders; the typical addict is thin, wan, and undernourished. Severe constipation is common, as is severe itching. The addict suffers from nervousness, insomnia, and depression, and suicidal attempts are not uncommon, especially during the typical postjag depression. Because of the anxiousness of the addict to experience the drug and because dilution by those who sell it is so common, the addict frequently does not know

how much is being taken. As a result, serious toxic reactions and even death may occur from an overdose. This is the most deadly complication of narcotic addiction. It is estimated to kill 1% of New York's addicts each year.

Even when not lethal, heroin excess can cause pulmonary congestion, edema, and fibrosis. Most complications, however, are caused not by the effects of the drug but by infections introduced through a contaminated needle or solution.[18,19] Prominent among these are viral hepatitis, bacterial endocarditis, pneumonia, syphilis, malaria, bacteremia, and various skin and subcutaneous infections at the site of injection. Viral hepatitis, occasionally fatal and frequently recurrent and severe, was observed in 42 out of 100 reported complications among New York addicts. Almost equally prevalent was bacterial endocarditis caused by a variety of microorganisms, the most common being *Staphylococcus aureus*. Contrary to the usual type of endocarditis, that of the heroin addict does not spare healthy valves or the tricuspid valve. Because of lowered resistance and malnutrition, the addict is much more susceptible than the average person to many other infections and organic diseases. Furthermore, one effect of the drug is to dull awareness to pain, fever, and other symptoms. All told, life expectancy is greatly shortened. Dramatic illustration of this is found in a 4-year follow-up study of 3,324 daily opioid users, both black and white, throughout the United States. Their death rate during the follow-up period was 15.2 per 1,000 person-years at a risk. When rates were adjusted for age, they were from 3 to 14 times higher than comparable age groups in the general United States population. Although deaths were attributable to a variety of causes, over three fourths of deaths among younger addicts were drug related or involved violence.[20]

The most unfortunate effect of narcotics is what they do to the morale, morals, and social behavior of those so unfortunate as to become addicted to them. The typical narcotic addict lives only for the next drug experience; nothing else really matters. As a result, anything will be forfeited to obtain the drug—job, social position, family, self-respect. The addict will beg, borrow, or steal to satisfy the craving, and considering the combination of lowered ability to earn and the high daily cost of the required drugs, much petty crime results. Male addicts commonly turn to picking pockets, shoplifting, burglary, dishonest gambling, and pandering. Women and girls frequently become prostitutes. Very frequently the addict becomes a willing "pusher" of the drug, the riskiest link in the delivery chain, to assure his or her own supply.

A particularly tragic consequence of heroin addiction has become evident within the past few years. Because of the increased prevalence of the use of this narcotic among women of childbearing age, an increasing number of infants are being affected. During the 9 years, 1960 through 1969, 384 infants were born to 382 heroin-addicted mothers in a New York hospital.[21] About one half of the infants weighed less than 2,500 grams. During the first 4 days of life, 259 of the infants had withdrawal signs, 178 of them severe enough to require treatment with chlorpromazine. Fourteen infants died during the neonatal period, 9 of them during the first 9 hours after birth. Most disturbing has been a sharp increase in such births, with more than 500 addicted infants born in New York City during 1970, increasing to over 1,000 in 1977.

Epidemiology

As with infectious disease or any other human malfunction, the problem of narcotic addiction may be approached from an epidemiologic point of view. This was well illustrated by Jacobziner[22] in connection with the program in the New York City school health program. In reviewing it, he said the following:

An epidemic of narcotic addiction must be studied in the same manner as any other outbreak of a communicable disease. The agent, host, and environment and their impact and interrelationship must be studied and investigated. In an epidemic of narcotic addiction the *agent* is perhaps of far lesser significance than the *host* and *environment*. It should be emphasized that drug addiction is not a primary disease entity, but merely symptomatic of an underlying deep-seated disturbance: narcotic addiction being only one of many forms of social maladjustment. Narcotic users are not definitely psychopathic, but in the main, products of an unhealthy and an unhappy environment. Therefore, the underlying causes and motivations must be investigated, discovered, and understood. It is not the *process of addiction* which is important to know, but what causes an adolescent to use a drug or to become socially maladjusted. . . . Two factors are needed for the production of addiction: There must be a vulnerable soil—the individual or host must suffer from a psychological or emotional disturbance—and the drug or agent must be capable of resolving the conflicts, tensions, and anxieties of the maladjusted individual.

The validity of this approach has been illustrated by Hughes and his associates[23] in relation to an almost classic epidemic of heroin addiction in the south side of Chicago.

From the standpoint of general and statistical epidemiology, a predilection for the young-adult component of the population is evident. The most susceptible age group since the end of World War II until the early 1960s was from 15 to 30 years, but the past decade has shown a downward shift to even younger ages of inception. Although males outnumber females (85% to 15%), it is interesting that the difference is not as great as among alcoholics. Narcotic addiction tends to be concentrated in large cities. New York City, Chicago, Washington, D.C., and Los Angeles account for over half of the nation's cases. In New York City, 60% to 70% of narcotic addicts are black, Puerto Rican, or Mexican-American; about 85% are males between 15 and 35 year of age; and from 40% to 60% also use amphetamines or barbiturates regularly. There is a tendency for narcotic addiction to coincide with substandard conditions that accompany or result from a low socioeconomic status. In this sense addiction becomes just another trap within a complex of traps.

The import of this was illustrated by an analysis of a sample of 400 individuals, in this instance in Chicago.[24] As the investigators summarized: "The potential for addiction is widely spread through the children of the migrants in the deprived areas of the city, and the ultimate use of drugs by any specific individual depends on many fortuitous circumstances. The high rates of mental disease, alcoholism and other social pathologies which are sown by thwarted desires are the harvest of the same social conditions." And to emphasize the infectiousness of these situations, they pointed out that the addict in such an environment becomes dehumanized and brutalized and in turn dehumanizes and brutalizes others. The terrible end result is indicated by the fact that in the addict population studied, the average addict between the ages of 10 and 25 years had spent 15% of his life in prison and that there was every indication that these persons would continue to spend about 2 months out of every year in a prison setting. They concluded that: "Once the addict enters the cyclical pattern of arrest, incarceration, release, and readdiction, the resultant personality makes the addict's role practically irreversible except through certain specific modes of therapeutic intervention, 'burning out' and/or active involvement in social change." It is the possibility of the alternatives to which attention is now turned.

Approach to the problem

Initially and traditionally, attempts to combat the narcotic problem in the United States have been based on legislation, prohibition, judicial action, and punishment. Simrell[7] has detailed the sequence of events well. A few highlights may be of interest. Police action goes back to 1885. In 1909 Congress passed legislation "to prohibit the importation and use of opium for other than medicinal purposes," the latter undefined, but to be regulated by the Secretary of the Treasury. An international convention was called in 1912 in the Hague that not only considered control of international commerce in opiates but also included national obligations to control domestic manufacture, traffic, and use. The Hague convention of 1912 was eventually superseded by a new convention adopted by the United Nations in 1961. The United States withheld signature until 1967, when it felt secure that certain controls stipulated in the earlier convention would not be weakened. Meanwhile, Congress, to implement its agreement with the Hague convention, passed the Harrison Act of 1914, administered by the Department of Justice through the chief federal policing agency for criminal narcotics activities, the Bureau of Narcotics and Dangerous Drugs. Based essentially on the taxing power, it strictly limited the importation, production, sale, and use of opiates with the specific exemption of the use of narcotic drugs by a registered physician as part of medical care. Since then, Congress has taken several actions to broaden the base to include such concepts as United States international obligations and the promotion of the public health, safety, and welfare. Throughout, the fundamental administrative tool has been the exercise of criminal sanctions. In 1929, however, Congress enacted legislation that added four important responsibilities to the Public Health Service:

1. Treatment and rehabilitation of federally convicted narcotic drug addicts
2. Prevention of federal narcotics offenses by means of treatment and rehabilitation of voluntary patients
3. Encouragement and assistance to states and local communities to provide adequate and acceptable facilities and methods for the care of narcotic addicts
4. Research and training in the causes, diagnosis, treatment, control, and prevention of narcotic addiction

One result of this was the establishment by the Public Health Service of a specialized hospital at Lexington, Ky., in 1935 for the study, treatment, and rehabilitation of addicted prisoners, probationers, and voluntary patients in circumstances described as "less prison-like than most prisons and more prison-like than most hospitals." In 1938 a second hospital for this purpose was established at Fort Worth, Tex., but this was subsequently closed. These activities led eventually to the passage of the National Mental Health Act on July 3, 1946, and provided the genesis of the National Institute of Mental Health on April 1, 1949. This is now part of the Alcoholism, Drug Abuse, and Mental Health Administration of the Public Health Service. The responsibilities and potentials of the institute in the field of narcotic addiction were significantly expanded by the passage of the Narcotic Addict Rehabilitation Act of 1966, which established a national policy of civil commitment for treatment and aftercare of addicts even if they are charged with or convicted of violating federal criminal laws. Added to this was the Comprehensive Drug Abuse Prevention and Control Act of 1970, which provided funds for additional research into the causes and prevention of drug abuse and dependence; additional funds for treatment and rehabilitation of addicts; and strengthening of existing drug abuse law enforcement authority. It also provided for the establishment of a Commission on Marihuana and Drug Abuse to report to the President and Congress. Subsequently, in December 1970, the Drug Abuse Education Act was added, which authorized funds for public education about the problem.

Fundamental to any planned approach to the drug abuse problem is some method of determining prevalence on some ongoing basis. This is particularly difficult because of the very nature of the problem, the materials involved, and the vagaries of human nature. An important step was the establishment in 1972 of DAWN, the Drug Abuse Warning Network. This is a data-collecting system sponsored jointly by the National Institute of Drug Abuse of the Department of Health and Human Services and by the Drug Enforcement Administration of the Department of Justice. Data on episodes of drug abuse are provided by emergency rooms and inpatient units of nonfederal short-term general hospitals, by medical examiners or coroners, and by crisis intervention centers. Already, DAWN is providing a valuable measure not only of the prevalence of drug abuse but also of the changes and fluctuations through time.

In recent years there has been a considerable reexamination of attitudes and methods.[2,25] Increasingly the addict is being regarded separately and differently from those who promote addiction for substantial economic profit. There has been occurring a gradual shift from a national philosophy and approach based on punitive action against addicts, who had been assumed to be intrinsically evil, hence criminal, toward an acceptance of the addict as a sick victim of an unfortunate social and physiologic phenomenon. In the process more enlightened legislation has been appearing in relation to the addict concurrent with a constant tightening of law enforcement and judicial action against those who promote narcotic traffic, who are still and must continue to be regarded as criminals.[26]

Any program designed to attack the problem of narcotic addiction must be multipronged and involve the understanding and cooperation of many disciplines, that is, religion, law and law enforcement, and education, to mention only the most obvious. The most logical first step is case finding. Police and other law-enforcement personnel are probably the primary sources of case finding; physicians, hospitals, and health centers are the secondary source. In addition, public health and visiting nurses and social workers occasionally learn of addicts from patients and clients. Regardless of the circumstances, on discovery the addict should be regarded primarily as an ill person and not as a criminal. Instead of being treated in a punitive fashion, the addict should be admitted promptly to an outpatient treatment center, or if necessary, to a hospital for evaluation and appropriate medical and psychiatric treatment.

As to chances of cure, studies of patients after discharge from the Lexington hospital are far from encouraging. Usual experience is that 3 out of every 4 addicts relapse at some time. Frequently the road to ultimate cure involves several relapses. A study[27] of the 43,215 patients treated at Lexington between 1935 and 1966 showed a total of 77,076 admissions. Some returned as many as six times. The overall patient readmission rate was about 38%. For white male voluntary patients under 21 years, the rate was 53%. The readmission rate for those discharged as cured was 37%, whereas for those who left against medical advice before 31 days it was 40%, and for those who stayed longer it was 42%.

The high relapse rate points to the most difficult part of the problem, that is, rehabilitation and follow-up. An important part of treatment is to make the addict aware of the underlying reasons for the addiction to assist the addict in psychologic and social rehabilitation. Many investigators have emphasized the importance of qualified field personnel—public health nurses or social workers—who may obtain pertinent family and environmental background information about the patient. Repeated visits to the home and neighborhood environment are suggested, not only before and after the discharge of the patient but also before the patient's admission for treatment. In addition to the patient, the family and the community need to be reeducated and prepared for the return of the patient. With special reference to the adolescent, the importance of a good parent-child relationship is emphasized; parents must be made to understand that a poor quality of parent-child relationship is responsible for many forms of social maladjustment. Those close to the patient should be forewarned of the possibility of a relapse and warned not to castigate the patient if this should occur but to contact appropriate professionals or institutions as soon as possible.

A variety of rehabilitative groups and organizations have formed throughout the country, especially in centers of high addiction prevalence. These facilities, which are called "halfway houses" and other names, play an increasingly important role in assisting in the return to community life. Since a sence of inadequacy and failure often plays an important role, efforts should be made to assist the discharged patient in obtaining employment to develop a feeling of fulfillment and confidence. Much remains to be done toward development of a willingness on the part of most potential employers to give the expatient an opportunity and to provide encouragement whenever possible.

During the past few decades, there has been much controversy about the validity of the so-called British system, wherein drug addiction is handled primarily by specially licensed members of the medical profession with controlled legal distribution of drugs to those who use them. The premise is that by removing the profit motive, there is no temptation to resort to crime to obtain the drug and there is no incentive to create new addicts. Variations of this approach are followed in several other countries, and it has been advocated on a selective and demonstrative basis by the New York Academy of Medicine.[28] In 1977 the Ohio state legislature, and subsequently several other states, considered limited trial under close supervision. However, none have been able to meet the strict control conditions established by the several pertinent agencies.

In addition, many investigators object on the basis that the procedure removes the incentive for real cure. The Study Group on Treatment and Care of Drug Addicts,[29] called by the World Health Organization in November 1956, discouraged this approach: "While complete withdrawal of the drug of addiction might be deferred in certain circumstances, the maintenance of drug addiction is not treatment." Similar reservations were reiterated in other terms by the World Health Organization Expert Committee on Drug Dependence, which pointed to a significant rise in the number of known narcotic addicts since 1964. The World Health Organization Expert Committee also noted that the number of drug-related complications and crimes has increased, despite the system.[30] That this may correctly be attributed to the system or to more complex sociologic changes is debatable. During the period a number of societal changes, including increased delinquency, drug addiction, and crime, have occurred in many parts of the world. In any case, it must be recognized that there will always be some who must be maintained on the drug as a medical management problem.

Methadone. The most significant event that has occurred with relation to possible solution of the narcotic and especially the heroin problem was the discovery by Dole and Nyswander[31] in the early 1960s of the effectiveness of methadone hydrochloride in the treatment and rehabilitation of addicts. Methadone is a synthetic narcotic drug with many of the properties of heroin, morphine, and other opiate drugs. For example, taken either orally or intramuscularly it is a highly effective analgesic. However, there are several unique and important differences when it is used properly to treat chronic opiate addiction. It does not lose effectiveness when taken by mouth. Its effects are longer lasting; a single dose suppresses heroin withdrawal symptoms for 24 to 36 hours. It suppresses the action of other opiates without itself producing sedation or euphoria, hence the addict ceases to have obsessive and compulsive thoughts about or craving for opiate drugs. As a result, the individual can renew interest in normal life and can return to school, maintain employment, and present no social problems.

Although a dependence on methadone is substituted for the heroin dependence, the individual develops a tolerance to most of the effects of the drug, which is remarkably free of side effects or complications when used properly. Sensitivity to pain is normal, and there is even a normal response to intramuscular morphine if its use should be indicated for medical reasons. Sleep, digestion, alertness, reaction time, and libido usually become normal. Infants of methadone-dependent individuals are born normal. DuPont, and Katon[32] have described it as one of the most important medical discoveries of the twentieth century, adding that "like Fleming's discovery of penicillin and Enders' discovery of virus tissue culture techniques, the Dole-Nyswander discovery enabled physicians to deal constructively with a major health problem that was previously unsolvable."

Methadone was first used by its discoverers in 1963 in New York City. The enthusiasm that resulted from its initial success and the accompanying publicity led to a rapid spread of its use throughout the country. By mid-1972 more than 50,000 heroin addicts (an estimated one fifth to one third of the total) were receiving the drug in about 300 clinics throughout the country, most of which had long waiting lists. Unfortunately the enthusiasm and available funds exceeded the number of available qualified personnel.

Despite its wide acceptance and many advantages, the use of methadone is not without problems.[33] It has no usefulness against nonopiate drugs. Taken in large, uncontrolled doses it can produce undesirable reactions and even death. Because of this, early in 1973 the Food and Drug Administration placed strict limitations on the method and circumstances of its use. Methadone maintenance programs have been permitted to expand, but prescribing of the drug is limited to heroin addicts who have been drug dependent for at least 2 years and who are over the age of 18 years, except in special circumstances. Methadone must be administered in the presence of an attendant, and the privilege of taking it home is severely restricted. This, of course, presents a problem for the patient, since daily doses are required.

Methadone programs typically are two phased. Initially there is an inpatient detoxification phase, during which the addict is detoxified from heroin and stabilized on methadone. This is followed by the outpatient maintenance phase, which involves the patient reporting to the methadone clinic to take the orally administered drug. Dole and Nyswander, on the basis of their experience, have claimed that 80% of new patients need not be admitted to a hospital for the first phase but can be supervised on an ambulatory basis. DuPont and Katon[32] found that methadone was so effective that many patients could not conceive of wanting heroin again. This led them to believe that the patients could be detoxified. However, every patient detoxified had some recurrence of drug hunger and almost all either resumed methadone treatment or returned to heroin.

This necessarily directs attention to cost. Methadone itself is inexpensive. However, the addict must be maintained on methadone for the remainder of his or her life. This is the minor part of the cost, since the drug must be administered in a controlled center with high costs for administrative overhead and medical personnel. Using 1978 figures, it cost about $36,000 per year to support a heroin addict. Most of this came from robbery and theft. Since each addict not under treatment lives an average of 28 years, the total value of thefts, discounted at 8%, was about $400,000, which, it is assumed would be avoided with the addict on methadone. Furthermore, assuming a productive or earning life of 28 years at a constant average of $8,000 per year, again discounted at 8%, the value of the future productivity of the individual on methadone would be about $100,000. The life-time gain, therefore, at 1978 values, from a lifetime expenditure of about $70,000 for methadone maintenance would be about $430,000 per patient ($400,000 + $100,000 − $70,000).

It should be emphasized that methadone provides supportive maintenance, not cure of addiction to opiate derivatives. As such, it must be regarded as one of several methods of treatment including, for example, various psychologic, social, and nutritional supports. Meanwhile, research continues for other, more effective and efficient substances, not so much to replace methadone but to serve as adjuncts or supplements. Among these are the narcotic antagonists *levallorphan* and *nalorphine,* which are useful in the presence of a strong narcotic effect. Both, however, may produce certain central nervous system complications such as hallucinations. Another useful synthetic, *naloxone* is essentially free of undesirable effects. It is rapidly effective but short lasting, requiring repeated doses. These substances provide addicts with a temporary chemical crutch, blocking the euphoria but not the tolerance.

Preventive measures. With reference to general preventive measures, several points should be considered. First, certain legislation is necessary (1) to control strictly the importation, production, distribution, and sale of all drugs that potentially may cause addiction; (2) to provide adequate organization and financing for carrying out preventive activities; (3) to provide for severe punishment of those found guilty of the illicit importation, handling, and sale of narcotics; and (4) to allow for addicts who are apprehended to be turned over to suitable organizations or institutions for necessary treatment without court action.

In the psychologic arena a number of "self-regulating" communities have been developing, the first founded in 1958 in California. Their conceptual basis is that the use of drugs is a symptom of an underlying character disorder or emotional immaturity that requires a restructuring of the individual's character and personality. Typically, new members are given the most menial or degrading tasks, from which they may advance to more desirable roles and greater responsibilities. Drugs and violence are strictly forbidden, and criticisms and punishments are deliberately harsh. This is offset, however, by a unique form of group concern for the individual that is rarely if ever found on the outside. Some communities have the advantage of assistance from professionals in mental health and public health as well as various social agencies. The value of such communities is subject to question. In a sense, they substitute one type of escape from reality for another.

Obviously, more adequate public education is needed to bring about better understanding and cooperation on the part of all those in society who may play a role in attacking the problem. This applies to physicians, nurses, public health workers, teachers, clergy, police, welfare workers, and many others. Most authorities, however, believe strongly that direct propaganda to young people on the subject of narcotics is not only of no value but may be detrimental. Thus H.J. Anslinger, former U.S. Commissioner of Narcotics, believes that it may only serve to awaken the interest or stimulate the curiosity of potential adolescent addicts. Similarly Artis, supervisor of the Chicago office of the U.S. Bureau of Narcotics, has stated: "We do not recommend or promote direct education on narcotic drugs. In this conclusion, we agree with the conclusions of the 68 nations of the United Nations who passed a resolution on this subject. Narcotic education is open to controversy and great objections. We prefer to educate at the parent-teacher level."

Experience in a number of schools that used various direct approaches to students appears to substantiate these negative views. On the other hand, some carefully designed courses to inform teachers have produced very discouraging results. In a great many instances either their preset biases or their apparent fear to be involved negated the expert information provided.[34] The educational dilemma has been summarized very well by McKee[35]:

There is far more, then, to the dilemma of drug education/prevention than a matter of identification and labeling. Many facts (legal, economic, social, etc.) surrounding drug use are usually quite clear from both sides of the using/nonusing fence. But the problems' exact meaning to each side (and therefore the behavioral consequence) is not at all as apparent. At present, we have in many communities a rather large problem with very few citizens adequately educating themselves and with

equally few organizations providing quality education. Past experience indicates that unbiased, informal self-education is at best sporadic and infrequent. With few opportunities for more formal, qualified, and objective education, many if not most of our citizens will probably remain ignorant and/or myth-filled.

Beyond the activities of adequate legislation and education, it is to be anticipated that, as in the case of alcoholism, increased and improved methods in mental health and their wider availability and acceptability will play a significant part in the prevention and amelioration of the narcotic problem. Added to this are the benefits that are sure to result from constantly improving and equalizing social conditions and opportunities. These in the long run may remove many (but not all) of the underlying factors that lead some to escape unpleasant realities through the insidious medium of narcotics.

Public and official awareness and concern are illustrated by the dramatic increase in facilities relating to narcotic and drug abuse. Thus in 1962 only 28 states had programs. Eight were operated by state health departments and most of the rest by state departments of mental health. In cities with populations over 100,000, only 4 local health departments reported programs, whereas 11 cities had programs under auspices other than the health department. Only 5 years later, in 1967, 110 governmental and 55 nongovernmental programs existed. Only 12 states reported no program, and in the interval since, most of them have instituted activities. Two thirds of the facilities sponsored by governmental agencies were in hospitals or clinics, usually under a department of public health, mental health, or public welfare. Services provided consisted variously of group and/or individual psychotherapy, medical treatment including detoxification and withdrawal, casework services and guidance, vocational and recreational therapy, referral, rehabilitation and treatment of unspecified types, and other services.

NONNARCOTIC DRUGS

A variety of substances, both natural and synthetic, although not addictive, should be included here. Among other reasons is the fact that many of them share certain characteristics with narcotics: they produce some unusual psychic effects; their use is not ordinarily socially acceptable in most cultures; commerce in them is ordinarily illegal and tends to attract certain socially undesirable types of individuals; and the majority of them have certain undesirable physical or mental consequences. Included are certain drugs with valuable legitimate medical uses.

Lipscomb[36] has categorized these many drugs into "ups" and "downs" (Table 27-2). The first he describes as having a centrifugal action on the human organism. Their effect is to elicit or enhance and sustain greater numbers of stimuli than the individual would ordinarily experience. Included in this group are the amphetamines, LSD, PCP (phencyclidine), DMT (dimethyltryptamine), marijuana, and caffeine. The second category is described as having a centripetal action on the human organism by diminishing, subduing, or reducing the number of stimuli that might be experienced. Included (in addition to alcohol and opiates) are tranquilizers and barbiturates.

Increasingly in American culture these substances, rather than being used singly, are used synergistically or, more commonly, "in tandem." Thus Lipscomb describes the all too familiar "sine curve individual," who takes a "wake-me-up" pill in the morning (caffeine or amphetamine), a midday "soother" (perhaps a martini), an evening "turn-me-down" (highball), and a nighttime "put-me-to-sleep" (barbiturate). To dispel any idea that the common use and abuse of many of these substances is limited to some insignificant "depraved" component of the population, it may be pointed out that hundreds of millions of prescriptions for psychoactive drugs, most of them to alleviate anxiety, frustration, agitation, boredom, and depression, are filled annually in the United States, despite the common realization that they will not solve any problems. In addition, of course, is the enormous amount of caffeine-containing and alcoholic beverages that are consumed in American and other societies. Obviously most of these materials are consumed by ordinary members of society who store much of it in overstocked "medicine" cabinets in their homes.

This profligate use has significance beyond the apparent. Children learn much from the examples of their parents. Studies in Canada,[37] for example, found that marijuana and other illicit drug use was more common among students who reported their parents to be users of both alcohol and tobacco, and if their parents used tranquilizers daily, the students were twice as likely to use illicit drugs.

It is unfortunate that so many consider these substances relatively safe as compared with narcotics. To the contrary, an analysis of the 35 most commonly named drugs that brought people to hospital emergency rooms in 24 Standard Metropolitan Statistical Areas, April 1974 to April 1975, showed the following[38]:

Drug	(%)
Tranquilizers	19.6
Sedatives	10.6
Alcohol in combinations	9.1
Analgesics	8.1
Opiate derivatives	7.2
Hallucinogens	4.1
Marijuana and hashish	2.1
Methadone	1.8

For purposes of discussion the various nonnarcotic substances will be considered in the four categories of depressants, stimulants, ataractics, and hallucinogens.

Depressants

Depressants include sedatives and hypnotics. Predominant in this group are the barbiturates, the most widely abused of the depressants. These substances are commonly used in medicine for their sedative or calming effect, especially for anxiety states, hyperthyroidism, and high blood pressure, as well as to allay pain and to control convulsions such as occur with epilepsy. When chronically misused, they may in some ways become more dangerous than narcotics. Physical dependence on them may develop, and tolerance is never complete. A person who is habituated to them shows evidence of slurred speech, staggering and even falling from lack of balance, quick temper, and quarrelsome disposition. Overdose produces coma, and pneumonia is not an uncommon complication.

When these drugs are withheld from habitué, the withdrawal symptoms may be as serious and dangerous as those of narcotic withdrawal. Central nervous system symptoms develop, leading possibly to epileptiform convulsions with subsequent delirium and hallucinations similar to delirium tremens. Indeed, this is becoming a serious aspect of the drug scene with increase in multiple drug use. Treatment for withdrawal from one type of drug, such as heroin, may lead to neglect of withdrawal stress from another, such as barbiturates, which may be fatal.

Persons who use these substances illicitly have a variety of colorful names for them, such as goof balls, peanuts, red devils, rainbows, and blue heavens, to mention only a few (Table 27-2). In any one year, enough amphetamines and barbiturates are medically prescribed to provide every man, woman, and child with a month's supply.

Stimulants

The second group of substances is stimulants, which includes drugs that directly stimulate the central nervous system, producing alertness, wakfulness, excitation, and sometimes a rise in blood pressure and respiration. The most common substances in this category are the amphetamines, which were widely used for years in the treatment of a variety of mental and personality disorders and as adjuncts in the correction of excessive weight, since they appear to have a specific effect on the appetite center in the brain. They are also valuable in the treatment of narcolepsy and Parkinson's disease. Because of their unusual stimulant action, amphetamines and related compounds have been greatly abused by individuals whose occupations require long periods of wakefulness or vivaciousness and by those who attempt to "burn the candle at both ends." A relatively high degree of tolerance can be developed to these substances without necessarily causing physical or psychic damage if dosage is gradually increased. In some instances, however, a true drug psychosis resembling schizophrenia may develop with delusions and hallucinations. Under ordinary misuse, however, the individual appears to be unusually excitable, talkative, and restless, with a tremor of the hands and an enlargement of the pupils, sleeplessness, and perspiration. Under certain circumstances a psychic or emotional dependence on these chemicals may develop.

As in the case of the depressants, these materials have many colloquial names, including bennies, copilots, peaches, cartwheels, hearts, and dexies. The economics of the illicit drug market is illustrated by amphetamines, which could be purchased wholesale for $1 per 1,000, sold in the illegal market for $30 to $50 per 1,000 and then to the individual for as much as 10 to 25 cents per tablet. The true medical need for oral amphetamines is not more than several hundred thousand units. However, the annual production in the United States is 8 billion doses! Effective March 1973, all the amphetamine-type drugs were banned from the open market and their medical use restricted to narcolepsy, minimal brain dysfunction in children, and short-term adjunctive management of exogenous obesity refractive to other measures.

Ataractics

The third category of nonnarcotic drugs that tend to be abused are the ataractics, or tranquilizers. These materials introduced during the 1950s are in one sense a type of nervous system depressant. They have revolutionized the treatment of many psychiatric disorders and, as such, represent a major advance in pharmacology and therapy. In fact, in Australia, a decline in the suicide rate between 1962 and 1973 has been attributed to the substitution of benzodiazepine (diazepam or Valium) for barbiturates. Suicide would require impractically enormous doses.

However, these substances have become the most abused medication in the United States. They now constitute the second most common pharmaceutical material prescribed and sold. More than 1 million pounds are produced, and over 60 million prescriptions are written for them each year in the United States. (In any given year, 20% of women and 14% of men in this country will use diazepam.) Although the use of ataractics is not apt to result in habituation, psychologic dependence is not uncommon. Similarly, although they appear generally to be lacking in toxic or other undesirable side effects, they can occur. It should be noted from the list above that they are the most commonly reported drugs requiring emergency treatment.

Some individuals who take these substances may actually become more aggressive instead of emotionally tranquil. One study showed that of 68 automobile drivers using diazepam over a 3-month period, 16 were involved in accidents. Others, especially older, organically ill persons, may develop tremulousness, impaired concentration and memory, insomnia, nightmares, depression, apprehension, and suicidal impulses. Undesirable effects are increased with alcohol. They are not "pleasant" drugs, and since they remain in the body about 48 hours, they generally have no withdrawal symptoms.

Hallucinogens

The fourth group of substances of a nonnarcotic nature and one that has been rapidly increasing in use are the various hallucinogens. Pharmacologically they are referred to as psychedelics or psychotomimetics. Prominent among them are LSD-25, a semisynthetic derivative of ergonovine; the seeds of some varieties of morning glory ("Ololiuqui," *Rivea corymbosa,* and *Ipomoea violacea*), the active principle of which is closely related to LSD; mescaline, a phenethylamine present in the buttons of a small cactus ("mescal," "peyote," or *Lophophora williamsii*), which has been used by Indians in southwestern United States and Mexico in certain accepted religious rituals of the Native American Church; psilocybin, an indole found in a mushroom ("teonanacatl," *Psilocybe mexicana*); PCP or 1-(1-phenylcyclohexyl)piperidine, a synthetic veterinary anesthetic; and DMT, a synthetic indole, also found in the seeds of a South American plant (*Piptadenia peregrina*). LSD is an extremely powerful drug, 100 times more potent than psilocybin and 7,000 times more potent than mescaline. Since it has been brought under legal control, however, the relatively newer synthetic DMT, with a shorter and stronger action, has appeared on the illicit market. An LSD "trip" or "experience" usually has a fairly gentle onset and lasts about 12 hours, whereas a DMT "trip" has a sudden "rough" onset and lasts only about 2 hours. One of the characteristics of these substances, especially the synthetics, is that eating, inhaling, or injecting only minute amounts, as little as 1/280,000 of an ounce of LSD for example, may produce severe and dramatic effects that sometimes may recur, even without taking the drug again.[39]

The illicit use of these substances, especially by certain psychosocial cults, by groups such as beatniks or hippies who attempt to withdraw from society, or by some misguided young people or older pseudosophisticates in search of a new and different "experience" or of their "identity," has been attributed to the mind-expanding effects of the drugs. It is true that many individuals may use them without serious effects and in the process experience a wide variety of stimulating and colorful hallucinations. Even in such instances the physical effects of LSD are usually disturbing. There is an increase in blood pressure and heart rate; the blood sugar level goes up; and there may be nausea, chills, flushes, irregular breathing, sweating of the hands, and trembling of the extremities. Sleep is virtually impossible until at least 8 to 10 hours after the LSD episode is over. The pupils of the eyes are widely dilated, so that dark glasses are often worn, even at night, for protection against the light. Beyond these more "usual" effects there is ample evidence of the development in some individuals of overwhelming fear and panic; paranoid delusions; distressing distortions of time, place, and position; and intense self-loathing. Unprovoked violence toward others, loss of sanity, and suicide are by no means rare.

At present there is much difference of opinion concerning possible genetic effects of hallucinogens, especially LSD. Observation of chromosomal damage was first reported in 1967 and since has been substantiated or discounted by various investigators in the United States and other countries. An especially provocative study[40] in 1968 reported 46 persons who ingested LSD and 4 persons who were exposed to the drug in utero. Fourteen drug-free controls had a chromosomal breakage rate of 6% to 16.5%, whereas among the drug users it was 8% to 45%. In addition to observed chromosomal breakage, several reports have been appearing in United States and British medical literature indicating possible relationships between LSD use and clinical teratologic malformations. A key problem is the concurrent use of a variety of other substances as medications, as additional drugs, or as foods that could conceivably cause or contribute to the phenomenon. The problem and its potentials are so significant as to encourage careful studies that separate clearly any effect on chromosomes produced by LSD from effects that might be attributed to other substances or factors.

PCP, popularly referred to an "angel dust," is a particularly dangerous hallucinogen of recent popularity. It was originally synthesized for use in curing rubber and as a powerful anesthetic for use on large animals in zoos and elsewhere. Many consider it the most dangerous illicit drug. Unfortunately it is easy and inexpensive to synthesize. Recorded use increased about 270% between 1975 and 1977, with an estimated 1 million persons possibly using it at least once a week. Currently it accounts for 38% of all drug arrests in Los Angeles, with other large cities experiencing similar case loads. The average user is in the teens. It caused 51 known deaths in Los Angeles during 1977, during the first half of 1978 an additional 54 persons had been using it at the time of death. Water appears to attract those who use it, but they lose their sense of depth and direction and sometimes drown, even in shallow water. Legislative measures have been taken to control the source and sale of the materials from which PCP can be made, but enforcement is difficult.

Marijuana

Because of the considerable publicity given to it during recent years, specific mention should be made of a much milder but more widely used hallucinogen, marijuana. Marijuana is a drug found in the flowering tops and leaves of the Indian hemp plant *Cannabis sativa,* which is related to the fig, hop, and nettle. It is used commercially in making rope, textiles, and birdseed. The consumption of cannabis in one form or another—marijuana, bhang, ganja, charras, maconha, kif, or hashish— has been known for at least 5,000 years. It was included in a Chinese medical compendium dated 2737 B.C. as a means of relieving pain during surgery. It was also regarded as a useful medicinal in ayurvedic and Arabic medicine.

It was introduced into western medicine in 1839 by Sir William O'Shaugnessy, a British physician who had served in India. He used it to treat rheumatism, tetanus, and seizures and described its use in an apparently rabid dog, which after dozing, "awoke, wagged its tail contentedly, ate greedily, and assumed a look of utter and hopeless drunkenness," after which it was perfectly well and lively! Its use spread, and many reports were published concerning its effectiveness in insomnia, dysmenorrhea, erysipelas, and numerous other ailments. Sir William Osler considered it the most satisfactory remedy for headaches, and in 1890 Reynolds wrote, "When pure and administered carefully, it is one of the most valuable medicines we possess." At that time it was also recommended as a treatment for opiate addiction. In 1941 it was removed from the *United States Pharmacopoeia* and *National Formulary,* but as recently as 1949, THC, a synthesized concentrate, was reported effective in preventing epileptic seizures, and it is being studied

as an antidepressant and analgesic, especially in terminal cancer patients, as well as a remedy for sunstroke and glaucoma.[41]

Marijuana was introduced to the United States as an intoxicating drug in 1920, and its use became especially well known among jazz musicians who attributed to it an enhanced ability to perform. In 1931 the Food and Drug Administration limited the importation of cannabis except for medicinal purposes and as birdseed. Largely to eliminate fears about its use by immigrants from Mexico, the United States government in 1937 passed the Federal Marijuana Tax Act. This was followed by strict laws and enforcement in every state. During the 1960s, apparently spurred by the examples and statements of several well-known personalities, a sharp increase occurred in its use, especially in college and university groups. This attracted greater law enforcement efforts, and arrests on marijuana charges more than doubled. This did not, however, diminish its use and indeed may even have contributed to its increase.

Dependable data on the extent of marijuana use are not available because of a number of variables, including unknown amounts grown domestically or smuggled into the United States, shared smoking, and the difficulty of defining terms such as *use* or *habitually.* The best information comes from carefully designed and conducted surveys that are also subject to unknown degrees of error because of boasts or reluctance. It is agreed that marijuana is the most widely used illicit drug in the United States. Dupont,[42] president of the American Council on Marijuana, estimates that 23 million people in the United States are regular smokers of the substance. According to a study of the problem by the National Academy of Sciences' Institute of Medicine,[43] 9% of high school seniors in 1980 reported daily or near-daily use. This represents a drop from 11% in 1978. The use of marijuana is most common in the late teen and early adult years and is twice as frequent among men as among women and among those who attended college as among those who did not.

Ordinarily when smoked, the active ingredient is absorbed through the respiratory system, enters the bloodstream, and acts on the brain and nervous system. The most obvious signs and symptoms include a rapid heartbeat, lowered body temperature, and reddening of the eyes. The blood sugar level drops; the appetite, especially for sweets, is stimulated; and the body is dehydrated. the user may become loud and loquacious, uncoordinated, or drowsy.

The effects on the emotions and senses vary, depending on the amount of strength of the marijuana, the social setting, and the experience, previous mood, and expectations of the user. Ordinarily its effects appear in about 15 minutes and may last from 2 to 4 hours. The effects may range from excitement and exhilaration to deep depression, and some users experience no change of mood. A common phenomenon is the distortion of time and distance. A moment may seem like an hour, hence musicians may think they are playing much more rapidly then they really are. Similarly objects nearby may appear distant and distorted in shape.

The Committee of the National Academy of Science[44] found that marijuana significantly impairs motor coordination and the ability to follow a moving object and to detect a flash of light, functions essential for safe driving and the use of machines in industry. It also hampers short-term memory, slows learning, impairs oral communication, causes inflammation of the lungs, increases the heart rate, decreases human sperm production, and may produce a gamut of mental phenomena ranging, as previously described, from euphoria to confusion and delirium. All of these effects appear to be short-term and reversible. Because no studies followed marijuana smokers for more than 5 years, the Committee found no conclusive evidence of long-term effects. Of pertinence with reference to the lack of long-term effects are earlier intensive studies of 30 long-term Jamaican cannabis users and 31 chronic hashish users in Greece who were noteworthy for the relative absence of pathology.

In consideration of its history, its widespread use, its mild reactions, and especially in relation to a long list of obviously more serious social offenses, legal sanctions in the United States in relation to marijuana have been unjustifiably harsh. Under federal law, to have, give, or sell marijuana in the United States is a felony. Federal and many state laws deal with the drug as severely as if it were a narcotic. In 1971, the American Public Health Association passed resolutions that "no punitive measures be taken against the users of . . . marijuana . . . when no other illegal act has been committed," and that federal and state drug laws exclude marijuana from the classification of narcotic drugs.

The report, "Marihuana and Health,"[44] issued in 1971 by the National Institute of Mental Health,

stated that current penalties for use and possession are much too severe and out of keeping with knowledge about its harmfulness. It is also interesting that the former Deputy Director of the Bureau of Narcotics and Dangerous Drugs of the Department of Justice accepted membership on the board of the National Organization for the Reform of Marihuana Laws, remarking that he had decided it was wrong to jail young people for smoking pot and that both liquor and tobacco have far more harmful effects. Numerous other professions, organizations, and individuals have been taking similar stands. The National Commission on Marihuana and Drug Abuse recommended in its 1972 report to the President that marijuana be "decriminalized." It also urged, however, that there be continued strong measures against the production, importation, or sale of marijuana. These modest yet practical recommendations, despite their coincidence with the recommendations of an international panel of experts convened by the World Health Organization,[45] are only gradually being accepted or acted on favorably.

At the present time a trend toward decriminalization of marijuana is underway in several states, notably California and Oregon, where possession has been changed from a felony to a misdemeanor. The penalty on citation is a fine and a notation on the individual's police record. A second citation, however, is dealt with more harshly. Consideration is also being given to changing the charge for growing marijuana for one's own use from a felony to a misdemeanor. The general feeling of enforcement officers concerning rigid enforcement is that it is a "bottomless pit" with no limit to the numbers that might become involved, that it is a victimless crime, that its effects are not especially detrimental, and that rigid enforcement and punishment place a tremendous drain on the police and judicial systems while demeaning them in the eyes of the public.

SOLVENT INHALATION

To shift to a more bizarre phenomenon, brief mention should be made of the use of several other substances by children and teenagers—airplane glue, lighter fluid, gasoline, nutmeg, and ether.[46] Smelling or inhaling these substances tends to provide a momentary sense of exhilaration, euphoria, and intoxication, but all of them have serious toxic side effects. An important aspect of the use of these materials by adolescents is the fact that frequently their use is by a group. Part of the reason is apparently a shared boredom, a lack of definite goals, a revolt against adult rules, and as a manifestation of wanting to belong to a group. Not uncommonly their use begins in a gang or party setting with one of the group introducing the material or practice and the rest responding for fear of appearing to be "chicken" or cowardly. Whereas some of these practices may on the surface appear innocuous, they may lead to criminal acts. For example, although there are no dependable data concerning the number of those who use these materials in the young population, there is mounting police and court evidence of violations of the law by juveniles after having engaged in the practice. These violations extend from breaking and entering and stealing of automobiles to more serious actions. In one instance the murder and rape of two small twin sisters was committed by a 15-year-old boy who had spent the afternoon sniffing glue. As is often the case, the boy remembered nothing afterward.

The solution of these problems is not easy, and as in the case of alcoholism or narcotic addiction, it requires the interest and joint action of several concerned groups. Public education, particularly in the schools, is important. In certain circumstances legal restrictions with reference to the sale of certain materials may have some effect. Development by industry of substitutes for dangerous chemicals that are nonetheless necessary for legitimate purposes may offer some hope. In addition to this is the need for persistent and consistent surveillance of the problem by public health officials, law enforcement officials, and other groups. There is also a critical need for the apprehension and presecution of any who are involved in the sale, dissemination, and use of the dangerous materials for improper purposes.

INTERNATIONAL EFFORT[47]

The history of international concern with narcotic and drug abuse began in 1909 with a conference in Shanghai of an International Opium Commission. This led to the Hague convention of 1917 to control opium, morphine, heroin, and cocaine. In 1948 international concern and control efforts relating not just to these substances but also to synthetic products came under the jurisdiction of

the newly organized United Nations and its specialized agencies. In 1961 a Convention on Narcotic Drugs was signed, followed in 1971 by a Convention on Psychotropic Substances. Within the Economic and Social Council are several commissions and boards concerned with policy, control functions, and project assistance. The World Health Organization has responsibility to evaluate drugs and to make recommendations for their control. In 1962 it established an international drug-monitoring program and in 1968 opened a center for this purpose in Alexandria, Va. In addition, The World Health Organization has actively sponsored expert committees, scientific meetings, and research on various aspects of the subject.

With specific reference to the circumstances under which control measures should be instituted, the World Health Organization's Expert Committee on Drug Dependence has stated[48]:

There are two main conditions, at least one of which must exist for a drug to be considered in need of control:

1. The drug is known to be abused other than sporadically or in a local area and the effects of its abuse extend beyond the drug taker; in addition, its mode of spread involves communication between existing and potential drug takers, and an illicit traffic in it is developing.

2. It is planned to use the drug in medicine and experimental data show that there is a significant psychic or physical dependence liability; the drug is commercially available or may become so.

If neither of these conditions is fulfilled, there is no need for an agent to come under consideration for control.

In reviewing international control activities, the United Nations Commission on Narcotic Drugs noted that efforts had long been directed mainly toward limiting legal narcotics to medical uses, controlling crops of narcotizing plants, licensing legal producers and accounting for their output, and tracking down illegal producers and smugglers. Little attention was being devoted to the medical and particularly to the psychologic problems of addiction. Although the Commission on Narcotic Drugs recognizes that efforts to eliminate illicit supplies constitute an effective and indispensable weapon in the fight against addiction, it considers realistically that even the most perfect regimen cannot completely accomplish this and that the more rigorous the action, the greater the probability of the development of a prosperous black market in illicit drugs. Accordingly, the treatment and rehabilitation of addicts, including studies of etiologic factors, and measures to meet the risk that addicts deprived of narcotic drugs by tight controls may turn to the abuse of other harmful substances have now become the principal items of deliberation and action by the commission. This shift in emphasis, it believes, has been so pronounced as to justify speaking of a new chapter of international collaboration in the field of drug abuse.

TOBACCO

One of the most significant events of history was the discovery of the Western Hemisphere. It was not devoid of drawbacks. Among others, two unfortunate curses were introduced into Europe and beyond—syphilis and tobacco. In addition to the use of tobacco as a symbol of peace and friendship, the American Indians attributed various medicinal values to it. These were transferred to Europe, and for a period its virtues were advertised for everything from deafness to problems of the womb and, ironically, even cancer. Its popular use was greatly accelerated when Sir Walter Raleigh brought some to Queen Elizabeth. From England and Spain it spread to the Middle East, Asia, and throughout the world. A measure of this is provided by the fact that during the American colonial period and the early years of the American republic, it was the leading export product.

In 1980 over 1,770 million pounds of tobacco were grown in the United States and about 6.5 times that amount elsewhere in the world. Each year about 3 trillion cigarettes are manufactured worldwide, and over 600 billion are consumed in the United States. This country also makes 5.5 billion cigars annually. Manufacture and sales of this magnitude generate billions of dollars in farm and industrial income. Because of this, many point to tobacco as a valuable economic asset, but this conclusion would seem subject to serious question in view of the lack of physiologic benefit, the use of large amounts of land that should be used for more important and less soil-destructive purposes, plus the costs of the devastating damage done to health.

Another measure of the magnitude of the problem is the annual consumption of tobacco. The number of cigarettes consumed per person per year in the United States was 49 in 1900; 1,365 in 1930; 3,522 in 1950; and 4,123 in 1975. Since then there has been a slight decline to about 3,900. This decline was especially significant among men—from 51% to less than 40%; in contrast, the decline among women was only from 33% to 30%. About 10 million people stopped smoking during the pe-

riod, whereas the percent of those who never smoked did not change significantly.[49] Smoking among teenage boys is no longer increasing but has remained stable during the past few years. Young girls, however, who traditionally were less likely to smoke, have caught up with the boys. Probability of smoking is inversely related to years of education.

Tobacco is in a somewhat different category from the other substances discussed in this chapter. Although its use commonly leads to a genuine habituation, its undesirability is not related to any psychic or ethical changes. Rather, it is because of its relationship to several chronic diseases of major significance. It can be stated unequivocally that cigarette smoking is the greatest preventable cause of illness and premature death in the United States. It is a prime causal factor for cancer of the lung, larynx, oral cavity, and esophagus; for chronic bronchitis and emphysema; for coronary heart disease; and for arteriosclerotic peripheral vascular disease. It is also associated with gastric ulcers and cancer of the urinary bladder and pancreas.[50] Maternal cigarette smoking is associated with retarded fetal growth, an increased risk of spontaneous abortion and prenatal death, and a slight impairment of growth and development during early childhood.[51] Cigarette smoking acts synergistically with oral contraceptives to increase the probability of coronary and cerebrovascular disease; with alcohol to increase the risk of cancer of the mouth and throat; and with asbestos and some other industrially encountered substances to increase the risk of cancer of the lung.[49] With reference to occupational exposure it has been found that for asbestos workers who smoke, the lung cancer risk is 8 times that of all other smokers and 92 times the risk for nonsmokers not exposed to asbestos. Similarly, the respiratory cancer rate per 10,000 person-years for uranium miners who smoke is 42.2, compared with 7.1 for uranium miners who never smoked.[52]

Cigarette smoking is associated with a 70% increase in the age-specific death rates of men and to a lesser extent of women. The total number of excess deaths causally related to cigarette smoking in the U.S. population has been calculated to be about 1 million each year. In general, the greater the number of cigarettes smoked daily, the higher the death rate. For men who smoke fewer than 10 cigarettes a day, the death rate is about 40% higher than for nonsmokers; for those who smoke 10 to 19 cigarettes a day, it is about 70% higher; for those who smoke 20 to 39 cigarettes a day, it is 90% higher; and for those who smoke 40 or more cigarettes a day, the death rate is 120% higher than for nonsmokers. In terms of increased mortality risk by cause, conclusions based on many different studies are consistent and clear. The total mortality for smokers in general is 1.84 times that for those who never smoked. For lung cancer, the rate is 12.14 times greater for smokers; for bronchitis and/or emphysema, 10.08; for coronary heart disease, 1.74; and for cerebrovascular disease, 1.52.[53]

When one considers the time lags that exist between the inception of the cause and the development of most effects attributable to tobacco smoking, the identifications represent true classics of long-term epidemiologic studies. As a result of these studies, several nations have taken steps to try to decrease the use of tobacco. In the United States the President established a Surgeon General's Advisory Committee on Smoking and Health. This committee led to the development of a National Clearinghouse on Smoking and Health within the Public Health Service, which has gathered, prepared, and disseminated data and information on the subject, carried out extensive public educational efforts in company with other interested organizations, promoted scientific and professional conferences, and was instrumental in the development and enactment of the Federal Cigarette Labeling and Advertising Act in 1965. This resulted in the requirement that all packages of cigarettes bear a warning of danger to health. In 1971 it was successful in having cigarette advertising banned from radio and television. These steps had already been taken in several countries, beginning in 1962 in Italy and New Zealand. Increasingly smoking has been restricted in restaurants, airplanes, and other public places.[54] To encourage these efforts, the World Health Organization has held numerous international conferences and has passed several pertinent resolutions on the subject.

Horn[55] has listed the following barriers to successful control programs: (1) gaps in medical and epidemiologic knowledge, especially better means of identifying those at greater risk; (2) economic and political conflicts that arise from agricultural, manufacturing, and marketing interests; (3) inadequate knowledge about smoking behavior and effective motivational methods to combat it; and (4) lack of communication and coordination among the groups, organizations, and nations concerned with the problem. He urges more extensive interchange of experts and advice, more exact monitoring of the extent of smoking and its consequences, better availability and exchange of information (especially with reference to public communications outlets), the search for and development of alternatives to the economic needs of tobacco-producing areas, and intensified research on all aspects of the problem.

Some progress has been achieved with regard to some of the obstacles that Horn has listed. The greatest advances have been in relation to medical and epidemiologic knowledge. Communication and coordination among concerned organizations and governments have been significantly improved. There has even been some success in dealing with the manufacturers and purveyors of cigarettes as indicated by laws and regulations about labeling, reduction of tar content, and establishment of nonsmoking areas. Efforts in the fields of education and motivation, however, have produced disappointing results so far. Many approaches have been tried: didactic teaching, group discussion, individual study, peer instruction, emotional role playing, desensitization, aversive conditioning, and all types of mass media. In reviewing the record, Thompson[56] found little evidence of success. Individual counseling and withdrawal clinics showed the most promise. Some of these techniques have value. However, it is notable that most former smokers, probably close to 95%, quit on their own without recourse to formal smoking cessation programs.[49]

SUBSTANCE ABUSE AND THE FUTURE

Substance abuse is not a transitory phenomenon. It is almost as old as mankind and unquestionably will always occur. The only variables are the nature of the materials, the extent of their use and abuse, and the vigor and imagination of efforts to control them. With this in mind it is difficult to improve upon a statement by Ayd:[57]

Science promises Utopia, a synthetic heaven on earth made possible by chemical, biological and technological developments. To achieve these objectives, drugs must and will be developed. Among these are drugs which will curb human reproduction, new chemical aphrodisiacs, drugs to induce hibernation and to ease the pains of hunger, drugs to transport man to mystical heights, drugs to combat boredom, drugs to raise intelligence to very high levels, drugs which will increase longevity, and drugs to produce temporary incapacitation of a population. These are only a few of the drugs which will be used to manipulate and control human behavior. Society must be aware of these trends and give serious consideration to them and their implications, good and evil, for the society before they are realities.

REFERENCES

1. Addiction-producing drugs, WHO Chron. **11:**81, March 1957.
2. Pattison, E.M., Bishop, L.A., and Linsky, A.S.: Changes in public attitudes on narcotic addiction, Am. J. Psychiatry **125:**160, Jan. 1968.
3. Drug addiction and drug habituation, WHO Chron. **11:**165, May 1957.
4. Dependence on alcohol and other drugs, WHO Chron. **21:**219, June 1967; Glatt, M.M.: Problems common to alcoholism and drug dependence, WHO Chron. **21:**293, July 1967.
5. Drugs, World Health (special issue), April 1971.
6. Musto, D.F.: A study in cocaine, J.A.M.A. **204:**125, April 1, 1968.
7. Simrell, E.V.: History of legal and medical roles in narcotic abuse in the U.S., Public Health Rep. **83:**587, July 1968.
8. Brotman, R., and Freedman, A.: A community mental health approach to drug addiction, DHEW (SRS) Pub. No. 9005, Washington, D.C., 1970, U.S. Department of Health, Education, and Welfare.
9. National Institute of Mental Health: A federal source book: answers to the most frequently asked questions about drug abuse, Rockville, Md., 1971.
10. Yost, O.S.: The bane of drug addiction, New York, 1954, Macmillan Publishing Co., Inc.
11. Drugs and the adolescent, WHO Chron. **25:**263, June 1971.
12. Dupont, R.L.: Profile of a heroin addiction epidemic, N. Engl. j. Med. **285:**320, Aug. 5, 1971.
13. Carson, D.D., and Lewis, J.M.: Factors influencing drug abuse in young people, Tex. Med. **66**(1):50, 1970.
14. Johnson, K.G., and others: Survey of adolescent drug use, Am. J. Public Health **61:**2418, Dec. 1971.
15. Johnson, K.G., and others: Surveys of adolescent drug use, Am. J. Public Health **62:**164, Feb. 1972.
16. Johnson, L.D.: Drug use during and after high school—results of a national longitudinal study. In the Epidemiology of drug abuse, Am. J. Public Health **64**(Suppl.):29, Dec. 1974.
17. Dealing with drug abuse; report of a task force of the Drug Abuse Council, New York, 1972, Frederick A. Praeger, Inc.
18. Louria, D.B., Hensle, T., and Rose, J.: The major medical complications of heroin addiction, Ann. Intern. Med. **67:**1, July 1967.
19. Cherubin, C.E.: The medical sequelae of narcotic addiction, Ann. Intern. Med. **67:**23, July 1967.
20. Joe, G.W., Lehman, W., and Simpson, D.D.: Addict death rates during a four-year posttreatment follow-up, Am. J. Public Health **72:**703, July 1982.
21. Zelson, C., Rubio, E., and Wasserman, E.: Neonatal narcotic-addiction, Pediatrics **48:**178, Feb. 1971.
22. Jacobziner, H.: Investigating narcotic addiction in school children, Am. J. Public Health **43:**1138, Sept. 1953.
23. Hughes, P.H., and others: The natural history of a heroin epidemic, Am. J. Public Health **62:**995, July 1972.
24. Abrams, A., Gagnon, J.H., and Levin, J.J.: Psychosocial aspects of addiction, Am. J. Public Health **58:**2142, Nov. 1968.
25. Koran, L.M.: American responses to heroin addiction and marijuana use. In Coelho, G.U., and Rubinstein, E.A., editors: Social change and human behavior, Rockville, Md., 1972, National Institute of Mental Health.
26. Geis, G.: Not the law's business: an examination of homosexuality, abortion, prostitution, narcotics and gambling in the United States. Center for Studies of Crime and Delinquency, DHEW Pub. No. (HSM) 72-9132, Rockville, Md., 1972, National Institute of Mental Health.
27. Ball, J.C., Thompson, W.O., and Allen, D.M.: Readmission rates for 43,215 narcotic drug addicts, Public Health Rep. **85:**610, July 1970.
28. Drug addiction. III. A statement by the New York Academy of Medicine, Bull. N.Y. Acad. Med. **41:**825, July 1965.
29. Treatment and care of drug addicts, WHO Chron. **11:**323, Oct. 1957.
30. Prevention and treatment of drug dependence; report of the Expert Committee on Drug Dependence, WHO Tech. Rep. Ser. No. 460, Geneva, 1970, World Health Organization.
31. Dole, V.P., and Nyswander, M.: A medical treatment of diacetylmorphine (heroin) addiction: a clinical trial, J.A.M.A. **193:**646, Aug. 23, 1965.
32. DuPont, R.L., and Katon, R.: Physicians and the heroin addiction epidemic, Mod. Med. **39:**123, June 1971.
33. Chambers, C.D., and Brill, L., editors: Methadone: experiences and issues, New York, 1973, Behavioral Publications.
34. Louria, D.B.: A critique of some current approaches to the problem of drug abuse, Am. J. Public Health **65:**581, June 1975.
35. McKee, M.R.: Drug abuse knowledge and attitudes

in "middle America," Am. J. Public Health **65:**584, June 1975.

36. Lipscomb, W.R.: An epidemiology of drug use-abuse, Am. J. Public Health **61:**1794, Sept. 1971.

37. Drugs, World Health (special issue), April 1971, p. 32.

38. Health, United States, 1976-1977, DHEW Pub. No. (HRA) 77-1232, Washington, D.C., 1977, U.S. Government Printing Office.

39. Dependence on LSD and other hallucinogenic drugs: Report of Committee on Alcoholism and Drug Dependence and the Council on Mental Health, J.A.M.A. **202:**141, Oct. 2, 1967.

40. Egozcue, J., Irwin, S., and Maruffo, C.: Chromosomal damage in LSD users, J.A.M.A. **204:**122, April 15, 1968.

41. Abel, E.L., editor: The scientific study of marihuana, Chicago, 1976, Nelson-Hall Publishers.

42. Dupont, R.L.: Marijuana smoking: a national epidemic, Bulletin of the American Lung Association, Sept. 1980.

43. Marijuana and health, Report of the National Academy of Sciences' Institute of Medicine, Washington, D.C., 1981, National Academy Press.

44. National Institute of Mental Health: Marihuana and health; report to the Congress, Rockville, Md., 1971.

45. The use of cannabis; report of the WHO scientific group, WHO Techn. Rep. Ser. No. 478, Geneva, 1971, World Health Organization.

46. Mullings, E.B.: Airplane glue, Mich. Health, Sept.-Oct. 1966.

47. Kahn, I., and others: Controlling psychotropic substances, WHO Chron. **32:**3, Jan. 1978.

48. Criteria for determining the need for drug control; report of the WHO Expert Committee on Drug Dependence, Tech. Rep. Ser. No. 407, Geneva, 1969, World Health Organization.

49. Smoking, tobacco, and health: a fact book, DHHS Pub. No. (PHS) 80-50150, Washington, D.C., 1981, U.S. Government Printing Office.

50. The health consequences of smoking: cancer, Washington, D.C., 1982, U.S. Government Printing Office.

51. The health consequences of smoking for women, Washington, D.C., 1980, U.S. Government Printing Office.

52. Adverse health effects of smoking and the occupational environment, DHEW Pub. No. (NIOSH) 79-122 Cincinnati, 1979, National Institute for Occupational Safety and Health.

53. Holbrook, J.H.: Tobacco and health, CA **27:**344, Nov.-Dec. 1977.

54. De Moerloose, J.: Legislative action to combat smoking around the world, WHO Chron. **31:**362, Aug. 1977.

55. Horn, D.: Smoking and disease: what must be done, WHO Chron. **31:**355, Aug. 1977.

56. Thompson, E.L.: Smoking education programs 1960-1976, Am. J. Public Health **68:**250, Mar. 1978.

57. Ayd, F.J.: Drugs and the future, Med. Counterpoint **1**(6):19, 1969.

CHAPTER 28

Suicide

To be, or not to be:—that is the question:—
Whether 'tis nobler in the mind to suffer
The slings and arrows of outrageous fortune,
Or to take arms against a sea of troubles,
And by opposing end them?

Hamlet III. I

HOW GREAT THE PROBLEM

Hamlet's question is one that many people ask themselves at some time, and many respond by some form of self-destructive act. Unquestionably, suicide is the most frequently concealed of the major causes of disability and death. Furthermore, as Shneidman[4] has emphasized, "Suicide is the first leading cause of *unnecessary* and *stigmatizing* deaths." Each year almost 30,000 suicides are reported in the United States.[5] This is equivalent to the number of deaths from all of the infectious and parasitic diseases including, among others, tuberculosis, influenza, meningitis, and the enteritides. Moreover, various authorities consider the true incidence to be two or three times the reported number.[6] This places its toll at more than that attributed to vehicular accidents, or possibly 2.5% of all deaths. Worldwide, the World Health Organization estimates that each year more than 500,000 successful suicides occur.[7] This is about the equivalent of the population of Pittsburgh, St. Louis, or Seattle. In addition, it is estimated that there are about 10 times as many attempts as there are successful suicides—the equivalent of the combined populations of Los Angeles and Philadelphia; or of Vienna, Paris, and Copenhagen; or of Buenos Aires and Caracas.

Official international death rates for suicides vary from 2 to 25 per 100,000 population. The highest rates for both sexes are reported from Germany (Democratic Republic), Hungary, Austria, Finland, Switzerland, Japan, and Denmark. The lowest rates are in Italy, Spain, Ireland, the nonwhite population of the United States, Columbia, and Costa Rica. However, such data must be regarded with considerable skepticism, since they are significantly affected by customs and mores, the quality and quantity of medical care, the frequency and accuracy of autopsies, official vital statistical procedures, and many other factors.[7] For example, as McCulloch and Philip[8] have pointed out, even in Great Britain, where public records are highly accurate, Northern Ireland has a rate one-half that of England, with Scotland and Wales between the two. As they indicate, it is probably not coincidental that the attitude of the law to suicidal acts over the years has tended to be punitive in Northern Ireland in contrast to indifference in England and Scotland. Whatever the reservations, the fact is that suicide now ranks as the second leading cause of death among persons 15 to 45 years of age in the 8 most industrialized countries of the world.

SUICIDE OR ACCIDENT?

A comparison has been made of suicidal and vehicular accident deaths. In this regard McCulloch and Philip[8] have stated:

Suicidal behavior, especially completed suicide, tends to be ignored as a public health or social action problem by all but a few bodies. It seems anomalous that death by suicide should be so treated, while road fatalities, which account for approximately the same number of deaths per

For a comprehensive review of the literature, see Farberow.[1] For excellent overviews of the subject, see Resnik and Hathorne[2] and Shneidman and associates.[3]

year, are combated by publicity campaigns and legislation which attempt to change people's attitudes and behavior. It is strange that road deaths, where the human factor looms no larger than it does in suicide and where in some cases there are suicidal connotations, strike people as being untimely and avoidable while these sentiments are felt less often about suicide and other forms of disease.

The question of the use of the automobile as a suicidal agent is therefore important.[9] A relationship has been suspected for some years, but only relatively recently has it been subjected to study by means of the technique of "psychologic autopsy."[10-12] This involves reconstruction of the life-style and personality of the deceased and a careful inquiry into recent events and behavior. Interviews are conducted with the spouse, mature children, parents, physicians, employers, friends, and others who knew the person well to determine on a probability basis whether death occurred accidentally or intentionally. Using this method, in combination with site and vehicle inspections and toxicologic analyses, several studies in American cities indicate that between 10% and 30% of fatal automobile crashes are conscious, goal-directed suicides. On these and similar bases it has been estimated that as many as 9,000 of the 46,000 deaths from motor vehicular accidents each year in the United States should be more properly attributed to suicide.

There appear to be some interesting similarities and differences between *true* suicides and *true* accidents. For example, it has been noted that in about one half of both fatal accidents and suicides the subjects had been drinking alcohol before their deaths and that drinking had been used frequently as a method of response to problems in their lives. One difference is that those who die by accident do not appear to have encountered any clearly psychologically traumatic situation just before the fatal event. This is in contrast with suicides who have suffered recent losses (death, money, affluence, status) and who tend to be more closely integrated and involved with others. However, it is interesting that true accident victims, more often than not, are involved in potential or recent moves to situations of greater responsibility. They also tend to be hypersensitive to criticism, relatively exhibitionistic and poorly integrated with others.[13]

The foregoing begs the question of definition or determination of suicide. This is not always simple. Frequently it can be established fairly easily that an injury or poisoning was deliberately self-inflicted. Whether or not actual death was the intended goal, however, is less easy to determine. Often the act is essentially a reaction to a crisis of despair or despondency and represents a dramatic appeal for help, an attempt to attract attention, or a means of spiting others or of submitting oneself to trial by ordeal. It should be recognized that many individuals engage in various forms of the last few of these, subconsciously if not consciously, while driving or engaging in certain sports or in choosing certain occupations. Then there is the dilemma that results from an individual *not* doing something necessary to the protection or preservation of life—not taking insulin or not wearing automobile seat belts. Certainly some deaths attributed to diabetes and certain cardiac and other ailments are actually willful suicides carried out by the simple expedient of inaction, the intent of which is unprovable. To place the problem in a rational context, Shneidman[14] pointed out that whereas deaths from a bullet, a vehicle, a poison, or an infection may be classified as a homicide, an accident, a suicide, or a disease, as far as the individual affected is concerned they are all simply threats to life or means to death.

THEORIES ABOUT SUICIDE

An important step forward in the understanding of suicide was taken by Durkheim[15] at the end of the last century. His was essentially the first major effort to study the problem as a sociologic phenomenon. His chief concern was with the forces in society that affect an individual's actions rather than forces within the individual. In 1897 he published his path-breaking book *Le Suicide,* in which he classified suicides into three sociologic categories:

1. *Altruistic suicide,* in which the customs and mores of a society demand and even facilitate the practice. There is an excessive integration of the individual with the society and, as described by Kramer and associates,[16] he sacrifices himself like a soldier in battle. Suttee or hara-kiri are examples.

2. *Egoistic suicide,* in which the individual is not strongly identified or integrated with the institutions of the society and must assume more responsibility that can be fulfilled. Individuals in this group typically have strong feelings of personal failure, unfulfillment, and guilt and may have an overwhelming unconscious drive to punish themselves. Parenthetically, some writers[17,18] have ap-

plied this concept to explain war as a form of mass suicide.

3. *Anomic suicide,* in which an individual's adjustment to or integration with society is suddenly disrupted or unbalanced as by financial, employment, or marital reverses or even as a consequence of sudden unexpected prosperity. Durkheim's outstanding contribution, as viewed by Kramer and associates[16] "was to show that suicide, like crime, neurosis, and alcoholism, is a factor that measures social pressure and tension."

Subsequent to Durkheim, Sigmund Freud[19] theorized that successful suicides represented the victory of an inborn drive toward death. Humankind's inner destructivity, like all instinctual tendencies, is rooted in the primordial struggle between the drive to live and the desire to return to the organic matrix of all life. It is not that a person who commits suicide has lost the desire to live—he or she merely wishes that life were different and thinks that by a fatal act he or she will approach happiness.

Although there are numerous other suggested explanations of suicide, one other may be mentioned here because of its relative comprehensiveness. The Dutch pyschiatrist, Meerloo,[17] has listed nine different categories or reasons for suicide as follows:

1. Suicide based on a magical or "inner call" to be killed
2. Suicide as a form of communication, a call for attention or help
3. Suicide as revenge, hopefully to make someone else regretful
4. Suicide as a magical murder or crime to partially destroy humanity
5. Suicide as unconscious escape from confusion, guilt, or inadequacy
6. Morbid or egoistic suicide to cheat illness or execution
7. Suicide as conscious escape from punishment or despair
8. Suicide as a necessary step toward magical revival or rebirth
9. Suicide as an altruistic sacrifice to an expected code of action

It will have been noted that none of the foregoing refers specifically to mental illness. Nevertheless, many have observed the common accompaniment of depression with suicidal thoughts and actions. But depression stimulated from a wide variety of real or imagined sources is a very common if not universal phenomenon. It is the nature, depth, and duration of the depression that is important. The consensus is that, although most individuals who commit suicide suffer from conflicts and ambivalence with many seriously disturbed by neurotic and character disorders, the majority are not insane in the popular sense. Only about one fifth fall in that category. The importance of this in relation to the potential for preventive anticipation and action is obvious. This and related aspects of suicidal individuals will be considered further in the discussion of motivation in suicide.

EPIDEMIOLOGY OF SUICIDE

Much is now known about the epidemiology of suicide. An interesting observation is that *actual* suicide presents a different age pattern from *attempted* suicide. The incidence of suicide increases with age, climbing from a rate of 0.3 per 100,000 among those 5 to 14 years of age to more than 40 per 100,000 in persons over 75 years. Suicidal attempts are most common in young people, being highest in the late teens and early twenties. However, the highest rate in the large Chinese population of San Francisco is between 55 and 65 years of age.[20] Litman,[21] codirector of the Los Angeles Suicide Prevention Center, in discussing the approximately 100,000 self-poisonings each year in the United States involving children between the ages of 6 and 17 years, estimated that not only were 75% intentional but more than 25% were attempted suicides.

This coincides with the findings of a similar study[22] of 1,103 poisoned patients, aged 6 to 18 years, admitted to the emergency departments of a group of midwestern hospitals. It concluded that self-poisoning in that age group is rarely accidental. Boys predominated in the 6- to 10-year group, but after 11 years of age girls showed an abrupt increase in self-poisoning. However, a significant relative increase was observed among boys 17 to 18 years old, entirely independent of drug use. The investigators noted that the histories of children and youths involved in self-poisoning, suicidal attempts, and suicide seemed to be patterned into what they called "the five Ps"—privation (either poverty or privilege), parents, peers, punctured romance, and pregnancy. The importance of pregnancy among certain groups as a factor in teenage suicidal attempts has been emphasized by several investigators.[23]

In the United States it is commonly estimated that about 1 out of every 1,000 teenagers attempts suicide.[24] Some investigators such as Jacobziner[25] and Ross[26] however, believe suicidal attempts by young people to be much more common, perhaps in the ratio of 1 out of every 100 individuals. In their detailed studies in Edinburgh, McCulloch and Philip[8] note that currently 1 teenager in every 250 deliberately poisons or injures himself or herself, a rate almost double that the mid-1960s! An adequate explanation is yet to be found.

Especially tragic is the incident of suicide among college students, for whom it appears to be the second leading cause of death (after accidents) and who are at a 50% greater risk than nonstudents of the same ages.[27] Enigmatically it is noted that texts on "college health" rarely give more than a few paragraphs' attention, if any to this important problem. In recognition of the problem, however, colleges increasing are establishing "hot lines" so that troubled or suicidal students can call for help or advice. Fox[28] has made the cogent observation that "the student who takes his life represents the tip of an iceberg of youthful distress. The more we can learn of it, the better we can understand the mass with emotional problems falling short of fatality. Furthermore, any measures designed to prevent suicide must serve also to relieve distress at other levels." Ross and others have pointed to the collegiate atmosphere of intense competition, rapid social mobility, and expectations greater than can be realized by many students.

There have been some indications that students who achieve high or even highest scholastic grades are more likely to attempt suicide, perhaps because they often place greater demands on themselves than do their professors, schools, or parents. Although depression is the most frequently noted precursor, Ayd[29] has pointed out that suicide in the young is usually an impetuous act that occurs soon after a real or imagined wrong or failure and at a time when the young person has been manifesting personality and behavioral changes. "Thus," he concludes, "prior to age 30 it is the tense, confused, and deluded schizophrenic and not the depressed person who commits suicide, whereas after age 30 it is primarily the depressed manic-depressives, in-

cluding the involutional melancholics, and the chronic alcoholics who take their own lives." The distinctions become greater in the advanced years of life. In his studies of the psychodynamics of suicide among almost 7,000 elderly patients, Seidel[30] found the following factors significant: an increasing failure of psychophysical capacity, affective changes associated with aging, poor integration, a tendency toward hypochondria and paranoia, a feeling of rapid passage of time and the nearness of death, the loss of influences that give life a meaning and value, and restricted social existence.

Suicide is observed three times as frequently among males as among females, although more women appear to attempt suicide than do men. In recent years the gap has been narrowing with a rise in female attempts. Possibly this is one of several prices to be paid by women for their increased emancipation, or liberation, and the resultant changing role of women in society. A similar increase is being noted with regard to hypertension, coronary heart disease, cancer of the lung related to smoking, and other stress-related conditions. Among the races, suicide is four times as common among whites as among blacks, although some investigators have noted more attempts among blacks. It should also be noted that suicide rates for blacks have begun to move upward in recent years. The phenomenon is highest among Orientals, although the Chinese of San Francisco have a rate only two-thirds that of the city as a whole.[20] This appears to be essentially culture linked.

If age, sex, and race are considered together, some interesting contrasts are seen. Among white males in the United States suicide death rates increase consistently with each age group from 9.3 per 100,000 males between 15 and 24 years to 65.1 per 100,000 in those 85 years and older. Among white females, rates peak at 12.5 per 100,000 among those 45 to 54 years, then decrease. The rate for nonwhite males peaks at 16.2 per 100,000 between ages 25 to 34 years, then levels off. For nonwhite females the peak is also between 25 and 34 years but is much lower, 4.7 per 100,000, and declines from there.

These figures are subject to further qualification, however. A disturbing phenomenon is the recent startling increase in suicide in young people, especially females. For example, death rates per 100,000 from known suicides in Los Angeles County increased between 1960 and 1970 as follows:

under age 19 years—for males, from 3.3 to 10.0 and for females, from 0.04 to 8.0; between ages 20-29 years—for males, from 18.3 to 21.3 and for females, from 6.3 to 26.2.[12] With reference to racial differences, recent studies in New York City have demonstrated that suicides among blacks are underestimated by 82% as compared to 66% underestimation among whites.[31]

There are significant variations depending on marital status.[32] Below the age of 35 years single women are more a suicidal risk than are single men, but after 35 years this is reversed. Although married women tend to have higher rates than single women of comparable age, this is not true of men. Under 35 years of age both single and married men have comparable rates, but among those over 35 years the suicide rate for single men is double that of those who are married. Contrary to what is often assumed, rates for those widowed are low, but among those who are divorced or separated the rates are extremely high. This difference may be related to some of the personality and behavioral characteristics involved in many divorces or separations.

Completed suicides are more common among the more affluent and better educated than among the economically and educationally disadvantaged. Laborers, miners, teachers, and clergymen have low rates in contrast with entertainers, artists, businessmen, the military, and professionals, especially dentists, lawyers, and physicians. It is interesting that rates among the military are highest during peacetime, but rates for them and most other groups drop sharply when confronted by a military emergency. Among the professions those in medicine, especially psychiatrists and psychologists, have the highest rate. Indeed, the annual suicide rate among physicians in the United States is at least 33 per 100,000 (equivalent to one medical school class per year)—three times the national average. Among psychiatrists and psychoanalysts the rate is an astounding 70 per 100,000 per year. Conjuctured reasons for these high rates are the tendency to suppressed and introspective personalities, confrontation and preoccupation with morbid situations, ready availability of drugs and poisons, and limitation of family and social life.[33]

Sainsbury and Barraclough[34] discovered an interesting contrast with reference to attempted suicides in Edinburgh. One tenth of attempted suicides occurred among families of professionals and middle management personnel, one tenth occurred

among families of skilled occupations, two tenths occurred among families of skilled workers, and four tenths occurred among families of unskilled workers (these are reported numbers, not rates). They recognize, however, that affluent individuals are more likely to be quietly treated in their own homes or even in hospitals than are the less affluent. Based on this and other observations, they conclude that social class is largely irrelevant and that potential or actual suicides resemble each other more than nonsuicidal persons of their own social class.

ENVIRONMENT AND SUICIDE

Many aspects of the environment appear to influence suicidal tendencies. The further west one goes in the United States the higher become the rates. The reason for this is not clear. Suicide rates are also higher in the temperate than in the colder or warmer climates. They also rise with altitude. An interesting study in Philadelphia showed a rise whenever the barometer dropped. Contrary to what many would expect, the phenomenon is more common in the United States during the months of May and June and on clear, sunny days. A similar contradiction is the more frequent occurrence early in the week, on a Monday or Tuesday morning soon after arising, rather than at the end of a possibly long and arduous week. Interestingly, in Edinburgh, April and November account for one fourth of all suicides, and weekends and holidays have particularly high rates with midweek the lowest. Wenz[35] suggests that people tend to review or audit their lives during holidays and that this factor merits more study. Obviously a knowledge of local time–occurrence relationships is important for effective program planning so that availability of resources will be related to suicide peak hours, days, and seasons.

Central cities generally have higher rates than suburbs, which in turn are more threatened than rural areas or small towns where it is less difficult to be unknown. Suicide is more common among immigrants than among the native born. Undoubtedly anomie and the frustrations of linguistic and economic problems are significant factors. This also applies to many native Americans, among some of whom suicide has been described as almost epidemic.[36] Religion, when it is practiced, plays an important role. Rates are highest among those who follow Oriental faiths, are next highest among Protestants and reformed Jews, low among Roman Catholics, and lowest among orthodox Jews and followers of Islam.

The effect of mass communications media on suicide also merits careful consideration. Although it did not address itself specifically to suicide, the Surgeon General's Scientific Advisory Committee on Television and Social Behavior[37] found evidence of some relationship between violent television programs and aggressiveness in children. Other studies have indicated that news media and so-called comic books may stimulate destructive action in young people by vivid and detailed portrayal and sometimes even glorification of various forms of aggression and violence. These factors seem to have played a role to some extent during the epidemic of campus violence during the late 1960s. If this can be true of externalized violence, why not internalized violence? It is significant that during the 268-day "news blackout" in Detroit between November 1967 and August 1968, the suicide rate in both sexes and all age groups dropped significantly.[38]

METHODS

Many methods are used by individuals intent on ending their existence. Women tend to use nonviolent or nondisfiguring methods, apparently maintaining some concern about their appearance even after death. An analysis[39] of the methods used by over 20,000 Americans who committed suicide in 1964 is shown in Table 28-1. Some question may be raised concerning the validity of the data for hanging and strangulation as well as for some of the other methods listed because of erotic implications in some instances.[40,41]

Be that as it may, an important consideration is the variation of methodology of the suicidal act through time and place. Studies have indicated a reflection of national attitudes in relation to predominant methods and changes over time as new drugs appear. The inexpensive and extensive production of barbiturates has resulted in these drugs being increasingly used throughout the world. In some parts of the United States and in Scandinavia they have replaced firearms and explosives as the most common method. Farberow[42] finds that in Los

TABLE 28-1. Methods used in successful suicides, United States, 1964

Method	Percentage
Firearms and explosives	47.2
Hanging and strangulation	14.7
Analgesics and soporifics	12.4
Gases	11.5
Other solid and liquid substances	3.6
Jumping from high places	3.6
Submersion (drowning)	2.6
Piercing instruments	1.8
Other and unspecified means	2.6
TOTAL	100.0

Angeles barbiturates are involved in 40% of suicides compared with 35% caused by guns and explosives. A somewhat similar picture was obtained by Ford and others[43] in their analysis of suicides in metropolitan Cleveland between 1959 and 1974. Asphyxia (drowning, suffocation, and hanging), which earlier had been the most common method, gave way to firearms among males and to poisoning among females. The use of both firearms and poisons increased significantly over the 17-year period. Firearm rates rose 62% among males and 125% among females, and poisoning rose 67% among males and 112% among females. The highest firearm rates were among young nonwhite city males (a 267% increase) and older white males. Suicide by poisoning increased among all subgroups except nonwhite city males. White city males had the greatest increase in poisoning rates (157%), but the highest rate of poisoning was observed among suburban white females.

SUICIDE AND THE LAW

The attitude of the law toward suicide depends on the prevailing ethics in a particular place at a particular time. Although most monotheistic religions prohibit suicide, they are sometimes inconsistent. For example, Buddhism forbids the killing of any form of life yet recognizes suicide as a religious practice under certain circumstances. Similarly, there may be social approval of suicide on the basis of national honor or security.[44,45] Generally, throughout history, governments and their laws have frowned on suicide. According to Blackstone, the great English legal commentator, in ancient Athens attempted suicide was punished by cutting off the hand that committed the forbidden act. Another approach was described by Plutarch in relation to an epidemic of suicides among women in Milesia, who for certain reasons preferred death to matrimony. The epidemic was brought to a stop by a decree that the bodies of those who committed suicide would be displayed naked in the public marketplace. Although it is unclear whether suicide was punishable under Roman law, an attempted suicide to evade trial for a crime was punished. Early Christians venerated martyrs who invited death, but the church prohibited suicide in AD 452, followed by an edict 250 years later that punished suicide by excommunication.

Suicide in England originally fell under the jurisdiction of the ecclesiastic courts, which condemned it. In AD 673 it became part of English common law, which made suicide subject to severe civil penalties including forfeiture of land and goods. For more than 1,000 years it was a felony, and at one time the punishment was ignominious burial in the highway without religious rites and with a stake driven through the body. The last crossroads burial of a suicide occurred in 1882 in London's Grosvenor Place. Meanwhile, the law had been amended to allow burial in church grounds, although unconsecrated and only between the hours of 9 PM and midnight! Blackstone himself regarded suicide as among the worst crimes, considering it a double offense—spiritual by invading the prerogatives by the Almighty, and temporal against the King by depriving him of a subject. Suicide is still considered a felony under English law, and one who aids and abets a suicide is a principal in the second degree to the crime of murder. Before 1916, imprisonment was normal punishment, but now the individual may be institutionalized, placed under guardianship, or still sent to prison.[46] When canon law spoke against suicide, both France and Italy made it a crime. However, when the French criminal code was written in 1810, it ignored suicide, and other countries of Europe followed suit, and it has not been punishable as a crime in continental Europe since the last half of the nineteenth century.

The harshness of English law toward suicide was never applied in America. However, as Curran[47] has indicated:

The current law in the 50 states is in hopeless confusion with some states still "punishing" suicide as a crime; some "punishing" attempted suicide, with or without punishing the "crime" itself; and some, with or without either of these, punishing a person who aids another in committing suicide. There is no pattern or purpose to the law which is at all discernible from a reading of the law and the last few law review commentaries published in recent years.

Diggory[48] in discussing some of the attitudes and laws concerning suicide in various cultures and religious groups, has emphasized the importance of consciously putting aside one's own value system, be it religious, philosophic, or scientific, when working with a suicidal person. He complains that an integrated value system involved in dealing with suicidal people has not been given the careful thought that is necessary if people are to develop functional concepts that are meaningful, both to the person who is contemplating or has attempted suicide and to those close to him. Such a value system, to the maximum degree possible, should be objective, empiric, and functionally oriented. Diggory concludes with the provocative question, "Do we value life in the sense of continued individual development of skill, knowledge, affiliations and achievements; or do we value it as a prolongation of vegetable metabolism?" In any case, to regard suicide or its attempt as self-murder is a curt way of justifying an indictment and trial of an unfortunate person who has succumbed to the stresses and exigencies of life. Such an act is neither sinful nor a crime. This person is a distressed sufferer from a severe emotional disorder and if a survivor, should be placed under expert medical and social care and not imprisoned. The implications of this go far beyond suicide and involve attitudes toward contraception, the limitation of treatment of those in extremis, and euthanasia.

SUICIDE AND THE PHYSICIAN

There has been a tendency even among members of the medical and health professions to regard suicide fatalistically, as if it were none of their concern or as if nothing could be done about it. Nevertheless, even the inadequate efforts that have been made to attack the problem provide sufficient evidence that suicides can be prevented. Some optimism seems justified. Potential suicide victims do not act impulsively; the majority of them talk about it or give other clues to their thoughts or intentions frequently for a long period of time. Specific statements are frequently made to family, friends, work associates, and often to physicians indicating preoc-cupation with death and the desire to die. Regret-fully, these warnings of impending suicide are often missed or ignored.

Kobler and Stotland[49] view "verbal and other communications of suicidal attempts, as efforts, however misdirected, to solve problems of living, as frantic pleas for help and hope from other people; help in solving the problem and hope that they can be solved. Whether the individual then actually commits suicide seems to depend to a large part on the nature of the responses by other people to his pleas." Havens[50] also considers suicidal efforts to spring from despair and helplessness. Illustrations of the extent to which these cries for help offer a challenge to the medical profession are frequent. In one study in New Hampshire nearly 50% of individuals who committed suicide consulted a physician a short while before for a wide range of illnesses considered as masks for underlying depressions or anxieties. In a San Francisco study 1 out of every 6 suicide victims was known to have seen a physician during the preceding week, and more than 2 out of 5 persons within the preceding 6 months. Shneidman and Dizmang[51] have main-tained that "a well-trained and skillful physician should be as able to identify a potentially suicidal patient on a routine examination as he can detect an early heart murmur or slightly enlarged spleen." Similarly, they indicate that a past suicidal attempt or history of suicide in a family "must be looked at just as carefully as a history of familial diabetes or previous history of glucose in the urine."

In other words, failure by physicians to prevent suicide is caused not so much by ignorance of the causes as by lack of awareness and failure to rec-ognize the signs and symptoms of impending sui-cide among those in their practices. Beyond this, many physicians are hesitant to report a death of-ficially as a suicide. This is especially true if they have known the patient and the family. Further-more, the fact that some life insurance policies re-fuse payment in the case of suicide not only causes many persons to mask the act but also leads some physicians to mask the diagnosis.

MOTIVATION IN SUICIDE

What, then, are the causes of suicide? The actual phenomenon appears to result from the interplay between (1) factors inherent in the patient and (2) factors in the environment. Of the two, the first is without question the more critical. Numerous stud-ies indicate that the most significant characteristic of those who attempt suicide is a state of frank psychosis. For example, Robins and associates[52] ob-served that 98% of the suicides they studied had been clinically ill and 94% of them psychiatrically ill. Of the group, 68% had been suffering from one of two diseases: manic depression or chronic al-coholism. None of the individuals in the study had an uncomplicated neurosis (anxiety reaction, con-version reaction, or obsessive compulsive reaction). It is of interest that 73% of the manic-depressives and 40% of the alcoholics had been under medical or psychiatric care for illnesses associated with their suicide during the year preceding their death.

To approach this question from a different direc-tion, evidence of the significance of mental aber-ration among would-be suicides includes the fol-lowing. Suicide is the most common cause of death among those known to be mentally ill. The method chosen for the actual suicide is often irrational. Thus individuals may hang themselves out of a high window instead of jumping. Related is a ten-dency to irrational response. Thus the suicidal per-son does not respond to reasoning or logic but may be influenced often by suggestion or threat. "Come in from that window ledge or I'll close the window!" or "Come aboard this boat or you'll catch a cold!" In such instances the response of course is merely temporary and unrelated to the heart of the prob-lem. Another significant observation is that rarely is insufferable pain a factor in suicide. More often it is an obsessive hypochondriac concentration on a trivial ailment or problem. Not infrequently the depression that precedes an actual suicide is out of proportion to the cause of the depression. This pro-vides the rationale for the prompt institution of an-tidepressant drugs or even electroshock therapy in some cases of emphatically threatened or attempted suicides.

Although, as indicated, some investigators point to high incidences of psychiatric disturbances among attempted suicides, not everyone agrees to its importance. Thus Kessel[53,54] states "distress drives people to self poisoning acts, and distress is not the exclusive province of the mentally ill." Sim-ilarly, there is no justification for assuming the ex-istence of a specifically suicide-prone personality. To do so would rule out such significant factors as acquired behaviorisms or undesirable environmen-tal and social conditions.[55]

The result of the combination of psychiatric, environmental, social, and acquired behavioral forces is illustrated by a study[8] of 50 men and 50 women after recovery from suicidal attempts. Almost 50% of each group were rated as character disordered. Forty percent showed other signs of psychiatric disturbance—one half of whom had personality disturbances, and the rest were of uncertain pathology. The remaining 12% showed no signs of psychiatric pathology. As would be expected, a higher proportion of psychiatrically disturbed individuals are found among those who attempt suicide repeatedly.

Many investigators have noted a close association between alcoholism and drug addiction on the one hand and attempted suicide on the other. It is important, however, to make certain distinctions. For example, a study of deaths involving psychotropic drugs in four major cities indicated 36% as "definitely suicide" and 44% as "nonsuicide."[56] "Suicide" deaths tended to be associated with barbiturates, analgesics, and/or sedatives, whereas "nonsuicide" victims usually died from an accidental overdose of narcotics, usually heroin. In about one fourth of the deaths in each category, alcohol played a significant role. It is significant that whereas only an estimated one fifth of those involved in first attempts are alcoholics or problem drinkers, almost one half of repeaters may be so classified. This points to a group at much greater than average risk that merits special community and public health attention. Essentially the same is true of those involved in drug abuse or addiction. Thus the apparent suicide rate for "mainlining" narcotic addicts is 50 times greater than that for nonaddicts. It is important to realize, however, the complexity of these situations in that alcoholics, addicts, and attempted suicide victims all tend to share many or most of the various precipitating or contributing factors such as inadequacy, escapism, loneliness, or dejection.

A fascinating sidelight of some studies of the behavior of dolphins is the discovery that these perceptive, affectionate, and intelligent mammals seem deliberately to commit suicide not only if they are sick or injured but also out of frustration and boredom. This perhaps provides further commentary on one of the consequences of a well-developed forebrain!

One of the greatest problems in the field of suicidology, as indeed it is in the mental health field as a whole, is the wish or tendency to oversimplify. Life—and death—are exceedingly complex phenomena. There is no easy answer or explanation

for either, and attitudes toward them have changed considerably throughout human history.[57] When death comes by one's own hand, the complexities are multiplied. Weisman[58] certainly had this in mind in a moving statement in which he distinguishes between the preterminal and the presuicidal person.

Some people begin the decline toward death calmly, while others feel apathetic or antagonistic about their fate. It is certain, however, that many more patients find death acceptable or appropriate than has heretofore been appreciated. Disinclination to live is not the same as the wish to terminate life, but some terminal patients acquiesce to death with something of the same quality that other patients display when they passively submit to lethal forces, or even when they take steps to hasten their demise.

I do not believe that pre-terminal patients have the same characteristics as pre-suicidal patients. Even the most superficial assessment of patients desperately sick with a life-threatening illness discloses that there is a wide difference between them and people who have attempted suicide and have inflicted grave organic impairment upon themselves.

Prominent among factors associated with suicidal attempts may be listed broken homes or frequent household moves during childhood, marital disharmony, emotional immaturity, cruelty to children, and jealousy bordering on the pathologic. Not infrequently these factors are coexistent, as indicated in Table 28-2. Handkoff[59] has placed the various suicidal conditioning or triggering factors into the following three categories: (1) stress, typically with heightened emotionality and reactivity; (2) crisis, based on a seemingly insoluble situation of very recent or acute nature; and (3) disorder of a psychopathologic nature.

Loneliness has been noted as highly significant. Indeed, it has been claimed that of all factors associated with suicide, isolation and loneliness may be the most significant. This would seem to justify special community effort toward identification of such persons and provision of easy and multiple channels of social communication and involvement for them. Organized "befriending" or "buddy" systems have been effective in this regard.[60] In men an important factor is anxiety related to inability to obtain and retain employment or advancement. This is worthy of particular concern at this time in view of the current rapid changes in science and technology, fears of automation, and the decreasing time-value of specialized training and education. Concern applies especially to middle-aged men who, coincident with real or feared decline in economic values, begin to observe the independence of their children and the waning of their own physical and sexual strength. It is suspected that the much vaunted shorter work week may exacerbate these problems. Some studies have indicated that about one third of men who attempt suicide have frequent or prolonged periods of unemployment unrelated to work capability or availability. To emphasize this further, unemployment has been noted as a precipitating factor in one third of male suicidal attempts and as a contributing factor in one half of male and one fourth of female suicidal attempts. In terms of elicited precipitating factors, it stands fourth, after financial difficulties, alcoholism, and marital discord, and often all four factors combine to form a vicious chicken-and-egg cycle.

The foregoing has been well summarized by Cautela,[61] who indicates that in essence three factors are determinants in suicidal attempts: (1) aversion stimuli, such as acute pain or rejection; (2) absence of adequate reinforcement; and (3) escape conditioning as a learned response. He adds that it is noteworthy that all three factors tend to be present in the elderly man. Not only do more elderly men take their own lives as compared with younger men and with women of all ages but the gap between attempts and completions narrows alarmingly. As some investigators have emphasized, "Suicidal old men seldom miss!" One is reminded of the comment by Weisman[62] that one aspect of terminal behavior is an attempt to create a distance between oneself and a noxious situation, and as he notes, the suicide, if successful, achieves this in a most complete way.

DIAGNOSIS OF IMPENDING SUICIDE

In most instances the presuicidal state is temporary. If the condition is recognized and the patient is protected from self-destruction through this critical period, there is a good chance of the suicide being prevented. This also provides time for appropriate treatment.

How may the potential suicide be diagnosed? Shneidman[63] has stated that the suicide syndrome is a constellation of symptoms and lists them as depressed, disoriented, defiant, and dependent-dissatisfied. This provides some indication of behaviorisms that should be watched for. As for the type of person to watch, the potentiality of suicide should be kept in mind with reference to (1) all depressed persons, (2) all manic-depressive patients, (3) especially all those who have previously attempted suicide—no matter how long ago, (4) those who often speak of suicide with apparent seriousness, and (5) those who have suddenly lost interest in previously important and valued things and events.

A question commonly asked is, "What about those who *think* of suicide?" This in itself would not appear to be dangerous. Several studies indicate that suicide is considered by the majority of individuals at one time or another. Fortunately, however, only a minor proportion act on the idea and action is based on deep psychologic problems. A number of warning signals merit attention. Among these are evidence of depression, especially with manifestations of guilt, tension, or agitation; insom-

TABLE 28-2. Rates of occurrence of certain social variables in attempted suicides, Edinburgh

Variable	Rate per 1,000 for attempted suicides	Rate per 1,000 for Edinburgh
Overcrowding	294.7	93.0
Rented accommodation	389.5	193.6
Divorce	73.7	9.7
Separation	94.7	25.3
Persistent truancy	684.2	2.1
Court prosecutions	410.5	39.6
Children in care	200.0	3.4
Referrals for child cruelty	105.3	6.6
Repeated attempted suicide	442.1	0.5

From McCulloch, J.W., and Philip, A.E.: Suicidal behavior, Oxford, 1972, Pergamon Press, Ltd.

nia, especially if great concern is expressed about it; severe hypochondriasis; expressions of fear of losing self-control; frequent discussion about and apparent preoccupation with the idea of suicide or death; and, of course, previous attempts. The depths of depression may be judged by an otherwise inexplicable loss of weight, appetite, and sexual desire; a slowing and blurring of speech and action; an unusual hesitancy or unwillingness to meet people; an attitude of hopelessness, often indicated by a drawn and wrinkled facial expression and dullness of the eyes; chronic low back pain that does not respond to appropriate medical treatment; chronic recurring headaches with elusive etiology; vague and frequent gastrointestinal complaints; and interestingly, as Ross[64] has observed, not only peculiar vague sensations and a bad taste in the mouth but actual dental pain and discomfort. Among the social and transitional changes to be noted are a history of a broken home or disorganized family life, lack of friends, or significant losses in an individual's life. Ross gives a good general word picture of such people:

One's first observation may be of a pale faced sallow person sitting huddled in a waiting room chair evidencing little or no spontaneous activity. Further inspection may reveal evidence of weight and sleep loss, perhaps accentuated facial wrinkles and eyelid folds, and lacklustre hair. There may be careless or unkempt grooming.

Ross also calls attention to the manner in which such individuals present complaints to physicians or others. For example, a highly anxious patient may tell his or her story rapidly without interruption or be preoccupied with minutiae. "Immobility of facial expression and body," he says, "can communicate underlined discouragement," and notes that "it is remarkable how often the patient presents the notion that things are different for him: his world, his life, his bodily function, his outlook and his habits."

MANAGEMENT OF THE IMPENDING SUICIDE

An important question is how best to handle the individual with apparent or frank suicidal intent. If contact is possible, every effort should be made to continue conversation while eliciting as much meaningful information as possible and alerting appropriate sources of assistance.[65] The patient should be encouraged by "gatekeepers"[66] (spouse, friends, neighbors, clergyman, policeman, barten-

ders, employer, etc.) to be examined by a physician. The physician in turn should give the patient an opportunity to talk out troubles and problems, great or small, real or imagined, in the patient's own way.

The reality of the intent or attempt to commit suicide should be accepted and discussed forthrightly and the patient encouraged to discuss thoughts, problems, reactions, and motivations. A complete medical examination should be performed since many would-be suicides have physical as well as mental complaints that are sometimes interrelated. This also provides the patient and the physician with a specific physical focus of attention and goal. Those who are mildly troubled should be given helpful suggestions. Single and lonely persons should be encouraged to participate in group and religious activities. On the other hand, agitated and depressed patients and those who have previously attempted suicide may be given antidepressant medications and should be referred promptly to a psychiatrist rather than to rely, as so often is the case, on the police or prison or on the county or municipal general hospitals.[67,68] It is the consensus that such individuals should be immediately referred by physicians for hospitalization in a closed psychiatric service.[52] This provides the best opportunity for further clinical and psychiatric study, psychotherapy, and whatever drugs or shock therapy might be indicated. After the acute episode is past and the patient is considered eligible for release, provision should be made for appropriate follow-up in the community by a competently staffed community mental health program.

SUICIDE PREVENTION PROGRAMS

Recent years have seen a slow but growing interest in the problem of suicide and its prevention. Initially, various essentially nonprofessional volunteer groups; then social workers, psychiatrists, public safety officers; the legal, medical, and public health professions; and finally the public became interested and willing to consider the problem. The trend bears out Dublin's[69] view that although all the questions are by no means answered, the practicality of developing effective programs has been well demonstrated in many communities and nations. Suicide is now recognized as a problem of great significance that lends itself to intelligent public health effort.

The first effort goes back about three quarters of a century to the Anti-suicide Bureau of the Salvation Army.[70] This was established in London in 1905 and in purposes and method bore many similarities to the programs of today. The work of the Samaritans[71] in England also merits special mention in view of this group's length of service and pioneering in the blending of the forces of theology, medicine, psychiatry, and social work. Similar organizations exist in Vienna, Berlin, Milan, and several other European cities.

Most notable in the United States for its leadership has been the Los Angeles Suicide Prevention Center.[72] In an address to state and territorial mental health authorities in 1966, Shneidman[73] predicted, "Now at the end of 1966, we stand on the threshold of an efflorescence and burgeoning of suicide prevention activities." He illustrated this by the fact that whereas in 1958 only 2 states had programs, by the time of his address 15 states were included. Within the following half year, 4 more states were added, and in the interval since, great progress has been made toward the goal of anti-suicide activities in all 50 states. Similar growth has occurred on the local level, and by now there are more than 200 suicide prevention programs in cities throughout the nation. Obviously many more are needed. These centers are conducted by a variety of agencies, including hospitals, medical centers, mental health facilities, official and voluntary social service agencies, religious organizations, and some health departments. They operate under a variety of names, often chosen for easy identification and an implication of empathy—Hotline, Life Line, We Care, Help, Call for Help, Rescue, Crisis Service, Crisis Intervention, and many others. It is regrettable that many are little more than telephone answering and referral services, which accomplish little but delay. Thus Kiev,[74] of Cornell University Medical Center, states that current programs that rely on receiving calls and referring have shown no evidence of reducing the suicide rate. He notes that whereas suicides are most common among men, most patients in psychiatric clinics and office practices are women. Because of this, he urged that active links be established with industry, schools, prisons, alcohol rehabilitation facilities, and similar institutions. Welu[75] has voiced similar concerns and recommendations, warning that

we have artifically served the phenomenon of suicide from the habitat in which it exists. Thus our suicide prevention efforts have been quite parochial. We have disassociated suicide prevention from the bigger arena of suicidogenic constituents, namely, society's rejection of the aged, retirement, social readjustment, social isolation, society's growing disregard for life, and other factors or elements existing and/or exhibited in a society which may have a causal relationship to suicide or be a condition which predisposes the individual to begin travelling on the suicidal continuum.

Welu proposes that suicide prevention programs should be based on the concept of a suicidogenic continuum that depicts movement, not necessarily causality, and includes suicidogenic constituents—a prodromal phase and a terminal phase. These views are subscribed to and have been presented in depth by many of the current leaders in suicidology.[76]

On these premises a suicide prevention program may be visualized as follows:

A. *Primary prevention.* This should be aimed, as Stengel[77] views it, to eliminate or reduce all factors that tend to increase the incidence of suicidal acts and to strengthen all those that tend to reduce it. This is recognized as going far beyond suicide and involves a "drastic reorientation of society to the social needs of its members."
   1. Preservation of the family
   2. Active membership in a religious community or some other social group
   3. Fight against alcoholism and drugs
   4. Improved mental and physical health
   5. Improved medical services
   6. Employment for all to the extent of their ability
   7. Improved medical and social care for the elderly

B. *Secondary prevention.* This should be aimed, as Welu[75] views it, in terms of the public health model, at early discovery, diagnosis, and prompt treatment to prevent progression and, hopefully, repetition.
   1. An active outreach program to contact the older population who exhibit prodromal clues
   2. Identification of the suicide-attempt population and initiation of follow-up treatment and continuity of care after discharge
   3. Education of professionals and the public

concerning prodromal clues and emergency and antisuicidal resources

4. Improvement of treatment facilities to assure prompt, correct, and adequate response to suicidal attempts

5. Mobilization of the entire community to recognize the magnitude of the problem and the community's role in its solution

6. Provision of a 24-hour crisis intervention service including efficient coordination of all pertinent resources

7. Development of a continuous research effort in all aspects of the problem and its solution

There are many sources of input for a suicide prevention program of this nature. Earlier, for example, the term *gatekeeper* was used to describe the types of individuals who are in a position to observe and be alert to the potential suicide and who might refer such an individual to adequate sources of assistance. In addition, there are the important roles of private physicians, outpatient clinics and hospitals, mental health programs, poison control centers, accident prevention programs, agencies that deal with juvenile delinquency, alcoholism, and narcotic addiction programs, and many other agencies and groups in the community. Generally speaking, on the basis of preventive philosophy, if suicide is essentially a psychiatric problem, it necessarily follows that the earlier the age at which emotional or mental problems are identified, the closer one comes to the interruption of the motivating factors for suicide. Because of this, particular emphasis should be placed on the care and training of young children.

Based on their various studies of suicide Tuckman and associates[78,79] have suggested the following suicide prevention program.

1. Evaluation and referral services for persons showing suicidal thinking and behavior

2. Consultation services for physicians, social agencies, and the community at large with respect to potential suicides

3. Community education, including the preparation of suitable educational materials with emphasis on diagnosis, prevention, and treatment, and the introduction of material on suicide in medical school curricula

4. Development of follow-up procedures for attempted suicides with special emphasis on children and young adults

5. Casefinding to obtain a more accurate estimate of

suicidal behavior in the community as well as to gather systematically life experience, personality structure, and environmental stresses

To these should be added the need for a type of 24-hour service on which the individual under stress can rely for help. This is perhaps best illustrated by the Nightwatch part of the Los Angeles program[80] or by the program of the Samaritans in England. Callers receive immediate sympathetic consideration with evaluation of the emergency, appropriate counseling, and referral. If indicated, appropriate individuals and teams may be sent to the caller on an emergency basis. Use of these services have been considerable with frequent successful results.

NATIONAL ACTION IN THE UNITED STATES

Of great significance in the movement to understand and do more about the problem of suicide was the establishment in 1966 of the Center for Studies of Suicide Prevention in the National Institute of Mental Health. Shneidman,[4] who organized it, considered it to have five basic functions:

1. To serve as the focal point within the Institute to coordinate and direct activities throughout the nation in support of research, pilot studies, training, information, and consultation aimed at furthering basic knowledge about suicide, and improving techniques for helping the suicidal individual

2. To compile and disseminate information and training material designed to assist mental health personnel, clergy, police, educators, and others in obtaining a better understanding of suicidal actions and learning to utilize research findings

3. To assist in developing and experimenting with the variety of regional and local programs and organizational models to coordinate emergency services and techniques of prevention, case finding, treatment, training and research

4. To maintain liaison with studies and programs on suicide prevention undertaken by other agencies, both national and international

5. To promote and maintain the application of research findings by state and local mental health agencies

More specifically, Shneidman listed 10 aspects of a comprehensive national suicide prevention program to include the following:

1. A program of support of suicide prevention activities in many communities throughout the nation

2. A special program for the "gatekeepers" of suicide prevention
3. A carefully prepared program in massive public education
4. A special program for followup of suicide attempts
5. An active NIMH program of research and training grants
6. A redefinition and refinement of statistics on suicide
7. The development of a cadre of trained, dedicated professionals
8. Governmentwide liaison and national use of a broad spectrum of professional personnel
9. A special followup program for the survivor-victims of individuals who have committed suicide
10. A rigorous program for the evaluation of the effectiveness of suicide prevention activities

This 10-point program for suicide prevention is indicated as a cooperative societal enterprise, which to be successful requires the active interest, support, and activities of many groups, individuals, and professions in communities throughout the country. Particularly important has been the development of a group of individuals labeled by Shneidman as "suicidologists," who focus on the problem as their chief interest. In this regard it is significant that in 1967 the first students of the new profession began a year's fellowship study at the Henry Phipps Psychiatric Clinic of Johns Hopkins University under a grant from the National Institute of Mental Health. Fellowships have been offered to qualified members of a variety of disciplines, including psychiatry, psychology, social work, anthropology, sociology, public health education, and psychiatric nursing. Also in mid-1967, the Center for Studies of Suicide Prevention inaugurated a *Bulletin of Suicidology*. After functioning successfully for several years, the center ceased to exist because of budgetary reasons. However, its functions were taken up by other programs and agencies. Most notable has been the American Association of Suicidology, founded by Shneidman in 1968. This organization publishes the successor to the *Bulletin of Suicidology* in the form of its journal, *Suicide and Life-Threatening Behavior,* as well as a variety of other very useful publications.

In view of the accelerating interest in the subject of suicide and the progress that has occurred in recent years, there is good reason to anticipate that at last a forthright and intelligent attack will be launched against this major cause of disability and death.

REFERENCES

1. Farberow, N.L.: Bibliography on suicide and suicide prevention, 1897-1970, DHEW Pub. No. (HSM) 72-9080, Rockville, Md., 1972, National Institute of Mental Health.
2. Resnik, H.L.P., and Hathorne, B.C., editors: Suicide prevention in the '70s, DHEW Pub. No. (HSM) 72-9054, Rockville, Md., 1973, National Institute of Mental Health.
3. Shneidman, E.S., Farberow, N.L., and Litman, R.E.: The psychology of suicide, New York, 1970, Science House, Inc.
4. Shneidman, E.S.: The N.I.M.H. center for studies of suicide prevention, Bull. Suicidol., July 1967, p. 2.
5. National Center for Health Statistics: Monthly Vital Stat. Rep. **31:**9, Washington, D.C., April 16, 1982.
6. Farberow, N.L., MacKinnon, D.R., and Nelson, F.L.: Suicide: who's counting? Public Health Rep. **92:**223, May-June 1977.
7. Brooke, E.M.: Suicide and attempted suicide, Geneva, 1974, World Health Organization.
8. McCulloch, J.W., and Philip, A.E.: Suicidal behavior, Oxford, 1972, Pergamon Press, Ltd.
9. Litman, R.E., and Tabachnick, N.: Fatal one-car accidents, Psychoanal. Q. **36:**248, April 1967.
10. Curphey, T.: The role of the social scientist in the medico-legal certification of death from suicide. In Farberow, N., and Shneidman, E., editors: The cry for help, New York, 1961, McGraw-Hill Book Co.
11. Weisman, A.D., and Kastenbaum, R.: The psychological autopsy: a study of the terminal phase of life, New York, 1968, Columbia University Press.
12. Allen, N.A.: Suicide in California 1960-1970, Sacramento, 1973, California Department of Public Health, p. 29.
13. Tabachnick, N., Litman, R.E., Osman, M., and others: Comparative psychiatric study of accidental and suicidal death, Arch. Gen. Psychiatry **14:**60, Jan. 1966.
14. Shneidman, E.S.: Suicide, sleep and death, J. Consult. Psychol. **28:**95, Feb. 1964.
15. Durkheim, E.: Le Suicide (Suicide), Glencoe, Ill., 1951, The Free Press. (Translated by J.A. Spaulding and G. Simpson).
16. Kramer, M., and others: Mental disorders/suicide, Cambridge, Mass., 1972, Harvard University Press.
17. Meerloo, J.: Suicide and mass suicide, New York, 1962, Grune & Stratton, Inc.
18. Brophy, B.: Black ship to hell, New York, 1962, Harcourt, Brace, & World, Inc.
19. Freud, S.: Beyond the pleasure principle, New York, 1950, Liveright.
20. Bourne, P.G.: Suicide among chinese in San Francisco, Am. J. Public Health **63:**744, Aug. 1973.

21. Litman, R.E.: Presuicidal states in adolescents, Am. J. Orthopsychiatry **39:**315, 1969.

22. McIntyre, M.S., and Angle, C.R.: Is the poisoning accidental? Clin. Pediatr. **10:**414, Oct. 1971.

23. Gabrielson, I.W., and others: Suicide attempts in a population pregnant as teen-agers, Am. J. Public Health **60:**2289, Dec. 1970.

24. Faigel, H.C.: Suicide among young persons, Clin. Pediatr. **5:**187, Jan. 1966.

25. Jacobziner, H.: Attempted suicides in adolescence, J.A.M.A. **191:**7, Jan. 1965.

26. Ross, M.: Suicide among college students, Am. J. Psychiatry **126:**220, Aug. 1969.

27. Peck, M.L., and Schrut, A.: Suicidal behavior among college students, HSMHA Health Rep. **86:**149, Feb. 1971.

28. Fox, R.: Suicide among students and its prevention, R. Soc. Health J. **91:**181, July-Aug. 1971.

29. Ayd, F.J.: Psycho-drugs as suicide inhibitors, U.S. Med. **4:**19, Feb. 1, 1968.

30. Seidel, K.: The independent internal dynamics of suicide in the aged, Bibl. Psychiatr. Neurol. **142:**42, Jan. 1969.

31. Warshauer, M.E., and Monk, M.: Problems in suicide statistics for whites and blacks, Am. J. Public Health **68:**383, April 1978.

32. Paffenbarger, R.S., and Asnes, D.P.: Precursors of suicide in early and middle life, Am. J. Public Health **56:**1026, July 1966.

33. Anonymous: High rate of suicide among physicians, Med. World News **4:**5, July 3, 1964.

34. Sainsbury, P., and Barraclough, B.: Differences between suicide rates, Nature **220:**1252, 1968.

35. Wenz, F.V.: Effects of seasons and sociological variables on suicidal behavior, Public Health Rep. **92:**233, May-June 1977.

36. Dizmang, L.H.: Suicide among the Cheyenne Indians, Bull. Suicidol., p. 8, July 1967.

37. Surgeon General's Scientific Advisory Committee on Television and Social Behavior: The impact of televised violence, DHEW Pub. No. (HSM) 72-9090, Rockville, Md., 1972, National Institute of Mental Health.

38. Anonymous: Suicide and the press, Lancet **7623:**731, 1969.

39. Felix, R.H.: Suicide, a neglected problem, Am. J. Public Health **55:**16, Jan. 1965.

40. Resnik, H.L.P.: Eroticized repetitive hangings: a form of self-destructive behavior, Am. J. Psychother. **26:**4, Jan. 1972.

41. Litman, R.E.: Eroticism, aggression and suicides in depressions. In Masserman, J.H., editor: Science and psychoanalysis, vol. 17, New York, 1970, Grune & Stratton, Inc.

42. Farberow, N.L.: Research in suicide. In Resnick, H.L.P., and Hathorn, B.C., editors: Suicide in the '70s, DHEW Pub. No. (HSM) 72-9054, p. 63, Rock-ville, Md., 1973, National Institute of Mental Health.

43. Ford, A.B., and others: Violent death in a metropolitan county. II. Changing patterns in suicides (1959-1974), Am. J. Public Health **69:**459, May 1979.

44. Silving, H.: Suicide and law. In Shneidman, E.S., and Farberow, N.L., editors: Clues to suicide, New York, 1957, McGraw-Hill Book Co.

45. Farberow, N.L., editor: Suicide in different cultures, Baltimore, 1975, University Park Press.

46. St. John-Stevas, N.: Life, death, and the law, Bloomington, 1961, Indiana University Press.

47. Curran, W.J.: Suicide: civil right or punishable crime? Am. J. Public Health **60:**163, Jan. 1970.

48. Diggory, J.C.: Suicide and value. In Resnik, H.L.P., editor: Suicidal behaviors: Diagnosis and management, Boston, 1968, Little, Brown & Co.

49. Kobler, A.L., and Stotland, E.: The end of hope: a social-clinical study of suicide, New York, 1964, The Free Press.

50. Havens, L.I.: Recognition of suicidal risks through the psychological examination, N. Engl. J. Med. **276**(4):210, Jan. 26, 1967.

51. Shneidman, E.S., and Dizmang, L.H.: In Discussion on suicide, M.D. **11:**93, Sept. 1967.

52. Robins, E., and others: Some clinical considerations in the prevention of suicide based on a study of 134 successful suicides, Am. J. Public Health **49:**888, July 1959.

53. Kessel, N.: Self poisoning, Br. Med. J. **5473:**1265, 1965.

54. Kessel, N.: Self poisoning, Br. Med. J. **5474:**1336, 1965.

55. World Health Organization: Prevention of suicide, Public Health Paper No. 35, Geneva, 1968.

56. McGuire, F.L., Birch, H., Gottschalk, L.A., and others: A comparison of suicide and nonsuicide deaths involving psychotropic drugs in four major U.S. cities, Am. J. Public Health **66:**1058, Nov. 1976.

57. Aries, P.: The hour of our death, New York, 1981, Alfred A. Knopf, Inc. (Translated by H. Weaver.)

58. Weisman, A.: Death and self-destructive behaviors. In Resnick, H.L.P., and Hathorn, B.C., editors: Suicide in the '70s, DHEW Pub. No. (HSM) 72-9054, p. 13, Rockville, Md., 1973, National Institute of Mental Health.

59. Hankoff, L.D.: Categories of attempted suicide: a longitudinal study, Am. J. Public Health **66:**558, June 1976.

60. Resnik, H.L.P., and Cantor, J.M.: Suicide and aging, J. Am. Geriatr. Soc. **18:**152, Feb. 1970.

61. Cautela, J.: Proceedings of the Annual Meeting of American Psychology Association, Washington, D.C., 1970.

62. Weisman, A.D.: Suicide, an attempt to reach for normality, U.S. Med. **7**:23, Jan. 1, 1971.

63. Shneidman, E.S.: Preventing suicide, Am. J. Nurs. **65**:111, May 1965.

64. Ross, M.: The presuicidal patient: recognition and management, Southern Med. J. **60**:1094, 1967.

65. Danto, D.L.: Assessment of the suicidal person in the telephone interview, Bull. Suicidol., Fall 1971, p. 48.

66. Snyder, J.A.: The use of gatekeepers in crisis management, Bull. Suicidol., Fall 1971, p. 39.

67. Litman, R.E.: Emergency response to potential suicide, J. Mich. Med. Soc. **62**:68, Jan. 1963.

68. Litman, R.E.: Acutely suicidal patients; management in general medical practice, Calif. Med. **104**:168, March 1966.

69. Dublin, L.I.: Suicide: a public health problem, Am. J. Public Health **55**:12, Jan. 1965.

70. Levine, M., and Kay, P.: The Salvation Army's Anti-Suicide Bureau, London—1905, Bull. Suicidol., Fall 1971, p. 57.

71. Varah, C., editor: The Samaritans, New York, 1965, Macmillan Publishing Co., Inc.

72. Shneidman, E.S., and Farberow, N.L.: The Los Angeles suicide prevention center: a demonstration of public health feasibilities, Am. J. Public Health **55**:21, Jan. 1965.

73. Shneidman, E.S.: State programs in suicide prevention, Address presented to the Surgeon General's conference with state and territorial mental health authorities, Washington, D.C., Dec. 6, 1966, National Institute of Mental Health.

74. Kiev, A.: United program urged to lower suicide rate, U.S. Med. **7**:8, April 1, 1971.

75. Welu, T.C.: Broadening the focus of suicide prevention activities utilizing the public health model, Am. J. Public Health **62**:1625, Dec. 1972.

76. Beck, A.T., Resnik, H.L.P., and Lettieri, D.J., editors: The prediction of suicide, Bowie, Md., 1974, Charles Press Publishers.

77. Stengel, E.: The complexity of motivations to suicide attempts, Bull. Suicidol., Dec. 1967, p. 27.

78. Tuckman, J., Youngman, W.F., and Bleiberg, B.M.: Attempted suicides by adults, Public Health Rep. **77**:605, July 1962.

79. Tuckman, J., and Cannon, H.E.: Attempted suicide in adolescents, Am. J. Psychiatr. **119**:228, Sept. 1962.

80. Litman, R.E., Farberow, N.L., Shneidman, E.S., and others: Suicide prevention telephone service, J.A.M.A. **192**:107, April 5, 1965.

CHAPTER 29

Aggression and violence

Have a heart that never hardens,
A temper that never tires,
A touch that never hurts.

Charles Dickens

The several chapters in this section have attempted to consider aberrant behaviorisms that are often referred to as "antisocial" or as "escapes from reality." All have a psychiatric base. The most evident are mental ill health, alcoholism, substance abuse, and suicide. To these should be added the various types of outwardly directed violent aggression.[1] A few words about the term *aggression* are indicated. Inherently, it is not necessarily bad or undesirable. Literally it merely means "to move actively"—and many actions are constructive. In fact, to be progressive, to achieve, one must have some degree of aggressiveness. Certain groups in society—racial, sexual, occupational—even obtain training in being aggressive. If this represents a self-assertive determination to improve and secure one's rightful status and opportunity, it is the proper thing to do. If, on the other hand, the concept of aggression is misdefined and misapplied by the inclusion of vengeful hostility or rage, the ultimate result can only be harmful to all concerned. Indeed, such action typically generates a reaction that usually or always makes things worse. It is important, therefore, to distinguish between appropriately aggressive self-determination on the one hand and hostility on the other.

Each of the types of hostile action considered here has at one time or another been the subject of various legal and criminal justice measures. Historically the legal profession has identified each of them with "the guilty mind." Even now there is much debate between those who advocate the legal or criminal justice approach to all such problems and those in the health and social service professions who regard those involved as frustrated or

disturbed personalities who either are calling for help or are attempting to escape from some personally unwanted and intolerable situation. Fortunately some rapprochement has been occurring. Matthews,[2] a lawyer and director of the project on mental illness and the criminal law of the American Bar Association has described its rationale:

If one observes both the persons who crowd our criminal courts . . . and the population of our mental hospitals, one is struck not by the differences between the two but by the similarities. Our preoccupation with trying to separate the "mentally ill" from the "criminals" may have led us to overlook a more central reality: both mental illness and criminality are tributaries of some deeper and more mysterious channel. Certainly there are differences between "criminals" and the "mentally ill" but it seems possible that the problems of mental illness and crime frequently lend themselves to similar if not identical methods of handling. This possibility is reinforced when one reflects to what extent entry into . . . and continued presence in the criminal process may be a result of what we call the "random factor"; that is, decisions based not so much on reason and scientific differentiation as on chance circumstances, social class, available mental health resources, divisions of political authority, and education and training levels of the officials whose responsibility it is to make decisions. There is a need for individualization at every step of the criminal process in order to neutralize the random factor as much as possible. If the wide range of alternatives available for handling persons thought to be mentally ill, especially alternatives in the individual's home community, should be made available to persons involved with the criminal law, then the accident of labels, whether civil or criminal, would be reduced. A wide spectrum of diagnostic and treatment facilities should be made available to the administrators of the criminal law to assist them in the related tasks of preventing crime and dealing

513

effectively with persons legally convicted of criminal acts. If mental health resources are available both in mental hospitals and correctional facilities, much of the sting of criminal convictions will have been removed.

Matthews concludes that an imaginative change in present competency procedures by prosecutors, judges, attorneys, and even defendants would lead to new dispositional alternatives to the criminal process. Many of these are or should be available at progressive mental health centers. He notes, however, the unfortunate reality of a limited supply of mental health resources as well as an inefficient use of those that exist.

This emphasizes perhaps that neither criminal justice nor public and mental health can stand or function alone. Each to a significant degree must depend on and work with the other.[3] It is significant that the major risks of death for young males in the United States are all violent: for white males, vehicular accidents, suicide, and homicide; and for black males, homicide, vehicular accidents, and drowning accidents (Table 29-1). Hall,[4] as president of the American Medical Association, pondered methods to prevent some of this tragic violent loss: the elimination of human judgment in driving by a complex computerized highway system, the tranquilization of all young men so they will not kill themselves or each other, the fencing of all lakes and rivers. Obviously, Hall notes, none of these are practical, much less acceptable, although it should be mentioned that the second, in the form of leucotomy (brain surgery in certain cases) or chemotherapy, has been attempted on a limited selective basis in several countries.[5] General reaction to such Orwellian approaches is negative, in part because of the macabre path down which they might lead civilization. To the contrary, the only practical approach is to attempt a better understanding of the underlying causes of hostility and violence and to seek effective methods to motivate the public to avoid or neutralize the causes.

HOSTILITY
Source of hostility

Underlying most if not all violence, whether directed toward oneself or others, is a deepseated sense of hostility, which the affected individual may or may not recognize. Hostility is a unique and

TABLE 29-1. Percent of deaths from violent causes, United States, by age, sex, and race, 1975, 1976, and 1977 averaged

Cause of death	10-19 years Male White	10-19 years Male Black	10-19 years Female White	10-19 years Female Black	20-29 years Male White	20-29 years Male Black	20-29 years Female White	20-29 years Female Black	30-39 years Male White	30-39 years Male Black	30-39 years Female White	30-39 years Female Black	40 years or over Male White	40 years or over Male Black	40 years or over Female White	40 years or over Female Black
Motor vehicle accidents	41.3	17.8	37.9	12.7	32.4	13.6	24.2	7.8	15.6	8.0	9.2	3.6	5.5	3.9	3.6	1.6
Nonmotor vehicle accidents	19.0	22.7	9.8	11.6	16.7	12.2	7.6	7.6	11.9	8.6	4.6	3.7	5.2	5.1	2.6	2.1
All accidents	60.3	40.5	47.7	24.3	49.1	25.8	31.8	15.4	27.5	16.6	13.8	7.3	10.7	9.0	6.2	3.7
Suicide	8.1	3.4	4.6	2.9	15.5	6.5	12.6	4.7	12.3	3.5	10.3	1.9	5.7	1.4	5.2	0.5
Homicide	4.9	25.2	5.2	17.1	8.4	37.0	7.1	21.0	7.6	22.7	3.8	9.6	2.6	10.1	1.1	3.3
All violent deaths	73.3	69.1	57.5	44.3	73.0	69.3	51.5	41.1	47.4	42.8	27.9	18.8	19.0	20.5	12.5	7.5

much misused term. In an attempt to describe it precisely, Saul[6] has defined it as "a motivating force—an impulse, urge, tendency, intent, motivation or reaction—toward injury or destruction of some kind or degree, toward an object which can be animate (including oneself) or inanimate, usually accompanied in humans by the feeling or emotion of anger." To elucidate, Saul emphasizes that hostility is not merely aggression, anger, or hatred, although any or all of these may be components or manifestations of overt hostility. Hostility may be manifest in many ways and for many purposes, varying in intensity from a simple unnoticed glance, a fixed stare, or facial tenseness, to active vindictiveness in the form of malicious gossip, the smashing of objects, brutality toward animals or other humans, and in the extreme, murder or suicide. Mere anger should not be confused with hostility, since typically anger is transient and often is expressed toward a loved one. A storm of sudden anger quickly passes usually leaving in its wake some degree of remorse. With hostility there is no place for remorse. It is the inherent Cain—or as some have said, the essential evil in humanity.

Some may find this an objectionable or unpleasant thought, but it must be realized that everyone, to varying degrees because of complex circumstances, is pulled by two opposing forces—strong social and self-satisfying motivations and strong asocial or antisocial motivations that may be equally or even more satisfying. An understanding of these opposing forces or motivations and the social application of that understanding offers the only ultimate hope of headway against individual or collective brutality and violence, which constantly threaten us and our societies. It is significant that toward the end of his life, Sigmund Freud[7] wrote, "I can no longer understand how we could have overlooked the universality of non-erotic aggression and destruction and could have omitted to give it due significance in our interpretations of life." Then he added that "those who love fairy tales do not like it when people speak of the innate tendencies of mankind toward aggression, destruction and cruelty. . . . The tendency toward aggression," he concluded, "is an innate, independent, instinctual disposition in man and . . . it constitutes the most powerful obstacle to culture."

In his classic studies of behavior and conditioning, Cannon[8] observed that an animal confronted with a threat, irritation, or frustration is physiologically stimulated and prepared for either of two

maximum responses—to fight or to flee. In our own special development in competitive biologic circumstances this was necessary for survival. It may still be observed in some primitive people. But in supposedly cooperative and civilized contemporary societies this automatic physiologic response, if misunderstood and uncontrolled in relation to existing stresses and problems, is likely to flood the mind with unwise and unwarranted feelings of fear and hostility and result in destructive reactions against others or oneself. This is unfortunately common, as a reading of history or any current newspaper gives ample testimony. This tendency, this characteristic seems almost unique to our species. Almost all animals have some form of organization based on protective and productive aggregations—hives, flocks, herds, and the like. So do we, but with an additional significant use—purposeful aggressive attacks on and destruction of our own kind. Thus Allee[9] has noted, "One species of animal may destroy another, and individuals may kill other individuals, but group struggles to the death between members of the same species, such as occur in human warfare, can hardly be found among nonhuman animals," To this, one may add the observation that only a human could have written Thanatopsis. Only a human could have conceived and composed a Götterdämmerung. And only a human could have attempted it.

Hostility—a disease

Because of such considerations, Saul[6] regards hostility as the central problem in human affairs and urges its recognition in its many forms. He provides health workers with the challenge in these terms:

Hostility is a disease to be cured and prevented like cancer, tuberculosis or smallpox, . . . its cure will result in healthier, better living—not only for society in general but for each individual in particular. . . . Hostility cannot be passed off as something we inherit and hence can do nothing about. The fact is that hostility is a disease of the personality, transmittable from person to person and group to group, and, basically, by contact from parents to children, from generation to generation. . . . Indeed if the major motivating forces in each of us could develop normally, healthily, without interference or coercion from the outside, friendly social cooperation would be the result. Only when this development is disturbed during the earliest formative years of infancy and childhood, by active mismanagement or by gross neglect (whether unconscious and well meaning or conscious and willful) does the fight-flight reaction, with its resulting hostility, flower into full strength.

To this Saul adds the pertinent health-related observation that through all the various forms of physical, physiologic, and psychologic reaction—withdrawal, depression, manic episodes, hysteria, phobias, compulsions, perversions, addictions, paranoias, schizophrenia, and the rest as well as the psychosomatic conditions in which emotions play a role—ulcers, hypertension, stroke, thyroid disease, and some allergies and arthritis—"however prominent the element of flight, invariably the power of the fight reaction with its rage, hate and hostility is also unmistakable." He concludes that "The elucidation of hostility in its causes, effects, transformations, connections, and the means of reducing and preventing it, could well be the great contribution of this generation of students of the human mind and human motivations."

Extent and form of hostility

Cannon's choice between flight or fight therefore has special implications for modern survival. There now exist awesome weapons with which to fight. Furthermore, they are not limited to physical form. Saul[6] has pointed out that aggression may now range from direct overt action to indirect hidden, subtle, and even masked forms disguised as justice, righteousness, and love: "It can be acted out within or outside the law by single persons on their own, by unorganized crowds or mobs, or by highly organized gangs or armies. It finds easy expression in crime, delinquency and warfare, the prevalence of which serves as an index of how widespread the problem is."

Obviously the true dimensions of the problem elude determination because of a variety of factors including failures to report, erroneous recording, population shifts, and variable criminal justice definitions and systems. However, some indications do exist. In the United States, for example, about 13 million serious crimes are reported each current year, and the rates have been increasing several times more rapidly than the population. In addition to more than 20,000 murders, there are over 1

million nonfatal violent crimes against persons, including about 60,000 reported forcible rapes, 500,000 instances of aggravated assault, and more than 500,000 robberies. Add to this 10 to 12 million crimes against property.[10] But this is not all. There are estimated to occur annually more than 1,200,000 cases of physical child abuse of whom over 2,000 die,[11] 2 million cases of spouses beaten or attacked by their partners,[12] 1,200,000 divorces, many of which are based on hostile actions,[13] and 1,500,000 children labeled "delinquent" by courts. Many of the latter involve familial hostility, and one third of them are held in adult jails and lockups, often with serious physical and mental consequences.[14]

In the world arena, one can point to the more than 130 wars of varying intensities since the end of World War II, with a minimum of 25 million people killed and several times that number injured. A large proportion if not most of these were civilian noncombatants. In addition, it is interesting to note our attitude toward the physical environment, which we "conquer," "subdue," "exploit," and "rape" (note the words commonly used) in the name of productivity and development.

CRIMINAL HOMICIDE

Every hour in the United States 15 or more people are stabbed, clubbed, or shot. A significant number of them die. During 1978 felonious murders and nonnegligent manslaughter accounted for over 21,000 deaths, or 1 every 25 minutes with a constant increase. Homicide decreased through the early 1950s, but about 1958 it began to increase again. Since then, the average annual increase has been about 6% with a total increase of about 100%. These, of course, are only the incidents known to the police and do not take into consideration the unknown numbers of individuals whose deaths are classified erroneously as accidents. The statistical chance of an American being murdered in any one year is about 1 in 20,000. The risk varies considerably, however, among different components of the population (Table 29-1).

Differences among racial and ethnic groups far outweigh differences by sex, with homicide rates for the nonwhite population 8 to 10 times greater than for the white population. When data are limited to men, the differences are even greater. Age adjustment further emphasizes the disparity, especially for nonwhite men, whose rates are raised about an additional one fourth. Homicide occurs most frequently in persons between the ages of 25 and 44 years, for whom the rate is twice the national average. At these ages racial differences are most pronounced, with a nonwhite level 10 to 12 times higher than that found in the white population.

The male to female homicide rate is a ratio of about 3 to 1. With reference to residence, rates are higher in urban areas, especially center city circumstances, as compared with rural areas. Some changes are taking place, however, in all of these dimensions. During the past decade, for example, the age-adjusted homicide rate for all ages combined increased nearly 30% among whites as compared with a 10% increase among nonwhites. The ratio of male to female homicides declined slightly, as did the average age, with an increasing number of homicides occurring in suburbs.

It is important to distinguish murders from other homicides. The term *homicide* includes not only "murder and nonnegligent manslaughter" but also "justifiable homicide" (such as the killing of a felon by a policeman in the line of duty and some other types of killing in self-defense). It also includes legal executions. Practically speaking, homicide includes any violent death that is neither a suicide nor an accident, although as pointed out previously, some of each of these are actually conscious or subconscious homicides. *Murder, or criminal homicide,* is a more restricted term. Most criminologists consider a murderer as "one who kills a fellow member of his society not by accident or negligence but with purpose or to defend himself in connection with an attempt to commit another crime, such as robbery, or to shield himself from accusation by a person whom he has offended or abused."[15]

Homicides therefore may be considered to fall into three categories. The best known and the type toward which the criminal justice system, as well as the public in general, has centered their attention is planned killing that is consciously acceptable to the perpetrator at the time. Contrary to popular belief, this type of killing, criminal homicide, represents only a small fraction of the total homicides in American society. By far the most common type of homicide is a form of resolution of conflict that usually has extended over a significant period of time. In these instances, which comprise about 80% of the total, often an insignificant provocation may develop an intense emotional response leading to the homicidal act, which was not deliberately planned. The perpetrators of such acts apparently do not have the ability to satisfy their aggressions

consistently and, as a result, on occasion may do so impulsively and explosively. The third type of homicide consists of justifiable acts taken by a law enforcement officer or an individual in self-defense.

It is notable that with reference to the most common type of homicide, that arising from attempted conflict resolution, a relationship either by birth or choice exists between the victim and the murderer. As stated by the noted criminologist, Wolfgang,[16] "Criminal homicide is probably the most personalized crime in our society." This has been detailed in the staff report to the National Commission on the Causes and Prevention of Violence.[17] It points out that although a large proportion of violent interactions involve strangers, the extent varies greatly in terms of type of aggressive action. The percent of nonprimary group relationships steadily rises from homicide (16%), to aggravated assault (21%), to forcible rape (53%), and to armed (19%) and unarmed (86%) robbery. The popular fear that an attacker will be a stranger, although strongly justified for robbery and relevant for rape, is much less valid for aggravated assault and generally inappropriate for homicide.

With these facts in mind it must be recognized that in a great many instances there are two active parties to a murder, the killer and the victim, and the latter by no means necessarily plays a passive role. As Houts[18] describes, many murders are the result of antagonisms that have gone on for years with the victim teasing, taunting, blaming, goading, or suppressing the eventual murderer until a breaking point was reached.

The foregoing facts prompted Judge George Edwards of the National Commission for Reform of Federal Criminal Laws, in an address before the American Psychiatric Association in 1971, to deflate what he referred to as the "four myths about murder." They are that the average citizen is justified in living with a top priority fear of being murdered, that most murderers are premeditated killers for money, that the most likely murderer is a stranger, and that you can protect yourself from murder by keeping a pistol handy. None of these myths, he emphasized, is true. As a consequence, murder is the least suppressible of crimes. Greater police visibility and more sophisticated police techniques have little effect on homicide because it occurs most often in the privacy of the home, with an existing prior relationship between victim and killer. This means that murder is almost always an act of blind rage or illogical violent passion that cannot be anticipated. It has also been pointed out by Pasternack,[19] a psychiatrist and a specialist in violent behavior, that perhaps as many as 40% of murders of passion are actually victim precipitated, wherein one person taunts another beyond endurance or where a philandering husband parades his mistress in front of his wife, daring her to do anything about it. This type of situation, says Pasternack, is far from rare and when it happens, the killer as well as the killed is the victim.

PREVENTION OF HOMICIDE

The question arises, "Can anything be done to reduce this significant loss of life?" For one thing, those in the health professions must recognize, as many still do not, that an individual killed with a weapon is just as dead and just as tragic as one who has succumbed to tuberculosis or cancer and that most if not all criminal homicides involve some degree of mental ill health. This is not the place for a detailed discussion of the psychiatric measures, individual or collective, that are needed. There are two aspects of prevention, however, that deserve mention.

The first is social conditioning. Banay[20] pointed out 2 decades ago that the American public is conditioned to murder, that it is no exaggeration to consider that except for maintaining the traditional legal penalty (in itself a form of homicide) for taking another's life, "the society we live in almost reaches out to encourage murder." Violence is the most common topic in children's so-called comic books, the focal point of mystery and adventure stories that are sold by the millions each year, and the stock-in-trade of television, radio, and motion picture "thrillers." Typically it receives the top headlines in American news media. More than one murderer has stated a wish for a day in the public eye.

The gun is probably the most common toy sold and encourages the most popular form of play, especially among boys, which takes the form of mock killing. In 1976, the American Public Health Association passed a strong resolution calling for legislation to prohibit the manufacture, assembly, sale, transfer, or possession of handguns or handgun ammunition for private use. Interestingly, a Gallup poll

(Feb. 3, 1980) showed overwhelming support for further handgun control—75% of the electorate, including 65% of the nation's gun owners—and only 6% wanted the laws relaxed. Offsetting this is the unfortunate fact that the National Rifle Association, which consistently and staunchly opposes any limitation or even registration not merely of rifles but even of handguns not used in hunting is one of the strongest and financially best supported political lobbies in Washington with an annual budget of $30 million. Banay concluded that "a psychologist studying our culture might fairly deduce that we are obsessed with the idea of sudden, violent and retributive death."

Washburn,[21] in his discussion of aggressive behavior and human evolution, goes even further. After considering development in several mammalian species, he observes that "all the evidence would indicate that evolution has built into man a propensity for learning to be aggressive. Our early ancestors' way of life was not easy . . . the group was defended by the young adult male who hunted and formed the army. The order of killing was very high." It has been estimated "that in many primitive tribes about 25 percent of the males were killed off in combat. This of course does not mean that humans must continue to be aggressive, but it does suggest the importance of institutional controls over aggression."

In contradistinction, Endleman,[22] as a result of his studies of street violence and riots, believes strongly that although violence is prevalent, it is not endemic or necessarily natural to the human condition and that preconditions of violent behavior must be sought in social rather than in our genetic or instinctual characteristics. This appears to be borne out by the current epidemic of homicides among black men, aged 18 to 35 years. In this group homicides doubled between 1970 and 1976, and homicide now ranks as the leading cause of death—12,000 annually, or one half of the nation's total. Dennis[23] has indicated that the civil rights movement of the 1960s, while achieving significant progress, itself discredited or swept away many of the institutions that had up to then provided support—black schools, churches, organizations, and even the family. Even the blacks' "functional leaders," she points out, are disappearing, leaving the way open for socially undesirable role models. Recognizing the three dominant and increasing causes of death among young blacks—homicide, accidents, and suicide—as violent reactions to social stress, the National Medical Association, a Black organization, has called the situation a public health problem requiring national action.

Recently much attention has been focused on the influence of television on aggressive behavior in the United States. As pointed out by the Surgeon General's Scientific Advisory Committee on Television and Social Behavior,[24] 96% of American homes have one or more television sets and the average home set is turned on for more than 6 hours per day. Most of the studies inquired into by the committee indicated positive relationships between exposure to television violence and aggressive tendencies, although most were of low magnitude. However, the observation raised other questions: (1) Does violence viewing lead to aggression? (2) Does aggression lead to violence viewing? (3) Are both violence viewing and aggression products of a third set of conditions? The studies tended to support the first and third of these propositions.

Gerbner[25] has emphasized that "there is now sufficient evidence conclude that television alone (as well as in combination with other social and cultural factors) makes a significant difference in the way viewers deal with reality." Violence on television, he points out, is different from any other medium:

It is accessible from cradle to grave; you don't have to go anywhere to see it, and you don't even need to know how to read. It comes home to all classes and groups everywhere in the industrialized world. And it is used nonselectively; most people watch by the clock, not by the program, and the TV clock is on over six hours a day in the average U.S. household. Television is like the environment; it's everywhere and it's indivisible.

Gerbner's group, which has been monitoring and scoring television programs since 1967, found that after 10 years of hearings, investigations, and presidential commissions 8 out of every 10 network programs (9 out of every 10 cartoons) still contain violence, with a rate of 5 violent episodes per program and 10 per children's cartoon: "About 65% of all leading characters (85% in children's programs) are still involved in some violence . . . and about 10% in killing." During the past few years, although killing in "family hour" programs declined from 28% to 1%, it increased after the family hour period from 9% to 23%. Also, violence in weekend daytime children's cartoons increased from 65% to 85%. Of great significance is Gerbner's observation that "for every incident in which a male is violent, there are

1.19 male victims, but for every incident in which a female is violent there are 1.32 female victims. Similarly children; lower-class, foreign, and non-white characters of both sexes; and older women are more likely to fall victim than to be perpetrators of violence. Old, poor, black women are cast for violent parts only to be killed." One must consider this in relation to child abuse, spouse beating, and the frequent mugging and robbing of aged women. Gerbner concludes that "potential incitement to mayhem among a minority of viewers is bad enough but the cultivation of fear and rigidity among many is scarcely less damaging in its long range effects."

An interesting observation[26] that has been made is that countries or cultures with high homicide rates tend to have low suicide rates and vice versa. Thus in Mexico, where 18.7 out of every 100,000 persons were murdered in 1966, only 1.6 killed themselves. This is in contrast with West Germany, for example, where only 1.3 murders per 100,000 were recorded in contrast to 25 suicides per 100,000 population. The question is raised whether a country is homicidal or suicidal depending on the level of its labor force status integration, that is, the degree of certainty among individuals about what society expects of them in view of their age, sex, and other factors. In rigid societies where roles are well defined and people have little freedom of choice in directing their lives, homicide rates are high. Dennis' studies[23] of homicide in young black men is a case in point. This is in contrast to societies where people have the opportunity to choose their lifestyle from a variety of alternatives and where suicide rates tend to be high.

There is a second important area for preventive action in relation to homicide. Experts in the field almost unanimously agree that the most urgent need is effective gun control. Thus Burka[19] says firmly:

The single most effective step we can take is to ban hand guns and to use stringent methods to make the ban work. A hand gun is meant for police work and that is the only place it belongs—not in the hands of criminals and would-be criminals, not in the pockets of frightened citizens, and not in the home. Anyone who thinks possession of a gun protects him and his family is deluding himself.

King,[19] of the International Association of Chiefs

of Police, who has studied the problem extensively, is equally emphatic:

By far the greatest number of homicides are shootings, so reduction of homicides starts with elimination of hand guns. Nobody denies that people are also murdered with every imaginable weapon besides guns—knives, fists, rocks, clothes lines, 2 by 4s, and so on. . . . but a gun is the most lethal of weapons; it has a range far greater than an attacker's arm, and recovery from a bullet wound is much rarer than recovery from a knifing or beating.

There is an obvious need to extirpate the almost juvenile avid retention by many individuals of the primitive urge to destroy other species long after the necessity to fear them or require them for sustenance. In the process all sorts of specious justifications are presented: the guns are needed not only for hunting but also "to protect one's castle," "that guns do not kill, people kill." The variety of illogical themes are many. "We are victims of the mystique of the gun," according to Pasternack,[19] "Who in his right mind could dispute that if there were no guns in the home or in the streets there would be a dramatic reduction in killings. Murders of passion would certainly diminish greatly with no chance for the impulsive, irreversible pulling of a trigger before passion can cool; street killings would plummet if the criminal had no gun to hide behind to draw false courage."

The late J. Edgar Hoover, director of the Federal Bureau of Investigation, stated, "The easy accessibility of fire arms is a significant factor in murders committed in the U.S. today." Approximately 2 million guns are sold in the United States each current year—many by mail. Far too many are purchased by the deranged, the hardened criminal, the convict, the addict, and the alcoholic. It is unreasonable to expect such individuals to be prudent in their use. Bakal,[27] in his book *The Right to Bear Arms* speaks of a plague of guns that sweeps over our land and points out that between 1900 and 1960 more than 750,000 American civilians were killed by domestic gunfire—a higher toll than all of the Americans killed in battle since the American Revolution. Only seven states at present even require a permit or a license before purchase of a pistol or revolver, and as Bakal indicates, almost every place one can purchase a rifle more easily than getting a dog or cat license or even a hunting permit. The

total result is about 100 million guns in the hands of private individuals in the United States.

CHILD ABUSE

A type of violence of special concern to the fields of public health, medicine, and social service is the "battered child syndrome." The term was applied in 1962 by Kempe[28] in the first comprehensive survey of child abuse. Throughout most of history children have been misused and abused, regarded as inherently evil or at least as the fruits of evil, and treated as replaceable chattel.[29,30] Thus the historian deMause,[31] on examining 200 statements of advice on child rearing, found that "virtually every child rearing tract from antiquity to the eighteenth century recommended the beating of children." The tradition was widely accepted. John Calvin preached that breaking the will of the infant at the earliest possible age was a parent's duty to God. Similarly the wife of John Wesley, writing about child rearing, states "when turned a year old (and some before) they were taught to fear the rod, and to cry softly."[32] The inception of the industrial revolution accentuated the overt aspects of child abuse. In England, wagonloads of unsuspecting children were gathered from the countryside and delivered to impatient factory and mine managers. Sir William Petty, the "father" of vital and health statistics advocated free maternity hospitals for unmarried women, whose resulting children, he said, would become wards of the state and their labor available for 25 years.[33] In the United States, the evils of child industrial labor were multiplied by the textile needs of the Union and Confederate armies, which also had diminished the supply of adult labor.[34] During the twentieth century, the organization of societies for the protection of children in company with other socially minded groups has resulted in the elimination of many of the evils of the industrial employment of children in the United States, Great Britain, and some other countries.

However, the problem of "the battered child" within the home remains a much less evident and more elusive aspect of child abuse—one that has attracted increasing attention during recent decades as a significant cause of disability and death in children. Usually the battered child is a rejected child, not infrequently the only one of several children in a family who is subjected to abuse and often the most recently born. Various reasons for rejection have been noted. Prematurity or small birth size seem to be significant, as are very frequent pregnancies close together.[35] Poor marital adjustment or resentment of a marriage forced by pregnancy or by other persons also plays a role. Postpartum depression with confusion of the identities of mother and child, resulting in outwardly directed hostility arising from feelings of guilt or self-deprecation, may be an important and sometimes fatal factor.[36] Other causes may be mental illness in one or both parents,[37] social and economic frustrations, unusually young and immature parents who may treat an infant like a doll or toy and mistreat it during a tantrum to "teach the other parent a lesson," jealousy in one parent over the attention given the child by the other parent, jealousy on the part of older children in relation to the new child in the family, or sexual aberrations on the part of one or both parents, older children, other relatives, or family acquaintances. Not infrequently, the child abuser believes that children exist primarily to satisfy parental needs, that the needs of children are unimportant, and that those children who do not fulfill parental needs deserve punishment.[38]

One characteristic of child abusers stands out. Practically all who have studied the problem have noted it as an intergenerational phenomenon, almost as if it were a communicable behavioral aberration. "It would appear," says Kempe, "that one of the most important factors . . . is 'to do unto others as you have been done by.'"[28] Among the many pertinent studies is one in the United States in which three generations of child abuse have been documented.[39] Another in England describes a family with five generations of known child abuse.[40] Wolfgang[41] states the case poignantly:

Perhaps the most malignant outcome of child abuse, however, is the seed of violence so often sown in the heart and mind of the young victim. Centuries ago, the sage Ben Sirach observed: "The branch sprung from violence has no tender twig." His observation has now been confirmed repeatedly by investigators who find an unusually high rate of violent behavior, including juvenile delinquency and crime, among children abused earlier by adult parents and guardians.

The number of such untender twigs in American society is proliferating at an alarming rate. While violence in general has been steadily increasing in our society, recent years have witnessed an especially remarkable spurt in the incidence of violent behavior among the young. Violent crimes committed by children of all ages have been increasing between three and four times faster than they have in the general population.

Abuse of children may run the gamut from overprotection in the form of isolation to general neglect with poor hygiene and malnutrition, constant nagging and scolding, sexual abuse, and severe and often irrational punishment, sometimes leading to death. It is these latter instances that have been given the name *battered child syndrome.*

Reliable statistics are understandably difficult to obtain. The annual incidence is estimated at 10 per 1,000 live births, resulting in about 33,130 significantly injured children, of whom 2,000 are killed. Ten percent of emergency room admissions of children below 5 years of age are the result of abuse. Mortality from abuse in children 1 to 6 months of age is second only to the "sudden infant death" syndrome, but even some of these must be in the abused category.[36] Among children 1 to 5 years of age, it is second only to accidents. Fathers are guilty of child abuse more often than mothers, but sometimes both parents actively participate. Battered children are not limited to any particular socioeconomic group, and not all abused or battered children are found among the very young. Thus a study in 1968 of 6,617 abused children showed 8.1% under 6 months of age; 5.5% between 6 months and 1 year; 10.8% between 1 and 2 years; 9.4% between 2 and 3 years; 19.9% between 3 and 6 years; 15.1% between 6 and 9 years; 12.2% between 9 and 12 years; 10.8% between 12 and 15 years; and 5.6% over 15 years of age, with 2.6% of age unknown.

The highest fatality rate is in the very young, commonly those under 3 years of age, who are too young to explain their bruises, fractures, and swellings. Among older children, many are too frightened or convinced of some accused or imagined guilt to discuss what actually occurred. It is estimated that 5% of battered children are killed outright and another 30% eventually suffer permanent injury. Furthermore, of those who are not killed outright, it is estimated that one of every two dies after being returned to the parents. This is extremely important especially for emergency care personnel to bear in mind. If physically abused children do survive, their intellectual and psychologic functions appear to be impaired. Money[42] has described what he terms *psychosocial dwarfism,* in which the endocrine system of the severely abused child fails to produce adequate growth hormones. Often such physically and mentally stunted children are misdiagnosed as psychotic or mentally retarded. Removal from the abusing environment may restore normal development. The extent to which this is possible, however, is subject to question. In a follow-up study of 31 children who had required hospitalization, Elmer and Gregg[43] found no serious long-term disabilities from bone injuries, but emotional and mental retardation as well as growth failure were significant problems. Among 20 of the children selected for longer term study, nearly all had speech defects. Of the 10 no longer living with their families 7 had developed normal intelligence but only 3 of the 10 who had been returned to their families had normal IQs.

Lacking an opportunity for normalization, progressive undesirable changes occur. Understandably, a state of constant hypervigilance develops, extending even beyond the home and the childhood period into the entire world about them and carried on through life. Beyond this, as Bakan[44] points out, the psychoanalyst Sandor Ferenczi concluded more than a half-century ago that severely abused children often lose even the willingness or desire to survive. As a group, they do have a decreased life expectancy. Ferenczi also noted that abused and rejected children tended to be frigid and impotent as adults.

Regretfully it is estimated that very few cases of battered or abused children, perhaps as low as 1%, are brought to the attention of appropriate authorities. Since most incidents occur in the home, all but the most serious tend to go unnoticed even by neighbors. Physicians represent a critical point of first suspicion and action. However, even here reporting tends to be limited and varies by type of practice or specialty.[45] The physician's concern may be so much with clinical signs that little thought is given to their source. If there are suspicions, they are difficult to prove and the parent's word is accepted about accidents, clumsiness, or other children. Furthermore, most people, including physicians, find it difficult to believe that any parents would injure their own children. In this regard Sanders[46] has expressed the opinion that most parents have both hostile and negative attitudes as well as warm and loving feelings toward their children and that the members of the medical profession also often have ambivalent childhood memories, which make them reluctant to deal with parents of battered children. In addition,

some may fear becoming involved in time-consuming legal processes. These reactions, Sanders points out, overlook the possibility that although few abusive parents are actually psychotic, most are immature, impulsive, and suspicious; and although frightened by the medical and legal professions, they recognize that something is wrong and want help themselves.

In 1963 the Children's Bureau and the American Humane Association developed a model law[47] to provide for mandatory reporting of suspicious cases of child abuse by physicians while protecting them against criminal or civil liability. Reporting would lead to investigation and if suspicions were confirmed, appropriate steps would be taken to protect the child and rehabilitate the family if possible. Meanwhile, the Committee on the Infant and Preschool Child of the American Academy of Pediatrics made the following recommendations.[48]

1. Physicians should be required to report suspected cases of child abuse immediately to the agency legally charged with the responsibility of investigating child abuse—preferably the county or state department of welfare or health or their local representatives, or to the nearest law enforcement agency.

2. The agency should have ample personnel and resources to take action immediately upon receipt of the report.

3. Reported cases should be investigated promptly and appropriate service provided for the child and family.

4. The child should be protected by the agency either by continued hospitalization, supervision in home, or removal from home through family or juvenile court action when indicated.

5. The agency should keep a central register of all such cases. Provision should be made for the removal of case records from the register when it is found that abuse did not, in fact, occur.

6. The reporting physician or hospital should be granted immunity from suit.

By now all 50 states have enacted laws based on either a combination of the proposed model law or the American Academy of Pediatrics recommendations. These laws and increased professional publicity concerning the problem have led to a significant increase in reports. It is notable that the state of California, which enacted its law in 1963, was a party to a court settlement in 1970 that involved the establishment of a $600,000 trust fund paid by insurers of four physicians and a police chief who had been accused in a $5 million damage suit for failing to report a "battered child syndrome" that resulted in permanent brain damage of a 3-year-old boy.

These various efforts crystallized in the passage of national legislation on January 31, 1974—The Child Abuse Prevention and Treatment Act (P.L. 93-247). It established a National Center for Child Abuse and Neglect in the Department of Health, Education, and Welfare to (1) compile, analyze, and publish an annual summary of research on child abuse and neglect; (2) act as a clearinghouse for information; (3) publish training materials for personnel in fields dealing with child abuse programs; (4) provide technical assistance (by grant or contract) to public and nonprofit organizations; and (5) conduct research in the area of child abuse. The center is also authorized to make grants and contracts for state and local demonstration programs designed to identify, prevent, and treat child abuse and neglect.

Obviously others, in addition to physicians and health and welfare agencies, have important roles to play with reference to the abused or battered child. Murdock[49] has made the following points with reference to the responsibility of school systems, based on his experience in Syracuse, N.Y.:

1. The reluctance of school personnel to report suspected cases (of child abuse) for fear of legal involvement and court appearances can be overcome by a proper presentation of the problem, especially in those states where reporting is mandatory.
2. Maximum cooperation between the school systems and the investigating agency is of extreme importance. A frequent exchange of information between the two organizations should be encouraged, not only in the initial reporting but also in the continued observation of these cases.

In addition, of course, is the extremely important contribution made by the social work profession and by many of the social service agencies throughout the nation. It is obvious, however, that none of the professions of organizations alone—health, legal, social service, education, or any other—can solve this tragic problem.[50] It presents a classic example of the necessity of interdisciplinary teamwork. This is emphasized by Gray[51]:

The problems of the battered child and his family are multiple and varied, and, therefore, hospital personnel who become involved in their solution must have varying backgrounds, abilities, and assets. This concept has led to the establishment of hospital-based battered child teams so that physicians, medical social workers, and pub-lic health nurses are all available for consultation regarding the most beneficial manner to help a battered child and his family.

SPOUSE ABUSE

A social and public health problem similar to child abuse is the aggressive behavior of some adults toward their marital partners. As with child abuse, the adequate solution of such occurrences often requires joint action by the social work, legal, and health professions. It has been estimated that of the approximate 50 million couples who live together in the United States, about 2 million spouses are attacked each year by their partners with a gun or a knife, and an equal or greater number are subjected to physical beating. In fact, one eighth of all murders in the nation are husband-wife killings.[52]

As Straus[12] points out, violence between husband and wife is by no means a one-way affair. In his national survey, 12.1% of husbands had acted violently against their wives during the preceding year, and 11.6% of wives had acted violently against their husbands. Furthermore, acts of violence by wives were somewhat more frequent and more severe in nature. Greater social concern for abused wives is justified, however, because of generally greater male strength, the large number of attacks by husbands when the wife is pregnant, and the generally greater economic and social dependence of the woman. Gelles[53] suggests several additional considerations. Some women are raised to be subservient to men and some for various reasons believe they deserve to be abused. Similarly, some men are raised to believe that "a man's home is his castle" and that no one has the right to question anything he may do inside it. This ignores the legal fact that physical violence against another person is a crime regardless of any relationship that may exist. However, in practice, only 2% of men who are known to physically abuse their female living partners are ever prosecuted. It is also significant that more police personnel are killed as a result of answering domestic violence calls than from any other aspect of their duty. About one out of every five police deaths occurs under such circumstances.

Spouse beating may occur in all races and socioeconomic classes. It has been noted, however, that the phenomenon occurs somewhat more frequently in families with socioeconomic difficulties, hence greater worries and frustrations. Education appears to play an interesting role. Thus while Parker and Schumacher[54] found no significant differences in the education of battered as opposed to nonbattered women, the husbands of battered women had less education than did those of nonbattered women. They also found that if a wife's mother had been a victim, the wife herself had a significant probability of being battered by her husband. Also, the more a beaten wife had been struck as a child, the more likely she was to remain with an abusive husband—in fact, as Gelles[55] suggests, the more likely she was to marry a violence-prone man. Parker and Schumacher concluded that "women who did not observe violence in their family of origin found wife battering inconsistent with their role and were able to cope with and avoid further violence."

Regretfully, little has been done up to now to ameliorate this serious physical and mental health problem. Many police personnel regard such episodes as an annoyance of relatively little importance. Hospital emergency room personnel tend to treat the injuries but not the essential problems. Neither they nor the police, much less neighbors, want to be caught in the middle of a domestic struggle, especially if they may end up being blamed or injured. The spouse, if a woman, when released usually has no place of refuge and can only return to the person who abused her. This, of course, reinforces the undesirable behavior and encourages repetition.

Some community agencies, including a few health departments, have been instrumental in the establishment of temporary refuges for battered women. Usually similar to halfway houses, such refuges should be developed in all communities of significant size and should have related to them the necessary health care, social services, counseling, and legal assistance that this serious problem warrants. In addition, much more effective interdisciplinary professional education and planning for health personnel is obviously indicated.

JUVENILE DELINQUENCY

Brief consideration should be given to delinquency in youth, since it also has certain relationships to public health. Unrest is part of youth. The problem is the degree and type of manifestation of unrest in relation to the social mores of the culture, place, and time. On the basis of police reports, juvenile delinquency rates are highest in cities, lower in suburbs, and lowest in rural areas. In 1968, for example, the rate for urban areas was three times that for rural areas. As would be expected, slums of large cities produce the largest number of offenders. That is where satisfaction of the normal needs of youth is most lacking. On the surface it appears that where the individual lives is more significant than whether the family is broken, poor, or socially deprived. During recent years, however, this premise has been increasingly questioned as a result of a dramatic rise in delinquency rates in all types of communities. There are probably four reasons for this: improved detection and reporting systems, the increase in the number and proportion of the population under 18 years of age, the peculiar conflicting interplay between the material benefits to today's youth combined with certain social limitations and restrictions placed on them, and an increased antiestablishment feeling. As a result, the increase in arrests of juveniles has outstripped the increase in their population increment. In 1960 with 25.4 million individuals between the ages of 10 and 17 years, there were 510,000 cases of juvenile delinquency handled by the courts in the United States, a rate of 20.1 per 1,000 population in the age group. By 1974, the population of the group had increased to 33.4 million, the cases to 1,252,000 with a rate of 37.5 per 1,000 population in the same age group.

Boys are referred to juvenile court four times as frequently as girls. However, girls now are becoming more aggressive. It is predicted that one out of every six boys today will end up in court for other than a traffic offense some time before his eighteenth birthday. The charges at present consist of theft, 25%; breaking and entering, 11%; violation of curfew, loitering, and runaways, 16%; vandalism, 9%; auto theft, 4%; violation of liquor laws, 2%; violation of drug laws, 1%; and all other charges, 32%. Girls are most often sent to juvenile court for running away, ungovernability, larceny, and sex offenses.

These differences indicate that in the United States people refuse to recognize certain basic physiologic and psychologic differences between boys and girls. Most schoolbooks deal with "children" rather than "boys" and "girls." Children through their teens are consistently put into the same school classes and presented with the same curricula and teaching methods as well as behavior requirements, ideals, and systems of rewards and punishments that in general are geared to the girl and not to the boy. Certain shared experiences are certainly important, but insistence on uniformity "across the board" has resulted in 10 times as many behavioral problems among boys as girls—stammering, bed-wetting, reading problems, and delinquency. Comparatively speaking, few youths are involved in violent offenses against the person, such as murder, assault, or robbery, although, as discussed in the preceding section on violence, this recently appears to be changing somewhat for the worse.

The attitude of youth itself toward delinquency is interesting. A comprehensive study,[56] the first of its kind, of an entire birth cohort involving almost 10,000 boys who were born in Philadelphia in 1945 revealed the following. By the time they had reached 19 years of age, about 35% had had at least one officially recorded contact with police for delinquent behavior. However, a group of only 627 boys (6%) accounted for more than one half of all of the delinquent acts and about 70% of the robberies, aggravated assaults, and homicides committed by the entire cohort. It was also notable that the juvenile justice system apparently had no subsequent effect on reforming the chronic offenders. It is especially significant that 90% of the teenagers interviewed confided that they had committed an act for which they could have been brought before a juvenile court. Fewer than 3% of the acts were detected by the police, and fewer than 1% of these were recorded as delinquent. It appears that teenagers themselves apply more rigid standards to their behavior than do the police or the courts.

Wolfgang,[57] a renowned sociologist who served as Director of the Center for Studies in Criminiology and Criminal Law at the University of Pennsylvania, in discussing delinquency in youth has emphasized that relatively few commit serious acts of violence as compared with adults. According to him, "Not yet arrived at positions of power where responsibilities are shared, youth cannot be blamed for a society that yields to violence because it fails to make automobiles and highways safer, fails to reduce inordinately high rates of infant mortality, to move more vigorously to reform cities of blight and organized crime, or to control the manufacture and sale of guns."

Whether it is boys smashing windows and tele-phones in the slums or their campus counterparts seizing university facilities, each group is expressing through action that they are attacking what they consider is not of fundamental value, especially since they are not allowed to participate in the conduct and rewards of the system. The delinquent in the slums wants to obtain by whatever method at least some part of what he is being deprived; whereas the student, although desirous of education, is opposed to the manner in which he must obtain it and the purposes for which he sees it being presented. Each group is deliberately and delinquently disruptive as a means of showing his disdain.

Wolfgang indicates that "for all their protest against their established elders, youth in a sense relies on the patience, understanding, tolerance, and responsibility of the older generation to check their escalating demands." Unfortunately, all too often in recent years well-considered checks have tended to be absent. "It is the task of those in power," says Wolfgang, "to be alert, to listen to the messages from the mouths of those once in our wombs. The older generation cannot retreat into the pit of their age. The education we offer youth must link the best of our traditions with the imagination and humanity needed to cope with the future." However, "Our model has been faulty and youth today will not trust our advice like a child who takes refuge in obedience. We should respect their caution, yet learn how to warn them."

The question still remains: How should society meet the challenge of the delinquent acts of youth? The traditional approach has been arrest and arraignment before a juvenile court. However, the juvenile justice system as it now exists has been described at its best as having no effect on the subsequent offensive behavior of youths, and at its worst it has a deleterious effect. "Not only do a greater number of those who receive punitive treatment . . . continue to violate the law, but they also commit more serious crimes with greater rapidity than those who experience a less constraining contact with the judicial and correctional systems.[56] It is shocking to note that the President's Crime Commission reported in 1967 that one half of the juvenile court judges in the United States had not even graduated from college and one fifth had no college-level education at all.[58] There is good reason therefore not to expect too much from many juvenile courts as now staffed. The uniqueness and potential value of juvenile courts, however, is that they are based on the philosophy that children are not to be considered criminals but rather immature individuals in need of help and guidance. Ordinarily the courts have access to consultation from psychiatrists, clinical psychologists, pediatricians, social caseworkers, and other professional specialists. Unfortunately in many places these resources have been minimally used.

Juvenile courts usually hold hearings in conference rooms with the proceedings essentially conversational. Pleas of guilty, not guilty, or nolo contendere should not be made or permitted in a juvenile court, and the proceedings should not lead toward a conviction or acquittal. The privacy of the juvenile should be respected, with the public excluded, and the publication of names and photographs prohibited. The juvenile should be advised of the right to legal counsel. Often juveniles are not told of their rights and do not even know what legal counsel means. If the juvenile or the court wishes, representation by counsel should be provided. The youth has the right to face the accusers, to cross-examine them and witnesses, and to introduce evidence that the youth believes might be pertinent. Disposition of juvenile delinquency cases varies from institutionalization to placement in a foster home or assignment to relatives. Usually, however, the juvenile returns to the home of the natural parents. Since so many juvenile offenders come from homes where the parents are failing in their roles and where other social and mental problems may exist, this represents in far too many instances the development of "revolving door cases."[41,59] Childhood abuse plays an important role. As high as 80% of juvenile offenders fall into this category.[32]

Health personnel and facilities have a far greater role in the field of juvenile delinquency than they have recognized or practiced. The physician and health officer should regard it as a public health problem, an endemic disorder that constantly threatens the community. The hard fact is that juvenile delinquents in general have more ills and die earlier than their nondelinquent peers. Just as health workers would not hesitate to provide or seek help for a case of communicable disease, they should, in behalf of the youth, the family, and the community, take the responsibility for assuring that available health resources are brought to bear on a family with a problem of delinquent behavior. Frequently in attempting to direct the delinquent child into the proper hands, they will find that necessary facilities will be inadequate or absent in the community. It is here that responsibility as a citizen will become an important aspect of the physician's or health officer's role.

A special characteristic of American psychiatry beginning in the late nineteenth century was the child guidance movement and its offspring, child psychiatry. "In this area," said Campbell,[60] "the emphasis has shifted to a study of the child's instinctive and emotional life, of his groping for satisfaction and for a grasp of the outside world and his urge towards self expression." This philosophy led to the establishment at the University of Pennsylvania in 1896 by Witmer of the first clinic where children with behavioral, emotional, or social problems were examined psychologically and medically. Subsequently the idea spread to Chicago, Boston, Allentown, Pa., and elsewhere, where a psychiatric perspective was brought to bear on juvenile delinquency not only from the standpoint of treatment but especially with an eye toward understanding and possibly prevention.[61] In addition, there has been a growing recent trend for more enlightened juvenile courts to refer delinquent children to new types of foster homes with small groups of children (six to eight) living together essentially normally under the guidance of substitute parents who are responsible to the court and backed to the extent necessary and available by community mental health centers, child guidance centers, and visiting health and social workers.

CONCLUSION

Hopefully what has been presented makes clear that much or most of crime, delinquency, and violence are essentially mental and social health problems and have their genesis within the family. In his essay on the family and mental disorder, Cumming[62] provides an excellent basis for this viewpoint in his delineation of family roles.

All families are divided along two great axes. Because of the generational differences which exist in any family, and because of the state of helplessness of the human infant, it is obvious that the father and mother can be designated as having more power than the children. A second axis of role differentiation corresponds with sex-categories. The male members play predominantly instrumental roles, that is, they provide for the family's needs in a practical way and relate the family to the surrounding community. They represent the family as it strives to achieve its goals, and defend it from any threat from outside. The women of the family play predominantly socio-emotional roles and are primarily responsible for dealing with the tensions which arise within the family and thus with defending the system against internal threats to its integrity. These two axes, taken together, yield four descriptions of the roles within the family. They give us the dominant role characteristics of the father, instrumental and powerful; the mother, powerful and socio-emotional; the son, less powerful and instrumental; and the daughter, less powerful and socio-emotional. According to this scheme, important disruptions in family functioning would occur if one or another member did not fulfill his or her appropriate function, or if competition for roles arose between family members.

This statement appears to explain well what is occurring today along both axes, not only in the United States but in many other nations. Both the respective age-related and sex-related roles are undergoing considerable change, giving rise to significant unaccustomed familial and social stresses manifest by marital discord; increased divorce and separation rates; jealousy, suspicions, and fears; sexual aberrations; youthful revolt, and increased delinquency, both juvenile and adult. Urban life today with its complexity and demands for conformity, yet rapid role change, places great stress on all participants but especially on those who are basically rigid and those who for socio-economic reasons are not able or permitted to cope. The frustrations of such groups result in threats of self-esteem and meaningful existence. This in time produces deep and continuing anxieties, which perhaps is the most fundamental or ultimate base on which antisocial behavior rests. This is especially likely to be true of those entrapped in the poverty "syndrome." As Chilman[63] has indicated, many of the very poor can find at least temporary escape only in fantasy, dramatic behavior, psychosomatic illnesses, impulsivity, alcohol, and drugs. Yet, she points out, the higher rates of child neglect and abuse, delinquency, crime, vandalism, and general social deviancy among the lower socio-economic classes cannot be merely accepted in a society that values the rights of the individual to protection from and for himself. She continues:

These behaviors especially cannot be accepted in an urban society where, for instance, one man's undisposed garbage becomes the neighborhood's rat problem, or where one impulsive, hostile, aggressive youth can become a menace to his family, neighborhood, community, and—with the aid of a gun—the nation. And, where a neglected, abused child can grow into such a youth. Of course, such behaviors pose a danger to the individual and to society in whatever social class they occur; these behaviors simply are—or appear to be—most prevalent in very poor groups.

This relates to much of what is discussed in Chapters 3 and 4. Poverty is indeed the germ of many social and biologic diseases. (And is there really any difference?) In view of this, there is ample justification for members of the health and social professions to address themselves to this complex of problems. However, to do so successfully requires the development of deep and genuine empathy and understanding, to look beyond the antisocial manifestations and see the social causes.

REFERENCES

1. Hovey, J.E.: Violence: is it a public health problem? Am. J. Public Health **71**:319, Mar. 1981.
2. Matthews, A.R.: Mental illness and the criminal law: is community mental health an answer? Am. J. Public Health **57**:1571, Sept. 1967.
3. Solomon, P.: The burden of responsibility in suicide and homicide, J.A.M.A. **199**:99, Jan. 30, 1967.
4. Hall, W.W.: Am. Med. News **14**:4, April 17, 1971.
5. Crime and medicine, MD **9**:120, Nov. 1965.
6. Saul, L.J.: The hostile mind, New York, 1956, Random House, Inc.
7. Freud, S.: Civilization and its discontents (1931). In Strachey, J., and others: The complete psychological works of Sigmund Freud, London, 1955, Hogarth Press, Ltd.
8. Cannon, W.B.: Bodily changes in pain, hunger, fear, and rage, New York, 1929, Appleton-Century-Crofts.
9. Allee, W.C.: Cooperation among animals, New York, 1951, Henry Schuman, Inc., Publishers.
10. Federal Bureau of Investigation: Uniform crime report, U.S. Department of Justice, 1980.
11. Gelles, R.J.: Violence toward children in the United States, Am. J. Orthopsychiatry **48**:580, Oct. 1978.
12. Straus, M.A., Gelles, R.J., and Steinmetz, S.K.: Behind closed doors: violence in the American family, New York, 1980, Doubleday Publishing Co.
13. National Center for Health Statistics: Births, marriages, divorces, and deaths, U.S. 1981, Monthly Vital Stat. Rep. 30, DHHS Pub. No. (PHS) 82:1220, Hyattsville, Md., Mar. 1982.
14. Editorial: Many people in jails don't belong there, Nation's Health, p. 8, June 1981.

15. Gillin, J.L.: Murder as a sociological phenomenon, Ann. Am. Acad. Pol. Soc. Sci. **284**:20, Nov. 1952.

16. Wolfgang, M.E.: Patterns of criminal homicide, New York, 1958, John Wiley and Sons, Inc.

17. Mulvihill, D.J., Tumin, M., and Curtis, L.: The interpersonal relationship between victim and offender. In Crimes of violence: a staff report of the National Commission on the Causes and Prevention of Violence, vol. 2, Washington, D.C., 1969, Superintendent of Documents, U.S. Government Printing Office.

18. Houts, M.: They asked for death, New York, 1970, Cowles Book Co., Inc.

19. Pizer, V.: Murder and the tyranny of fear, Washington Star, May 7, 1972.

20. Banay, R.S.: Study in murder, Ann. Am. Acad. Pol. Soc. Sci. **284**:26, Nov. 1952.

21. Washburn, S.L.: Aggressive behavior and human evolution. In Coelho, G.V., and Rubinstein, E.A., editors: Social change and human behavior, DHEW Pub. No. (HSM) 72-9122, Rockville, Md. 1972, National Institute of Mental Health.

22. Endleman, S.: Violence in the streets, Chicago, 1968, Quadrangle Books, Inc.

23. Breo, D.: Prolonged social stress linked to increase in black homicides, Am. Med. News, Sept. 6, 1976.

24. National Institute of Mental Health: The impact of televised violence; report of the Surgeon General's Advisory Committee on Television and Social Behavior, DHEW Pub. No. (HSM) 72-9090, Rockville, Md., 1972.

25. Gerbner, G.: Television violence: measuring the climate of fear, Am. Med. News, Dec. 13, 1976, p. 1.

26. Psychogenic death rates, Am. J. Public Health **60**:790, April 1970.

27. Bakal, C.: The right to bear arms, New York, 1966, McGraw-Hill Book Co.

28. Kempe, C.H., and others: The battered child syndrome, J.A.M.A. **181**:17, July 7, 1962.

29. Radbill, S.X.: A history of child abuse and infanticide. In Helfer, R., and Kempe, C., editors: The battered child, Chicago, 1973, University of Chicago Press.

30. Aries, P.: Centuries of childhood: a social history of family life, New York, 1962, Alfred A. Knopf, Inc.

31. deMause, L., editor: The history of childhood, New York, 1974, Psychohistory Press.

32. Segal, J.: Child abuse: a review of research. In Corfman, E., editor: Families today, vol. 2, DHEW Pub. No. (ADM) 79-815, 1979.

33. George, M.D.: London life in the eighteenth century, New York, 1925, Alfred A. Knupf, Inc.

34. Spargo, J.: The bitter cry of the children, New York, 1906, Macmillan Publishing Co., Inc.

35. Elmer, E.: Child abuse: the family's cry for help, J. Psychiatric Nursing **5**(4):332, July-Aug. 1967.

36. Asch, S.S.: Crib deaths: their possible relationship to postpartum depression and infanticide, J. Mt. Sinai Hosp. (New York) **35**:214, May-June 1968.

37. Elmer, E.: Studies of child abuse and infant accidents. In The mental health of the child, Washington, D.C., 1971, Superintendent of Documents, U.S. Government Printing Office.

38. Steele, B.F., and Pollock, C.B.: A psychiatric study of parents who abuse infants and small children. In Helfer, R., editor: The battered child, Chicago 1968, University of Chicago Press.

39. Silver, L., Dublin, C., and Lourie, R.: Does violence breed violence? Am J. Psychiatry, **126**(3):404, Sept. 1969.

40. Oliver, J.E., and others: Five generations of ill-treated children in one family pedigree, Br. J. Psychiatry, **119**:473, Nov. 1971.

41. Wolfgang, M.E.: Child and youth violence. Quoted in Segal, J.: Child abuse: a review of research. In Corfman, E., editor: Families today, vol. 2, DHEW Pub. No. (ADM) 79-815, 1979.

42. Money, J.: The syndrome of abuse dwarfism, Am. J. Dis. Child. **131**:508, May 1977.

43. Elmer, E., and Gregg, G.S.: Developmental characteristics of abused children, Pediatrics **40**:596, Oct. 1967.

44. Bakan, D.: Slaughter of the innocents, San Francisco, 1971, Jossey-Bass, Inc., Publishers.

45. Chang, A., and others: Child abuse and neglect: physicians' knowledge, attitudes, and experiences, Am. J. Public Health **66**:1199, Dec. 1976.

46. Sanders, R.W.: Resistance to dealing with parents of battered children, Pediatrics **50**:853, Dec. 1972.

47. Children's Bureau, U.S. Department of Health, Education, and Welfare: The abused child—principles and suggested language for legislation on reporting of the physically abused child, Washington, D.C., 1963, U.S. Government Printing Office.

48. Maltreatment of children: recommendations of Committee on the Infant and Preschool Child of the American Academy of Pediatrics, Pediatrics **37**:377, Feb. 1966.

49. Murdock, C.G.: The abused child and the school system, Am. J. Public Health **60**:105, Jan. 1970.

50. Nagl, S.: Child maltreatment in the United States: a challenge to social institutions, New York, 1977, Columbia University Press.

51. Gray, J.: Hospital-based battered child team, Hospitals **47**:50, Feb. 16, 1973.

52. Friedman, K.: The image of battered women, Am. J. Public Health **67**:723, Aug. 1977.

53. Gelles, R.: The violent home, Beverly Hills, 1972, Sage Publications, Inc.

54. Parker, B., and Schumacher, D.: The battered wife syndrome and violence in the nuclear family, Am. J. Public Health **67**:760, Aug. 1977.

55. Gelles, R.J.: Abused wives: why do they stay? J. Marriage and the Family **38**:659, 1976.

56. Wolfgang, M.E., Figlio, R.M., and Sellin, T.: Delinquency in a birth cohort, Chicago, 1972, University of Chicago Press.

57. Wolfgang, M.E.: Aggression in youth, lines of communication, Philadelphia, Jan. 1973, Mental Health Association of Southeast Pennsylvania.

58. Curran, W.J.: Due process, jury trials, and juvenile justice, Am. J. Public Health **61:**1901. Sept. 1971.

59. Eisner, V.: Effect of parents in the home on juvenile delinquency, Public Health Rep. **81:**905, Oct. 1966.

60. Campbell, C.M.: Destiny and disease in mental disorders, New York, 1935, W.W. Norton & Co. Inc.

61. Rosen, G.: Madness in society, Chicago, 1968, University of Chicago Press.

62. Cumming, J.H.: The family and mental disorder: an incomplete essay. In Causes of mental disorders, New York, 1961, Milbank Memorial Fund.

63. Chilman, C.S.: Growing up poor, SRS Pub. No. 109, Washington, D.C., 1969, U.S. Department of Health, Education, and Welfare.

Public health and health care services

Historically, one of the most significant events in the development of public health in the United States was its separation from medical care. Although much of the early history of public health involved the provision of personal health care services, the activities were usually a part of the police power functions of government to prevent the spread of dangerous communicable diseases. Governments at the state, county, and city level have been involved in medical care, but until recently that involvement has been through separate agencies concerned with corrections, welfare, or mental health. Public hospitals more often than not were operated under some other authority than that of the local health department.

Health officers have customarily been physicians selected for their jobs by boards of health, which were dominated by physicians. Many state and local health officers have long maintained that public health has no business providing medical care. The argument over the role of medical care in public health and vice versa has been deeply entwined in the history of the American Public Health Association, whose Medical Care Section rose to prominence because the Health Officers' Section had maintained, predictably, that medical care was not a public health service. However, in the seventies, the Health Officers' Section renamed itself the Health Administration Section and began to broaden its sphere of interest. Although it remains difficult in many states to obtain the consensus of the official health officers that personal health care services are a proper concern of health departments, many of the nation's most effective departments have extensive personal health care delivery systems, and several either operate public hospitals or participate in their operation.

Several generations of public health workers and physicians have been practicing both public health and medical care without either realizing it or openly acknowledging it. Even though many clinics have been ostensibly limited to tuberculosis, venereal disease, prenatal care, or well-child care, there has been more continuity and breadth in those services than is apparent at a cursory glance. The trend toward more personal health care delivery is continuing, not because health officers are trying to expand their domains but because the needs are there and the public expects their public agencies to do something about unmet needs for essential services. The public policy theme for 2 decades has been to move those without access to dependable health care into the mainstream of private practice. However, although this was partially accomplished, it is apparent that a vigorous public system of health care exists, is growing, and must continue to meet the needs of a large number of people who cannot obtain access to private services.

Part eight will describe the principal components of that system: nursing, social work, dental public health, the organized systems of medical care and the special field of emergency medical services.

CHAPTER 30

Community nursing services

America's two greatest contributions to public health were the Panama Canal and the public health nurse.

William H. Welch

HISTORICAL DEVELOPMENT

Among all of the various professional persons engaged in public health work, one group, nurses, merits particular mention. Aside from the fact that they constitute a considerable proportion of the professional public health work force, nurses are of special significance in that, considered as a group, they have closer personal contact with greater numbers of the public than does the rest of the professional staff of the health department. To many citizens the nurse represents the health department: that person who reduces the work of the organization to its lowest common denominator—direct service to the individual. Many health departments owe their start to communities' becoming convinced of the value of the services rendered by one or two visiting nurses. One old but still pertinent review[1] of the subject has stated it in this way:

It is precisely in the field of the application of knowledge that the public health nurse has found her great opportunity and her greatest usefulness. In the nationwide campaigns for the early detection of cancer and mental disorders, for the elimination of venereal disease, for the training of new mothers and the teaching of the principles of hygiene to young and old; in short, in all measures for the prevention of disease and the raising of health standards, no agency is more valuable than the public health nurse.

Since that time, nurses have taken a leadership role in planning, program development, policy formation, and administration, both in the community as well as in the institutional setting.

The community health nursing movement owes its inception to William Rathbone of Liverpool, who in 1859 was impressed by the care and comfort given by a nurse to his fatally ill wife. A philanthropist, he promoted the establishment of a visiting nurse service for the sick poor of his city. Despite the enormous existing demand for therapeutic nursing of the sick, the first nurse, Mary Robinson, was directed not only to give direct care to her patients but to instruct them and their families in the care of the sick, the maintenance of clean homes, and other matters that contribute to healthful living. As stated in the previously mentioned review[1]:

This went far beyond mere nursing, and the work of the visiting nurse was thus bound up with and made part of a general health movement—the nurse herself becoming perforce a social worker as well as a nurse. And the highly constructive educational work all this involved put new life and vitality into the age-old charity of visiting the sick poor, gave it enormously increased importance, and brought about its later amazing development.

So that qualified nurses would be available for the work, Rathbone enlisted the assistance of Florence Nightingale and established a training school in affiliation with the Royal Infirmary of Liverpool. Interestingly, Miss Nightingale from the beginning referred to the graduates who engaged in home visiting as "health nurses."

Early in 1873 Bellvue Hospital in New York City opened the first school of nursing in the United States. It was patterned after Miss Nightingale's principles. One of its first graduates, Frances Root, went out to work with poor patients in their homes and thus pioneered community nursing in the United States.[2] In 1877 the first visiting nurses were employed by a voluntary agency, the Women's Branch of the New York City Mission. The idea soon spread to other communities. Meanwhile official health organizations were being established, and they soon recognized the unique contribution that nurses could make to their programs. At first, resort was made to the visiting nurses of the voluntary agencies. Thus the nurses of the New York City Mission carried out the orders of the school medical inspectors, visited the pupils' homes, instructed the mothers in general health and infant care, and took sick children to the dispensary.[3]

The first visiting nursing associations per se were established in Buffalo in 1885 and in Boston and Philadelphia in 1886. Originally, those of Buffalo and Philadelphia were named District Nursing Societies and that of Boston was referred to as the Boston Instructive District Nursing Association. Eventually all their names were changed to visiting nurse associations. They depended on lay contributions for their support, and small service charges where indicated. At the beginning not only were they administratively under the direction of lay boards but the actual work of the nurses themselves was supervised by lay persons. Within a short time, however, the Philadelphia organization led the way by providing for a supervising nurse. These three early voluntary nursing organizations are still active.

With the expanding concept of public health, it was inevitable that nurses be employed directly by official health departments. The first city to do so was Los Angeles in 1898. The initial purpose was to provide visiting nursing care to the sick poor rather than to engage in educational or health promotional activities. The first official community health nurse, although paid with tax funds and responsible to the health officer, was assigned to the Los Angeles Settlement Association. As more nurses were added, however, there was established in 1913 a bureau of municipal nursing in the health department.

In earlier days of public health work, it was easier to focus public attention on special individual problems and to obtain public and private funds for their solution than it was to gain support for a broad, general program. As a result, most community health nursing programs were originally organized on a specialized basis; nurses were employed specifically as tuberculosis nurses, school nurses, maternal and child health nurses, communicable disease nurses, and, later, industrial nurses. This trend

was given further strength by the activities of the National Tuberculosis Association, by the passage of the Sheppard-Towner Act, and by the growing interest of school officials in the health of the schoolchild. On the other hand, the demonstration of the value of county health units sponsored by the Public Health Service and the Rockefeller Foundation and of the Town and Country Nursing Service sponsored in many parts of the nation by the American National Red Cross indicated distinct advantages to the generalization of visiting nursing activities.

The argument over specialization has continued into the present. At first, it was argued by many that a specially trained nurse could be more effective, especially in such settings as the tuberculosis clinic. Others argued that people and families, not a specific disease, were the focus of community health nursing and that the specialist might deal effectively with specific organs and pathology but poorly with the person. Initial training usually took place in the hospital setting. Those nurses who wished to work in the community setting had to acquire additional training. Over the past 2 decades two trends have emerged in community health nursing: more rigorous training for the generalist, usually at the baccalaureate level but increasingly at the master's level, and, at the same time, a growth in nurse practitioner training programs, including those with a specialty emphasis such as nurse midwifery, pediatric nursing, geriatrics, family planning, and industrial nursing. Some of the turmoil surrounding these developments is discussed later.

Bullough[4] has described three phases in the evolution of nursing in the United States. The period from 1900 to 1938 involved the legalization of the process of registration. This did not limit what people could do but limited the use of the title "registered nurse" to those who had been approved by a board. Beginning in 1938 the practice of nursing began to be limited to those who could demonstrate special knowledge, skill, and training to their state licensing boards. This necessitated the definition of nursing so that the laws could be specific about what those who were not nurses could not do. In most states, nursing practice acts avoided such terms as *diagnosis* and *treatment*, which were considered medical acts, and either required or inferred that nurses carried out the orders of a physician. The third phase began in 1971 with an Idaho statute that broadened the practice of nursing to include the diagnosis and treatment of problems under certain circumstances. Since then most states have rewritten their nursing practice acts to provide for similar extensions. The New York law, for example, states that

the practice of the profession of nursing as a registered professional nurse is defined as diagnosing and treating human responses to actual or potential health problems through such services as case finding, health teaching, health counseling, and provision of care supportive to or restorative of life and well being.*

Efforts to define nursing in a manner acceptable to the practitioners proved to be difficult, and the American Nurses' Association[5] had taken until 1955 to provide the following definition:

the performance, for compensation, of any acts in the observation, care and counsel of the ill, injured or infirm or in the maintenance of health or prevention of illness of others, or in the supervision and teaching of other personnel or the administration of medications and treatments as prescribed by a licensed physician or a licensed dentist; requiring substantial specialized judgment and skill and based on knowledge and application of principles of biological, physical and social science. The foregoing shall not be deemed to include any acts of diagnosis or prescription of therapeutic or corrective measures.

By the time the Association had adopted this definition, it was out of date. Although they often called the process "assessment" and "planning," nurses had of necessity been engaged in diagnostic and therapeutic practices for some time. Until fairly recently such practices had occurred as part of an elaborate physician-nurse game ritual that involved the nurse calling the physician's attention to a particular problem or set of symptoms and asking if it was all right to start a particular treatment. The many games developed over the years are still engaged in frequently, but the evolution of extended roles for nursing and the independent practice of nursing[6] indicate that the compulsion to do so is less common. Soares[7] has defined a nursing diagnosis as one that is amenable to nursing intervention—an answer that raises a question. (Simply put, a physician might make a diagnosis of diabetic coma and prescribe insulin, whereas a nurse might diagnose a subconscious state that requires assistance with eating, eliminating, moving, and possibly breathing.)

*New York State Education Law, Section 6902, Article 139.

There have been numerous other attempts to define nursing, but these attempts have been complicated by the fact that the practice of medicine was licensed before the practice of nursing; physicians staked out the whole field of health care, making it necessary for all other professional groups to work around the medical practice acts, either nibbling off small bits (such as dentists, optometrists, and podiatrists) or working in a dependent relationship to a physician. The American Nurses' Association has defined *community nursing* as "a synthesis of nursing practice and public health practice applied to promoting and preserving the health of populations."[8] Another term, *distributive nursing,* has emerged in recent years and may further confuse the nonnurse.[9] Originally coined to differentiate community nursing from the direct delivery of nursing services to the acutely or chronically ill person, the term has begun to take on an ethical hue involving the concerted attempt to distribute health services according to need rather than the ability of people or communities to pay for the services.

The phrase *community health nursing* became popular during the 1960s when a number of private, not-for-profit community agencies developed to provide health services that the community members felt should have been provided by the existing public health agencies. To indicate that they were not part of a governmental effort but rather a more indigenous and less bureaucratic enterprise, the workers used the adjective *community* instead of *public,* and the term has continued in use in training programs. *Community health nursing* is used in this discussion to indicate both official health agency programs as well as those in school settings and private, not-for-profit organizations.

There probably have been more conferences to discuss the role of the nurse in recent years than the roles of all other health professionals combined. The significance and possible direction of this search for specificity is explored later.

THE SUPPLY OF NURSES
Supply versus need

In 1970 the National League For Nursing[10] estimated that there were 850,000 nurses in the United States but that only 530,000 of them were in active practice. By 1980, the Bureau of Health

Professions estimated that there were 1,662,382 licensed registered nurses in the United States and that 1,272,851 of them (76.6% of the total) were employed in nursing.[11] That represents a 76% increase in the ratio of nurses to population during the 1970s (from 418 per 100,000 to 745 per 100,000). During the 1960s it was believed that there was a growing shortage of nurses, and federal support for nursing education increased rapidly. The Nurse Training Act of 1975 limited that support and required the Department of Health, Education, and Welfare to develop work force projections that were more reliable. Both the Department and the Congressional Budget Office estimated that there would be between 1.467 million and 1.541 million nurses by 1990, and the congressional report concluded that supply and demand would be in balance through that period with no new initiatives.[12,13]

Whether "demand" will equal "need" is not known. The concept of work force needs is just as complex as the concept of the need for hospital or nursing home beds, and for many of the same reasons. The health industry has an astonishing degree of elasticity in that it can and usually will use resources as they become available without any apparent relation to an objective assessment of need or the usual law of supply and demand. Moreover, the need or demand for the services of one particular professional group will vary with the supply and role of other professional groups. Physicians, various kinds of physician assistants, and nurses cannot be defined usefully independently of each other, which is exactly what most needs-assessment methodologies attempt to do. The dynamics of the interrelationships and what they portend for health work force planners and health economists have not been explored in sufficient detail to provide a realistic base for calculating "need."

There are several estimates of the number of nurses who are employed in community health programs. In an overview of a 1980 survey, the Bureau of Health Professions estimated that there were 65,449 registered nurses who were working full time in community health settings and 16,745 who were working part time.[11] Combining the two figures produces an estimate of 73,693 "full-time–equivalent" nurses employed in such settings. In a different project, the Bureau developed estimates

of the number of community health nurses who were working in different types of agencies in 1979.[14] Bureau personnel believe that the former set of figures provides a better count of the total numbers but that the latter study provides a more accurate picture of the distribution of the nurses by sponsoring agency. Applying that distribution to the total of 73,693 derived from the 1980 survey produces the estimates shown in Table 30-1.

Until the 1920s, the majority of community health nurses were employed by voluntary agencies. Since that time, the distribution has changed considerably with a large increase in the number of nurses employed by local health departments and boards of education. Slightly more than 92% of all community health nurses are working in local agencies. Slightly more than half of those working for home health agencies are employed by not-for-profit organizations, and the remainder are working for proprietary home health organizations. As noted earlier, it is difficult if not impossible to indicate whether these numbers are sufficient for the work that needs to be done. Elliott and Kearns developed a model in a 1978 report[15] that indicated a need for approximately 103,217 community health nurses by 1982: 20,403 in home health agencies, 52,308 in general public health, and 30,506 in school health work. These two different series of calculations result in a more conservative estimate of the gap between need and supply than is ordinarily suggested by health workers. They should not be considered a realistic appraisal of the current situation because of the methdologic problems inherent in health work force planning and analysis.

TABLE 30-1. Distribution of registered nurses employed in community health work, by full-time–equivalent positions and type of agency, United States, 1980

Type of agency	Number of full-time–equivalent positions
National	1,345
University	1,420
State agency	2,979
Local health agency	26,146
Community health centers	1,474
Home health agencies	15,797
Boards of education	22,036
Other	1,474

Even with that warning, it is tempting to refer to a very old suggestion that there ought to be one community health nurse for every 2,500 people, which results in a "need" for 90,602 nurses! It is also tempting to note that the entire "deficit" could be overcome by moving 3% to 4% of hospital nurses from that setting to community nursing.

Education and training

Most nurses working in community health programs are graduates of diploma programs usually sponsored by a hospital and not affiliated with a college or university. Community health nursing directors generally believe that it requires at least baccalaureate-level training to qualify as a community health nurse, and many would require additional training—either formal academic or planned in-service training. Only about a third of the staff nurses working in community health nursing have received 1 year or more of academic training. At the supervisory level and above a majority have had 1 or more years of such training. Some significant steps have been taken during recent years to extend the effectiveness of community health nursing staffs by the training and use of a variety of auxiliary personnel. Several thousand practical or vocational nurses are employed in public health agencies, and nursing aides have been employed with increasing frequency. In view of rising health care costs generally and the increasingly sophisticated skill training that occurs in aide and vocational nurse programs, it is anticipated that many more such individuals will be employed in nursing programs in the future. This influx will result in continued role changes for registered nurses. In addition, much of the burden of epidemiologic case finding and follow-up is being taken off the shoulders of the public health nurse by disease control investigators.

In nursing generally 70.8% of the employed registered nurses were graduates of diploma or associate degree programs in 1980, whereas only 23.3% were graduates of baccalaureate programs. The American Nurses' Association has resolved that baccalaureate-level training should be the minimum entry requirement for professional practice by 1985.[16] It is difficult to predict the effect of the growth of various "nurse practitioner" programs on the credentials of community health nursing in the future. Nurse practitioners were relatively new in 1970, but by 1978 there were 144 nurse practitioner programs.[17] Approximately 5.3% had master's or doctoral degrees.[11] (Most of the master's degrees were in nursing or public health, but many of the doctoral degrees were in education.) This is a marked change from 1974, when 81% were graduates of diploma or associate degree programs, 16% were graduates of baccalaureate programs, and 3% had master's or doctoral degrees.[12] This trend toward higher levels of academic preparation is expected to continue with concomitant changes in the roles that nurses expect to play in the health care system.

Whereas some nurse practitioners are generalists or specialize in primary care, many (about 13,000 of the 17,000 working in 1980) followed specialty training programs. The differences between nurse practitioners and community nurses are often debated, and at least one program titles itself *Clinical Nurse Practitioner Training in Community Health Nursing.* In general, nurse practitioners provide more depth in the management of selected cases, whereas community health nurses provide greater breadth and engage in individual, family, and community educational efforts more frequently.

Some of the changes in training and titles make evident much of the turmoil going on in nursing, a profession under considerable pressure. As Archer and Fleshman[18] point out, community nurses are caught between physicians who oppose their attempt to function as an independent professional group; other professional workers, such as social workers and rehabilitation workers, who feel that their turf is being invaded by the nurse; other nursing groups, such as nurse practitioners and clinical nursing specialists, who have fostered specialization of their practice just as did physicians before them and with the same zealous notion that generalists are not well qualified; and client and community forces who want better access to a more caring health worker at less cost. A few short years ago it appeared that these conflicts would continue to evolve in the direction of a stronger role for nursing in primary care, but as Aiken[19] has pointed out, circumstances have changed rapidly: there is a decline in the rate at which resources are being added to health care, there are enough providers to meet present and future needs (although they are not always where they are needed), most people can get the health care that they need now, those who cannot obtain necessary health care require additional monetary resources, not more providers, and nursing so far appears not to displace or reduce costs but to add to them (whether that produces an increased benefit has not been determined). Given that impression, it is unlikely that nursing can progress rapidly in the development of primary nursing care unless there are major structural reforms in the health care system generally.

NURSING AGENCIES

In the evolution of community health programs, the contribution of nurses has been increasingly recognized on all levels.

National level

In the past, on the federal level several programs of the Public Health Service conducted activities in public health nursing. They operated by providing grants-in-aid and consultation service to the states and through them to local health departments and by participating in the development of proper standards and qualifications. For a period of years the Office of Indian Affairs provided direct nursing service by means of public health field nurses stationed on the various reservations. In 1953 this activity was transferred to the Public Health Service and has been significantly expanded. Among other activities it promotes nursing as a career among young Amerindians. The Division of Nursing is now in the Bureau of Health Professions of the Health Resources and Services Administration of the Department of Health and Human Services. Three private organizations that are active on the national level are the National League for Nursing, the American Nurses' Association, and the new Council of State Boards of Nursing.

State level

By 1937 all of the states employed community health nurses in their state health organizations. The manner of their placement in the organization varies. The majority of state health departments have had separate bureaus or divisions of public health nursing. Recently the trend has been to place nursing personnel in the operating programs such as maternal and child health, preventive medicine, or local health administration. The organizational placement of nursing in a state health department has involved a considerable amount of

conflict. Nursing, as an organizational unit, is not usually a program; rather, it is a service. Nursing staff members are involved in many health department programs. The historical role of community nursing in public health agencies and the natural desire of a group of workers sharing a common background, training, and commitment to form a unit has long left both state and local agencies in an awkward organizational position. Many public health administrators have believed that the nursing staff of the agency should be distributed into the major program areas, but community nursing leaders have feared that such dispersal would lead to inattention to the integrity of the nurse's role, a loss of skills, and a gradual decline of the impact of the nurse on public health planning. The advent of more professional administrators in decision-making positions within official health agencies seems to have encouraged the gradual movement toward dispersal of the nursing staff. There are three ways to avoid the loss of nursing concepts in public health program development: (1) maintain a bimodal organizational structure in which nurses can belong to a nursing organization within the agency while also serving as members of a program team; (2) place trained community health nursing administrators into key program management positions within the agency; or (3) reestablish an identifiable community health nursing program by explicitly changing the role of the nurse in favor of a more independent practice—independent, that is, from the control of the physician. The most recent report of the Association of State and Territorial Health Officials[20] does not list a separate program of community health nursing, although it indicates that all state health agencies provide public health nursing services.

The functions and responsibilities of nurses in state health departments depend on the legislative basis of the department. In the majority of instances they act as advisors to local health departments, boards of education, voluntary health agencies, and other state agencies. In a few state health departments that have been given broader responsibilities and powers, the nurses may actually supervise and administer certain direct services, local as well as state, and may have regulatory responsibilities related to nursing practice, nurseries, day care, nursing homes, and hospitals. Other important activities of state health department nurses include demonstrations of particular services or of total community health nursing programs, the development of home health services programs and agencies, and the conducting of in-service training courses.

All state health departments are active in the promotion of community health nursing services for prenatal and postnatal care, infants, and preschool children. To do so, they function either through the direct assignment of state nurses to local areas, through the loan of state nurses to specially selected local communities, or through subsidy of local nursing programs.

Local level

Generally speaking, community health nurses today may be placed into two general categories—those employed by official health agencies primarily to carry out preventive and promotive health functions, and those engaged by voluntary or commercial agencies primarily to render home nursing care to the sick. In addition, a large number of nurses have been employed by boards of education as school health nurses, and in recent years a number of community health nurses have been employed by neighborhood health centers and community mental health centers. It has been difficult to make a durable distinction between community health nurses and visiting nurses. Generally, it has been held that those who provide preventive and promotive services are practicing community nursing, whereas those who provide nursing care to the sick are providing visiting nursing services. The functional differences have become increasingly obscure. The visiting nurse often engages in health promotive activities while in the home, and the community nurse may help with a dressing change, either because it needs to be done or because some member of the family needs to learn how to do it. Increasingly, both activities are being provided by the same nurse; the only useful distinction that can be made is that visiting nursing services are often reimbursable whereas community nursing services usually are not.

The employment and supervision of school nurses has always been a source of friction. Many school officials feel that the personnel working in the school system should be a part of that system, whereas public health administrators claim that teachers cannot adequately supervise nursing personnel and that nurses working for school officals will be relegated to first-aid tasks rather than play a role in health promotive activities and counseling. Community health nurses working for boards of education have generally been paid better and/or have worked less than their counterparts in public health agencies, and this has often added to the friction. The determining factor will probably be fiscal. Boards of education have their own tax base and until recently were able to obtain the personnel they wanted. Since public health administrators had a more difficult time getting support for community health nursing services, the school board could and did hire its own nurses. The property taxpayer has become increasingly concerned about the rising cost of the educational system, however, and school boards have elected to decrease nursing and counseling services to retain their teaching personnel. The result has been a gradual decline in the amount of community health nursing service available in the school setting—a valuable environment for assessment and diagnosis and for planning, implementation, and evaluation of group and individual health programs.

The American National Red Cross nursing program began in Ohio in 1912 and spread to many parts of the country, particularly in rural areas. From the beginning its policy was to promote and assist in the establishment of local public health nursing programs and of full-time local health departments to which it eventually turned over its work. The American National Red Cross also played an important role in the promotion of public health nursing units in state health departments.

Two other groups that until recently provided visiting nursing services should be mentioned. Some of the larger insurance companies, particularly Metropolitan Life and John Hancock, for many years offered home nursing service to persons holding certain types of policies. The manner in which this was done varied, depending on the size of community, the number of policyholders, and the existence of other qualified nursing agencies in the community. In some areas nurses were employed directly by the insurance companies, whereas in others the service was purchased on a cost per visit or on a contract basis from local private nursing agencies. These programs were phased out some years ago on the basis of the services' having become readily available from other sources.

Another source of nursing service that has played an important role in some parts of the country is the large private occupational medical and health

programs, many of which employ not only industrial or occupational health nurses but also nurses
whose function it is to attend sick employees and
sometimes members of their families in their
homes. With the broadening scope of occupational
health and safety and the interests of labor unions
in health services, such programs often include
health protection and promotion activities provided
by industrial clinic and home visiting nurses. A
guide to nursing assessment in the industrial setting has been developed by Serafini.[21]

The National Organization for Public Health
Nursing did not render direct service to the public
but played a dominant role in the advancement of
the field. It was organized in 1912 as the national
professional society for those engaged or interested
in public health work and became recognized as
the voice of the profession. No other single agency
contributed so much to the improvement of educational and service standards and to the promotion
of the public acceptance of and respect for the work
of the community health nurse. By 1952, however,
concern developed about the growing number of
nursing agencies and the need for coordination. As
a result, in that year the National Organization for
Public Health Nursing joined the National League
of Nursing Education and the Association of Collegiate Schools of Nursing to form the National
League for Nursing. At the same time the bylaws
of the American Nurses' Association were changed
to provide for cooperation with the new National
League for Nursing. Meanwhile the National Association of Colored Graduate Nurses also went out
of existence, and its functions were integrated into
the other organizations.

FUNCTIONS AND RESPONSIBILITIES

The statement of functions and responsibilities
for community health nurses, first prepared in 1931
by the Subcommittee on Functions of the National
Organization for Public Health Nursing, has undergone several revisions. The most recent statements of standards for community nursing practice
have been developed by the American Nurses' Association.[8] The original listing of functions included
assessment (collecting and analyzing information
about the individual or the community), planning
(for intervention), implementation, and evaluation
of the intervention. More recently, the task of di-

agnosis has been added. The functions are described in these standards as follows:

Standard I: The collection of data about the health status of the consumer is systematic and continuous. The
data are accessible, communicated and recorded. . . . .
Standard II: Nursing diagnoses are derived from health
status data. . . .
Standard III: Plans for nursing service include goals
derived from nursing diagnoses. . . .
Standard IV: Plans for nursing service include priorities and nursing approaches or measures to achieve the
goals derived from nursing diagnoses. . . .
Standard V: Nursing actions provide for consumer participation in health promotion, maintenance and restoration. . . .
Standard VI: Nursing actions assist consumers to maximize health potential. . . .
Standard VII: The consumer's progress toward goal
achievement is determined by the consumer and the
nurse. . . .
Standard VIII: Nursing actions involve ongoing reas-
sessment, reordering of priorities, new goal setting and
revision of the nursing plan.*

Some very significant concepts are contained in
the above. The term *consumer* is used rather than
patient or client. That was not done in the spirit of
the consumer movement of the 1960s but in the
more sophisticated sense that a consumer-provider
contract is being developed by two equal partners.
The plan will be developed in the context of this
partnership. That is, the nurse will discuss possibilities with the consumer, but the consumer will
ultimately be the one to select the goals and objectives, on which the two partners will work together.
Periodically progress will be reviewed, the plan will
be evaluated, and new goals and objectives may be
agreed on. This contract-negotiating process is a
unique concept in American health care and is of
fundamental importance to the clinician and the
administrator, whether dealing with an individual
consumer or an entire community.

Ruth Freeman, one of the most articulate and
thoughtful nursing leaders and authors, said simply that "the traditional function of community
health nursing is to help others help themselves."[22]
It is not a solo practice but a care system. Accepting
Freeman's description, there may be no such thing
as a "community health nurse," rather there is a

*Reprinted with permission from Standards of community
health nursing practice, Kansas City, Mo., 1974, American Nurses' Association.

variety of nursing practices that go together to make up a community nursing program. The term *independent practice* may be used to describe a professional nursing practice that is not dependent on the direction or orders of a physician, or it may be used to describe a private nurse practice that is not part of private or public agency. In this discussion, the adjective *independent* will be used to characterize professional nursing as a distinct form of practice in contrast to a physician-dependent practice. The term *private practice* is better suited to distinguish individually provided patient care services from nursing that takes place under the auspices of a nursing agency.

Nurses, in their practice relationships, may focus their efforts on one or more of the following[18,19]:

1. Disease or diagnostic categories such as tuberculosis, diabetes, or mental illness
2. Primary care
3. Population groups such as mothers and children or the aged
4. A place such as a specified community served by a community health center
5. Management (supervision) and teaching
6. Administration and the maintenance of the system

ADMINISTRATIVE RELATIONSHIPS

An important administrative consideration influencing the value and efficiency of community health nursing programs is the nature of the relationships that exist among the various nursing and social agencies in the community, the public, and the members of other health professions. The need for community health nursing services is so great that it is important for agencies engaged in this work to cooperate and coordinate their respective programs as much as possible for maximum efficiency.

Relationships within the health department

The professional relationships of nurses in community health agencies take place in two areas: (1) within the agency itself and (2) in contacts with other agencies and individuals in the community. Within a health department the relationship between the community health nursing staff and the administrator of the agency or department is of paramount importance. All too often satisfactory relationships between the nursing staff and the administrator are falsely assumed to exist. It is not unknown for health officials merely to support the

nursing program quantitatively and to neglect to participate in the planning and organization for the effective delivery of nursing services.

Some health officials follow the path of least effort by allowing the nursing unit to proceed almost as if it were an independent agency. Inevitably this policy leads to difficulty both within and outside the department. The agency administrator is ultimately responsible for all phases of the health program of the department, and, to a considerable extent, of the community as a whole. With respect to the nursing aspects of the program, the health director, who may be a nurse, should carefully select a well-qualified director of nursing services, provide adequate administrative support, and see that general policies and interagency relationships are developed by the nursing services director rather than perhaps haphazardly and inadequately by staff nurses and the workers of other agencies. The health agency director needs to maintain constant interest in the nursing program and endeavor to learn enough about it to assist the nurses in their efforts to fit into the total community health picture. If nursing is a service unit rather than a program, the nursing services director may be relegated to a role that exists outside of the policy-making group within the health agency. The agency director may discuss problems and policies frequently with directors of maternal and child health programs and environmental health directors, but the nursing services director may be excluded from such discussions. The conceptual framework and the value system of community health nursing should permeate virtually all discussions about programs and policies. If the nursing services director cannot maintain that sort of involvement in a productive manner, then the agency administrator either has the wrong person in that job or has not allowed the nursing services director sufficient intellectual exercise within the agency to maintain a forceful role. Most of the local health agency directors in the United States are physicians, and the traditional physician-nurse relationship can seriously weaken the potential effectiveness of the nursing services director. Only a fraction of the physician directors of local health agencies have had any training in public health or public health administration, and their vision of community problems is often narrow, whereas the nursing services director may have had training and experience in community health programs that exceed that of the department director.

The community health nurse and the staff working in environmental health may on the surface seem unrelated. However, they are part of the same organization and should work in a helpful as well as cordial relationship. In the course of daily field visits, the alert community health nurse is certain to become aware of many insanitary situations. Often they have a direct or indirect bearing on the nurse's professional interests and activities. A policy of prompt and effective intra-agency referral should be developed to handle such situations. The same applies conversely to the engineer and sanitarian. The problem becomes more difficult in communities that have separated environmental health from the rest of public health.

Consolidation of nursing services

There is little if any justification for more than two community nursing groups in any given community: (1) the community health nurses working as employees of the official health department and (2) the staff of a visiting nursing association. The trend has been to explore ways of effectively merging these two groups. Regardless of the number involved, the coordination of the work of all agencies providing nursing services in a community is necessary to best serve the needs and interests of the public. Since there is no one answer as to how this may be accomplished, each community must work out a solution best suited to its particular needs and background. The number and variety of possible arrangements in a given community may be somewhat as follows. If there are several voluntary or nonofficial agencies that render nursing services in the community, they may (1) remain completely independent of each other; (2) retain their individual identities but coordinate their programs by means of a central nursing advisory committee in which each agency participates; or (3) combine their programs to form a single community health nursing agency. (Once common, the delivery of nursing services by voluntary health associations such as tuberculosis or cancer is now rare, except for the visiting nursing association.) The voluntary agencies singly or united may limit their activities to bedside care, leaving most or all educational, promotional, and legal control measures to the nurses of the official health department. On the other hand, the health department may delegate some or even all of its community health nursing responsibilities to the voluntary nursing agency. In the few communities where this procedure is followed, it is usually attributable to two influences: the existence of a long-established, well-supported, and accepted visiting nursing association, and a weak official health department.

The completely satisfactory consolidation of community nursing services is as yet relatively rare, usually strongly resisted, and in some situations premature. One of the most successful solutions developed up to the present time was effected in Seattle, Washington. The official and voluntary nursing agencies agreed on a cooperative, completely generalized community health nursing program that includes all preventive, promotive, educational, and bedside services but retains the board of directors of the voluntary nursing agency as an advisory committee that controls its own contribution to the total cost of the program by means of an annual contract with the official health department. When carefully prepared and put into effect, this plan has worked well and has brought about increased efficiency and economy, and both groups of nurses have found more professional job appeal and stimulation from it.

As of 1979, 1,290 or 45% of the 2,873 certified home health agencies were official agencies, 512 were visiting nurse associations, and only 50, or 2% of the total, were combined agencies. The remainder were hospital-based agencies (351), other private, not-for-profit organizations (440), and proprietary organizations (163) or organizations of some other type (67).[23] There are many other organizations that provide home health services but are not certified. Certification means that the agency's standards and practices have been reviewed and are in compliance with federal standards for participation in the Medicare program.

Physician relationships

The nurse in community health work has traditionally served under the direct or indirect orders of the physician. As noted earlier, licensure of a professional group is a process that involves declaring particular activities to be illegal and then specifying a procedure whereby certain individuals can be authorized to carry out those activities. The boards that issue licenses are traditionally composed of members of the profession licensed. Physicians were successful in getting licensure programs established before other health professionals in the United States could do so, and their definition of medical practice was global. The license to practice medicine and surgery is still the most unrestricted grant of authority any government can give to a citizen. The effort to license nurses, which began in 1938, of necessity had to be more restrictive in its definition of nursing practice and made that practice a dependent practice of medicine; that is, whatever a nurse could do depended on what a physician ordered done for the patient. This relationship has dominated and retarded the development of nursing for decades.

The relationship of nurses in community health agencies with locally practicing physicians was carefully circumscribed and designed in such a way as to reduce the effectiveness of the nurse, although it has also offered considerable protection. Traditionally, no health officer, who usually worked for a board of health dominated by physicians, could allow the expansion of the nurse's role with impunity. A primary function of the community health nurse was to interpret medical advice and guidance when asked to do so by the physician of the patient. The nurse was expected to assist people in obtaining medical care when they needed it or wanted it and then to assist them in carrying out the physician's orders. In doing this, the nurse was explicitly forbidden from recommending a particular physician, from advising patients to change physicians if the care they were getting was obviously unsatisfactory, or from offering advice about their treatment or other actions they might consider unless that advice could be considered the carrying out of the physician's orders. To be sure that this was done properly, it was common to appoint a medical advisory committee to discuss, clear, and implement policy. The members were usually appointed by the local medical society. Such committees were of obvious help to the health officer and the nursing service director when a local physician felt affronted by nursing advice given to a patient that seemed to be at variance with what the physician had prescribed because the medical committee often would intervene to suggest to the physician that he or she might have erred.

In most cases the nurse did not enter the home without first discussing the matter with the private physician and obtaining permission and direction. The nurse was expected to report observations and findings about the patient's progress to the physi-

cian, but if the nurse thought that the diagnosis or management of the patient was incorrect, it became a very difficult matter to deal with, usually involving consultation with the supervisor and often with the physician health director, who might try to find some tactful way to remedy the situation without offending the private physician. It is clear that the feelings and well-being of the physician took precedence over the best interests of the patient. It is also clear that the entire charade was, and to some extent still is, based on the political vulnerability of the health department to the concerns of organized medicine. The ethics of professional practice preclude one professional criticizing the work of another professional in front of a client. There is some virtue as well as some self-interest in this ethic, but its observance requires that special consideration be extended to the rights of the consumer or client involved in the whole transaction. Some of the issues involved in this complex series of relationships are discussed at the conclusion of this chapter, but reality dictates that health agencies and their community nursing staff continue to pay attention to the difficult problem of serving the community while maintaining the support of the principal provider organizations.

In many instances, the nurse is serving as an assistant to the physician in carrying out the latter's prescriptions. In such cases a traditional supervisory relationship exists, and good professional practice will dictate the manner in which that relationship works for the benefit of the client. Sometimes the community health nurse will be asked for a reference to a physician. Standard practice in the past has been to advise the client to call the medical society for a list; or, if approved by the medical society and the agency director, the nurse may provide the patient with a list of physicians in the area whose field of practice is pertinent to the needs of the patient. In reality, such attempts to be nonpartisan often do not work. The nurse may have good reason to doubt the competency of some of the physicians on the list and may also know that a particular physician will not take any new patients or any new patients who depend on certain insurance or welfare programs for payment of their medical bills. Experienced nurses often find ways to signal the client in such a way as to get a particular message conveyed. It is important that personal biases, which may not be useful, do not enter into such transactions. It is often helpful for the nurses practicing in a given area to compare notes and update their unofficial list so that it reflects judgments about competency and social attitudes rather than personal preferences. Occasionally community health nurses have been criticized for referring low-income patients to the county or city hospital instead of to private practitioners; and faced with such criticism, agency and nursing service directors have sometimes prohibited those referrals. Such a policy would be a mistake. It is very hard for some people who do not have a personal physician relationship to establish one, especially when they are low-income and minority group members. The local public hospital or health department clinic is frequently the best place to refer such individuals, since the staff is usually adept at dealing with such problems and have the social support services available that are often needed by their clients.

In some areas a community nursing council exists to assist in studying, planning, improving, and coordinating all of the nursing activities in the community. Its membership is usually fairly large, including representatives from all official and nonofficial agencies that provide nursing services; from organized professional groups such as medicine, dentistry, nursing, and social work; and from the public at large.

More recently the trend has been to develop a council of social agencies. The council plays a most important role in the development of joint analyses, planning, and implementation by all of the many social agencies that exist in the typical community. It usually functions by means of several standing and ad hoc committees with representatives of various interested and pertinent agencies. The health committee, which is almost universally one of the standing committees, may serve effectively in the absence of a community nursing council.

NURSING AND OTHER COMMUNITY SERVICES

The association of the official health nursing program with the other social agencies in the community emphasizes the fact that in a certain sense the nurse in a community health agency is part of a social service system. The approach to individual and family problems differs depending on the provider's training. Social workers, nurses, and nutritionists may all describe the same problem differently and plan a different approach. Nevertheless, because of the complex nature of all social problems, of which illness and its prevention are one, mutual understanding and cooperation between the groups are of great importance. The more they know about each other's special training and abilities, the better will be their individual and joint performance. The role of social services in public health is considered in Chapter 31. The nurse should be familiar with each of the social agencies in the community and know what each does and where its interests and contributions cut across, supplement, or complement those of the nursing program. Both the nurse and the social worker should have available for ready reference a directory or file indicating the interests, resources, location, and leadership of each social service agency.

Usually the social welfare programs consist of child welfare services, family services, medical social services, psychiatric social work, public assistance, and in- and out-of-home care services. Occasionally most or all of these are found in a single agency. However, the usual pattern is for several official and nonofficial agencies to be involved. One of the important practical reasons for familiarity with the social agencies of a community is for purposes of referral. A case of tuberculosis, for example, may appear to be primarily the concern of the health department. However, problems of hospitalization and its costs, family support in the absence of the breadwinner, the placement of dependent children, and rehabilitation, to mention a few, will usually arise. The nurse cannot solve all of these singlehandedly and should refer certain aspects of the total family problem, which has been crystallized by the appearance of tuberculosis, to other appropriate community resources.

At one time many communities tried to establish a social service exchange system that was essentially a registry of clients of various official and voluntary health and social service agencies. Their purpose was to enable workers to be sure that they were not duplicating the efforts of some other agency and to find out what other problems might exist in the family and who was doing what about them. Without computers, the maintenance of the registry was too difficult for most communities and their popularity declined. The need still exists, but computerized systems are costly. Moreover, considerable attention has to be paid to the problems of confidentiality. Mental health workers, alcoholism and drug abuse counselors, and venereal disease investigators are understandably and properly concerned about the problems. If all potential users are involved in the design of the system and thoughtful attention is given to the concept of "need to know" and what is clearly in the client's best interest, such sophisticated clearinghouses are possible and useful.

ADMINISTRATIVE AIDS IN COMMUNITY HEALTH NURSING

As in other professional areas, community health nursing has found it practical to apply certain well-proved administrative aids.

Supervision

Unquestionably the most valuable administrative aid is the supervision provided at each level within a community health nursing agency. Supervision is necessary for the properly balanced development of the nursing service in public health programs and for the maintenance of its standards. Total responsibility for such supervision rests on the nurse administrator and, depending on the size of the agency, assistants and one or more supervisors. At the staff level, supervision ensures the quality and quantity of the service through both administrative and educational processes. With a ratio of 1 supervisor to every 6 to 8 staff nurses, it should be possible for the supervisor to offer sufficient guidance and counsel to the field or staff nurses to maintain the standard of the service offered and to encourage them individually to develop their ability to serve the patient and the family. The nursing supervisor is also a liaison person who serves as a two-way link between the staff nurses and the administrative officers of the agency. The supervisor interprets policies and methods of application and may also transmit the impressions of the staff, together with suggestions for additions or changes in policies, to the administration centers of the agency. In this way it is possible for the field staff to play an important role in the formation or modification of policies and program. Knollmueller,[23] in an editorial comment, has decried the shift of the supervisor from the important functions of teaching, counseling, and problem solving to management. It is a pertinent observation as more community agencies become involved in collective bargaining, often separating staff nurses from supervisors in a traditional labor-management arrangement.

Standard procedures

In any situation where several persons perform similar work toward a common purpose, it is desirable that they each follow the same procedures with regard to certain aspects of their work. To avoid misunderstanding and confusion, it is helpful, even in the smaller agencies, to have available a manual that sets forth clearly the policies of the agency and the procedures that are used. This should include statements of the exact responsibilities and authority of the personnel, standing orders used by the agency, and descriptions of techniques that are considered safe, effective, and ethically acceptable. Although each agency will find it necessary to develop its own manual, attention is directed to the *Manual of Public Health Nursing*, which has been prepared and is periodically revised by the National League for Nursing (formerly the National Organization for Public Health Nursing). Many state health departments have also prepared excellent nursing manuals for use by local health departments. There also should be a record manual in which the purpose and proper use of each record used by the community health nursing staff is explained and illustrated. It must be remembered that, valuable as these administrative manuals are, they quickly become useless unless continually kept up to date.

Nursing records have been transformed in recent years as a result of the problem-oriented approach first developed by Weed.[24] Its application to nursing practice has been well described by Woolley[25] and in *Problem Oriented Systems of Patient Care,* published by the National League for Nursing.[26] An ongoing audit process is important to assure high quality and staff development.[27]

Clerical staff

Although much of the recording, particularly that relating to details of field visits, must of necessity be done by the nurses themselves, there is much clerical work that is more efficiently carried on by an office clerical staff. Despite this, it is by no means uncommon to find the professional nurses of many organizations devoting large proportions of their work time to details of record keeping and analysis in the office. This is particularly unfortunate in the face of a shortage in community nursing personnel. The false reasoning appears to be prevalent that, as long as nurses must be employed in the community health nursing program, they might as well do all or most of the clerical work involved. It should always be realized that the records are also a necessary part of the program and that proper personnel for their handling is wholly justified. Furthermore, one may do well to remember that the use of the relatively expensive time of a professionally trained nurse for office work, which may more efficiently and effectively be turned over to lesser trained employees in lower salary scales, is poor administration.

THE FUTURE OF COMMUNITY NURSING

It should be evident from the preceding sections of this chapter that nursing is in a continuing state of flux and evolution. Chaska[28] collected and edited an outstanding collection of papers on nursing that have been published in a book titled *The Nursing Profession: Views Through the Mist*. The papers deal with the topics of professionalization, education, research, nursing theory, practice, relationships, and the future of nursing. The ferment within the profession is obvious. Chaska describes three role possibilities: (1) primary care as a lower level practitioner (that is, lower than the physician), (2) a combination of medical activities with nursing assessment and teaching, or (3) a concentration on nursing's primary role. She asks if nursing should compromise or develop its own unique role. She makes a strong case for the latter.

As noted earlier, there have been marked changes in licensure, in education, and in the definition of nursing in recent years. New and more autonomous roles for nurses have been described in virtually every field of health care, including the management of diabetes, the practice of pediatrics, family planning, and, of course, midwifery. Perhaps the most striking departure from the past has been the development of independent nursing practices. Started by Kenline in Maryland and almost an underground movement at first, this concept was the topic of a special conference in December 1975.[6] These developments, scarcely whispered about a decade ago, suggest that a stronger role for nursing may be emerging, much to the benefit of society.

It is unfortunate that many of the new nursing practice efforts have found it necessary to develop a fee-for-service system since it is probable that such systems will direct the new providers into the same entrepreneurial practices that have increased the costs and diminished the value of medical care. It is important that nursing become more aware of health care policy issues, economics, and administration if the profession is to avoid becoming part of the problem rather than part of the solution.

The practice of medicine is a high-technology form of practice. Most problems that cause people to seek help are low-technology problems. When a low-technology problem is managed in a high-technology system, money is wasted and harm may ensue because high-technology diagnostic and treatment procedures are also relatively high-risk procedures. Moreover, the selection, recruitment, education, and training of physicians orient them toward the management of organ-specific pathology, whereas most health problems have multisystem (physical, emotional, and social) involvements and causes. Nursing practice is more oriented to multisystem assessment and planning techniques and relies more on interpersonal skills than on high technology. It is likely that some nurses, physician extenders, physicians' assistants, aides, and other technicians will become the new working group that will serve to carry out the physician's prescriptions in the high-technology system of medical care, whereas professional nurses, and those with public health training particularly, may develop an entirely new low-technology system of holistic primary care. Such a system is badly needed, and no other professional group is as well equipped to develop it. Public health agencies will find it difficult to aid in this development because it is likely to be resisted by other professional groups, especially physicians, but the change is necessary; and, looking through Chaska's mist, it can be seen.

REFERENCES

1. Department of Philanthropic Information, Central Hanover Bank and Trust Co.: The public health nurse, New York, 1938, reprinted by the National Organization for Public Health Nursing.
2. Birth of nursing at Bellevue, MD **17:**68, April 1973.
3. Waters, Y.: Visiting nursing in the United States, New York, 1909, Charities Publication Committee.
4. Bullough, B.: The law and the expanding nurse role, Am. J. Public Health **66:**249, March 1976.

5. A.N.A. Board approves a definition of practice, Am. J. Nurs. **55**:1454, 1955.

6. Jacox, A.K., and Norris, C.M., editors: Organizing for independent nursing practice, New York, 1977, Appleton-Century-Crofts.

7. Soares, C.A.: Nursing and medical diagnosis: a comparison of variant and essential features. In Chaska, N.L., editor: The nursing profession: views through the mist, New York, 1978, McGraw-Hill Book Co.

8. Standards of community health nursing practice, Kansas City, Mo., 1974, American Nurses' Association.

9. Hall, J.E., and Weaver, B.R., editors: Distributive nursing practice: a systems approach to community care, Philadelphia, 1977, J.B. Lippincott Co.

10. The need for nurses, New York, 1971, National League for Nursing.

11. Bureau of Health Professions: The registered nurse population: an overview, Bureau Rep. No. 82-5, Hyattsville, Md., 1982. U.S. Department of Health and Human Services.

12. First report to the Congress, Feb. 1, 1977: Nurse training act of 1975, U.S. Department of Health, Education, and Welfare, PHS Pub. No. (HRA) 78-38, Washington, D.C., 1978.

13. Congressional Budget Office: Nursing education and training: alternative federal approaches; budget tissue paper for fiscal year 1979, Washington, D.C., 1978, U.S. Government Printing Office.

14. Bureau of Health Professions: Public health personnel in the United States, 1980, U.S. Department of Health and Human Services Pub. No. (HRA) 82-6, Hyattsville, Md., 1982.

15. Elliott, J.E., and Kearns, J.M.: Analysis and planning for improved distribution of nursing personnel and services: final report, U.S. Department of Health, Education, and Welfare Pub. No. (HRA) 79-16, Washington, D.C., 1978.

16. The American Nurse **10**:7, July 15, 1978.

17. A directory of programs preparing registered nurses for expanded roles, 1978, Department of Social and Preventive Medicine, State University of New York at Buffalo, and the U.S. Department of Health, Education, and Welfare.

18. Archer, S.A., and Fleshman, R.P., editors: Community health nursing: patterns and practice, ed. 2, North Scituate, Mass., 1979, Duxbury Press.

19. Aiken, L.H.: The practice setting: an overview of health policy issues. In Aiken, L.H., editor: Health policy and nursing practice, New York, 1981, McGraw-Hill Book Co.

20. National Public Health Program Reporting System: Public health agencies, 1980, Washington, D.C., 1981, Association of State and Territorial Health Officials.

21. Serafini, P.: Nursing assessment in industry, Am. J. Public Health **66**:755, Aug. 1976.

22. Freeman, R.B., and Heinrich, J.: Community health nursing practice, Philadelphia, 1981, W.B. Saunders Co.

23. Knollmueller, R.N.: What happened to the public health nurse supervisor? Nurs. Outlook **27**(10):666, Oct. 1979.

24. Weed, L.: Medical records that guide and teach, N. Engl. J. Med. **278**:593, 652, 1968.

25. Woolley, F.R.: Problem oriented nursing, New York, 1974, Springer Publishing Co.

26. Department of Home Health Agencies and Community Health Services: Problem oriented systems of patient care, Papers presented at the 1973-1974 workshop series, National League for Nursing, New York, 1974, The League.

27. Flynn, B.C., and Ray, D.W., Quality assurance in community health nursing, Nurs. Outlook **27**(10):650, Oct. 1979.

28. Chaska, N.L., editor: The nursing profession: views through the mist, 1978, McGraw-Hill Book Co.

CHAPTER 31

Social work in public health

You see clearly that something more
than a microbe is needed to make us ill,
since we so often find the organism and
so rarely the disease.

Louis Pasteur

THE SOCIAL FACTOR IN HEALTH

It is a paradox that the great era of bacteriologic discovery actually resulted in delaying broad effective progress in public health. The discovery that highly specific living organisms are related to plague, anthrax, and many other disease conditions and that these clinical syndromes could not occur in the absence of their respective causative organisms brought about a great flush of enthusiasm and hope. An unfortunate result, however, was the development of an attitude by many that effective bacterial exposure was the alpha and omega of disease causation. Indeed, this had much to do with the broad acceptance and support of certain sanitary measures in the late nineteenth and early twentieth centuries, since it became recognized that bacteria could invade the town house and the palace through the servants' quarters and that *Corynebacterium diphtheriae* could strike the children of the wealthy and privileged as well as the children of the poor.

As long as etiology was still indeterminate or uncertain, men tended of necessity to cast about widely in their search for causal relationships. Once a scientific or, better yet, a laboratory answer was forthcoming, there was a tendency to close the issue with a Q.E.D.

In recent years, however, it has been increasingly realized that man is a combination of physical, psychologic, social, and cultural factors. If the recognition and acceptance of this is to be meaningful, practitioners of public health and medicine must cease to evaluate and treat man by the first of these factors alone. Sir Farquhar Buzzard,[1] regius pro-

fessor of medicine at Oxford, stressed that the aim of workers in public health should be:

to expose the sources and bases whence arise ill health and disability, by investigating the influence of social, genetic, environmental, and domestic factors on the incidence of human disease . . . [taking into consideration] . . . such varying agents as heredity, nutrition, climate, and occupation . . . [as well as] . . . the part played by the individual and mass psychology.

A similar conclusion was reached by Ryle,[2] who after 30 years as a student and teacher of clinical medicine accepted the chairmanship of the first Department of Social Medicine (Oxford, 1942). He observed that during those 30 years he saw disease studied ever more thoroughly and mechanically, but not more thoughtfully, as if through the high power of the microscope. He commented:

Man, as a person and a member of a family and of much larger social groups, with his health and sickness intimately bound up with the conditions of his life and work—in the home, the mine, the factory, the shop, at sea, or on the land—and with his economic opportunity, has been inadequately considered in this period by the clinical teacher and hospital research worker. [And may I add—by a large number of health workers!]

In his prefacing statement Ryle avers:

We no longer believe that medical truths are only or chiefly to be discovered under the microscope, by means of the test tube, and the animal experiment, or by clinical examination and increasingly elaborate pathological studies at the bedside. Psychological and sociological studies have as important a part to play. Even so, it is not yet appreciated how intimately disease and social circumstance are interrelated. The whole natural history of disease in human communities, as well as in individuals, is ripe for a fuller and more exhaustive study.

This comparative attitude was well put by Stern[3] in a discussion of living conditions and health:

In contrast with the narrower focus of public health work after the modern science of bacteriology had developed, the objective of the pioneers of public health included demands for better housing conditions, nutritious food, unpolluted water, cleaner streets and improved working conditions. These men anticipated the fundamental truth of modern preventive medicine, that the health of the individual is intimately and indivisibly tied up with the social as well as the physical environment in which he resides.

Leavell also had this in mind when he wrote:

Two major types of changes with which public health must deal are going on in the modern world: "public" changes and "health" changes. Our professional training helps us most with the health changes. . . . The public changes that are so important in public health work are in many respects more difficult for us to appreciate. Most of us have limited backgrounds in the basic social sciences—sociology, anthropology, psychology, economics, and political science—that might help us understand better the people with whom we must work. Yet public changes are often of even greater importance than health changes. . . . When we meet a health problem, we must recognize that two kinds of diagnosis and treatment are necessary. We must understand and deal with the health problem. We must also understand and treat the social or public part of the situation. Our pharmacopeia in both fields must be strong. It is no longer sufficient to prescribe drugs and neglect the social factors in a given case.

SOCIAL MEDICINE

As far back as 1847, Solomon Neumann in Berlin had propounded that "medical science is intrinsically and essentially a social science, and as long as this is not recognized in practice we shall not be able to enjoy its benefits and shall have to be satisfied with an empty shell and a sham." Only recently, however, have medicine and public health become widely recognized as applied social sciences. The enigma of the delay in acceptance of this relationship has been well analyzed by Rosen[5]:

In Great Britain, as in the United States, interest in the development of a concept of social medicine is a recent phenomenon. The social relations of health and disease had been recognized by physicians and laymen, but owing to a number of causes no concerted effort had been made to organize such knowledge on a coherent basis and thus

make it available for practical application. In part this was due to the dominant role that laboratory sciences and techniques had come to play in medicine, in part to the concurrent rise and expansion of medical specialism, and in part to the limited view of public health that had been current in both countries. Furthermore, the bias created by these factors was reinforced by powerful social ideologies still rooted in the nineteenth century version of natural law.

During the past few decades, however, influences within medicine itself and in society as a whole have acted to overcome these factors. The development of such branches of medicine as endocrinology, nutrition and psychiatry tended to break down the compartmental thinking of the physician, and to bring back into mental focus the sick person, the patient. Moreover, within society as a whole, the ideology of the complacent individualism was wearing thin, and the consciousness of social problems, including those involving health, became exceedingly acute.

The terms *social medicine* and *social pathology* have been used* but are much better known and understood in Europe than in America. There have been numerous attempts to define social medicine and social pathology. One of the earliest and still one of the best definitions is that of Grotjahn,[9] who listed the following principles necessary in the proper study of a disease:

1. The social significance of a disease is determined primarily by its frequency. This emphasizes the importance of accurate medical statistics.

2. The most common form of a disease, its sociopathologic prototype, is also of social significance—more so than its unusual or complicated rarer forms.

3. The etiology of every disease includes both biologic and social factors. The latter may affect a disease in several ways—they may be causative or predisposing, or they may influence the transmission or the course of illness.

4. The prevalence and outcome of disease may be influenced by attention to social and economic factors as they relate to the individual and to the group.

5. It is important to determine the influence of

*For historical review the reader is referred to *The Concept of Social Medicine as Presented by Physicians and Other Writers in Germany*, 1779-1932 by Kroeger,[6] *Social Pathology and the New Era in Medicine* by Ryle,[7] and *The Meaning of Social Medicine* by Galdston.[8]

successful treatment of a disease on the subsequent prevalence and on other social factors.

6. Diseases may themselves affect social conditions for the individual or for the group through recovery, predisposition to other illnesses, chronic infirmity, degeneration, or death.

The British journal *Lancet* attempted to clarify the issue editorially in 1947 by the following statement[10].

Social medicine is that branch of science which is concerned with: (a) biological needs, inter-actions, disabilities, and potentialities of human beings living in social aggregates; (b) numerical, structural and functional changes of human populations in their biological and medical aspects. . . . Social medicine takes within its province the study of all environmental agencies, living and non-living, relevant to health and efficiency, also fertility and population genetics, norms and ranges of variation with respect to individual differences and finally, investigation directed to the assessment of a regimen of positive health.

The importance of statistics of mass phenomena and relationships is again stressed by Wolff[11] in his definition of social pathology:

The relation between disease and social conditions is the content of social pathology; its method is necessarily a sociological description of this relationship which, for simplicity's sake is mostly based on a statistical analysis of the quantitative findings.

In the discussion so far, the terms *social medicine* and *social pathology* have been used almost interchangeably. Although similar and related, they are different. The following definitions are therefore suggested in an attempt to synthesize and simplify the several statements to which reference has been made and to indicate the relationship and the difference between the two terms:

1. *Social pathology* is a state of community imbalance evidenced by significant prevalence of disease and its related social disorders.

2. *Social medicine* is the study of the manner in which disease may result from, cause, or accentuate social problems and of the ways in which medical and public health efforts may contribute to their solution.

HEALTH AS A SOCIAL PHENOMENON

One of the most interesting aspects of the medical and public health movements has been the progressive use of sociologic methods to understand the etiology and epidemiology of disease. For a long time, disease was considered to be punishment for sins; thus it was regarded as an individual phenomenon rather than one that involved interpersonal or group relationships. As time passed, this interpretation became inadequate for explaining the spread of disease, and the concept of communicability developed. This led to a beginning awareness of social processes. Efforts were made to deal with the sanitary problems of towns, the practice of quarantine, the development of hospitals, and the provision of medical care. The era of microbiology stimulated great public interest in health problems; but, as has been mentioned because of its specific and unitary nature, it caused a delay in understanding the true importance of the social environment.

Increased urbanization, industrialization, and specialization forcefully revived an awareness of the significance of social factors in relation to disease. Health problems that developed in crowded industrial centers pointed clearly to the interrelationships of social problems and disease and to the necessity for instituting new approaches to disease prevention that involved social effort. Special attention was given to health problems of the poor and of the working class. Malnutrition was common, infant and maternal mortality high, tuberculosis and typhus rampant, housing pitiful, and other conditions of life generally unsatisfactory.

Toward the end of the nineteenth and into the twentieth century, various governmental and voluntary programs were established to provide needed community social services and to educate the public. Child welfare programs were expanded, school services for children were instituted, public health nursing was established, and other important health programs were developed. The study of social processes was recognized as fundamental in considering both physical and mental diseases, which were now attributed to multiple causes. In our present society this is especially pertinent because of the shift in importance from infectious to chronic illness. The high social and economic costs of these conditions have brought about greater concern for the welfare of patients and their families; the need for more and better facilities for medical, nursing, rehabilitative, and custodial care; and more effective health education of the public through organized social effort.

It is interesting to review the motivations during each period of societal health effort. Originally the

motivating force was essentially fear born of ignorance. This was followed by the provision of refuge
and care of bodily needs for the afflicted destitute
by ecclesiastic groups seeking salvation by good
deeds. From the eighteenth to the early twentieth
century, the gradually more extensive health and
social services were determined largely by a social elite motivated by noblesse oblige and enlightened self-interest. During the midtwentieth
century leadership passed to a professional elite on
the basis of the great scientific achievements of the
period. The supremacy of knowledge and technology provided the motivation.

This, however, has had its shortcomings as
Frankel[12] observed:

> The growth of technical problems and technical knowl-
> edge seems to have evicted the citizen . . . placed him in
> the hands of a new class of experts . . . who stand between
> him and his experience, . . . we have more knowledge
> than ever before, and so strangely enough, the open so-
> ciety seems to be less possible than ever. The effort to
> achieve it has led now only to the conviction that they do
> not and cannot understand the world in which they live.

This turn of events has led to an increased recognition of the social as well as the scientific complexities of health and illness and a strong move
toward a consideration of both. Spurred by the dis-
illusions and consequent activist movements of the
mid-1960s, based partly on a sense of little personal
control over one's destiny, there developed what
Levin[13] has referred to as the "era of de-profession-
alization," which challenged the established order,
including professional domination over health policies and programs. One result was "to place health
decisions into the larger context of competing
needs and interests," allowing individuals to determine their priorities and risk mix: "choosing to live
according to their interests and expectations rather
than according to the medical—public health mo-
rality of a totally disease-free world where 'keeping
healthy' is life's highest goal." Paradoxically, this
has provided impetus to the concept of health as a
human right and to concern about more effective
organization and management of the health care
field. Greater public or consumer participation in
policy determination as well as cost containment
and quality surveillance is now replacing the traditional unilateral elitist control. In the process,
public health is now very clearly recognized as an
applied social field.

Dana[14] has summarized the joining of the issue
of human rights to health and the shift from concern simply for the needs of the socioeconomically
disadvantaged to the broader question of meeting
the health needs of society as a whole. During the
1960s, she notes, there came about (1) a more exact
definition of the social costs of poverty and racism,
including health status discrepancies; (2) the documentation of the social inequities in health care,
in the education and employment of health personnel, and in the conduct of biomedical research
with reference to ethnic minorities and the poor;
(3) the disclosure of social deficits in the provision
of ambulatory care services; and (4) the exposure
of the system's indifference to sociocultural and
psychologic needs, especially of the disadvantaged.
She notes also the well-intentioned but unfulfilled
legislative promises and false starts during the decade, which nevertheless did institutionalize the
roles of government and of consumers in health
affairs. This led to the shift during the 1970s to
legislation aimed at benefitting the entire population: Medicare and Medicaid, Health Maintenance
Organizations, health-manpower development programs including the National Health Service Corps,
and measures to assure availability of and accountability for services for all. Although throughout the
issue has been health, the instruments have been
social.

THE FAMILY AS A SOCIAL FOCUS

Traditionally, social action to remedy the various
types of social problems has been substantively
fractionated. This was natural, since the recognition of each specific problem and the espousal for
public action usually were caused by the interests
and efforts of visionary individuals. Sometimes
these persons had had some personal or familial
experience with a particular problem. The result
was a parochialism of interest and action with separate reforms for health, housing, working conditions, welfare, prisons, or other specific social problems. Gradually a relationship among all these apparently discrete social problems was recognized.

Another very significant development was a re-
focusing of concern and attention from the individual alone to the family. Thus it is now accepted
that the individual cannot be considered apart from
the family or from the many forces in the physical
and social environment that may influence the family. Hence it is recognized as usually futile to attempt to treat an individual problem without taking

into consideration the family situation and all the forces that may affect it. This even applies to single individuals on the basis of their having come from a family, living in a family substitute, and subsequently entering or establishing a family or some type of partnership-living relationship. Richardson[15] emphasized this many years ago in his well-known book, *Patients Have Families:*

> The individual is a part of the family, in illness as well as in health . . . the idea of a disease as an entity which is limited to one person . . . fades into the background, and disease becomes an integral part of the continuous process of living. The family is the unit of illness, because it is the unit of living.

It is important to consider the multiple functions of the family. To begin with it provides the means of continuity and development of the human species. It accomplishes this by providing a socially supported group pattern for the sexual union of man and woman and a stable situation that encourages a quality of parental partnership essential to the care of the resulting offspring. It presents a setting for the proper emotional development of children and of their parents, for the guided evaluation of personal identities, for the development of normal and acceptable sexual patterns, for the establishment of social and ethical standards and the ability to accept social responsibility, and for the acquisition of knowledge and creative ability.

Children who grow up in a family setting acquire not only the general patterns of the culture of their particular society but also their parents' unique interpretation of it. Thus although children of the same generation of a society develop in a more or less similar manner, the children in each family are somewhat different from those in other families. Part of the role of the family therefore is not only to nurture a new generation that can thrive in a society but also to provide the great variety of personalities necessary for the biologic and cultural evolution of the society.

Many psychiatrists and sociologists have emphasized that one of the greatest values of the family is as a stabilizing force for the individual member, on the one hand, and for society, on the other. It accomplishes this by means of two apparently conflicting mechanisms. For purposes of long-term security the family tends to resist change. However,

in times of trouble or emergency it provides a psychic and social cushion, a means for sharing difficulty, and a basis for accommodation to change. Unfortunately, all family structures are not such as to ensure this. As Ackerman[16] has said, "In the meeting of new problems and crises, some families are weakened and others grow in solidity and emotional strength. Some families grow and learn from experience; others seem unable to do so because they are too inflexible and tend to disintegrate." This will be further discussed later.

A subject for particular concern is the tendency toward small, urban families. Bossard[17] stated this graphically: "The very size of the family unit is important to the child . . . for the same reason that the size of the ledge from which we view the precipice below affects our sense of security." In families with one or two children and no other relatives, the child has few people on whom he or she may depend, and a single or a few difficulties may spell disaster. This problem is greatly magnified in the single-parent household, the number of which is increasing. It has been observed by Freeman and her coworkers[18] for example that in a group of 400 urban black teenaged girls, those who lived in single-parent homes were three times more apt to become pregnant than those who lived with two parents. They also had sex more frequently and wanted a first child before their twentieth birthday.

A small number of people in the home tends to increase the frequency and intensity of emotional reactions because there are fewer people to absorb impacts and frictions. For the single parent, support tends to be concentrated in one wage earner, since there are few if any other people to contribute to the family needs. Household duties and responsibilities of the wage-earning homemaker are increased in a relative sense since such work must be done whether there is one or a number in the house, and in an absolute sense, since there are fewer people to share the work. Compounding this are the numerous extrafamilial distractions and demands on parents in the urban situation. When illness occurs in the small family, the burdens and risks are greatly increased. One result of ever-increasing consequence is an increased need and demand for homemaker services, day care centers, and personal care institutions. Thus it has been suggested that the growth and increasing use of hospitals is not merely a result of advances in medical knowledge and technology but is also a response to a shift in family structure, which incidentally is often linked to the occupational structure.

INTERRELATIONSHIP OF SOCIAL PROBLEMS

It is clear that neither we nor our problems exist in vacuums. By virtue of being a product of a family and a participant in a society, innumerable external factors, both good and evil, impinge on the individual. Some cause difficulty and problems, others provide support and solutions to problems. Thus it is now recognized that the state of personal or familial health or illness is the result of many interacting biologic, physical, and social factors. Any one of these may be primary and the others contributory. Furthermore, given a state of disease, these same factors are involved in the chances for and mechanism of recovery and rehabilitation. This has led increasingly to the consideration of disease in the individual as a social phenomenon involving several people and especially those immediately related to and around the patient.

This leads to an even more significant consideration—the interrelationships that may exist among a number of seemingly diverse types of social problems that may affect an individual, a family, and a society. An example is the case of a man suffering from pneumonia who is brought into a hospital. Physical and radiographic examinations may conclusively determine the clinical diagnosis. Sputum examination may clearly implicate *Diplococcus pneumoniae* as the causative organism. However, is it that simple? Several questions remain unanswered. It is known, for example, that many more people are exposed to this organism than become clinically ill. Why did this particular individual become ill with pneumonia? True, he could not develop this particular disease in the absence of the organism. Nevertheless, a valid question may still be raised as to what actually caused the illness. Investigation may elicit the following: The patient suffered from overexposure because the preceding night he slept on a park bench in the rain. He slept on a park bench because he did not know what he was doing. He did not know what he was doing because he was under the influence of alcohol. He indulged in an excess of alcohol because of discouragement and despondency over a bitter argument with his wife. She complained because her husband was unemployed and had no income. He may have been unemployed because of inadequate training, a disagreement with a superior, or some complex interplay of business eco-

nomics. Which of these factors caused his pneumonia? Obviously they all did.

Similarly, consider the case of an adolescent apprehended by the police as a juvenile delinquent. The immediate circumstance may have involved being caught while breaking into a store. Was the child intrinsically antisocial, and was the fault exclusively his? Investigation may show that he is only one of a group of similar adolescents who have formed an antisocial club or gang. It may be discovered that the group is sexually promiscuous, that venereal infections and abortions are common, and that alcoholism and narcotic addictions are present or incipient. In fact, the crystallizing storebreaking incident may have occurred to obtain money for alcohol or drugs. Why did this boy or, for that matter, any of the others belong to the gang and engage in such antisocial behavior? A parent may say "I just can't do anything with him." Inquiry, however, may bring out several other causative factors, most of them relating to the family and the social environment. Often the family bonds are discovered to be frayed or parted. The home may have only a single parent because of illegitimacy, divorce, separation, illness, or absence of one or both parents because of their employment. In such instances the gang is often a substitute family situation to provide a sense of security and belonging, a place in which to socialize and to exercise self-expression.

On the other hand, both the parents and the children may live together. However, the home, because of economic stringencies caused by ignorance, misfortune, or other reasons may consist of just a few crowded rooms of substandard quality with little or no privacy, ample opportunities for bickering and quarreling, and few facilities for cleanliness. Such a situation offers little incentive for the development of a sense of dignity, pride, or responsibility. The most intimate personal and sexual acts may be commonly observed, which encourages a cynical attitude toward them; there is little opportunity or reason to develop respect for the property of others even within the family; education, virtue, frugality, and social responsibility may be derided; dependence on public welfare and public assistance may be the cornerstone of the family finances; parental bouts of alcoholism and physical and verbal abuse may be so common as to

Public health and health care services

establish themselves as the standard of behavior. Under such circumstances one may properly ask: Why did this boy attempt to steal? Why was he sexually promiscuous? Why did he have gonorrhea? Why, perhaps, was he on his way to being an alcoholic or a drug addict? Why had he no respect or use for the concepts of family and society? Obviously none of the answers to these questions can stand alone; they are all interlinked. And they all devolve into the three fundamental questions: Where and how did it all begin? How can this chain be broken? How can similar complex situations be prevented from occurring in others?

One of the conclusions indicated by such cases

is that the primary diagnosis of a situation is not always in the same field as that under immediate or initial consideration. Social problems tend to exist together like different vegetables in stew, as it were, and occasionally a particular problem erupts on the surface, which, if regarded singly and momentarily, gives a limited and false impression. To appreciate the total situation, one has to stir the stew, sample it, and observe it over a period of time. In terms of such an analogy, it is important to realize that although each vegetable when dredged up and examined appears to be discrete, it flavors the rest and is meaningful only in relation to the total stew. If spoiled, it can affect all other parts of the stew.

Simmons and Wolff[19] have presented some of these interrelationships in tabular form. The es-

TABLE 31-1. Interrelationships of undesirable physical, social, and cultural factors

Undesirable sources or events	Consequences		
	Physical	Social	Cultural
Physical			
Disease or injury	Facial deformity	Inability to obtain employment	Misanthropy Condemnation of parenthood
Social			
Industrialization	Increased venereal disease	Free sexual relationships and promiscuity	Changes in attitudes toward marriage and family
Cultural			
Urbanization	More accidents and insanitation	Overcrowding Development of gangs Alcoholism	Breakdown of kinship and family bonds

TABLE 31-2. Interrelationships of desirable physical, social, and cultural factors

Desirable sources or events	Consequences		
	Physical	Social	Cultural
Physical			
Improved nutrition, public health, and medical care	Less illness and longer life	Greater productivity	Stronger family and social responsibility
Social			
Social security plans	Fewer complications	Less pauperization of sick and aged	Changed attitude toward aged
Cultural			
Improved education	Earlier diagnosis, prevention, and treatment	Demand for better public health and medical care	Rational understanding of sickness and health

sential point made by them is that physical, social, or cultural events or forces may constitute either or both sources and consequences of strength or weakness, good or evil. Thus a particular physical source, event, or force may have physical consequences, social consequences, or cultural consequences singly or in combination. This is similarly true of social and cultural sources, events, or forces. It is also important to recognize that the resulting consequences may in turn become sources of forces themselves.

With regard to the interrelationships among negative or undesirable sources, events, or forces and consequences, the following examples may be considered as *sources:*

1. *Physical:* Disease, congenital defect, or injury to the face
2. *Social:* Sudden industrialization with an influx of young adult workers
3. *Cultural:* Development of an urbanized living pattern

Each of these may have undesirable physical, social, and cultural *consequences* (Table 31-1).

In a similar manner sources, events, or forces may be of a positive nature and result in desirable consequences. To illustrate this the following *sources* may be used:

1. *Physical:* Improved nutrition, public health, and medical care
2. *Social:* Development of social security and medical care plans
3. *Cultural:* Provision of improved education

Each of these may have desirable physical, social, and cultural *consequences* (Table 31-2).

MULTIPROBLEM FAMILIES

People and families in difficulty tend to be concentrated geographically, especially in urban situations, and difficulties seldom occur singly. In recent years this phenomenon has been described in several ways, one of them by the use of the phrase, *disease-delinquency-dependency syndrome.* At any time in a society there are a certain number of individuals and, more significantly, families who get caught in a vortex of contributory social problems, each of which complicates the others, making it more and more difficult to escape. For some, the situation becomes so extreme and hopeless that there results an eventual condition that has been referred to as *cumulative degradation.*

Based on their many community social surveys, Voiland and Buell[20] have developed the following interesting classification of multiproblem or disordered families:

1. *The perfectionist family.* Their pathologic social functioning is manifested by overemphasis on perfection. Such self-imposed demands for good behavior allow no place for human error; as a result, marital relationships, child-rearing practices, and child development become fraught with anxieties and doubts that distort personal and family living. Prognosis is generally favorable if diagnosed and adjusted early.

2. *The inadequate family.* This is marked by constant dependence on others for encouragement, continued support, guidance, and help in solving problems in social living. They live "hoping for the best," and are incapable of coping with sacrifices or stress. Prognosis is relatively good, provided the situation is diagnosed accurately and agency caseworkers have the time, patience, and teaching ability to build a basis for rehabilitation.

3. *The egocentric family.* The members of this type of family are characterized by self-seeking motives in family interpersonal relationships and social conduct. Its pathology lies in an excess of self-interest and an overemphasis on social status or personal prestige. Prognosis is guarded. Often the husband and wife may consciously recognize the problem and their need for guidance but reject the prospect of receiving advice from "experts."

4. *The unsocial family.* Both partners lack social rapport with other people and with their social environment and have strong tendencies toward acting-out behavior, delinquent conduct, and/or regression into psychosis as a pattern of adjustment to problems or dislikes. They lack two essential qualities of good family functioning—a capacity for meaningful personal relationships and a normally functioning conscience to guide and stimulate social behavior. This affects marital relationships, parental roles, work habits, and total community relationships. Prognosis is poor. It is noted that from the community's standpoint such families comprise a substantial proportion of its public health and welfare agency loads.

Sometimes and possibly often the type of social pathology indicated in this fourth group passes on through generations. This has been found true, for example, of both child and spouse abuse (see Chapter 29). McCulloch and Philip[21] have described a remarkable example in their study of suicidal behavior. They present a dramatic pedigree of 12 members of a family who in three generations committed more than 35 suicidal attempts.

Another way of considering multiproblem families is on the basis of the degree of ability to respond affirmatively to assistance. One type of multiproblem family is self-sufficient under ordinary circumstances and goes along reasonably well until some catastrophe or crisis (medical, economic, or otherwise) sufficient in magnitude to throw the family off balance occurs. This crisis, if unsolved, eventually gives rise to problems in other areas. Unless some assistance is forthcoming, this type of family is in danger of irreparable damage and may become a permanent multiproblem family. If, on the other hand, significant assistance is rendered with regard to the original or to each of the several accumulated and related problems, this type of family is able to rehabilitate itself and assume and maintain its proper and desired role of self-sufficiency.

A second type of family is somewhat similar to the first. It has good intentions and wants to be self-sustaining but lacks good management and staying power. As a result, every once in a while it slips below the surface. If appropriately aided, it is able to climb back and operate on a relatively even keel until some new crisis occurs. Then it slips again and must be helped back again.

A third type of family is the most discouraging to deal with. Either because of overwhelming crises and catastrophies for which it has received no help, insufficient help, or, important to this discussion, unilateral help, or because the family unit lacks sufficient integrative strength, no extent or type of assistance seems to enable it to recover. The desire for recovery for a different way of life may be lacking, unacceptable, or incomprehensible. The roots of the difficulties of these so-called hard-core problem families go very deep. They are almost irretrievably caught in an exceedingly difficult situation that might be referred to as the *syndrome of the seven Ds:*

Disease
Deficiency (often both nutritional and mental)
Destitution
Dependency
Despondency
Delinquency
Degeneracy

Since it may have taken several generations to get to that point, it clearly takes concentrated and persistent effort to reverse the situation.

The same situation with regard to England is summarized by Williams[22] in the following terms:

After the Industrial Revolution with its child labor, cheap alcohol, poor wages, and bad landlords, there must have been a much higher proportion of our working-class families living under conditions far worse than anything we see today.

As social amenities become more readily available to the people so the great majority took advantage of the benefits and improved their conditions of life. . . . Yet one finds a small minority, either through a temperamental instability or a mental defect, who fail to keep pace with the advancing times.

Williams cites five surveys conducted by the Eugenic Society of Great Britain, which found an average incidence of such hard-core families to be 3 per 1,000 families. According to him, "a large number of these people are in early middle life, able-bodied and capable of regular manual work, who have difficulty in adjusting themselves to the recognized standards of life."

In the United States several significant investigations of this problem have been carried out. They too have clearly indicated the importance of the family as the basic unit of social significance, the simultaneous or successive occurrence of social problems, and the existence of a small hard core of multiproblem families.

Analysis of the reasons for multiproblem families is even more difficult than analysis of the problem. Almost all observers agree on one thing: family stability and cohesiveness are usually weak in such situations. Foster[23] has itemized four factors that make for family solidarity: (1) stability of location, with the development of an empathy with and a stake in the surroundings; (2) frequent contacts among the members of the family; (3) homogeneity resulting from common or shared experiences; and (4) an intangible dynamic element or life principle within the fabric of the family itself. Foster makes the important point that this appears first as an ideal or common purpose shared by the two people who marry and establish the family. He also expresses the opinion that all four of these basic factors have been subjected to weakening influences during recent years. The foregoing considerations provide cause to be concerned about future social instability and its effects on health.

As McNeil and Pesznecker[24] point out in their

study of the effects of life-change crises, a person's tolerance to change and the ability to cope with it vary among people. "Community workers," they feel, "are in a unique position to identify the persons who may suffer an illness following significant life changes. To reach people before illness strikes should be our focus in health education and in the prevention of illness and accidents in the community."

It has also been observed by many that a multiplicity of problems tends to occur among recent immigrants to nations and communities. In addition to the usual displacement adjustments, there are frequently other stresses resulting from racial, ethnic, and religious prejudices; language barriers; a different climate; as well as unaccustomed behaviorisms, food, and dress. Nonacceptance by the new and different society, especially of school age children of races or nationalities different from the local majority, can result in various anxiety states.[25,26] This is not surprising. Simmons and Wolff[19] have observed:

When peoples migrate, many elements of the new homeland's culture are rapidly adopted while large parts of the original culture survive in the family or small mobile group. Striking examples are found in first and second-generation immigrants . . . who because of contemporary patterns of prejudice may be barred from full participation . . . and become, in a sense, "marginal men" trapped between two cultures and subject to the conflicts arising from both.

Their statement continues in a sense that gives some hint regarding the development of multiple social problems in another group, those in the older ages subjected to the stresses of "the generation gap" and essentially ignored or abandoned physically and socially:

Furthermore, a person in the same physical surroundings . . . may continue to cling to attitudes, habits, and goals acquired in his youth, while the cultural norms are changing rapidly, with the result that he is not in harmony with the newly evolved patterns within his own society. He may be left as one stranded with his own personal and outmoded cultural values and attachments. The sweeping tides of cultural change frequently produce new areas of stress in personalities and not seldom leave their marks on the organism.

All human beings engage to varying extents in a search for status and goals. In recognition of this, Simmons and Wolff[19] have presented a graphic picture describing the genesis of a third type of individual who tends to become enmeshed in a triangle of multiproblem situations. Approaching the subject from the standpoint of medicine, they describe this person in the following manner:

Clinicians will often find, at the other type-extreme from the creature of culture, the socially deviant individual who also strives, although perhaps unconsciously, for "wayward" goals and who follows his own atypical and partly false clues in response to his life situation. His adaptations are out of harmony with socially approved behavior, as well as inappropriate on a physical basis. Under such circumstances social penalties are added to the physical injuries, and stress may be compounded in a kind of "vicious cycle," for the more the subject reacts the worse becomes his plight. Following his false clues, he simultaneously impairs his body and his social relationships, perhaps even alienating the very persons best qualified to help and support him and whose rejection leads to further deviation.

The last sentence of this statement might well be reread occasionally by persons engaged in social improvement, including those in the field of public health. Too often, it is feared, the spontaneous reaction to confusion and despondency in others is condemnation of them as intrinsically bad or worthless. A study of attitudes of chronic addictive drug users by McKee[27] illustrates this. He concluded that much of the approach, based on descriptions and warnings of the dangers and consequences of continued drug use, will not dissuade addicts from further drug use. The basic premise is wrong, he contends, in that many chronic drug users "have a drug-oriented self-definition, perceiving who and what they are as being intimately connected with drug use and drug effects." The typical evaluation of such individuals is that they are hopeless.

Another human reaction that should be borne in mind is the frequent use of illness as a response to social difficulty or dissatisfaction. Some individuals who cannot achieve satisfaction and fulfillment in positive or socially acceptable channels turn to negative, escapist, or antisocial channels. These may take the form of alcoholism, drugs, violence, sexual deviation, dependency, or crime. This is discussed in Chapters 25 to 29. For some individuals, still another solution is illness. Feigned or genuine sickness has the advantage of being the most socially acceptable and of eliciting the most sympathy and ready assistance among the various escape mechanisms. Furthermore, it provides other individuals and groups in society an opportunity for the achievement of their sense of fulfillment and self-satisfaction.

One other aspect of the subject should be mentioned. It is entirely possible that excessive zeal on the part of public health workers may sometimes give rise to social problems in families and may contribute to the establishment and continuation of a vicious social cycle. For example, the public health worker knows that tuberculosis is communicable and may insist on prompt hospitalization of an infected wife and mother. This may be the scientifically correct thing to do. It is best for the patient, for her family, and for society—best, that is, from the public health viewpoint. If however, at the same time that hospitalization of the wife and mother is arranged, the public health worker neglects to work intimately with the total family and with other sources of assistance in the community, especially social workers, good intentions may lead to considerable difficulty for the family, even to the point of its destruction.

Public health workers must recognize the hospitalization of a parent interferes with family structure and relationships. Removal of maternal care and guidance may result in decreased family cohesiveness and supervision, which may lead to delinquency on the part of the children. Prolonged absence of wifely companionship compounded by concern over increased expenditures for medical care and housekeeping may lead to alcoholism and philandery on the part of the husband. This in turn may lead to lowered income. Eventual dissolution of the family with firm establishment of a disease-delinquency-dependency syndrome is by no means an impossibility. If the woman's tuberculosis is successfully arrested or cured, the pleased staffs of the institution and health agency may discharge her to a grim future with an excellent chance of relapse. Worst of all, the undesirable set of circumstances that has been set in motion may well carry over into several future generations.

Therefore, at the risk of redundancy, it must be emphasized that public health workers should be most circumspect when considering any measure that may interfere with the social and economic integrity of the family. Public health workers should always ask themselves if a program or an action might in any way contribute to the disintegration of the family, even though it might aid the family

or society in other ways. Such situations call for careful consideration of all possible alternatives. In this, close working relationships with members of the social work profession can be of critical value.

RELATIONSHIP OF PUBLIC HEALTH AND SOCIAL WORK

To this point, attention has been focused on the health worker. Social work and social workers in turn merit consideration. Their perspectives also have been somewhat limited, with almost exclusive concentration on social casework approaches to the consequences of societal discrepancies on individuals and families. In this sense they are comparable to therapists who exclusively address ailments that have been allowed to develop in individuals. Granted, individually oriented remedial caseworkers are needed in both the health and the social work field; but this should not preclude professionals of both fields addressing the larger issues of prevention and long-term strengthening of the total society. In another vein, professional provincialism has in some instances tended to limit the potential of social workers in the health field. To whatever extent this is true, it is strange, since representatives of each field contributed notably to the early development of the other. Both Rosen,[28] a physician, and Brody,[29] a medical social worker, have emphasized that social work and public health evolved essentially from the same roots. Indeed, as described later, social work began in the health field. This is not surprising. The National Conference of Social Work in 1971 concluded that ill health, both community and individual, is the most important single factor in maladjustment, hence in social work. Similarly, illness and poverty are widely recognized as reinforcing social phenomena—each can be a cause or an effect of the other.[30]

Recognition of the relationship between health and social work is evidenced in the definition of social work adopted by the National Association of Social Workers in 1970:

Social work is the professional activity of helping individuals, groups, or communities enhance or restore their capacity for social functioning and creating societal conditions favorable to this goal. Social work practice consists of the professional application of social work values, principles, and techniques to one or more of the following ends: helping people obtain tangible services; counseling and psychotherapy with individuals, families, and groups; helping communities and groups provide or improve social and health services; and participating in relevant legislative processes. The practice of social work requires knowledge of human development and behavior; of social, economic, and cultural institutions; and of the interaction of all these factors.

An ever more intimate partnership of social work and public health should be fruitful. It would help health personnel to understand better the relationship of social processes to the etiology and epidemiology of disease and to develop more effective action to cope with the exigencies that arise. It has been indicated that all public health problems involve economics, education, cultural attitudes, and many other factors. In the normal conduct of their activities, public health workers must involve themselves to an increasing degree in the solution of these other aspects of the problems with which they deal. Public health nurses have been particularly active and successful in this regard. However, the recognition and adequate handling of such problems and the dealing with certain types of individuals and agencies often require special training and skills that the traditional health worker has only partially acquired in training and experience. Only relatively recently have public health agencies, especially official health departments, realized the great potential value of social workers to the public health program.

Public health and social workers should understand and relate to each other with relative ease and to mutual advantage, since both groups are concerned with overlapping aspects of the multifaceted problems of individuals and families. To be successful, both professions must be family and society oriented rather than merely individual oriented. Social casework, public health nursing, health education, and in fact public health activities in general attempt to assist individuals or groups in the understanding and solution of their problems. Far more could be accomplished if these professionals were trained to work as members of a team.

On the basis of experience in a housing project, Robinson[31] has suggested that critical attention be given to the effectiveness of intensive medical, nursing, and social work as a unit in obtaining maximum return on the development of scarce personnel, facilities, and especially in multiproblem communities. An extension of this has been described by Ebie[32] in relation to solving the sociomental problem of families in Edinburgh, Scotland, where the facility is actually a multidisciplinary social casework center with social workers backed by psychiatrists, psychologists, marriage counselors, and others as necessary.

Health legislation enacted during recent years in the United States has forced public health workers to take a much broader view than in the past, including a greater realization of the importance of social work in the achievement of health goals. Barnett[33] has stated the case clearly:

If health is perceived to include more than medical or biologic entities, and is a by-product of social systems, then social work is intimately related to public health. Family planning, alcoholism, suicide and drug addiction are public health and social problems. The major social problems of today—juvenile delinquency, racial discrimination and violence, poverty, crime, child neglect, marital incompatibility and divorce, deterioration of the inner city and expanding suburbia relate to health and to welfare. These are social and health problems. These situations are crucial. In planning it is recognized that health and social problems are interrelated and have interwoven etiologies. Thus far, social problem intervention has been carried out through one social system and health problem intervention through another. There has not been consensus on social-health issues, problems, and decisions either by the people in need, the professional service groups, or the decision makers.

DEVELOPMENT OF THE PROFESSION

Social work originated in England in 1895 as a means of relieving physicians and other hospital-based professionals of concern with the financial situation of patients. Subsequently, in 1905 Dr. Richard Cabot and Ida Cannon at the Massachusetts General Hospital introduced the concept of medical social work. Their philosophy was that beyond what the physician and hospital might do, the patient's understanding and cooperation were needed to overcome illness. They recognized that many other factors were involved in recovery, including family economy, living conditions in the home and neighborhood, social relationships, and the life. They recognized also that there were usually available in the community numerous resources that might be tapped for the best ultimate solution of all aspects of the case, provided the physician or someone had time to seek them out. In a very real sense, the social caseworker assumed the role of advocate for the patient. Social work and its involvement in health and medical programs has therefore progressed considerably as a profession since it was presented to hospitals as an economy measure to preclude giving free care to people who might be able to pay.

Social workers in the medical or hospital setting must now understand the significance of an illness or infirmity to a patient—the fear and loneliness it may cause and the adjustments needed and possible within the limitations of the patient and the ailment. Beyond this, as indicated by Wittman,[34] the emphasis is increasingly on prevention, and the social worker's role on the health team is to seek out potential sources of difficulties that lie within the personality of individuals or within family relationships and attempt to modify the situation favorably. This may involve working with a child in a family rather than directly with the disturbed mother, or with a wife rather than with her sick husband. In other words, the emphasis now is often as much on strengthening the supporting factors as on helping to treat the individual who is ill. Under such circumstances, as Rice[35] has indicated, the social worker is confronted with a difficult decision as to the most effective balance between the nature and extent of services to give to persons who already have problems and need immediate help as against those who are in situations or groups that may make them vulnerable to potentially harmful societal stresses. In the latter role the emphasis must be on analysis, anticipation, and neutralization or at least diversion of the undesirable social forces. This indicates the difference between social casework and social work. But as Hamilton[36] has warned:

Case work and collective action can be equally dangerous if viewed as the only method of social problem solving. One may isolate and the other overwhelm the individual. This is only to say that if the modern physician must be both clinically and public health minded, so the modern case worker must also be a social worker. The profession is not case work but social work.*

It is interesting to note that a Sociological Section was established in the American Public Health Association as early as 1910. At that time John M. Glenn,[37] director of the Russell Sage Foundation,

*Copyright 1977, National Association of Social Workers, Inc. Reprinted with permission from *Encyclopedia of Social Work,* 17th Edition, Washington, D.C.: NASW, Inc., p. 19.

pointed out that already "many social workers have recognized the value of the American Public Health Association and felt that acquaintance and close alliance with its members was essential to the success of their work."

Rosen[38] has described with regret the subsequent struggle of the Sociological Section to find a meaningful place and role in the organization. Despite active support and participation by several of the leading medical figures in the American Public Health Association, the section finally faded away by 1923. However, according to Rosen, considering the period, it was a product of unusually progressive thinking, whose day had not yet come. In the time since, many social workers have become active members of the professional public health society but have done so by joining a variety of specialized sections. Perhaps in terms of ultimate effect, this process of unintended infiltration of other disciplines has produced the greatest result. For several years a Conference of Social Workers in the American Public Health Association met in conjunction with the annual meeting of the association, leading to the establishment in 1971 of a Social Work Section.

Meanwhile, in 1918 the American Association of Hospital (later "Medical") Social Workers was organized. In 1958 it was incorporated into the new National Association of Social Workers as the Medical Social Work Section and later became the Medical and Health Section. The National Association of Social Workers also has a flourishing Mental Health Section. Overall, more than a third of the membership of the National Association of Social Workers are involved in some part of the health care system. It is hoped that health professionals other than social workers will increasingly participate in these organizations.

In 1973 there were an estimated 190,000 professional social workers in the United States. Only 29,500, however, were employed in health and related settings. About 75% worked in hospitals or convalescent institutions and only 29% in all other health programs or agencies.[39] Despite the emphasis on institutional practice, that field is far from covered. Of 6,614 hospitals that reported in 1974 to the American Hospital Association, 3,671 or 56% stated that they had social work departments. Even this represents a significant increase during the past decade, attributable in part to the emphasis by Medicare on greater use of extended care facilities for the elderly and chronically ill, which has necessitated social services in hospital discharge and placement planning. The employment distribution of social workers in the health field is probably transitional. Increasing emphasis is being placed on ambulatory care, prevention, and health maintenance. Phillips[40] has predicted that although the main administrative and specialized aspects of social services will remain in hospitals, comprehensive care, including direct social work services, will be carried on for the most part in community health centers.

By 1981 there were 299 undergraduate programs in social work in the United States accredited by the Council on Social Work Education. Four others were in candidacy status. Combined, they grant about 1,800 baccalaureates each year. A number of other educational institutions grant degrees that are not accredited. On the graduate level in 1981, 86 schools of social work were accredited to grant master's degrees, with 2 others working toward accreditation. Each year they graduate more than 8,800 students. Beyond this, 34 schools currently offer accredited post-master's programs and grant about 160 degrees annually.

ROLE OF THE SOCIAL WORKER IN PUBLIC HEALTH

The range of the social worker's activities in a health agency is necessarily determined by the size, scope, and changing purposes and priorities of the agency, the vision and understanding of its administration, and the availability of social work personnel. On the individual casework level, and especially with young families, Rice[35] has cited the usefulness of social workers in the following situations:

1. Experience of families in crises, such as the birth of a congenitally handicapped child, acquired handicapping conditions due to trauma or disease, the birth of a premature baby, a patient newly diagnosed as having tuberculosis or cancer, a death, or a miscarriage. These all are crises in families to which individuals will react intensely. Knowing this and working with them at the time of crisis, or preferably in advance of an anticipated crisis, will help to lessen the impact on the individual and family.

2. Early years of marriage and pregnancies at an early age.

3. Separation of the child from the family or separation of the parent from the child. Hospitalization of a parent often results in unfortunate experiences for the child.

4. Assumption of a new responsibility, such as becoming a spouse, a parent, or meeting the difficulties of widowhood.

5. Pressures on both mothers and children because mothers are working.

6. Siblings of sick, disabled, or handicapped children.

7. Supportive services to adolescents who are trying to make their adjustments to adult life.

8. Children who leave school early, to become often unemployed in the labor market, or marry young, or who frequently are added to the group of our juvenile delinquents in a community.

A basic question must be answered with respect to the role of social workers in a health department. What is the extent of direct service through personal contact with individuals in need of assistance, in contrast with working essentially through other members of the staff, especially the public health nursing staff? An ancillary factor here is the extent to which other members of the staff have been prepared to understand and accept the potential professional contribution of the social worker and are willing to accept this person as a specialized consultant. This highlights the importance of social work and health personnel sharing some of their educational experience. In most instances in which social workers have been brought into programs of local health departments, many individual and family contacts were initially anticipated and emphasized. Repeatedly, however, it has been found that the most fruitful use of the limited number of social workers is as staff consultants, fellow program planners, and as liaisons with the many other pertinent community agencies. Despite the limited number of social workers active in public health agencies, a substantial literature is developing to describe the many areas in which social workers are already contributing significantly. Among the many examples that could be mentioned are in child health, family planning, mental health, child or spouse abuse, alcoholism, drug abuse, suicide, chronic disease, geriatric and genetic programs, as well as in relation to health insurance plans and health maintenance clinics.

The increased need for and employment of social workers in public health programs led the Committee on Professional Education of the American Public Health Association in 1962, in collaboration with The National Association of Social Workers, to develop not only statements of qualifications for the several levels of social work in health agencies* but also the following statement of social work functions in health and medical programs.[41]

*Currently under review and reedition.

Public health and health care services

1. **Social work consultation services.** Consultation is a major responsibility of social workers in public health. It is often available on any aspect of the health department's program. More commonly it is related to the social problems of an individual or family, to problems met by other agencies, to social needs within the community, to coordination of the services of the health department with other community services, to agency administration, and to program and policy development within the department. Depending on the situation, the social worker may provide consultation service alone or as a member of an interprofessional team, as in evaluation of particular aspects of a community or institutional program.

2. **Program planning, implementation, and policy formulation.** Social workers in public health usually have responsibility for participating in program planning and policy development in the agency. On the basis of their professional equipment and the cumulative evidence from day-to-day activity, they are generally in a position to know how policies affect individuals or groups, or what standards and programs need to be strengthened, modified, or developed.

Social workers participate, with other personnel, in the development of joint projects; in the stimulation of activity on problems which fall within the jurisdiction of the health agency; and in the determination of program priorities. As a member of an interprofessional staff, social workers have the added responsibility of conferring with and advising health officers and program chiefs and su-

TABLE 31-3. Social components in health department programs: a guide developed by the social service

Analysis	Planning
Analyzing the social needs of people in the community and the resources available as they affect the total public health program	Planning programs with consideration of social factors in health department services and how people are affected by the ways in which the services are given
Program determination	
Who are the people mainly served by the health department? From what economic, national, and racial groups do they come? To what health problems do these factors contribute?	Determining through evaluation by health department personnel what problems, such as resistance to care, exist in tuberculosis, crippled children's services, and maternal and child health and determining whether solutions should be found within the health department and/or in cooperation with other agencies
Economic factors	
Where can families and individuals served by the health department turn in times of financial stress? What are the prevailing community attitudes toward giving and receiving help? What are legislative and administrative policies and how are they interpreted?	Ascertaining how interpretations of special needs in relation to health should be done if economic deprivation or transiency is a major community problem and stringent policies are in effect
Psychosocial aspects	
What facilities (casework services, foster homes, day care, vocational rehabilitation, psychiatric, housekeeping, etc.) are available and how adequately are these provided? Are there gaps or duplications?	Considering, over and above financial assistance, what services people want, what seem needed, and what cooperation and leadership the health department can give in using or developing services having a bearing on the maintenance of health
Community participation	
What are the working agreements and relationships between the health, social, and education agencies in the community?	Deciding with which agencies there is need to work on a continuing basis concerning referral procedures and cooperative services to people

Modified from Editorial: Social components in health department programs, Am. J. Pub. Health **45:**97, Jan. 1955.

pervisors in other professional areas on appropriate matters, or help in determining the most satisfactory solutions to social problems.

In most health agencies, administrative and supervisory responsibilities for the social work services are assigned to one person, who is often designated chief social worker, director of social work, or chief social work program consultant.

In some instances, primarily in mental health agencies, social workers carry out the major administrative responsibility for development of the total program of the agency.

3. **Social work services to individuals and families, social case work.** Social case work in public health involves social study and evaluation leading to services for individuals or families who are having difficulty in social functioning, primarily as it affects their health and their ability to use health services. The problems may be those "which impinge upon the family unit or individual from the social or physical environment" or those "which the individual brings into being, in whole or in part, by modes of behavior and interaction between himself and other persons and situations." Individuals or families needing social case work may be brought to the attention of the social case worker by the members of the health team, by other agencies, by the individual or family, or they may belong to a group already identified, needing social case work on the basis of diagnosis or the type of situation. Persons within selected categories may be routinely referred for the purpose of identifying social factors

staff, California State Department of Public Health

Operations	Research
Maintaining a public health program that recognizes and deals directly or indirectly with concomitant social problems	Investigating through research psychosocial and economic factors related to the maintenance or breakdown of health and to the use of health facilities by such projects as:
Carrying out policies and procedures in health department programs that consider basic needs of children and adults as well as individual and group differences, including staff and community education around these concepts	Studying the use of health department facilities by various groups such as migrant, national, and ethnic
Referring patients to agencies for financial assistance and having a continuing relationship with these agencies, bringing regularly to their attention case situations where restrictions aggravate public health problems, and encouraging appropriate referrals from these agencies	Studying the incidence of a specific disease in relation to socioeconomic status
Helping individuals and groups served by the health department to use existing services, within or outside the health department, which best meet their health, social, and emotional problems	Studying normal and premature births in relation to marital stability, planned or unplanned pregnancy, fear of childbirth, reasons for delayed or no prenatal care, etc.
Bringing to the attention of the community the need for modification and extension services and programs and reaching an understanding with agencies as to types of referrals and exchange of information that will be mutually helpful	Studying cases to determine if there is a need for a proposed resource or if existing facilities are meeting current needs

which affect the individual's health problems or his use of needed health and medical services. The social worker initiates case work services in instances where resolution of social and emotional problems helps to prevent problems or facilitates care. Collaboration with other professional staff is an essential part of the case work process.

Social case work service may be provided temporarily for the purposes of demonstration, in order to develop methods of effective referrals to appropriate agencies, or to facilitate more comprehensive study and treatment by the health agency.

Opportunity for direct case work services is most often provided in local agencies, less frequently in state programs, and least often in programs at the national level.

4. **Social work services to groups.** Increased use of the group process in resolving social problems is a definite trend in social work in public health. The social worker in public health may act as leader of groups of patients or family members, or as a consultant or resource person to groups or to their leaders. This group process may be used by social workers with patients in a single diagnostic category, with relatives of patients who have the same health problem, or with other groups where there is a health need.

Social group workers, especially trained in social work methods, have been used more frequently in hospitals and mental health programs than in other public health programs, although the opportunities in all are apparent.

5. **Social work services to the community.** All members of the public health team contribute to the provision of community services. In public health, the social worker places a major emphasis on the activity, in which he applies his social work knowledge of individuals, groups, and communities and of community process, his understanding of social welfare as a social institution, and his knowledge of social work organization to the task of community planning.

The social worker in public health is in a strategic position to identify, evaluate, and document social problems relating to health needs, to discover ways of preventing them, and to plan new services or to strengthen those already in existence. He serves also as an interpreter of social resources to other team members and of health services to social agencies. He thus assists in improving collaboration and in coordination of programs for health and social welfare, and in modifying or developing services to meet new needs.

Social workers especially trained in the social work method of community organization have been used more often in voluntary health programs than in public health departments.

6. **Research, studies, and surveys.** Research is carried on by social workers, both independently and in collaboration with other professions in public health, mental health, and medical care programs.

7. **Educational responsibilities.** The social worker is responsible for the supervision of social work students assigned to the agency for field instruction. He also participates in the preparation of students from other professions with respect to promoting an understanding of the social and health needs of individuals, groups, and communities, and ways of preventing and meeting these needs. He contributes to and benefits from the educational program of the health agency by participation in programs of staff education within the agency and in the community.

In an effort to reemphasize for all public health personnel the relationship between psychosocial factors and public health practices, the social service staff of the California Department of Public Health organized the various social work roles into a functional guide.[42] This guide (Table 31-3) stresses the integration of social work and public health through the use of social work knowledge and techniques in preventive and administrative public health programs on the state and local levels. Since health agencies vary, as do social problems and available resources, the guide was made brief, broad, and general. Although developed some years ago, it merits presentation as a useful administrative and supervisory tool in program planning and development, in evaluation of current activities, and in staff education. It is probably most productive when a social worker participates in its use.

As evidence of the intent and ability of social work to contribute significantly in efforts to combat the multifaceted problems of ill health, Corwin[43] has stated that "any referral may be in the form of a request for consultation or for direct service. Subsequently a decision can be reached with the other staff members as to future management. In addition, some conditions are so fraught with social implications that, by their very nature, some type of social work intervention to alleviate distress, limit disability, and assist in rehabilitation seems indicated." Phillips[40] has expressed somewhat the same broad view in looking ahead, concluding that "social work, along with the other health professions, faces the challenge of being innovative in offering service within today's complex health system to a population of unprecedented magnitude while at the same time maintaining its values and knowledge base."

THE SEARCH FOR SOLUTIONS

It appears that two things are important in solving these complex problems: first, application of the principles and methods of epidemiology to chronic diseases, disabilities, dependency, and maladjustment; second, cooperative planning and action by representatives of the various human services professions and organizations: specialists in health, family services, mental hygiene, social casework, and other related fields. What is called for is a synthesis of philosophy, interest, resources, and effort to be applied to total social problems of the community through its families. Certain specific suggestions may be made. Health departments and health centers could provide space for liaison personnel from certain other public and private agencies and in turn could assign public health personnel to other agencies for the same purpose. Multidisciplinary and multiagency committees or councils for *case* planning and review should be established, as well as committees concerned with *program* planning and review. Some of the community agencies and services that might be included or at least consulted are health, welfare, public assistance, hospitals, police, courts, fire protection, voluntary health agencies, and the social service agencies. Beyond this, it is advantageous to include in the program and service planning process representatives of those who are to be served and who know their problems only too well. Reporting and filing systems should be on a family rather than an individual basis whenever possible.

A valuable source of help is a Social Service Referral Center to which representatives of member agencies (and sometimes others) may refer cases for specific investigations or services. A common difficulty is that individuals and families sometimes get lost in the referral system. Sometimes they are never referred back to the initiating agency for follow-up or for resumption and completion of care that may have been instituted but were interrupted to provide time or opportunity for solution of a secondary or contributory problem. An unfortunate practice occasionally indulged in consciously or subconsciously is to avoid referral of cases for needed auxiliary services because of a sense of proprietorship over the case and a fear that it might be lost, reflecting poorly on the agency when it is time to publish an annual report or to engage in a fundraising activity based on case load. Obviously such an attitude, however rare, is totally unwarranted and inexcusable if it detracts in any way from the earliest possible and most satisfactory solution of a family's problems.

Since social problems, including health problems, are so often family problems and since most multiproblem situations have their roots in the early period of married life, health and other social agencies should make greater use of marriage reports as a means of contact with certain individuals and groups before difficulties have an opportunity to occur. Undoubtedly some relatively limited assistance in the establishment of a household, alerting a newly married couple as to sources of assistance and counseling, would prevent the unimpeded progression of numerous problem situations. From an overall community standpoint, concentration of multiproblem families in one area, whether the problems are incipient or fully developed, should be avoided. Segregated or concentrated, they tend to accentuate or exacerbate each other's problems. Separated, they have more opportunity and incentive to learn and improve by contact with more stable families.

A statement by Koos[44] summarizes very well the concepts that have been presented here:

Community organization for health is in no sense an activity divorced from other forms of activity for community welfare . . . all community organization is interwoven in a common effort. Health, says modern research, is not to be found apart from a general welfare of the individual and the community. It consists not only of an absence of disease but also of a sense of general well-being, of adjustment to all of the forces that make up the intricacies of the society in which we live.

REFERENCES

1. Buzzard, F.: The place of social medicine in the organization of health services, Br. Med. J. **1**:703, June 6, 1942.
2. Ryle, J.A.: Changing disciplines, London, 1948, Oxford University Press.
3. Stern, B.J.: The health of towns and the early public health movement, Ciba Symposium **9**:871, May-June 1948.
4. Leavell, H.R.: New occasions teach new duties, Public Health Rep. **68**:687, July 1953.
5. Rosen, G.: Approaches to a concept of social medicine, Milbank Mem. Fund Q. **26**:7, Jan. 1948.
6. Kroeger, G.: The concept of social medicine as presented by physicians and other writers in Germany, 1779-1932, Chicago, 1937, Julius Rosenwald Fund.
7. Ryle, J.A.: Social pathology and the new era in medicine, Bull. N.Y. Acad. Med. **23**:312, June 1947.
8. Galdston, I.: The meaning of social medicine, Cambridge, 1954, Harvard University Press.
9. Grotjahn, A.: Soziale pathologie, Berlin, 1915, August Hirschwald Verlag.

10. Editorial: Social medicine, Lancet **1:**458, April 5, 1947.
11. Wolff, G.: Social pathology as a medical science, Am. J. Public Health **42:**1576, Dec. 1952.
12. Frankel, C.: The democratic process, New York, 1962, Harper & Row, Publishers, Inc.
13. Levin, L.: The layperson as the primary health care practitioner, Public Health Rep. **91:**206, May-June 1976.
14. Dana, B.: Health care: social components. In Encyclopedia of social work, ed. 17, Washington, D.C., 1977, National Association of Social Workers, Inc., p. 546.
15. Richardson, H.B.: Patients have families, New York, 1945, Commonwealth Fund.
16. Ackerman, N.W.: Psychological dynamics of the family organism, Public Health Rep. **71:**1017, Oct. 1956.
17. Bossard, J.H.S.: The sociology of child development, New York, 1954, Harper & Row, Publishers, Inc.
18. Freeman, E.W., and others: Never-pregnant adolescents and family planning programs: contraception, continuation, and pregnancy risk, Am. J. Public Health **72:**815, Aug. 1982.
19. Simmons, L.W., and Wolff, H.G.: Social science in medicine, New York, 1954, Russell Sage Foundation.
20. Voiland, A.L., and Buell, B.: A classification of disordered family types, Soc. Work **6:**3, Oct. 1961.
21. McCulloch, J.W., and Philip, A.E.: Suicidal behavior, Oxford, England, 1972, Pergamon Press, Ltd.
22. Williams, H.C.M.: Rehabilitation of problem families, Am. J. Public Health **45:**990, Aug. 1955.
23. Foster, R.G.: Effect of mobility on the family, Am. J. Public Health **46:**812, July 1956.
24. McNeil, J., and Pesznecker, B.L.: Keeping people well despite life-change crises, Public Health Rep. **92:**343, July-Aug. 1977
25. Dinnerstein, L., and Reimers, D.M.: Ethnic Americans, New York, 1975, Harper & Row, Publishers, Inc.
26. Hashmi, F.: Immigrants and emotional stress, Proc. R. Soc. Med. **63:**631, June 1970.
27. McKee, M.R.: Drug abuse knowledge and attitudes in "Middle America," Am. J. Public Health **65:**584, June 1975.
28. Rosen, G.: Social and health problems are inseparable, (editorial), Am. J. Public Health **61:**2311, Nov. 1971.
29. Brody, S.: Common ground: social work and health care, Health and Social Work **1:**16, Feb. 1976.
30. Piore, N.: Health as a social problem. In Encyclopedia of social work, ed. 17, Washington, D.C., 1977, National Association of Social Workers, Inc., p. 534.
31. Robinson, D.: Effectiveness of medical and social supervision in a multiproblem population, Am. J. Public Health **58:**252, Feb. 1968.
32. Ebie, J.C.: A multidisciplinary social casework center with a staff psychiatrist, HSMHA Health Rep. **86:**863, Oct. 1971.
33. Barnett, E.M.: Social work training needs. Background paper prepared for Third National Conference on Public Health Training, Washington, D.C., Aug. 1967, U.S. Department of Health, Education, and Welfare.
34. Wittman, M.: Preventive social work—a goal for practice and education, Social Work **6:**19, Jan. 1961.
35. Rice, E.P.: Concepts of prevention as applied to the practice of social work, Am. J. Public Health **52:**266, Feb. 1962.
36. Hamilton, G.: Development of the case work idea. In Encyclopedia of social work, ed. 17, Washington, D.C., 1977, National Association of Social Workers, Inc., p. 19.
37. Glenn, J.M.: Sociological section; report of the section committee, Am. J. Public Health **3:**645, Nov. 1913.
38. Rosen, G.: The sociological section of the American Public Health Association, 1910-1922, Am. J. Public Health **61:**2515, Dec. 1971.
39. U.S. Department of Health, Education, and Welfare: Health resources statistics, DHEW Pub. No. (HSM) 73-1509, Rockville, Md., 1974.
40. Phillips, B.: Social workers in health services. In Encyclopedia of social work, ed. 17, Washington, D.C., 1977, National Association of Social Workers, Inc., p. 624.
41. Educational qualifications of social workers in public health programs, Am. J. Public Health **52:**317, Feb. 1962.
42. Editorial: Social components in health department programs, Am. J. Public Health **45:**97, Jan. 1955.
43. Corwin, R.: Some new dimensions of social work practice in a health setting, Am. J. Public Health **60:**860, May 1970.
44. Koos, E.L.: New concepts in community organization for health, Am. J. Public Health **43:**466, April 1953.

CHAPTER 32

Dental public health

There was never yet philosopher that could endure the toothache patiently.

Much Ado About Nothing, v. 1

MAGNITUDE OF THE PROBLEM

Studies of the prevalence of dental disease during recent decades have placed problems of dental health in a position of major importance with regard to national health needs. Fortunately the same interval has seen the dramatic development of the field of preventive and public health dentistry—something which at the beginning of that period could not have been forecast. To put what has occurred into perspective, in 1938 two of the major contributors[1] to the progress that has since been made stated:

Inasmuch as the etiology of dental caries is unknown, prevention of the disease causing these defects is still in the experimental stage. It is generally acknowledged, however, that the treatment of early carious lesions by the proper placement of chemically and physically stable filling materials will largely prevent carious teeth from terminating in tooth loss, or tooth mortality. A primary purpose of dental health programs becomes, therefore, the promulgation of procedures whereby the early detection and treatment of carious teeth is accomplished, and tooth mortality thereby prevented.

Fortunately it became possible for one of those same contributors to state before the American Public Health Association in 1953, "I look back over the past ten years and conclude that more has been accomplished during the decade than during the previous fifty years."[2] By the 1980s it is appropriate to label dental caries as a preventable disease. In fact, in one experimental program in Sweden, the incidence of dental caries in children has been reduced almost to zero.[3]

Three factors in particular contributed to the tremendous change that occurred during this period. First was the generally progressive attitude of the dental profession in the United States. This was exemplified by its many inquiries into ways of preventing dental ailments and methods of providing dental care of good quality to large numbers of people. Second was the tremendous impact that resulted from the drafting of a fourth of American dentists during World War II and particularly the shocking results of the physical examinations of inductees. One of the most startling findings was that, of the first 2 million men examined for service in the armed forces, more were rejected because of dental defects than for any other physical reason. The third contributing factor in the progress of recent years is to be found in the brilliant research by various investigators and particularly by dental officers of the Public Health Service, the Eastman and Forsyth Dental Institutes, several of the schools of dentistry, and some community dental health programs. These inquiries into the incidence and prevalence of dental disease, dental physiology and pathology, the relationship of various dietary factors (particularly sugars), and the studies of the relationship of fluorides to mottled enamel and the prevention of caries are considered epidemiologic classics.[4,5]

To appreciate the magnitude of the problem that confronts public health, one must consider the incidence and prevalence of dental disease. The National Center for Health Statistics[6] surveyed the United States Population in 1971 to 1974 and found that:

- Twenty percent of children aged 1 to 5 had at least one untreated, decayed primary tooth.
- This increased to 31% of children aged 6 to 11 with at least one untreated, decayed permanent tooth, 54% of youths aged 12 to 17, and 47% of adults aged 18 to 74.

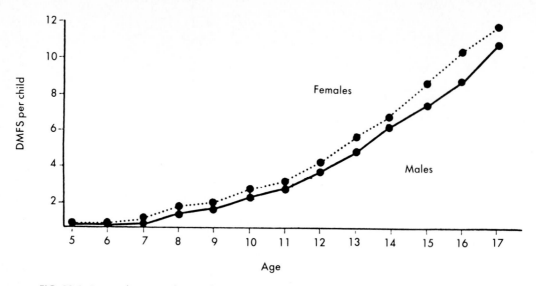

FIG. 32-1. Age- and sex-specific prevalence of dental caries in permanent teeth for United States, 1979-1980. (From National Caries Program, National Institute of Dental Research: The prevalence of dental caries in United States children, 1979-80, NIH Pub. No. 82-2245, Dec. 1981, U.S. Department of Health and Human Services.)

• Children between the ages of 12 and 17 averaged 6.2 decayed, missing, and filled teeth (DMFT) per person (1.8 were untreated, decayed teeth) and adults aged 18 to 74 averaged 16.9 DMFT.

A 1979 to 1980 survey of children aged 5 to 17 indicated a substantial improvement had occurred[7]: from 7.06 decayed, missing or filled surfaces (DMFS) to 4.77, a reduction of nearly 33% (although the study designs were not strictly comparable). The survey showed an increase in the prevalence of caries with age and a slightly higher rate among girls than boys (Fig. 32-1). Nearly 37% of children aged 5 to 17 had no caries at all, but 7.7% of the children had nine or more DMFT (Fig. 32-2). Adults were not studied in the 1979 to 1980 survey, but, based on the improvement in adult disease between a 1960 to 1962 survey and the 1971 to 1974 survey mentioned, it seems likely that dental health among adults has also improved.

Periodontal disease, which affects the gums and the supporting tissue surrounding the teeth, affects at least 15% of adults aged 18 to 44, 36% of those aged 45 to 64, and half of all adults aged 65 to 74.[8]

Although the prevalence of dental disease is de-creasing, it remains one of the most common health problems, resulting in pain, disfigurement, and considerable expense. Freeland and Schendler estimated the 1981 dental bill at $18 billion, of which $12.7 billion was paid as an "out-of-pocket" expense.[9]

The terms used in measuring dental disease can be confusing. For children and persons up to about age 35, the DMF count is a reliable indicator of the prevalence of dental caries. It is a count of decayed, missing, and/or filled teeth (DMFT) or surfaces (DMFS). The DMFS count is always higher than the DMFT count because there may be more than one decayed or filled surface on the same tooth. In the 1979 to 1980 survey, the 5- to 17-year-olds averaged 4.77 DMFS and had an average DMFT count of 2.91. In reviewing the dental health problem in any community, it is important to ascertain exactly what is being counted. By the age of 35, periodontal disease begins to be more important as a cause of tooth loss, and the DMF index is less useful. The National Center for Health Statistics used a periodontal index (PI) to develop its estimate of the prevalence of periodontal disease. The PI appears to have the virtue of consistency and reli-

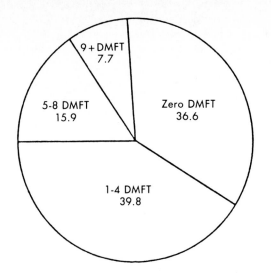

FIG. 32-2. Percent distribution of United States children according to DMFT status, 1979-1980. (From National Caries Program, National Institute of Dental Research: The prevalence of dental caries in United States children, 1979-80, NIH Pub. No. 82-2245, Dec. 1981, U.S. Department of Health and Human Services.)

ability, but it does provide a much lower estimate of the prevalence of periodontal disease than other studies.

FACTORS INVOLVED IN DENTAL DISEASE

Before considering public health dental programs, some of the factors involved in the development of dental disease should be reviewed. Dental caries constitute by far the major proportion of the total dental problem.

It is a disease of the calcified tissue of the teeth that begins with a softening of the enamel caused by acid. Once the enamel surface is penetrated, decay begins in the softer subenamel tissue, spreading out beneath the enamel surface. If unchecked, it can spread to the pulp in the center of the tooth and, from there, down into the root and out into the supporting tissue, causing abscess formation.

The development of caries is caused by host factors, the presence of microorganisms, the existence of a substrate (sugars), and the time during which the factors are allowed to interact. Host factors include the composition of the saliva, the configuration of the teeth (fissures and crevices accumulate debris), the nutritionally based composition of the tooth, including the availability of the fluoride

ion, and probably some as yet undefined genetic factors. Microorganisms prevalent in the mouth work on food, primarily simple sugars such as sucrose, to produce acid, which begins the softening process within hours after eating.

Most diets in the United States have sufficient calcium and vitamins to support normal tooth growth, but fluoride supplements are often needed. It is common practice to worry about dental health during pregancy, but pregnancy appears to have little or no effect on the mother's teeth: calcium is not withdrawn to support fetal growth.

Attention has been given to the possibility of inherited susceptibility or immunity to dental caries. This has been approached by (1) animal breeding studies, (2) human family studies, and (3) twin studies. By selective breeding, caries-resistant and caries-susceptible strains of hamsters and rats have been developed. Family studies in the United States and Sweden indicate fewer caries in the children of caries-free parents. Twin studies show less intrapair difference in the incidence of caries than among children selected at random. Many investigators have reported the existence of families that appear to experience few or no caries. Despite these various studies, the general belief is that inherited or acquired susceptibility or immunity to dental caries, if a reality, plays a minor role in the total caries picture.

Racial differences exist, with white children having more caries (4.89 DMFS per child) than children of other races (4.15 DMFS per child), but these differences have to be interpreted with caution. The DMF count consists of three actions: decayed, missing, and filled teeth or tooth surfaces. Access to dental care is income related, and white children have more filled surfaces and fewer decayed surfaces than black children. Since there is a tendency in dental treatment, as there is in medical treatment, to find and repair pathology if at all possible, access to dental care results in an increase in the number of filled surfaces.

As a result of highly successful commercial marketing, it is widely accepted that various oral hygienic practices and products will reduce the probability of development of dental caries. Included is the use of the toothbrush, dentifrices, dental floss, miscellaneous mouthwashes, lozenges, medicated chewing gum, and professional dental prophylaxis.

Whereas these agents and procedures may be worthwhile from the standpoint of general oral hygiene and cosmetic effect, no evidence exists to indicate that their use bears a relationship to the suppression of caries. Although toothpastes do not appear to reduce the incidence of caries, the fluoride now contained in most products does have a beneficial effect. However, it should be noted that this disappointing finding is related only to caries formation. As will be shown later, brushing and flossing regularly have a significant effect on the later development of periodontal disease and therefore remain a valid part of the health education effort in the home and in the school.

Sealants have also proven effective in reducing caries. Like topical applications of fluorides, sealants are temporary but may last for many years. They require individual application treatments and careful technique, particularly to "etch" the surface of the tooth to enable better bonding of the sealant. Sealants work well in fissures and crevices, whereas topical fluorides work better on flat surfaces, making the two techniques additive in value.

Systemic and topical fluorides and sealants will not eradicate caries. Although they are more efficacious and efficient than dental care in the office, regular check-ups are still beneficial. As previously mentioned, one Swedish study has shown that professional prophylaxis, topical fluorides, continuing oral hygiene education, and water fluoridation can reduce the prevalence of caries to virtually zero.[3] Given the heterogeniety of the United States, that is an unlikely outcome for many years to come but is certainly a reasonable goal.

Of particular interest is the finding that even professional dental prophylaxis cannot remove all bacterial plaques from the surfaces of the teeth, and that even when they are removed they tend to reform in a matter of days.[8,10] Plaque does play a significant predisposing role in the development of both caries and periodontal disease. Plaque is a soft, adherent, mucinous substance composed of bacteria, epithelial cell, leukocytes, and debris. Acid-producing bacteria in the plaque erode the tooth substance, causing caries, whereas calcified salts at the gingival line may irritate the soft tissues, causing gingivitis, which may result in periodontal disease.

Considerable research has been carried on to determine the relationship between various microorganisms and the development of dental caries. Most attention has been given to the streptococci (*Streptococcus mutans*). This research has brought investigators much closer to the goal of understanding the mechanism of dental caries development and of devising practical preventive measures. It is clear that streptococci present in the mouth are an essential part of the etiology of caries. Efforts to either reduce the bacteria count or to increase host resistance to the bacteria appear promising. Some researchers have concentrated on the development of a vaccine against the strain of bacteria involved while others have attempted to increase the presence of antibodies to the streptococci in the saliva. There is optimism that this research will prove successful during the 1980s, but it may result in a reexamination of some of the ecologic issues involved in artificially increasing the antibody-forming efforts of the host. As in any consideration of a vaccine, the total costs and benefits will need to be considered before adopting the practice as a general prevention technique. Other research has focused on different types of carbohydrates and carriers of free sugars. For example, those fed free sugars in the form of toffee develop significantly more caries than those fed chocolate, which is less adherent and is swallowed more quickly.

Given a susceptible surface, the ubiquitous presence of streptococci, and the ingestion of a suitable substrate in the form of such simple carbohydrates as sugar, it does not take much time for the mixture to result in acid formation and enamel softening. The brevity of time makes toothbrushing less effective as a caries prevention practice than might be anticipated. It appears more practical to concentrate on host factors, techniques to reduce the prevalence of the bacteria, and educational efforts to modify diet. Efforts to modify diet are treated with some skepticism by dental health experts, but eating habits are changing in the United States, and a longer view of the problem suggests that a strong and persistent attempt to improve nutrition will have significant benefits in reducing caries in the next generation of children as well as in reducing the prevalence of periodontal disease in the present generation.

Next to caries, periodontal disease is the most common dental health problem and the most frequent cause of tooth loss in adults. Plaque and calculus formation are strongly related to periodontal disease. It involves gingivitis (inflammation of the gingiva, or the soft, fleshy tissue surrounding the teeth) and periodontitis, which occurs when the inflammation attacks the subsurface supporting structures, including the alveolar bone. Pockets of food and other debris may be lodged beneath the gum line. Calculus formation separates the gum from the teeth, allowing this to happen. These pockets are always infected, and the slow process of decay attacks not only the root of the tooth but the supporting tissues as well. Gingivitis is common even in children. Thirty-two percent of adolescents aged 12 to 17 have some gingivitis and approximately 1.3% have periodontitis.[8]

Plaque and calculus formation are important to the development of periodontal disease and are best controlled by individual effort. Brushing and flossing, of little importance to caries prevention, are very important in the prevention of periodontal disease, as is the regular use of professional dental care to remove calculus (which is not amenable to brushing once it has formed) and to restore carious lesions.

FLUORIDATION

Although only one aspect of the prevention of dental disease, fluoridation has had such a dramatic impact on public health practice, from health education and sanitary engineering to ethics and marketing, that it merits special emphasis.

Teeth blackened by minerals or, more correctly, hypoplastic teeth, which in areas of high fluoride concentration develop posteruptively a characteristic brown stain, were first described two thirds of a century ago by Eager,[11] who studied the condition in a localized area of Italy. Not long afterward, in 1916, Black and McKay[12] presented the first of an outstanding series of reports on what was called "mottled enamel" in children in certain areas of Colorado. Repeated searches for the cause of mottled enamel culminated in the report by Smith and associates[13] in 1931, which definitely implicated a relatively high amount of fluorides in the soil and water. Up to this time and for several years thereafter, mottled enamel was looked on exclusively as a pathologic condition and fluorine as its undesirable causative agent.

During the 1930s, however, some investigators, not only in the United States but also in Argentina, China, Japan, and South Africa, began to notice a possible relationship between high fluoride content of soil and water and mottled enamel on the one hand and apparent resistance to caries on the other.

In their 1937 report on dental caries in American Indian children, Klein and Palmer[14] raised the question of the possible benficial effect of a certain amount of fluoride in the drinking water. They noticed that children of some tribes in the southwestern part of the United States had much lower caries attack rates than those living elsewhere. Noting that the section involved had been found to be an endemic fluorosis area, they suggested the following:

This fact may have important implications, and would seem to justify some discussion. Fluorides are well known as enzyme inhibitors, and it may be suggested that perhaps a measure of the responsibility for low caries attack rates in the southwestern area may be the result of the drinking of fluoride water. Such water may provide an enzyme inhibitor which will operate to limit the chemical degradation of tooth-impacted carbohydrates to organic acids, so reducing the production of local acidity about the teeth, and so limiting an important vector in caries initiation.

There followed a large series of investigations by many scientists who compared the fluoride content of the enamel of teeth from different areas and of carious as against noncarious teeth, animal feeding experiments, and many comparative community studies. All substantiated the thesis that whereas an excessive amount of fluoride in water would produce mottled enamel, a certain amount, as low as 1 part per million of fluoride in water consumed during the period of tooth calcification, resulted in a significantly lower incidence of dental caries.

The first step to be taken for the practical use of the new knowledge was to apply fluorides directly to the teeth in the early 1940s. The success of these studies, which were widely publicized, led to a $1 million nationwide demonstration program sponsored by the Public Health Service to disseminate knowledge about the technique. The National Institute of Dental Research was established in 1948. The Institute provided funds and facilities for research, research grants, and fellowship programs.

Meanwhile, studies demonstrated that fluorides in the concentrations being considered were nontoxic. The Kettering Laboratory and the Institute of Industrial Health listed over 8,500 carefully analyzed and accepted scientific reports on the subject. The result was summarized by the statement[15]:

"The question of public safety of fluoridation is non-existent from the standpoint of medical science." More recently, prompted by continued false accusations of antifluoridationists, a large study of 24 major communities, 12 with and 12 without naturally fluoridated water, showed no evidence of any adverse effect on overall mortality.[16] By now the subject has been explored from so many vantage points and over such a long period of time that the safety and efficacy of fluoride as a natural additive for the prevention of dental caries is beyond dispute, although there are still those who do dispute the fact.

During the 1950s, sanitary engineers and waterworks chemists and operators developed policies and procedures for maintaining within extremely narrow limits the fluoride levels in water. A number of carefully controlled community studies were initiated in which fluorides were added to the public water supplies. The results indicated conclusively that the addition of fluorides up to a concentration of about 1 part per million of the drinking water supply resulted in up to two-thirds reduction in the incidence of dental caries in children who consumed it from birth. If they began to drink it when they were 5 or 6 years of age, the reduction was still 22%.[17] Current data indicate that, overall, a 60% reduction in caries will be maintained with fluoride concentrations ranging between 0.7 and 1.2 parts per million. The lower concentrations are used in hotter climates where more water is consumed on a daily basis.[8]

The acceptance of the fluoridation of public water supplies as an exceptionally safe, effective, and inexpensive procedure was disappointingly slow. Nevertheless, by 1980, more than 60% of all children had fluoridated water available. Every state now has some communities with fluoridated water, and many states have passed statewide fluoridation laws. Most communities with populations over 50,000 have added fluoride to their water.

Despite the evidence, a relatively small group—the antifluoridationists—have retarded progress. The characteristics, motivations, and methods of these people have interest and meaning for public health workers far beyond the subject of fluoridation.[18-20] They are the same type and often the same individuals who tend to oppose many progressive advances, be they immunization procedures, pasteurization of milk or international technical assistance. Their motivations vary. As Paul[21] has pointed out, the arguments of antifluoridationists fall basically into three categories: its benefits are uncertain, it may be injurious, and it violates individual rights. In addition, some object on the basis of added public cost, ignoring the fact that the measures they oppose almost always result in considerable savings. A simple calculation to compare the per capita, per family, or community cost of fluoridation with the tremendous expenditures required to repair carious teeth makes the economic argument absurd. An analysis was conducted 20 years ago that compared the costs of dental care for children in nonfluoridated Kingston, N.Y., with those in fluoridated Newburgh, N.Y.[22] The mean cost per child for initial dental care in Kingston was $27.61 as opposed to $11.92 for Newburgh.

Perhaps more serious is the charge that fluoridation constitutes enforced medication and violates individual rights. In 1966 the Michigan branch of the American Civil Liberties Union considered the issue and concluded that there was no basis on which to consider a violation of personal or civil liberties.

The issue remains active today, as the report by Dolinsky and his colleagues shows.[20] The referendum process has been used in many communities to prevent water fluoridation. Many prevention programs are faced with the axiom of political imbalances: a small number of zealous campaigners can often negate the wishes of the majority, if the majority has a broad but shallow interest in the matter. The same phenomenon has occurred with abortion and gun control. Repeated studies have indicated that the majority of people in the United States favor gun control and legalized abortions, yet a relatively small group of people who are willing to make the contrary position their dominant concern in life have been able to thwart progress. The people who are against an issue cannot be dismissed simply as irrational zealots, since they are often literate, well-educated men and women and because they will continue to play a major role in the dissemination of prevention information. Although the process is often frustrating, it does protect the concept of community self-determination and does force a continued debate about and the evolution of an ethical base for public health.

CHANGES IN THE DENTAL WORKFORCE AND IN DENTAL PRACTICES
Dental health workforce

The dental health workforce has increased substantially both in size and in productivity since 1950. There were approximately 75,000 active, civilian dentists in the United States in 1950. Partly because of support from Congress for health professions education, 18 new schools were formed and existing schools increased their enrollment. By 1980 the number of practicing, civilian dentists had increased to 121,240.[23] They tend to be concentrated in the Northeast and in the Pacific States with ratios in excess of 60 per 100,000 people, in contrast to ratios as low as 40 per 100,000 in the East South Central States. Similar to other health professionals, they prefer urban areas with a ratio of 60 per 100,000 in metropolitan areas compared to 37.4 per 100,000 in nonmetropolitan areas.

Women have increased as a proportion of entering dental classes from 3% until 1970 to 1971 to 18% in 1979 to 1980. Enrollment of minorities increased only slightly during this same period (about 9% in 1970 to 1971 to 12% in 1979 to 1980).

Most dentists are in private, fee-for-service practices (87%) with the remaining mostly in a variety of public programs including the armed forces and public health agencies. The practice setting appears to be changing dramatically with the advent of a variety of alternatives such as department store practices, corporate practices for employees, franchise practice systems, hospital-based dental services, and health maintenance organizations.[24]

The form of dental practice is also changing. Not too many years ago most dentists worked alone or with one assistant who worked at the chair side and handled office clerical chores. By 1978 about 95% of all dentists used one or more auxiliary workers, including dental hygienists, dental assistants, and laboratory technicians.[23] The dental hygienist is a licensed dental health educator and operative who can perform many direct care services. The extent of their practice varies from state to state. They generally have a minimum of 2 years of training and, with an expansion in their preparation, can function as primary dental care providers, performing assessments and preparing and even filling cavities. Their expanded role has been resisted by the profession, and this resistance will probably become stronger because the supply of dentists is now greater than effective demand partly as a result of

fluoridation and other preventive strategies. In 1977 there were 32,200 practicing dental hygienists in the United States, many of them working part-time in several offices. A few have moved into private practice, but this development has also been resisted by the dental profession.[24]

Because of the growing public and professional awareness of the importance of dental health, and because of several practical measures that could be taken for the solution of those problems, the specialty of public health dentistry was established. A Dental Health Section of the American Public Health Association was formed, which by 1945 had defined the field of public health dentistry and had established educational qualifications for public health dentists. About the same time the American Association of Public Health Dentists came into being, along with a Dental Health Section of the American Dental Association. Annual professional and official conferences of those most directly concerned with programs of dental health were instituted with the establishment of the Conference of State Dental Directors with the Surgeon General of the Public Health Service and the Chief of the Children's Bureau, on the one hand, and the Council on Dental Health of the American Dental Association, on the other. The specialty was formally recognized in 1952 through the establishment of the American Board of Dental Public Health.

Forms of practice

The growing concern of the dental profession for the size of their market has resulted in attempts to curtail the development of alternative forms of practice. Dentistry is unique in that over 90% of all practicing dentists are members of their local, state, and national association (the American Dental Association) compared to only 37% of practicing physicians who are members of their parallel tripartite structure.[25] In 1981 the American Dental Association's Council on Dental Education urged that only the clinical disciplines (those involved in the direct treatment of patients) be recognized as a proper dental specialty.[26] Only about 14% of all dentists specialize, mostly in orthodontia (about 40% of specialists), followed by oral surgeons (20% of specialists), and periodontists and pedodontists (about 10%), with the remainder made up of non-clinical specialists in prosthodontics, oral pathology, and public health.[23] In many other countries, non-doctoral-level–trained dental technicians have taken over a large part of the routine, primary dental care, but this appears to be an unlikely development in the United States given the decline in dental disease because of prevention, the increased supply of dentists, and the strong role played at the state legislative level by dental associations.

Dental insurance and payment plans

A number of private insurance companies have extended medical prepayment plans to include dental care. Several labor unions, beginning in 1945 with the St. Louis Health Institute,[27] have sponsored prepaid dental plans with some success. Of particular interest is the prepaid dental insurance package in the 1974 contract agreement between the United Steelworkers of America and the major steel companies. The program, which took effect on August 1, 1975, is paid for by the employer and covers 100% of preventive services for children under 19 and half the cost of orthodontics for children. Dental insurance now represents one of the fastest growing fringe benefits in labor contract negotiations.

Since 1942, the American Dental Association has sponsored numerous studies of prepayment mechanisms. Its original plan[28] proposed to provide dental service to low-income groups and involved the payment by the subscriber of $1 each month plus an additional $1 monthly for the first dependent and 50 cents a month more for additional dependents. Thus the total fee for a subscriber with two or more dependents amounted to $2.50 a month. Certain services, such as orthodontics and the construction of crowns, bridges, and dentures, were not included. It must be remembered that the suggested fees applied to the year 1944. In 1953 the House of Delegates of the American Dental Association adopted a set of principles in relation to prepaid dental health plans.

Although the medical profession has been opposed to capitation as a form of payment, the dental profession faces a more elastic demand market. That is, although many people get regular dental check-ups and restorative and cosmetic care, a large proportion of the population will not spend money on dental care unless they have considerable pain. Capitation represents a way to broaden the base of economic support for dental practice and to stabilize use. Schoen[29] points out that a capitation rate for a population has to be based on its need for dental resources and the cost of supplying them. Factors requiring consideration are the amount of dentists' and hygienists' time required, which is affected by the need for initial care as opposed to maintenance care, stability of the population, use of services, family size, age of eligible persons, fluoridation, and socioeconomic variables. Provider time and cost are also affected by the type, quantity, and use of facilities and auxiliary personnel. Schoen has devised a method that takes these various cost factors into account and provides a realistic basis for arriving at a capitation rate per person or family for a given population. The method is applicable to populations with differing dental requirements and financial capabilities, since the pertinent formulas and priorities include numerous variations. For example, to lower the capitation rate, members of families may be phased into treatment. Also, surcharges or copayments can be placed on patients for all services or only for specific ones. He considers that if this method is used to provide care under a rational system of priorities, capitation group practice of dentistry can achieve results not obtainable under the fee-for-service solo practice system. Schoen also believes that in prepaid group practice there are incentives for using expanded-duty auxiliaries, containing costs, and improving the level of dental health of the eligible population through both treatment and prevention.

PUBLIC HEALTH DENTAL PROGRAMS

In summing up the dental public health situation as it existed in 1954, Knutson[2] stated:

The nature of accomplishments during the past 10 years made this a decade of beginning in the field of dental public health. Water fluoridation, topical fluorides, oral cancer detection and control programs, the team approach to the diagnosis and treatment of cleft lip and cleft palate cases, orthodontic care programs, utilization of chairside assistants, the National Institute of Dental Research, approaches to the epidemiology of dento-facial deformities and periodontal diseases, and principles of prepayment for dental care services—all these are no better than well begun and several are in the budding stage. The objectives of all and the merits of most of them have been firmly established . . . .

In view of this, it can readily be understood that present-day public health agencies and the relatively few but well-qualified public health dentists on their staffs are in a different situation from that which existed 30 years ago, when all they could do was try to devise ways and means of reducing by dental therapy the discouraging flood of accumulating dental needs. A practical approach has unfolded, with some clearly defined and proved preventive measures that, if properly applied, hold promise of reducing the needs for caries correction to a point at which it may be handled reasonably adequately along with the prosthetic, orthodontic, and dental surgical needs of the community.

Dental public health programs focus on primary, secondary, and tertiary prevention, with the emphasis necessarily on primary prevention. All state and territorial health agencies report the existence of dental health activities of some kind.[30] In 1980, they reported a total expenditure of $32.3 million, of which $14.8 million (45.9%) was for prevention. Approximately 9,142,000 people received dental health services from official state and territorial health agencies.

Although dental care is inexpensive as compared to medical care (because of lower professional income [partly a function of lower demand], higher productivity through the use of auxiliary personnel, and the more standardized nature of most office encounters), it would nonetheless be impossibly expensive for a public agency to take on the task of treating dental pathology generally. Even though many citizens urge that local public health agencies provide free services, the resources are simply not there, given the prevalence of caries in children and periodontal disease in adults. However, public pressure may force the issue. If so, the program's limitations should be carefully demarcated. If possible, it should be limited to young children at first, expanding upward in age eligibility only as the prevalence of dental disease declines, making such services economically feasible.

By using available knowledge, it is possible (1) to prevent and control most dental caries; (2) to prevent or control soft tissue inflammation and disease of the supporting tissues of the teeth; (3) with specialist cooperation, to correct maloccluding teeth and prevent a relatively small number of the gross tooth irregularities that may interfere with mastication, with the health of the supporting tissues, and with the emotional stability of the individual; (4) with specialist cooperation, to treat the problems arising from anomalies of the oral cavity, for example, the cleft palate, congenitally missing

teeth, supernumerary teeth, hypoplastic teeth, and other developmental dental abnormalities; (5) to treat and restore teeth involved in accidents; (6) to detect oral cancer in the early stages; and (7) to prevent and eliminate oral infection that may contribute to systemic disease.

Because the fluoridation of water supplies will decrease dental caries prevalence by 60%, it is obvious that a basic goal of a public health dental program should be the acceptance and development of this procedure. To accomplish this, several steps are suggested. Probably the first should be to obtain a positive statement of policy on fluoridation by the state dental society and the state health agency. After this it will probably be advisable to promote the establishment of a state fluoridation committee to work with the state public health dentists and the state dental society. Such a group may be of considerbale value in providing information and data on fluoridation to the general public and the press, to local dental societies, and to state and local nonprofessional organizations and officials. It may also assist by drawing up a sample fluoridation ordinance in conformance with state legislation and by collecting information on costs. On the local level the local dental society might preferably provide the leadership in organizing a local committee and should play an active role in the planning and establishment of the local program.

Many communities have apparently felt that the job was completed once the water supply was fluoridated, but surveys by the U.S. Public Health Service have revealed that a large number of systems are improperly maintained and that necessary concentrations of fluoride are present in the water only intermittently. Maintenance of the equipment and training of the personnel have become important components of health department programs.

Many people live in rural communities where public water supplies are not available or in small towns where the effort to fluoridate the water supply has been successfully resisted. One alternative is fluoridation of the water supply of the school system. This requires the support of the health department and the board of education. The concentration of fluoride in a school system is necessarily greater than in a community system, since the children use the water only part of the day and do not start using it until they are 5 or 6 years old. When the small systems are properly maintained, they result in a 40% reduction in caries at a cost (1980) of about $1.50 per child per year.

Despite its greater cost and more difficult method of use, topical application of fluoride to the teeth of children has a place in many if not all public health dental programs. This is especially true in rural areas or where there is misinformed but effective opposition to fluoridation of public water supplies. Another reason for retaining the topical fluoride procedure is that, since water fluoridation is most effective during the years of enamel calcification, it is advisable that children whose teeth were already calcified when fluoridation was begun have topical fluoride applications. Subsequently, as the benefits of fluoridated water become effective, topical fluoride applications may be discontinued gradually, beginning with the younger age groups. The extent to which the topical procedure is carried out in the offices of private practicing dentists, on the one hand, or through public facilities, on the other, will depend entirely on the local situation.

Topical applications can work effectively in group settings without the necessity for relatively expensive one-on-one dental care. Fluoridated mouth rinses, gels, and gel-packs that fit around the teeth, bathing them in a fluoride solution for a short time reduce caries by 20% to 50%, depending on whether the area already has fluoridated water. The cost may be as low as $1.50 per child per year. These programs can be managed very simply especially when volunteer support is available. Children have been taught to rinse to music in a highly social peer-driven environment. The Public Health Service has developed an excellent guide to the development of a self-applied fluoride program, including background information, brochures and pamphlets, and excellent suggestions for developing community support.[31]

There probably always will be a need for some remedial treatment of caries. For this and other reasons, an essential part of the public health dental program should be the promotion of regular dental supervision. With a major proportion of caries subject to prevention, it may be possible to repair the backlog of caries on an incremental basis. Even in the face of vast accumulated dental needs, it has been found practical and fruitful in several places to restrict caries corrective programs to children in a limited age span. For example, some programs that began by caring for children from 5 to 10 years of age have found it possible during the second year of the program to add the new crop of 5-year-old children and, in addition, to continue with the 11-year-old children who were in the original group the year before. As each year goes by, new 5-year-olds have been added, and all children previously cared for are continued.

The part of a community dental health program that relates to the remedial treatment of dental and other oral defects, including orthodontics, prosthetics, and dental surgery for congenital defects, would seem to rest largely in the hands of private practicing dentists aided to whatever degree may be possible by the services, facilities, and contributions of public clinics for indigent or low-income groups, philanthropic agencies, and prepayment dental care plans. Significant numbers of underprivileged children with oral and dental defects that ordinarily would be uncorrected have been cared for through the provisions of the Economic Opportunity Program, Head Start, the Maternal and Child Health Programs, and the Comprehensive Health Care provisions of the Social Security legislation. These programs were all either reduced or eliminated in 1981 as a result of budget cuts.

Underlying all the other activities should be a carefully planned dental health education program. On the state level public health dentists should work closely with state departments of education, dental schools and teachers' colleges. An extremely important area for dental health education is in the school health program. Those responsible for the community dental health program should work particularly closely with the board of education, classroom teachers, and physical education personnel, assisting them in preparing sound and practical information in the field, in screening classroom teaching aids, and in obtaining material for them from the various dental and public health associations.

Most dental health researchers are skeptical about the efficacy of dental health education, but it is likely that they are looking for the same sort of relatively quick results that are obtained in prevention efforts based on biochemical technology. Significant differences have not been found between classrooms exposed to dental health education and those unexposed, but dental health education has been notoriously prone to fads, changing from moment to moment. Many educators have made brushing technique a big issue, but brushing in any fashion is both so uncommon and so important that teaching children to brush at least once and preferably twice each day is much more important than teaching them to brush in a particular manner.

Another area worthy of particular attention is the school lunch program. The public health dental personnel in collaboration with teachers of nutrition and home economics and with the school lunchroom managers should attempt to bring about a change in lunch and snack habits, particularly with regard to the intake of carbohydrates. With this in mind, a great many school systems have discouraged the availability of candy and soft drinks in their lunchrooms and elsewhere on school premises. Although it is recognized that schoolchildren may obtain these products elsewhere, this is at least a partial step in the right direction to bring about a change in the habit pattern at mealtime. Food habits change slowly and appear to start with older children and adults who are better able to conceptualize long-range benefits from present-day actions. As noted in Chapter 17, dietary practices are changing and generally for the better. Although the evidence is not available to support the contention, anecdotal information from both parents and dentists indicates that many more children are brushing and using dental floss regularly now than they did 20 or 30 years ago. More well-trained public health dental professionals are badly needed to help shape technically sound and epidemiologically oriented dental health education programs. There were only 1,600 public health dentists and 800 dental hygienists practicing in public health in 1979. There were only 44 graduates of dental health programs in schools of public health in 1979 to 1980 and one third of these were foreign students who will presumably return to their own countries.[32]

SUMMARY

Dental public health is certainly not the most important area of concern for a modern industrialized nation, but it is important both for what has been accomplished and what can be learned.

The prevalence of dental disease has decreased and will continue to decrease as a result of deliberate preventive efforts, a strong program of research, good dental care, an increased supply of practitioners, and general changes in diet, income, and self-awareness. Although dental disease cannot be eradicated, it is clearly controllable. The vast reservoir of caries and periodontal disease is decreasing in size, making it possible for the dental workforce to clean up the remaining pathology.

The result of these changes is better dental health and the possibility of a lower dental disease bill both for individuals and for society. The result also is likely to be more competition among dentists, stronger efforts to control the competition emanating from alternative forms of practice, and some retreat by the dental profession into a narrower approach to community dentistry. It is likely that as the prevalence of dental disease continues to diminish, more dental providers will attempt to market more services of marginal value. These likely changes have been summarized by Wotman and Goldman[33] and offer some interesting opportunities to speculate on the future of other traditional health professions.

REFERENCES

1. Knutson, J., and Klein, H.: Tooth mortality in elementary school children, Public Health Rep. **53**:1021, June 1938.
2. Knutson, J.: Dental public health accomplishments and predictions, Am. J. Public Health **44**:331, March 1954.
3. Axelsson, P., and Linhe, J.: The effect of a plaque control program on gingivitis and dental caries in school children, J. Dental Res. **56**(special issue C):142, 1977.
4. Federal Security Agency: The epidemiology of dental disease: collection of papers of Henry Kelin and others, 1937-47, Washington, D.C., 1948, U.S. Public Health Service.
5. Law, F.E.: Highlights of research in dental public health, 1956-1960, Am. J. Public Health **51**(6):825, June 1961.
6. National Center for Health Statistics: Decayed, missing, and filled teeth among persons 1-74 years, United States, U.S. Department of Health and Human Services Pub. No. (PHS) 81-1673, August 1981.
7. National Caries Program, National Institute of Dental Research: The prevalence of dental caries in United States children, 1979-80, NIH Pub. No. 82-2245, December 1981, U.S. Department of Health and Human Services.
8. Schoen, M.H., and Freed, J.R.: Prevention of dental disease: caries and periodontal disease, Ann. Rev. Public Health **2**:71, 1981.
9. Freeland, M.S., and Schendler, C.E.: National health expenditures: short-term outlook and long-term projections, Health Care Fin. Rev., **2**:97, Winter 1981.

10. Voker, J.F.: Dental science. In Contributions of the biological sciences to human welfare, Proceedings of the Federation of the American Society for Experimental Biology, vol. 31, II, Bethesda, Md., Nov.-Dec. 1972, The Federation.

11. Eager, J.: Chiaie teeth, Public Health Rep. **16:**2576, 1901.

12. Black, G.V., and McKay, F.S.: Mottled teeth: an endemic developmental imperfection of the enamel of the teeth heretofore unknown in the literature of dentistry, Dent. Cosmos **58:**129, 1916.

13. Smith, M.C., Lantz, E., and Smith, H.B.: The cause of mottled enamel, Science **74:**244, 1931.

14. Klein, J., and Palmer, C.: Dental caries in American Indian children, PHS Bull. No. 239, Washington, D.C., Dec. 1937.

15. Campbell, I.R., editor: The role of fluoride in public health: a selected bibliography, Cincinnati, 1963, Kettering Laboratory, University of Cincinnati.

16. Tokuhata, G.K., Dignon, E., and Ramaswamy, K.: Fluoridation and mortality, Public Health Rep. **93:**60, Jan.-Feb. 1978.

17. Ast, D.B.: Effectiveness of water fluoridation, J. Am. Dent. Assoc. **65:**581, Nov. 1962.

18. Evans, C.A., and Pickles, T.: Statewide antifluoridation initiatives: a new challenge to health workers, Am. J. Public Health **68:**59, Jan. 1978.

19. Dwore, R.B.: A case study of the 1976 referendum in Utah on fluoridation, Public Health Rep. **93:**73, Jan.-Feb. 1978.

20. Dolinksy, H.B., and others: A health systems agency and a fluoridation campaign, J. Public Health Policy **2**(2):158, June 1981.

21. Paul, B.D.: Fluoridation and the social scientist, J. Soc. Issues **17**(4):1, Oct. 1961.

22. Ast, B.D., and others: Time and cost factors to provide regular periodic dental care for children in a fluori-

dated and nonfluoridated area, Am. J. Public Health **57:**1635, Sept. 1967.

23. Office of Health Research, Statistics, and Technology: Health: United States, 1981, U.S. Department of Health and Human Services Pub. No. (PHS) 82-1232, Dec. 1981.

24. Rovin, S., and Nash, J.: Traditional and emerging forms of dental practice: cost, accessibility, and quality factors, Am. J. Public Health **72**(7):656, July 1982.

25. Lipscomb, J., and Douglass, C.W.: A political economic theory of the dental care market, Am. J. Public Health **72**(7):665, July 1982.

26. Allukian, M., Jr.: Dentistry at the crossroads: the future is uncertain: the challenges are many (editorial) Am. J. Public Health **72**(7):653, July 1982.

27. McNeel, J.O.: Dental program of the St. Louis Labor Health Institute, Am. J. Public Health **44:**878, July 1954.

28. American Dental Association: Proposed plan for prepayment of dental insurance, Chicago, 1944, The Association.

29. Schoen, M.H.: Methodology of capitation payment to group dental practice and effects of such payment on care, Health Services Rep. **89:**16, Jan.-Feb. 1974.

30. National Public Health Program Reporting System: Public health agencies, 1980: a report on their expenditures and activities, Washington, D.C., 1981, Association of State and Territorial Health Officials.

31. Horowitz, A.M.: Preventing tooth decay: a guide for implementing self-applied fluorides in school settings, NIH Pub. No. 82-1196, revised Dec. 1981, U.S. Department of Health and Human Services.

32. Bureau of Health Professions: Public health personnel in the United States, 1980, U.S. Department of Health and Human Services Pub. No. (HRA) 82-6, Jan. 1982.

33. Wotman, S., and Goldman, H.: Pressures on the dental care system in the United States, Am. J. Public Health **72**(7):684, July 1982.

CHAPTER 33

Medical care delivery

Accuse not nature! She hath done
her part. Do thou but thine.

John Milton

The delivery of medical care services is an extraordinarily complex subject that is poorly understood by most practitioners and analysts. This chapter is not intended to supplant complexity with simplicity, nor is it meant to serve as a complete description of programs and problems. Its purpose is to provide a perspective on medical care that is based in epidemiology and the obligations of government "to promote the general welfare." For further information the reader is referred to some of the books devoted to the subject of medical care from a variety of perspectives.[1-5]

THE RELATIONSHIP BETWEEN PUBLIC HEALTH AND MEDICAL CARE

Public health involves the contributions of many different kinds of professional, technical, and clerical workers. The medical profession is one of the most important contributors as well as one of the most important problems in public health. Many programs in public health require the work of physicians: the management of tuberculosis and venereal disease, prenatal and early childhood care, and clinical work in ambulatory care programs. Beyond that, physician involvement is desirable although not mandatory in planning, organizing, and managing public health programs. In many instances it is helpful if not actually necessary to have public health physicians who can negotiate effectively with private practitioners, but the work of public health is not inherently medical work as that term is ordinarily understood. Even in tuberculosis and venereal disease control, the essential components of the program are case-contact investigation and follow-up. Treatment of an active case is essential and ethically obligatory, but it is a rel-atively minor part of the process. The purpose of the public health agency, unlike the purpose of the private physician, is not to cure a disease but to prevent disability and the spread of the disease to other members of the community. If that could be done without the use of medical care, most public health agencies would change their programs quickly. Medical care is relatively expensive and inefficient, but there are some occasions when there is simply no alternative. When viewed from a social policy perspective, medical care is one of the technologies employed by public health to solve problems, but it is not the controlling technology.

EVOLUTION OF MODERN MEDICINE

Before the Industrial Revolution, which is usually considered to have begun about 1750, the social and economic structure of the Western Hemisphere was relatively simple. Few large cities existed, and the economy was essentially agrarian. The provision of medical service in a public sense was in its most embryonic form. As early as the thirteenth century, a few European towns employed town surgeons. Town physicians, on the other hand, are not encountered historically until the sixteenth century. Whatever care was provided for the sick poor, aged, and homeless, the Church, not the government, was its source in the occidental world. Later, during the sixteenth, seventeenth, and eighteenth centuries, these responsibilities gradually began to shift from the Church to the state. As pointed out by Shryock,[6] however, "This humanitarianism, like the clerical form of earlier centuries, largely expressed the benevolence of the upper classes rather than any demand for reform from below."

Public health and health care services

With the Industrial Revolution, the social and economic center of gravity shifted from the agrarian to the urban scene. Rural areas themselves were directly affected. The populations of industrial cities were not self-maintaining, because of their appalling death rates. They therefore required continuous replenishment from the rural population.

It was during this period of cruel industrialization that the search for scientific knowledge received a much needed impetus. Although the primary incentive was the development of new techniques for greater economic gains, the emphasis on science spilled over into human biology. The character of the practice of medicine began to undergo some improvement. A trend toward logical experimentation and observation developed. A system of medical training by apprenticeship came into vogue.

Gradually social reforms began; these reforms dealt with working conditions, welfare, housing, the care of orphans and the insane, education, and sanitary conditions. Scientific and technologic investigations that had formerly been conducted largely from the point of view of industrial development now began to be pursued for their own sake and for the benefit of humanity as a whole. Despite these trends, economic welfare was still insecure. The greatest handicap to industrial expansion was that distribution of goods lagged far behind techniques of production. The solution of this was dependent on the invention of the steam locomotive, the internal combustion engine, and the construction of paved, all-weather roads.

During this period of social revolution, the contributions of the natural scientists to the social science of public health were very important. Athanasius Kircher,[7] who may have seen bacteria as early as 1658, formulated an animate theory of contagion. John Snow[8] stopped an outbreak of cholera in London in the 1850s by removing the pump handle from the source of disease. The work of Pasteur in the 1870s marked the beginning of modern immunology. Rudolf Virchow made the first real contributions to the understanding of pathology during that time. Lister[9] published his first paper on antisepsis in 1867, and Robert Koch[10] first set down his famous postulates in 1882. The rapidity of discovery must have seemed breathtaking at the time, and it was. So extraordinary were the findings of the late 1800s that Sir William Osler[11] wrote:

For countless generations the prophets and kings of humanity have desired to see the things which men have seen . . . in the course of this wonderful 19th century. To the call of the watchers on the towers of progress there has been the one sad answer—the people sit in darkness and in the shadow of death. Politically, socially and morally the race has improved; but for the unit, the individual, there was little hope. Cold philosophy shed a glimmer of light on his path, religion in its various guises illumined his sad heart, but neither availed to lift the curse of suffering from the sin-begotten son of Adam. In the fullness of time, long expected, long delayed, at last science emptied upon him from the horn of Amalthea blessings which cannot be enumerated, blessings which have made the century forever memorable, and which have followed each other with a rapidity so bewildering that we know not what next to expect.

With this new knowledge, public health moved out of the darkness and into the grime of industrial metropolitan life.

Medical education became formalized with the establishment of schools with increasingly higher standards. Although the general practitioner was still the prototype, many medical specialties began to appear.

The scientific discoveries coincided in time with changes in the welfare system that led to the formation of hospitals. Before the mid-1850s public welfare was handled as "out relief," much as it is today. That is, paupers were given a certain amount of money to spend on their own needs. The welfare commissioners (known as the Guardians in London) became concerned over the rising cost of this form of relief and began a program of "in relief," which resulted in the formation of large workhouses. Instead of money, paupers were given shelter and some food, and they were expected to work for it. The process was not only cheaper but the stigmatizing effect of living in the workhouse was throught to be a beneficial social lesson. Such concentrations of the poor, the disabled, and the incompetent resulted in the aggregation of a population group at high risk of disease. It became necessary to separate the infirm in a space called the infirmary. With the rapid succession of scientific discoveries previously described, teachers of medicine needed places with sick persons to show students what diseases looked like and how to treat them. The workhouses were a natural source of such "teaching material," and they quickly became the teaching hospitals of London, affiliated with the major schools. This was true in the New World as well. Bellevue Hospital in New York began as a workhouse and Philadelphia General, now closed, began as an almshouse.

Despite the remarkable medical discoveries of the late nineteenth century, such as improved diagnostic and therapeutic techniques; the development of anesthesia, antisepsis, and asepsis; and the study of cellular physiology and pathology, medicine as practiced by the average physician was still very primitive. Until the close of the century treatment consisted mostly of blood letting and the evacuation of "ill humours" by physicking, sweating, diuretics, vomiting, and the formation of blisters.

Characteristic of the American physician of this period was Dr. Hiram Buhrman, who practiced in small towns in Maryland and Pennsylvania in the 1870s. His regular fee was 25 cents for an office call. This included medicines unless expensive drugs were necessary. A house visit within the township was 50 cents without medicine, 75 cents with medicine. The physician compounded his own prescriptions. In case of death there was a $3 fee, for which he did most of the work of the present-day mortician. All obstetric cases, regardless of the length of labor, were $5, as were abortions, whereas miscarriages were billed at $1.50. Dr. Buhrman also functioned as a dentist. A tooth extraction cost 25 cents, except when several in a row were removed at the same time, in which case the fee per tooth was reduced. In this unspecialized small town practice, conducted with few instruments and drugs on a limited number of diseases, the hospital did not enter into the picture at all.[12]

With the beginning of the twentieth century, and especially as a result of the Flexner report on medical education, the practice of medicine began to mature as a science and as a result became much more effective. The speculative theories and traditional practices of the physician of the nineteenth century had failed to win the confidence of the public, and as a consequence many medical cults flourished. It has been said that 1912 was a turning point in the United States: a patient finally had a 50% chance of a correct *diagnosis*. With the acceptance and application of newer scientific knowledge by the orthodox physician in practice and as a result of more widespread public education and understanding, the medical profession has since risen high in public esteem.

This has not occurred without complications. Improvements in diagnosis and treatment have required the development of highly trained specialists and costly diagnostic and therapeutic tools with a corresponding increase in the cost of medical care. In the decade following 1910 it was not uncommon for a complicated illness to be treated in a hospital by one physician, possibly an intern, and a consulting pathologist-bacteriologist. The complete record would rarely cover more than two to three pages and the cost for 10 days in the hospital including medical care would amount to about $30. By the 1980s the same patient would commonly be seen by 3 to 5 primary physicians, several interns and residents, 5 consultants, and from 10 to 14 technicians. The record would commonly cover 80 pages with as many as 100 laboratory tests and x-ray films. The total bill would range between $5,000 and $8,000, depending on whether or not surgery was performed. The use of laboratory tests alone has increased by 500% in the last 20 years, with laboratory and x-ray work representing about 25% of the total hospital bill.[13]

The scientific progress that did so much to make medical care effective had an even greater impact on the practice of public health. Although many principles of sanitation had been established through empiric observation, they were largely embodied in the requirements of organized religion or folklore. Even Jenner's use of the cowpox virus was based on empiric rather than scientific investigation. The work of Pasteur, Lister, Koch, and others changed that dramatically. Contagion could now be understood, its mechanisms could be unraveled for each disease, and preventive steps could be taken. The work done in protecting water and milk supplies was particularly striking. But other social action programs had an equally important impact on the changing patterns of morbidity and mortality in the United States.

At the turn of the century influenza and pneumonia, tuberculosis, and diarrhea and enteritis were the three leading causes of death in the United States—ahead of heart disease. By 1980 only influenza and pneumonia remained on the list of the 10 leading causes of death. The striking changes in mortality from communicable diseases can be seen in Table 33-1. The seven disease categories listed were responsible for 393 deaths per 100,000 population per year from 1900 to 1904 but only for 1.3

TABLE 33-1. Decline in deaths from selected communicable diseases, United States, 1900-1980

Cause of death	Deaths per 100,000 population per year	
	1900-1904	1980
Diphtheria	32.7	0
Pertussis	10.7	0
Measles	10.0	0
Typhoid fever	26.7	0
Diarrhea and enteritis	115.3	0.2
Syphilis	12.9	0.1
Tuberculosis	184.7	1.0

deaths by 1980. Virtually all of this improvement was the result of the great discoveries of the nineteenth century, but very little of it could be attributed to the direct intervention of physicians treating individual sick persons.

Death rates for diphtheria, pertussis, measles, and tuberculosis began to decline before the advent of widespread specific treatment or preventive techniques. Although it is difficult to know exactly why these changes took place, most theorists believe that the general improvements in living conditions and nutrition were of great importance. Typhoid and the diarrheas (which particularly caused terribly high infant death rates during the summer months) were virtually eliminated as causes of death when water supplies were protected and chlorinated and milk became pasteurized. The public health emphasis on contact investigation, immunization, sanitation, better nutrition, and improved housing had more to do with the marked changes in disease and the rapidly lengthening life span of Americans than did the specific curative techniques of physicians.

The formation of the health departments in the United States began to take place at about the same time that the practice of medicine became better organized and more highly professionalized. The private practitioners saw a distinct difference between the practice of medicine and public health and were successful in keeping the latter out of the former. They did so by helping to pass the public health laws, by creating and controlling the boards

of health, and by insisting that health officers be physicians. Lacking any reason to differ with what seemed to be reasonable approaches to public health, legislatures readily agreed with such concepts and effectively placed the policies and practices of public health in the hands of the private practitioners. This allowed practicing physicians to refer all nonmedical problems to the public health department, and it certainly encouraged health officers to insist that public health stay out of clinical medicine.

Where medical care delivery systems did develop in the public domain, they were largely separate from health departments. The big municipal and county hospitals had their own separate history and, as we shall see, the major efforts to pay for the medical care of the poor in this country took the form of insurance systems administered through welfare departments, which paid private physicians for treating public patients. This division of public health and medical care in the United States took place between 1900 and 1920 and has confounded all efforts to develop a consistent public policy for health ever since.

THE COMPONENTS OF MEDICAL CARE

There are many different parts to a complete medical care system, ranging from ambulances to emergency rooms, ambulatory care programs, hospital or inpatient care units, laboratories, supply businesses, nursing homes, pharmacies, social work programs, physical therapy programs, mental health centers, blood banks, dental offices, and many more. The essential component is the encounter point between the physician and the patient. In the United States, although potential patients often seek advice from friends, family members, or other people known in their community for their knowledge about health, they do not usually enter into a care system until they meet with a licensed physician.

That encounter usually takes place in a private office in the United States. The average American makes 4.7 physician visits per year, and 3.1 of those occur in the office or clinic with the remainder of the contacts taking place in a hospital emergency room or outpatient department or by telephone. Once that initial contact has been made, the patient may have access to a variety of diagnostic and treatment procedures, either as an outpatient or as an inpatient in the hospital. Laboratory and x-ray services can be requested by an individual, but most pathologists and radiologists will not honor the request without the prescription of a physician; nor can a patient be admitted to a hospital without the request of a physician who has membership privileges in that hospital. Hospitals admit patients only in the technical sense that they process the admission by completing the papers and assigning the space: the admission is by order of the physician. To obtain the right to make such an admission, the physician has to apply to the board of directors of the hospital. The application is reviewed by the medical staff, which evaluates the training and qualifications of the applicant and then makes a recommendation to the board, which is generally accepted. The new member's privileges are restricted to those procedures that the credentials committee of the medical staff believes the applicant is qualified to perform. The new member agrees to abide by the rules of the medical staff, which are promulgated by the medical staff and adopted by the board. The physician staff member usually has no contractual responsibility to the hospital other than that, nor does the physician pay for the use of the hospital's services. The hospital, which is usually built with public funds or supported by tax-exempt bonds, provides a free working environment for the physician.

Most physicians (72% of those in practice) receive a fee for their services, often itemized so that a separate fee is paid for each of several different services that may be provided during the course of a single visit. Twenty-eight percent of physicians are paid by salary rather than by fee-for-service. The fee-for-service mechanism has been criticized for its incentive to provide additional and possibly unnecessary services, whereas fee-for-service advocates maintain that salaried physicians will not work as hard for their patients. The evidence indicates that patients seen by salaried physicians do spend less for their care, receive fewer high-cost services, but benefit from the encounter at least as much as do those who see fee-for-service physicians. The fee-for-service mechanism makes it very difficult to control costs. If a payment source, such as Blue Shield or Medicaid, reduces or does not increase the fee paid for a service, physicians tend to order more services for their patients, thus increasing their income to some predetermined level in spite of fee controls exercised by the payment sources.

Public health programs have had a difficult time obtaining an adequate supply of practicing physicians. Most public health programs do not have the funds necessary to compete with the income that can be earned in private practice, and civil service systems will not often allow salaries high enough to attract physicians even if the money is available. In the past, there have always been a few people who were interested sufficiently in public programs to keep the clinics operating, but in recent years private practice incomes have become so high that fewer people are willing to forego what can be earned privately for participation in the public health clinic. That appears to be changing once again as the increasing supply of physicians makes it necessary for many of them to work part-time in clinic activities to supplement their income.

Ambulatory care clinics are operated by health departments to aid in the control of specific diseases such as tuberculosis, sexually transmitted diseases, and addictive disorders. They are also common for such purposes as prenatal care and well-child care, although customarily they have been precluded from providing obstetric services in the hospital or from providing medical care for a sick child. Some health departments have operated general medical practice clinics for many years, primarily to serve the indigent and others who have a difficult time obtaining private medical care. In some instances these clinics have been part of a public hospital. Since 1965 more ambulatory care clinics have been built or acquired at public expense, and they often function as free-standing medical clinics. Well-developed systems of primary care are operated by the public health departments in Denver, Birmingham, Detroit, and several other cities.

Clinics function effectively as part of a health department. Many of the routine and traditional public health activities can be integrated into the work of a general clinic and, with good business management, effective, low-cost public health clinics can provide such categoric services as family planning, hypertension control, sexually transmitted disease control, and tuberculosis management alongside comprehensive pediatric clinics, obstetric programs, and general medical and surgical clinics. The cost of acquiring or constructing such clinics is high but affordable in most urban areas, and the staff can usually be employed in a civil service system. Properly designed and organized, they provide not only an outstanding service but a very satisfying professional experience for selected physicians, nurses, and other workers. It is important to have management personnel well trained in clinic functions and in the fiscal aspects of medical care. Negotiations with insurance companies, the Medicare carrier, and the state's Medicaid agency should be carried out before the clinic begins operation so that the elected officials as well as the public health board and director have a good understanding of the costs and revenues to be expected from the clinic. By carefully selecting medical personnel who are comfortable working in a general practice environment that discourages overuse of laboratory, x-ray, and other ancillary services, costs can be kept low. This is difficult, since most medical practice settings encourage the use of costly ancillary services to increase profits. Although the public clinic can bill insurance companies and Medicaid and Medicare for such services, they must also bill themselves or their local tax base when the patients are not covered by some other source of funds. Moreover, any effort to increase revenue by proliferating billings ultimately results in higher costs, often paid for by state and federal as well as local taxes. The gap between costs and revenue should be reduced by well-planned cost cutting and a conscious effort to deliver good medical care without overusing expensive and risky diagnostic and treatment procedures.

It is more difficult to operate a public hospital. A 100-bed hospital now costs between $15 and $20 million to build. Most public jurisdictions cannot capitalize such a venture. Nor for that matter can many existing voluntary hospitals without the use of governmentally endorsed tax-exempt bonds. Much of the new hospital construction currently under way is by private corporations, and that trend will continue with the voluntary and public hospitals faced with the burden of continually renovating old buildings in very expensive construction efforts. Management of the hospitals requires well-trained individuals who are aggressive in their search for revenue. Faced with a medical staff that insists on the latest in equipment and trained staff, public hospital managers cannot escape the 15% to 19% annual inflation in costs that has been customary over the past decade in the voluntary hospitals. Voluntary and private hospitals can recover most of the money they spend through insurance

receipts that are based on the costs incurred by the hospital. There is no effective brake on hospital spending, and they are quick to obtain new equipment when it enhances their competitive position with the physicians in the community. It is the physicians who are the real customers of the hospital, since they are the ones who admit the patients and write the orders for the services. If a public hospital tries to compete in that environment, it has to bill its own jurisdiction at higher and higher rates for those services provided to patients who do not have insurance or personal resources and who are not eligible for Medicare or Medicaid coverage. Operating costs usually dwarf the cost of the remainder of the public health department's programs and, as costs increase, disease prevention and health promotion activities are often reduced to meet the voracious needs of the hospital and its medical staff.

As will be noted later, the presence of a strong and effective public hospital and public clinic is needed throughout the United States, but the hospital especially presents constant management and policy problems for the public health agency. It may be more effective to operate a network of general medical clinics as a part of the health department and to establish the general hospital as an affiliated but separately governed public enterprise. In both programs it is essential to obtain managers who understand the financial management of medical care and are at the same time knowledgeable about public sector financial management and policy. The financial goals and management practices of the private medical care sector are not suitable to the attainment of public sector objectives.

SOCIOECONOMIC FACTORS INFLUENCING HEALTH STATUS

It is obvious that the socioeconomic status of a community plays a significant role in determining the degree of its health and illness, as well as its ability to provide public or private services.* Since many socioeconomic variables are not distributed uniformly, it follows that the health of a community or of a nation cannot be uniform. In a literal sense health and the treatment of illness are purchasable, but the ability to purchase them is not always present. The use of average figures to depict the pur-

---

*For recent data see Health of the disadvantaged, chart book II, U.S. Department of Health and Human Services Pub. No. (HRA) 80-633, Hyattsville, Md., 1980.

chasing power of a community of people obscures important differences.

Socioeconomic status is commonly measured in terms of income and less commonly in terms of type of employment or amount of education. It is also depicted by the racial composition of a neighborhood or community. It is hard to know just what comes first: education, wealth, employment, or minority status. Many health indicators are related to one or more of these variables. Are people less educated because they are black or because they are poor; are black people poor because they are black or because they are less well educated? This is not the place to attempt a lengthy exploration of such fundamental questions, but a hypothesis is beginning to form that suggests that the underlying variable in any society is education: that a society that has the advantage of a good, broad-based education system, with equity of access and individualized attention paid to the needs and resources of each participant, is not only a healthier society but a more humane one. Having stated an unproven nascent hypothesis, the remainder of this discussion will generally use proxy measures of human status, such as income.

Although the median family income in the United States is high, about $19,661 in 1979, there is considerable variation by region, race, degree of urbanization, and other factors. For example, the median family income for white families was $20,552 compared to $11,580 for black families. Table 33-2 presents the distribution of families by income, before taxes, in 1979 in the United States. It indicates, for example, that 33.1% of white families and 57.8% of black families had less than $15,000 in income.

The U.S. Department of Labor periodically calculates how much income a family of four needs, given current prices. It calculates three different levels: a lower budget, an intermediate budget, and a higher budget. In 1980 the totals were $14,044, $23,144, and $34,409, respectively.[14] The important feature of this model budget process is that the cost of medical care for the family of four is virtually the same among the three levels. In the 1980 calculations it increased from $1,298 in the lower budget family to $1,303 in the intermediate budget family, and $1,359 in the higher budget family. The budgeted items that varied most between the levels were such things as food, rent, transportation, clothing, and "other." Anticipated medical care costs would claim 10% of the after-tax budget of the low-income family, 7% of the after-tax income of the family with an intermediate level of income, and 5% of the after-tax income of the higher level family. These budget tables, well-known to welfare workers, dramatize the concept of medical indigency. A serious illness or accident could easily make it impossible for such families to meet any other expenditure requirements. Conversely, it can become very difficult for a lower budget family to voluntarily take steps to obtain medical care unless they believe that the problem is very serious.

The grossly uneven distribution of purchasing power is magnified still further when the nation is considered in terms of its constituent parts. Physicians tend to cluster in and around cities, especially the large metropolitan centers of population. The income of families in metropolitan areas is 21% higher than that of families outside of metropolitan areas. This factor, combined with another—regional wealth—brings about a geographic variation of considerable dimension. The more affluent states have the lion's share not only of physicians but also of specialists. Beyond this, the average age of physicians is significantly higher in the economically less privileged states and areas.

Another factor that accentuates the disparities that exist between regions is the proportion of older persons in the population. Persons 65 years of age and over require more medical attention and hospitalization than any other age group: about 2.9 days of hospital care per capita per year as compared

TABLE 33-2. Money income of families distributed by race, 1979

Money income	Percent distribution	
	White	Black
Under $5,000	5.4	17.9
$5,000-9,999	12.3	22.5
$10,000-14,999	15.4	17.5
$15,000-19,999	15.3	12.3
$20,000-24.999	14.9	10.2
$25,000-34,999	20.1	12.5
$35,000-49,999	10.9	5.4
$50,000 and over	5.7	1.8

From Bureau of the Census: Statistical abstracts of the United States, ed. 102, Washington, D.C., 1981, U.S. Government Printing Office, Table 725.

with less than 1 day per capita for persons aged 17 to 44. Furthermore, this is a period of decreased or absent earning power, hence much less ability to afford the needed care. Regionally this works especially to the disadvantage of the northeastern, central, and northwestern states.

The unequal distribution of resources would not be of such serious consequence if the socioeconomic factors causing it did not also have an adverse influence on the need for them. Although the average American suffers an injury or an illness about two and one half times a year, there are some who go through the year unscathed, whereas others far exceed the average expectation. In any average current year, out of each 1 million Americans 470,000 will suffer no serious illness, 320,000 will have one illness during the year, 140,000 will have two illnesses, 50,000 will have three illnesses, and 20,000 will have four or more illnesses.

For the general population it is possible to know in advance not only the total amount of illness but also the type. The continuing series of surveys and publications by the National Center for Health Statistics (U.S. Department of Health and Human Services, Public Health Service) have provided students, analysts, planners, and legislators with a rich source of valuable information. The data in Table 33-3 reveal the marked differences in activity limitation by age and family income in 1979. When this is correlated with the family budgets developed by the Department of Labor, the impact of income on health is obviously compounded. People in families with income below $10,000 per year have nearly twice as much activity limitation as do members of families with $25,000 or more per year.

Such data make it possible to predict the overall pattern of illness in the general population, but the forthcoming experience of the individual cannot be foretold. It is known that the lower individuals are on the socioeconomic scale, the more likely they are to experience one or more serious illnesses during any year. This is not surprising, since purchasing power determines the amount and quality of food consumed, the degree of exposure to or protection from the causes of illness or accidents, and the ability to obtain many medical as well as other types of services.

There is no convincing evidence that the availability of medical care services directly influences the wellness of a population group. Comparing life expectancy and the number of physicians per 1,000 persons in each of the 50 states does not result in a pattern that can illustrate any such correlation. Since virtually all other medical care expenditures depend on the number of physicians in an area, efforts to correlate the existence or nonexistence of other medical care resources with wellness or disability are also unenlightening. The important elements appear to be education, employment, housing, nutrition, and other environmental and socioeconomic factors. However, once illness or disability occurs, particularly in the acute phases, the availability of medical care services has a great deal to do with the rapidity and completeness of recovery. Medicare, Medicaid, and other government programs have had a significant impact on access since 1965. Low-income people now use more physician visits than do high-income people. Given the greater prevalence of disability among low-income people, it is not known whether the higher use rate is commensurate with need. Moreover, a high proportion of the physician visits con-

TABLE 33-3. Limitation of activity, according to selected characteristics: United States, 1979

Characteristic	Percent of population with limitation of activity
Age	
Under 17 years	3.9
17-44 years	8.8
45-64 years	24.1
65 years and over	46.0
Sex	
Male	14.8
Female	13.2
Race	
White	13.6
Black	17.7
Family income	
Less than $7,000	22.0
$7,000-9,999	17.8
$10,000-14,999	14.0
$15,000-24,999	11.7
$25,000 or more	10.0
TOTAL	13.9

From Office of Health Research, Statistics, and Technology: Health: United States, 1981, U.S. Department of Health and Human Services Pub. No. (PHS) 82-1232, Hyattsville, Md., 1981.

sumed by low-income people occur in hospital emergency rooms and outpatient clinics rather than in physicians' offices (21% for low-income people versus 9% for high-income people). This does not necessarily mean that the services used by low-income families are inferior, but it does indicate continued access problems.

Income has a marked effect on health status: it relates directly to wellness and to the ability to get medical care. The two income effects operate together to produce a continuing disparity, which tends to reinforce the difference. Although the ready availability of medical care when and where it is needed could help reduce this disparity, changing the environmental and socioeconomic conditions that determine health status would have a greater effect.

EXPENDITURES FOR MEDICAL CARE AND PUBLIC HEALTH

Warren and Sydenstricker[15] wrote in 1919 that with the costs of medical care rising into the "millions" of dollars annually, it was unlikely that legislative bodies would continue to support public health and other disease prevention activities. The cost pressures have become enormous. The data in Table 33-4 reveal the startling facts: from a total annual cost of about $13 billion as recently as 1950—representing 4.4% of the U.S. gross national product—the figure had increased to $247 billion—or 9.4% of the gross national product—by 1980.[16] It increased to $279 billion by 1981[17] and shows every sign of continuing to increase at a rate between 10.5% and 16%, as it has every year since 1966. At that rate of increase, the cost could exceed a half-trillion dollars by 1986! Of the $12 billion spent for health services in 1950, approximately $11.6 billion was spent for personal health care services and supplies and $400 million was spent for public health activities. Expressed differently, 97% of the total was spent for personal care services and supplies and about 3.3% was spent for public health. By 1980, 95.3% of the total was spent for

TABLE 33-4. National health expenditures according to source of funds: United States, selected years 1929-80

| | | Source of funds | | | | | |
| | | Private | | | Public | | |
Year	All health expenditures in billions	Amount in billions	Amount per capita	Percent of total	Amount in billions	Amount per capita	Percent of total
1929	$ 3.6	$ 3.2	$ 25.49	86.4	$ 0.5	$ 4.00	13.6
1935	2.9	2.4	18.30	80.8	0.6	4.34	19.2
1940	4.0	3.2	23.61	79.7	0.8	6.03	20.3
1950	12.7	9.2	59.62	72.8	3.4	22.24	27.2
1955	17.7	13.2	78.33	74.3	4.6	27.05	25.7
1960	26.9	20.3	110.20	75.3	6.6	36.10	24.7
1965	41.7	30.9	156.32	74.1	10.8	54.57	25.9
1970	74.7	46.9	224.68	62.8	27.8	133.22	37.2
1971	83.3	51.6	244.36	62.0	31.7	149.87	38.0
1972	93.5	58.1	271.89	62.1	35.4	165.88	37.9
1973	103.2	63.9	296.19	61.9	39.3	182.15	38.1
1974	116.4	69.3	318.18	59.5	47.1	216.44	40.5
1975	132.7	76.5	348.08	57.7	56.2	255.49	42.3
1976	149.7	86.7	390.63	57.9	62.9	283.51	42.1
1977	169.2	99.1	442.14	58.6	70.1	312.67	41.4
1978	189.3	110.0	485.29	58.1	79.4	350.27	41.9
1979	214.6	124.5	543.61	58.0	90.1	393.31	42.0
1980	247.2	143.0	617.10	57.8	104.2	449.96	42.2

From Office of Research, Demonstrations, and Statistics: National health expenditures, 1980. In Gibson, R.M., and Waldo, D.R.: Health care financing review, Health Care Financing Administration Pub. No. 03123, Washington, D.C., September 1981, U.S. Government Printing Office.

Public health and health care services

personal care services and supplies, but the amount available for public health activities had declined to 3%.[16,18] What has been described as America's *health care* crisis is really an *economic* crisis in the medical care arena.

Although most of the money spent for public health is tax money, a substantial proportion of that spent on medical care remains a personal obligation and often an unpredictable one. Of the $10.9 billion spent for personal health care in 1950, $7.1 billion (65.5%) was spent as a direct payment by the consumer. The rest was paid by insurance and some government programs. By 1980 the personal or out-of-pocket payments had increased 9.9 times, to $70.6 billion dollars.[16] Although this represented a smaller proportion of the total expenditure for personal health care (32.6% of the $218 billion), the problem of out-of-pocket payments for low-income families, even those with Medicare coverage, remains severe and is growing.

Expenditures for other needs and activities offer an interesting contrast to the amount expended for medical purposes. Table 33-5 presents a breakdown of personal expenditures of the American public in 1980. The public spent more on jewelry than it did on public health, and it spent $20.4 billion on tobacco and $42.8 billion on alcohol. These amounts are less than that spent on medical care to repair damage, but 5 and 10 times greater, respectively, than the expenditures for public health and disease prevention.

How is the medical dollar spent? Table 33-6 presents the breakdown of medically related expenditures for the period from 1960 to 1980. The amount of money spent in each category has increased, but significant shifts have occurred among them in relation to each other. The proportion of the personal health care expenditure dollar now being spent on hospitals has increased from 36% to 42%, whereas the proportions spent for physicians and drugs have decreased. This relative change has been used by organized medicine as a defense against the charge of high prices, but it cannot stand as a defense. It is clear that the cost of hospital care is both directly and indirectly influenced by the admitting physician. As a member of the medical staff, the physician is very persuasive in convincing the hospital administrator and the board of directors to build, expand, improve, and

TABLE 33-5. Personal consumption expenditures, United States, 1980 (in billions of dollars)

Item	Amount
Food	$302.9
Tobacco	20.4
Alcoholic beverages	42.8
Housing	272.0
Household operation	111.7
Transportation	63.8
Clothing and accessories	87.4
Recreation	106.4
Jewelry	10.3

From Bureau of the Census: Statistical abstract of the United States, ed. 102, Washington, D.C., 1981, U.S. Government Printing Office.

TABLE 33-6. Per capita national health expenditures, by type, selected fiscal years, 1960-1980

Type of expenditure	1960	1970	1980
Hospital care	$49	$133	$430
Physicians' services	31	69	201
Dentists' services	11	23	68
Drugs	20	38	83
Nursing home care	3	23	89

From Gibson, R.M., and Waldo, D.R.: National health care expenditures, 1980. In Health care financing review, U.S. Department of Health and Human Services Pub. No. (HCFA) 03123, Fall 1981.

replace. Since most hospital bills are paid by insurance or Medicare and Medicaid, the costs of these changes do not have to come out of profits, as they would in private industry or in the physician's office. When physicians suggest that they may have to start taking some patients to another hospital because it has a new computerized scanner or a new laminar flow operating room, board members and administrators are easily pressured to compete. Once the patient is admitted, it is the physician who decides how much of what will be done for or to the patient. The price of each service or test has already been predetermined by the demands of the medical staff for the procedures and the equipment, and the number of procedures to be performed are decided by the admitting physician as well as by any consultants called in on the case. Virtually all of the procedures and costs of an

TABLE 33-7. Annual rates of price increase, selected periods

Consumer price index	Pre-Medicare 7/59 to 6/66 (%)	Post-Medicare 6/66 to 6/71 (%)	Controls 8/71 to 4/74 (%)	Post-controls 4/74 to 12/74 (%)	1975 (%)
All services except medical care	2.0	5.8	5.2	9.5	7.7
Medical care services	3.2	7.9	4.9	12.1	10.3
Hospitals	6.0	14.8	5.7	16.9	14.7
Physicians	2.9	6.9	4.0	12.8	11.8
Dentists	2.3	5.9	4.2	9.6	7.8
Drugs	−0.7	1.0	0.7	7.8	7.4

Modified from The problem of rising health costs; staff report, Washington, D.C., April 1976, Executive Office of the President, Council on Wage and Price Stability.

episode of illness are under the control of the physician, and the distribution of average annual per capita costs shown in Table 33-6 can obscure that important fact.

When reviewing data such as the above, one must also bear in mind the general inflation that has affected all costs. For example, the costs of dental services and drugs have increased at a rate below that of inflation generally. This is particularly striking with regard to the cost of drugs: even with the high costs attributable to advertising, merchandising, and the unusually high profits enjoyed by pharmaceutical companies generally, the proportion of disposable personal income that goes for the purchase of drugs is approximately one half of what it was in 1940.

A more revealing look at the dynamics of price changes in the medical care industry is contained in a special report of the President's Council on Wage and Price Stability released in April 1976.[19] The council examined the effect of Medicare and Medicaid on medical care price boosts and then examined the effect of the wage and price controls that were in effect from 1971 to 1974. As shown in Table 33-7 the annual rate of increase in the consumer price index for medical care services was slightly greater than that for the rest of the economy in the pre–Medicare/Medicaid years; it increased much faster than the general economy following enactment of the two federal programs and fell off during the period of wage and price controls, only to accelerate at a still greater rate after the controls were taken off.

THE MEDICAL CARE PROBLEM

The data just discussed reveal several factors that indicate the nature of the problem of medical care in the United States. First, it is considered to be a private business, and, except for disease control activities and major public programs in mental health, most medical care is delivered in an environment that is considered to be a private place, even though it is heavily subsidized by public money. It is also clear that the availability of medical care and, more importantly, access to medical care are not distributed in proportion to need but rather in proportion to ability to pay. As Sager[20] and many others have pointed out, hospitals and the physicians who use them are reducing their presence in the inner-city areas where needs are greatest and relocating in more affluent and suburban areas. People with low income need more medical care than people with high income, but it is more difficult for them to obtain it, and current indications are that the disparity is worsening after nearly 2 decades of improvement. Government programs to support third-party payments for low-income and elderly patients are declining, as is federal support for the development of health centers in underserved areas.

While the disparity between need and accessible supply is growing, the cost of the supply has been rising faster than any other sector of the American economy. Reimbursement practices in the medical-industrial sector of the economy are particularly favorable to the manipulation of price by the producer. Physicians function effectively as price set-ters, even when the supply of physicians is increasing. Their performance fits the classic definition of monopoly.

As the interrelationships of health, disability, employment, family stability, and education and the inequitable distribution of the supply of health goods and services have become more apparent, the cost of the product has become so excessive that matters of equity have given way to concerns over the opportunity costs to society in general and to business and government in particular. Health has become a public good, but it is produced in the private sector, largely at public cost, with no ability of the public to control either the cost or the production of services. The difference between a privilege and a right is that the people must guarantee the latter through their government. How this may be accomplished in the present environment is and will continue to be the biggest dilemma in public health.

Rosen,[21,22] in his discussion of the early attempts to solve the problem, rightly highlights the propositions of three outstanding social thinkers of the times: Defoe and Bellers in England and de Chamousset in France. With the development of statistical methodology and the increasing accumulation and analysis of vital data, it became possible, at least in a crude way, to calculate certain types of risks. Marine and fire insurance were fairly well established and used. Life insurance companies were in the process of acceptance. It is not too surprising, therefore, that even at a relatively early date some thought was given to the possibility of applying this valuable social technique to the risk of illness. Daniel Defoe was apparently the first to make the suggestion, in 1697. In an essay he proposed that the insurance principle be applied to the social problems of the poor, including medical and institutional care and disability pensions.

Shortly afterward, in 1714, John Bellers[22] suggested a rather detailed plan for a national health service in England. He believed that the program should be sponsored by government, since "it is too great a burden to be left upon the shoulders, or to the care of the physicians alone, no private purse being able to bear the needful charges of it. . . . the State should bear a good part of the expense of it." He therefore proposed the establishment of government hospitals for teaching and research, a na-

tional health institute, and a plan to provide medical care to the sick poor. Going even further in his social thinking, de Chamousset in 1754 proposed a plan of hospital insurance with a broader population base. Here for perhaps the first time is encountered a concern for others than the traditionally dependent poor, that is, a concern for the bulk of the population comprising the middle class. He argued as follows:

There are asylums available to the destitute, and that is a resource useful to those to whom it is not humiliating to accept the free assistance which charity offers. (But there is) the class of the greatest number of citizens, who not being rich enough to provide sufficient aid at home or poor enough to be taken to an almshouse, languish and often perish miserably, victims of the propriety to which they are subjected by their class of society. Such are the industrious artisans, merchants whose trade is limited, and in general all those valuable men who live daily by the fruits of their labor, and who often for that reason have no recourse to treatment when a disease becomes incurable. The start of a disease exhausts all their resources; the more they deserve help, the less can they bring themselves to profit by the only resources that remain to them, and to find themselves in public asylums.

Unfortunately little came of these suggestions. Eventually, with no action forthcoming from other directions, workers themselves in some parts of England and a few other countries began to inaugurate schemes at their own expense for protecting themselves against the risks of illness and injury. Trade benefit associations and societies were formed to contract with physicians and surgeons for the care of the members of the group, and each worker was assessed a fixed sum for annual dues or fees.

To understand the differences between medical care in Europe and in the United States, one must recognize the difference in the origin of medical care insurance. The first attempts to organize some form of insurance against the risks of medical expenses in Europe were taken by consumers of care. They knew what they wanted and they organized to buy it on their terms. They employed the physicians and decided what services were to be covered by the programs. The first health insurance programs in the United States were organized by producers of medical services (first hospitals and then physicians), and the programs were designed to assure the producers that they would get paid for the services that they had chosen to provide. With very few exceptions (The United Mine

Workers until 1978 and some other group health plans), most medical care insurance programs in the United States were organized by providers and designed to help sell the services they wanted to produce. This difference has a great deal to do with the fact that insurance programs in the United States rarely cover preventive services and tend to pay the most for hospital-based services and for surgery.

By the beginning of the nineteenth century, there had been formed in England nearly 10,000 societies of this type with a total membership of close to a million workers. During the same period, there was much discussion in England concerning the possibility of requiring by law that all workers join privately operated benefit societies, and suggestions were even made that the government should bear part of the cost.

Meanwhile, the medical profession was not entirely inactive. Many steps were being taken to clean house by the development of standards, professional licensure, and the improvement of medical education. Public health measures, in the then ordinary but now narrow sense of state administration of quarantine and public sanitation, were generally supported by the medical profession. Opposition to public provisions for vaccination, however, was not unknown. Support was given to the extension of charity relief and medical care to the indigent. Beyond this, except for rare instances, little was attempted by the medical profession to solve the broader aspects of the medical care problem.

The most significant attempt was made in Germany during the second half of the nineteenth century. It took the form of a nationally sponsored and administered plan for compulsory, comprehensive social insurance. Although it took 9 years of debate in the Reichstag, the plan met with relatively little opposition from German practitioners of medicine. The plan provided for sickness, accident, and old-age benefits, supported by contributions from employees, employers, and the state.

Recognition of the problem and attempts to solve it spread not merely throughout the European continent but beyond to many other parts of the world. One nation after another adopted some form of compulsory health insurance, and at the present time almost every major nation has some plan in operation. No two plans are identical; every major aspect of them shows some variation, whether in comprehensiveness of service, population served,

type of administration and payment, or source of funds. Table 33-8 presents a listing of the years in which some of the major compulsory health insurance plans were enacted.

The National Health Service, which was initiated in England in 1948, attracted much worldwide attention. This plan, adopted by the government over the strong opposition of the medical profession, now claims 97% enrollment. From its inception it has been very comprehensive in its benefits and services. This resulted in considerable difficulty in its early years because of the public rush to remedy vast backlogs of dental and visual defects. Although it is still criticized on various counts by many outside as well as within the medical profession, there is general agreement that it has resulted in more widespread and generally better medical and related services for more people. During this time private health insurance and a small private practice industry have persisted in England. The Thatcher government began to encourage the growth of private plans in an effort to deflect expenditures from the nationally financed health service during the early 1980s. Although that effort could damage the

TABLE 33-8. Dates of enactment of compulsory health insurance, 1883 to 1948

Year	Country
1883	Germany
1888	Austria
1891	Hungary
1909	Norway
1911	Great Britain
1920	Poland
1922	USSR
1922	Yugoslavia
1922	Japan
1922	Greece
1924	Chile
1925	Italy
1928	France
1933	Denmark
1936	Peru
1938	New Zealand
1941	Costa Rica
1943	Mexico
1945	Brazil
1948	England

program if it acquires any significant growth, a certain degree of exit option for dissatisfied customers of the National Health Service could be beneficial.

One important difference among the prepaid medical care systems that have developed in various countries is the method of payment of physicians. As indicated by Glaser,[23] no generally accepted system can be found in Europe at the present time; the following are currently in existence:

1. Fee for service, as in West Germany
2. Salaried physicians, as in Russia, and, for specialists, in Great Britain
3. Capitation payments, as in Great Britain for family practice and in Turkey

The United States was slow to develop any explicit policy or pattern of thought with regard to a delivery system for medical care. This was quite unlike the approach to education, which was from the earliest colonial times considered a public responsibility. There were probably many reasons for this delay. Medical care at its best was crude. There was little chance that a patient would benefit from the work of a medical practitioner in the most advanced communities in Europe. There was a still smaller chance of a favorable outcome in the New World. Since medical care was so poor, it made little sense to the colonists to spend their money providing it to people who could not look after themselves. In addition, each successive wave of the poor represented new colonists, and it was likely that the more established settlers felt that these newcomers should and could make their own way, as had their predecessors. A settler could always find land; thus there was little accepted need for public charity.

Provisions for free medical care were simple and restricted to the very poor. The pattern that was followed varied from one town to another. In some instances a private physician would be engaged, perhaps because of a low bid, at a fixed stipend to provide care to the sick poor. In others stated fees were paid by the town treasurer when bills submitted by a physician were authorized. Not infrequently the fee for each case required a special vote.

From this amorphous beginning emerged the patterns that have been followed ever since. Medical services for the poor traditionally have been considered either as an act of self-protection against contagious disease or as an act of charity. The early benevolent hospitals were built by private citizens;

and, depending on the amounts of their individual contributions, the benefactors were provided with tickets of admission that they could give to the "deserving" poor. To the extent that the process took place in the public sector, a means test was required. On the other hand, public health programs that had as their main concern the prevention of contagious diseases had a rather spectacular growth. Mixed in among these activities were certain medical care responsibilities that the private sector either would not or could not provide.

The largest public sector enterprises were the big state hospitals for the mentally ill and for those with tuberculosis. The sanitaria were built out in the country to isolate the patients from society. In rural communities they were often the largest employers and the largest buyers of food and other commodities and services. Without a merit system of employment or the use of competitive bids, they became major centers of patronage and political control. They could and did house and confine those who were unfortunate enough to become troublesome to influential family members, as well as those who appeared eccentric. Although the large tuberculosis hospitals have given way to modern treatment practices, they are not completely unknown to this day. The big mental health institutions continue at the center of an increasingly heated debate about the role of institutions in treating and creating problems—a debate that has become entangled with arguments about social welfare, zoning, unionization of public employees, the economic development of many small and isolated communities, the role of the foreign medical graduate in providing backup to the private sector, etc.

It is hard to escape the conclusion that the public sector was enabled (or empowered) to become involved in what might otherwise be considered the "practice of medicine" only when the practice was unpalatable or unprofitable to the private sector. Although there has been (and is) great public pressure on health agencies to take more of a leadership role in providing medical care, the profession itself has been mixed in its attitude toward such involvement. Moreover, there has never been a clear mandate to do so or sufficient funds to accomplish what is needed in an acceptable manner. Public health has found itself caught between its past, the forces of organized medicine, hospital interests, private enterprise, public expectations, and its own training. The result has been an extremely heterogeneous array of localized systems and attitudes. The relationship of government and medical care is still evolving in the United States.

That relationship can be examined through three successive periods in history since 1900: the period from 1900 to 1940, which was a period of scientific development and private growth; the period from 1940 to 1960, which was characterized by consolidation and professionalization of the resources of medical care; and the period from 1960 to the present, which could be called the conception of medical mercantilism.

1900 to 1940: scientific development and private growth

The period of scientific development and private growth was characterized by inner direction, self-evaluation, and a gradual acquisition of scientific control that accelerated in its growth throughout the period. It was a time of professional self-determination with little governmental involvement. It was almost totally private.

During the nineteenth century more than 450 medical schools were in operation at one time or another. Most of them were proprietary schools. In conjunction with the Carnegie Corporation, the American Medical Association (AMA) sought an evaluation of the medical situation that resulted in Bulletin No. 4 of the Carnegie Corporation—the Flexner Report.[24] A frank and willful analyst, Abraham Flexner suggested in no uncertain terms that those medical schools that could not acquire the capacity for adequate instruction of a scientific form of medicine should close or be closed. That report marked the beginning of a sense of scientific integrity that has characterized American medical education ever since. As with many other landmarks, later-day historians find much to criticize in the report. Many feel that the Johns Hopkins–Harvard influence over medical education led to overspecialization of medical care in the United States and to some of the organizational and cost problems that now characterize the situation. If someone else had done the job, the report might have taken a different approach and the history of medical care in the United States might have been different—maybe better, maybe worse—but no one else did. The Flexner Report was instrumental in reforming medical education and thus medical care in the United States.

Postgraduate medical education was not common before 1910. Osler and Halstead at Johns Hopkins began to explore continued clinical training at the turn of the century and to model their curriculum on the already well-developed European medical schools. In 1923, 11% of physicians in practice were specialists. By 1979 this had increased to 85%.[25] This commonly stated change tends to be misleading, since many physicians who have specialized in internal medicine or pediatrics can be considered as generalists and are usually classified as part of the group of primary care practitioners. Together these three groups comprise 39% of all practicing physicians, and many general surgeons engage in general practice as well. Nonetheless, specialization is the norm in medical practice as it is in other professional fields in the United States. The emphasis on specialization and subspecialization has led a number of medical educators and political leaders to reemphasize general practice, resulting in the reestablishment of family practice and community medicine as essential parts of the medical curriculum. It has also led to a successful movement to call general practice a specialty, and the American Academy of Family Practice has become increasingly influential in continuing medical education and in the design of health personnel programs.

The evolution of social positions in relation to medical care also took place largely in the private sector during this period. The American Association for Labor Legislation was instrumental in bringing about the widespread enactment of worker's compensation laws. On achieving this success, the Association selected medical care insurance as its next cause. It established a Committee on Social Legislation, which at first was supported and participated in by the AMA. The Progressive Party and its presidential candidate Theodore Roosevelt supported a form of national social insurance that included health insurance. In 1916 the AMA Social Insurance Committee recommended compulsory, state-run health insurance, and in 1917 the AMA House of Delegates adopted principles for a governmental health insurance program.[26] However, with the end of World War I and awareness of the Russian Revolution, many Americans began to fear any form of social insurance. California voters defeated a referendum for a state health insurance program in 1918, and in 1920 under new leadership the AMA began to reverse its earlier position; this led to a 1932 editorial that stated:

Public health and health care services

The alinement [sic] is clear—on the one side the forces representing the great foundations, public health officialdom, social theory—even socialism and communism—inciting to revolution; on the other side, the organized medical profession of this country urging an orderly evolution guided by controlled experimentation which will observe the principles that have been found through the centuries to be necessary to the sound practice of medicine.[27]

In 1927 the Committee on the Costs of Medical Care was established. It was financed by six foundations and included 42 persons representing medicine, public health, institutions, economists, and the general public. Its many studies and reports between 1928 and 1932 resulted in a final report, the conclusion of which has been summarized by Falk[28] in the form of five basic recommendations:

1. Comprehensive medical service should be provided largely by organized groups of practitioners, organized preferably around hospitals, encouraging high standards, and preserving personal relations.
2. All basic public health services should be extended to the entire population, requiring increased financial support, full-time trained health officers and staffs, with security of tenure.
3. Medical costs should be placed on a group payment basis through insurance, taxation, or both; individual fee-for-service should be available for those who prefer it; and cash benefits for wage loss should be kept separate.
4. State and local agencies should be formed to study, evaluate, and coordinate services, with special attention to urban-rural coordination.
5. Professional education should be improved for physicians, health officers, dentists, pharmacists, registered nurses, nursing aids, midwives, and hospital and clinic administrators.

A minority report was submitted. It agreed with recommendations 2, 4, and 5 but took strong exception to recommendations 1 and 3.

In 1933 the American Hospital Association accepted the concept of hospital insurance, which led to the domination of the Blue Cross plans by hospital interests initially. This was a singularly American event. In most European countries health insurance programs were developed through consumer pressure. Although the provider groups became involved in the legislative developments, the purpose was basically to insure consumers for the services they wanted. In the United States,

troubled by the great depression, hospitals saw insurance as a way of increasing the likelihood that they would get paid for the services that they and their medical staffs had decided to provide. This private social action program was followed by a major public effort, the passage of the Social Security Act on August 14, 1935. At its inception the architects of Social Security meant it to be an incremental program growing to a comprehensive national system that would include protection against the costs of medical care as well as all of what has been developed subsequently as a welfare program. However, the impetus for social change began to weaken by the second half of the 1930s, and World War II stopped it altogether. In spite of repeated urgings by some advisors, President Roosevelt never again sponsored national health insurance. He referred to a right to "good medical care" in his State of the Union speech in 1945 but made no specific recommendations.

Public health was quiescent in the medical care arena. The cautious beginnings of public health helped guide the development of state and local health departments and, although the evidence suggested real growth in the movement toward universal public health services for all communities, medical care was not part of the effort. Many communities operated public hospitals and poor farms, and a substantial amount of charity care was actually provided, but most of this took place outside the boundaries of the state or local health department. Medical care was strictly a private affair.

This first period of scientific development and private growth ended as America entered World War II. It had been a period of astounding improvement in medical education and medical practice. American medical care had moved, in a few short decades, from disgraceful resemblance to a carnival, with its patent medicines and quacks, to a position of international eminence, but the nation's position on governmental involvement in the delivery of medical care remained both conservative and confused.

1940 to 1960: consolidation and professionalization

The period from the end of World War II to the early 1960s continued along uniquely American lines. It was a period marked by effective collaboration between the government and private medical care and by consolidation of the scientific and professional gains of the first half of the twentieth century. As Americans turned from war to peace, a number of beliefs and attitudes intermingled, guiding the development of both public and private policy. There was an exuberant sense of prosperity and self-confidence that was marred but not destroyed by the development of an atomic bomb by Russia and by the Communist witch-hunts of Senator McCarthy. There were periods of recession, and employment for returning veterans was a problem; but the general mood was one of relief, optimism, and a feeling that American productive genius could solve all problems.

There was a continued interest in national health insurance, but attempts to develop a program were unsuccessful. Legislation for a national health program was introduced in 1939 by Senator Robert Wagner, and extensive hearings were held. In addition to federal grants to match state expenditures for public health, the bill proposed to offer "services and supplies necessary for the prevention, diagnosis and treatment of illness and disability." This prompted the AMA to call an "emergency" meeting in St. Louis which lead to the formation of the National Physicians' Committee for the Extension of Medical Services. Subsequent action by this committee belied its name; whether because of great pressure from the National Physicians' Committee or for reasons of political expediency, President Roosevelt late in 1939 withdrew his support of the Wagner bill, and it died in Congress. Then the nation entered World War II. The large number of young men who were found unfit for military service because of physical defects obviously contradicted the claim that the American people were receiving adequate medical care. Furthermore, millions of young men and women who served in the armed forces were exposed to a system of medical care operated by the government that served their needs promptly and effectively. Beyond this, while the war was in progress, a public opinion poll by *Fortune* magazine in 1942 indicated that three fourths of the people of the nation were in favor of national health insurance.

Because of these and other factors, Senator Wagner, in company with Senator James Murray and Representative John Dingell, Sr., in mid-1943 sponsored another bill more far-reaching than the earlier one. It proposed comprehensive medical, hospital, dental, and nursing home care for almost the entire population, to be paid for out of a special fund based on equal contributions from employers and employees. The AMA called it "the most virulent scheme ever to be conjured out of the mind of man," and again was successful in causing the bill to die in committee. As the war approached an end, President Truman asked that a new health insurance bill be prepared with careful consideration given to the rights of both the public and the medical profession. As a result, a new Wagner-Murray-Dingell bill was filed, which according to the AMA would "mean the end of freedom for all classes of Americans." This bill, like its predecessors, was also killed.

In 1946, with the war at an end, Senator Robert A. Taft, widely known as a conservative, decided to solve the problem by means of a bill that would provide matching grants to states for medical care for those who on the basis of a means test could be proved to be indigent. The bill appealed to no one, and it is interesting that the AMA called even this tame gesture "socialized medicine." A year later another Wagner-Murray-Dingell bill was introduced. No one expected it to get any further than its predecessors. However, apparently on the basis of President Truman's reelection, the AMA declared a crisis and assessed every member $25 to establish a $3.5 million "war chest" to finance the largest lobby in American history. Despite its earlier opposition, the AMA now claimed that voluntary health insurance was meeting fully the needs of the citizens. Again the bill was defeated in Congress.

In the postwar years the United States began to invest heavily in medical research. The National Cancer Institute had been established in 1937. In 1948 Congress established the Heart Institute and in quick succession the rest of the institutes and centers of the National Institutes of Health—the world's largest medical research center. The extramural research programs sponsored by the institutes touch virtually every area of human physiology and biochemistry as well as every university and medical school in the nation and also in some other countries.

Biomedical research was by no means the only arena in which private medicine and government collaborated in easy comfort. The post-war buoyancy led to the Hill-Burton Act in 1946 and its expansion in 1954. This federal–state–private sector partnership invested nearly $16 billion in new hospitals and other health facilities. It sponsored nearly 11,500 projects and helped build nearly a half million hospital beds. Scarcely a community in the United States was left untouched by this program. By the 1970s the excess of hospital beds in the nation was being attacked as a principal cause of high costs.

Substantial public investments were made in medical education during this period. A program of traineeships established in 1953 had, by 1963, grown to include institutional grants for basic medical education and for the construction of medical schools. The initial investments continued to grow until about 60% of the cost of medical education in the United States was paid for by the federal government.[29] This program, too, came under attack in the 1970s, as a number of health personnel analysts began to question whether the increased production of physicians might serve to drive the cost of medical care still higher.

The Graduate Medical Education National Advisory Committee served as an advisory group to the Secretary of the Department of Health and Human Services from April 1976 to September 1980. Its 107 recommendations led to the conclusion that there would be a substantial oversupply of almost all types of physicians by 1990.[30-33] The general evidence supports the notion that the marked increase in supply has led to better distribution of physicians in urban and rural areas but that a greater number of physicians generally leads to higher rather than lower prices.[34]

During this period organized public health remained officially outside the realm of medical care, but some changes were occurring. The Medical Care Section of the American Public Health Association began to make heretic assertions that the public sector and public health agencies particularly had an obligation to provide medical services especially where they were not generally available. Some local health departments, under local leadership and within their own local customs and history, began to do just that. It was scarcely a movement and it did not influence the general theory about the proper role of public health, but a growing number of people, generally poor people with limited access, began to obtain needed medical services through the programs of their local health department. Although legislative bodies, organized medicine, and the official public health establish-

ment did not assume the responsibility was there, most citizens assumed that their health department was supposed to provide medical care services when they were needed and not otherwise available. Sometimes they could get it. In other communities, they were surprised to find the health officer uninterested and began to get the notion that if they needed a public medical care resource, they would have to turn elsewhere for leadership or do it themselves.

As the United States approached the 1960s and the end of the period of consolidation and professionalization, the public-private concurrence on goals and methods was nearing its end. The investments had been made that would later lead to what has been called the "crisis in American medical care." The crisis appears to have come about because the investments were structured in such a way as to drive up unit costs while decreasing productivity. Moreover, most of the investments were in the treatment and correction of disabilities rather than in their prevention. Rising expectations of what could be accomplished were soon to get dashed on the walls of reality, but the nation entered the next period with a strong and effective system of medical education, medical research, and medical practice. It appeared as if the American way was the right one.

1960 to present: the conception of medical mercantilism

The more recent years have been a period of mixed messages and frustration. The nation failed in its war on poverty but won its race for the moon. It failed in the war in Vietnam but survived a major presidential challenge to its Constitution. Most of all, it has been a period of inexplicable shortages. At times Americans have run out of gas, toilet paper, wheat, beef, oil, and even optimism and prosperity. The period began with continued optimism that has since given way to doubt. A prolonged period of economic stagnation, high interest rates, severe unemployment, and seemingly insoluble budget-balancing problems have caused many to recognize that the era of easy expansion is over. It has become as difficult to solve major social problems in the United States as it is elsewhere: more so, since the period of unblemished growth and expansion continued so long in the United States that most of the people currently alive never knew it could be any other way.

Growing concern about the problems of chronic

and degenerative diseases, especially among the older members of the population, caused the Senate Committee on Labor and Public Welfare to establish a Subcommittee on the Problems of the Aged and Aging. Senator McNamara was made chairman, and he proceeded to conduct public hearings in several cities throughout the nation. The attendance was considerable, and Senator McNamara followed a practice of first listening to experts and then making the microphone available to anyone in the audience. Large numbers of older citizens responded and told of their problems in dramatic and sometimes pathetic form. It became apparent to the nation through these firsthand statements that, contrary to the avowals of the AMA, their needs were not being met. When the subcommittee submitted its report to the Senate in February 1960, its first recommendation was that the Social Security program be expanded to include health service benefits for all persons eligible under the program. Congress now began to be deluged by letters concerning the Forand bill for Social Security beneficiaries, 2 to 1 in favor. This forced the Ways and Means Committee of the House to vote on it. Nonetheless, contrary pressures led to its defeat.

The Eisenhower Administration finally presented a bill of its own called the Medicare Program for the Aged. Viewed superficially, the administration bill seemed to go even further than the Forand bill. However, when the various deductibles and exceptions were considered, few elderly people could benefit much. As a result, it received little support from any quarter. Nevertheless, it served an unintended purpose: it indicated that by this time both political parties manifested an obligation on the part of the federal government to somehow provide medical care for the indigent and elderly. Meanwhile, the Forand bill was again defeated in committee.

Soon afterward, the House passed a bill introduced by Congressman Mills, empowering the federal government to make grants to states to provide medical care for the elderly poor. It was not, however, to be financed through the Social Security system. This was quickly followed by a bill in the Senate under the sponsorship of Senator Kerr, the intention of which was to assist the aged who were neither poor enough to be on welfare nor wealthy enough to pay their own medical expenses. Again, financing would be by federal grants matching state expenditures. Wilbur Cohen, who drafted the bill for Kerr, adroitly included in it much of the intent of Congressman Mills' bill. It passed both houses with little opposition, and in mid-September 1960 the President signed what became known as the Kerr-Mills Act. The new act lacked many things. It was estimated that actually only about 2 million persons would be assisted by it. Interestingly, whereas the AMA did not oppose it, apparently on the basis of the lesser of two evils, it included many principles to which that organization had been objecting over the years. It consisted of two parts: (1) extension of the Old-Age Assistance Program, which had originated with the 1935 Social Security Act; and (2) a new section known as the Medical Assistance for the Aged Program. The intent of this was to provide medical services for elderly citizens who previously were ineligible for aid—in other words the so-called medically indigent who were over 65 years of age and who, although not on relief, could not meet the cost of medical services. The legislation placed no ceiling on federal support for this part of the act; the federal government would pay a flat percentage of total outlays ranging from 50% for high-income states to 80% for poorer states. It was left entirely to the states to determine whether they wished to participate in the program. Furthermore, individual states could set not only their own income limits and deductibles but also all the conditions for the provision of care. The overall result was that many states did not elect to participate in the Kerr-Mills Act, and the conditions established by those that did presented all possible variations. Although the AMA during the next several years spent large sums of money to try to convince everyone that the Kerr-Mills program was actually meeting the needs, it became apparent very shortly that this was far from the truth.

When Senator John Kennedy became President-elect, he let it be known that one of the first items on the agenda for his administration would be the enactment of a health insurance bill for the aged. Shortly after he took office, Representative King and Senator Anderson served as cosponsors of what became known as the Medicare bill. Its provisions were extensive, and again it was proposed to be financed by an increase in Social Security assessments. It called forth the usual and expected accusations and cries of alarm from the AMA, which promptly established an American Medical Political

Action Committee to raise several million dollars with which to fight it. The bill had great support, however, not only from the public but also from organizations such as the National Council of Churches, the YWCA, the American Nurses' Association, the American Hospital Association, and the American Public Health Association. In addition, groups of physicians in several places in the nation disassociated themselves from the AMA to form endorsing groups. Despite this, the bill was defeated in the Senate by a close vote. It was reintroduced in 1963 at President Kennedy's request, but his assassination brought hearings on the matter to a halt. The Vice President, Lyndon Johnson, had made clear his support of the Medicare idea while he was the majority leader in the Senate.

After election in his own right, in his State of the Union address on January 4, 1965, at the opening of the Eighty-ninth Congress, President Johnson made a strong call for action on a Medicare bill as the first order of business. Promptly, Senator Anderson introduced S. 1, and Representative King introduced H.R. 1—identical bills that were very similar to those they had introduced in the previous Congress. In short order several other bills were introduced, among them one by Representative Byrnes, which provided for subsidies to pay for private health insurance policies, and one to expand and liberalize the Kerr-Mills Act. To the surprise of everyone, Representative Mills, as Chairman of the Ways and Means Committee of the House, suddenly resolved the problem by deciding on a meld of the King-Anderson bills, the bill to expand and liberalize the Kerr-Mills Act, and Representative Byrnes' bill. As he explained, this would provide a sort of three-layer cake: the expanded Kerr-Mills program making up the bottom layer to take care of those who were close to indigency; Medicare making up the middle layer to take care of the cost of hospital, nursing home, and home health care for the rest of the elderly; and the voluntary supplement making up the top layer to take care of physicians' fees, in and out of hospital. The bill to accomplish this was drawn up by Wilbur Cohen at the Ways and Means Committee's request and was finally approved by the House of Representatives by a vote of 313 to 115 and passed the Senate by a vote of 68 to 21.

On July 30, 1965, President Johnson flew to Independence, Mo., to sign the bill into P.L. 89-97 at the Harry S. Truman Memorial Library in honor of the former President, who had fought so valiantly for the principle of health insurance. Title XVIII of the act (Medicare) provided help for everyone 65 years or older through the Social Security program. Title XIX (Medicaid) extended eligibility to all persons who were eligible for federally aided public assistance programs—the aged, the blind, the disabled, and families receiving assistance through Aid to Dependent Children. For the aged, Title XIX (a welfare program administered by the states) could serve as a supplement to Title XVIII, the basic Medicare section, since it allowed states to pay both the deductibles and the voluntary medical insurance premiums for the aged who were wholly dependent on old-age assistance. The states were enabled to develop their own Title XIX programs, ranging from very comprehensive systems to none at all.

The Eighty-ninth Congress passed an astonishing array of social legislation, frequently rushing incomplete social experiments into national programs. Among the major pieces of legislation were the Community Mental Health Act (P.L. 89-105), the Regional Medical Programs (P.L. 89-239), the Health Professions Education and Assistance Act (P.L. 89-290), the Comprehensive Health Planning Act (P.L. 89-749), and the Model Cities Act (P.L. 89-754), in addition to Medicare and Medicaid. Since that time, a number of related acts have been passed: the Health Maintenance Organization Act (P.L. 93-222), the Professional Standards Review Organization law (P.L. 92-603), and the National Health Planning and Resources Development Act of 1974 (P.L. 93-641). If this legislation is reviewed in sequence, some trends and changes become evident. The Regional Medical Programs were in the tradition of the 1950s. Their purpose was to speed up the application of research through more or less traditional, university-linked methods, directed by the traditional academic and medical structure. Even so, it expressed discontent: how come, after billions of dollars had been spent on research, was there a continued epidemic of death and disability caused by heart disease, cancer, and stroke? The question was critical, but the answer seemed to be that the federally supported research effort had failed to make adequate provisions for the application of its findings. To speed this up, Congress turned to the medical schools and to the medical profession to bridge the gap.

Medicare and Medicaid were not overtly critical of American medicine. In fact, the legislation contained language specifically prohibiting any federal official from implementing the laws in such a way as to interfere with the traditional practice of medicine. But clearly something was wrong. Not only were congressional leaders concerned that their research efforts had not been more beneficial in more practical ways but they were now aware that a lot of people could not afford the medical care they needed and that some were being impoverished by illness. Moreover, they knew that organized medicine was strongly opposed to the federal government doing anything about these problems. Public criticism was becoming much more focused and audible.

The first health planning legislation (the Comprehensive Health Planning Act of 1966) was more overtly critical and pointed in its implications. The nation was concerned about cost and equity and did not like the way decisions were being made. To correct these problems, the law mandated the development of planning bodies that would limit the role of providers of medical care services. In addition, an important change was made in the definition of "need" as it related to the construction of buildings and programs. Up until that time, from an operational standpoint, the test of need for new health facility construction had been whether or not the providers needed it. The new test was to be whether or not the community needed it; and the community, represented by a majority of consumers, would vote on the issues. The success of this venture is still being debated, but its implications are unmistakable. The same criticism was apparent in the Model Cities Act and in the War on Poverty. It was both criticism and support at the same time—criticism of the medical care establishment and support for the ability of the people to make complex decisions.

There was a relative hiatus in such social experimentation until the 1970s, by which time there was considerable dissatisfaction with the new experiments as well as with the medical care establishment. Official public health agencies were included in this dissatisfaction. Medical care costs were increasing at an alarming rate; expectations, particularly in the inner cities, had risen far higher than Congress and the state legislatures were willing to go. The nation's health care bill, $3.6 billion in 1929, had risen to $163 billion by 1977—8.8% of the gross national product. Moreover, there were plenty of facts to suggest that the health status of Americans was not as good as that of the people of many countries who spent a far smaller proportion of their wealth on medical care.

Economists were seriously concerned about cost. They saw an industry that seemed to be functioning outside of normal market restraints—in fact, it seemed to operate in defiance of the rules of a free enterprise economy as they had been taught. Legislation led to the increased production of physicians, in part to increase competition and reduce costs. But the result seemed to be a decline in productivity and an increase in unit costs. Medicare and Medicaid were designed to increase the ability of the elderly and the poor to get needed medical care, but the result was a net transfer of dollars to the providers of care and away from everyone else. Costs increased at such a pace during the early 1970s that a straight-line projection pointed to a possible national cost of a half-trillion dollars by 1986. It was not just cost in terms of the number of dollars that was so alarming: it was the opportunity cost. As the percentage of the gross national product required to pay the nation's medical bill grew toward 10%, it reduced the opportunity to make investments in virtually all other areas—in education, in the construction of new factories, in the development of new sources of energy, in the maintenance of roads, in agriculture, and in human nutrition.

The next wave of legislation was more sharply critical than ever before of the established structure for providing medical care. The Health Maintenance Organization Act (P.L. 93-222), requested by a Republican president, was a direct attempt to change the market forces operating in the medical care industry in a specific direction. The knowledge that General Motors had a bigger contract with Blue Cross than with U.S. Steel had come as a shock to the business community. It was becoming clear that the cost of medical care was depressing wages, profits, and the ability to make capital investments in future production. Medical care clearly had a growing and significant impact on the economic development of the entire nation. That impact might not have been readily seen or realized by individual practitioners or most families, but union leaders, corporate managers, and economic analysts pored over the figures, trying to find out why costs were going up and employment was going down. Although no one would have suggested that medical care alone was responsible, the aggregate costs became apparent. It was an alarming situation: the private physician, practicing in what had been described as the "cottage industry" of medical care, was beginning to influence all other sectors of the economy. Some entrepreneurs were quick to take advantage of the situation—computer manufacturers, accountants, architects, students, and other health workers (the industry employed about four million workers)—but most people in business, in labor, and in government were worried.

In 1972, the Ninety-second Congress passed the Professional Standards Review Organization Amendment to the Social Security Act (P.L. 92-603). Ostensibly a measure to monitor and improve the quality of medical care, this amendment was clearly aimed at cost constraint—one of the new and popular phrases in the lexicon of social engineering. Another slap at the health establishment was taken by Congress when it passed the National Health Planning and Resources Development Act of 1974 (P.L. 93-641; see Chapter 11). This new act strengthened the basic concepts of the older Comprehensive Health Planning Act of 1966, even though that act had not been particularly successful, by limiting and making more complex the involvement of providers and by giving to successful Health Systems Agencies the authority to actually review and approve or reject local proposals for the use of federal project and formula grant funds. Although the law made it possible for local governments to form Health Systems Agencies, it was very difficult for them to do so, and most of the new organizations were formed as private, not-for-profit corporations tied to the Department of Health, Education, and Welfare for guidance and continued grant support.

While efforts were being made to bring the medical services industry under control, other efforts were being made to develop a stronger public delivery system. The neighborhood health center concept of the Economic Opportunity Program had become a standard part of the Public Health Service's repertoire, and urban and rural community health centers were developed in communities throughout the United States, often in conjunction with other categoric funding, private foundation support, and the revenue sources of the Medicaid and Medicare programs. The National Health Service Corps, which was designed to make trained health professionals available in medically underserved areas, was used to help staff the community health centers. The scaffolding for a nationally funded health service network of ambulatory care centers was in place by the late 1970s. President Carter promised to produce a national health insurance proposal as did Senator Kennedy, and their emissaries met to work out their differences with the Secretary of Health, Education, and Welfare, Joseph Califano, as a third participant in the process. However, nothing came of it. Costs were continuing to rise, and Congress began to develop an awareness of the size of their social programs and tried unsuccessfully to bring the cost-escalation process under control. They were unable to cap Medicare and Medicaid, and they were unable to block increases in hospital reimbursement. In that climate, it became apparent that a national health insurance plan would cost more than anyone was willing to pay.

President Reagan was elected on a platform that was plainly opposed to spending for domestic or human service programs and was supportive of the private economy to produce whatever reforms might be needed in health care. The mood of the country was, at least for a short while, congruent with the new President's attitude, and Congress proceeded to roll back 45 years worth of social legislation and make huge cuts in maternal and child health programs, community health center support, and the Medicare and Medicaid programs. The architect of the market competition approach to economic reform in health care was Alain Enthoven.[35] There were many different versions, but the basic elements included (1) a requirement that employers offer a choice of at least two distinctly different types of health insurance plans for their employees; (2) that the employer's contribution to the health plan cost be fixed at the same level for all types of plans and that, above a certain level, that contribution would be treated as taxable income to the employee; and (3) if the employee chose a plan that cost more than the employer's contribution, the employee would have to pay the difference with after-tax income. There were many different approaches to the use of tax incentives to modify both employee and employer attitudes toward health insurance and to the financing of health insurance for low-income and unemployed people, but the concept clearly espouses continued

reliance on private medical practice with less regulation by government as well as less federal support for the direct provision of health services by
public health agencies. This approach to the problem of assuring access to medical care is peculiarly
American and is either a quaint anachronism or a
remarkably prescient venture into the future.

THE FUTURE

While the executive and legislative branches
of government have moved away from tax financing of medical care and toward a market approach to delivery and reform, state and local
government and the private sector have been
moving in some contrary directions. Most local
health departments now consider the provision of
medical care services as a public responsibility and
many state health departments support the community health center movement.[36,37] States have
also developed sophisticated planning and regulatory control programs[38] and a number of creative
experiments in the use of the Medicaid program.[39]
Recent legislation makes it possible for the states
to obtain waivers and exceptions to the requirements of the Medicaid program and develop a public sector response to the unmet needs of the poor
and the medically indigent. Even so, with cuts in
federal support for the Medicaid program and difficulties in bringing effective controls to bear on
hospital costs and nursing home use, most states
have found it necessary to reduce their Medicaid
programs.

Miller and Moos[37] have reviewed the existing
data, and the overall picture is one in which approximately 20 million Americans receive part or
all of their health care through the infrastructure
of the health departments and community health
centers. They are not all uninsured nor are they all
poor, but most of those who use the public systems
would have a difficult time obtaining needed medical care were it not for such organized programs.
There are about 22 to 25 million uninsured people
in the United States at any time, consisting of about
18.2 million who are always uninsured and another
16 million people who are either uninsured part of
the time or all of the time for some services.[40] Whenever they are poor they turn to public organizations
for help. The public organizations are having a hard
time. In California, then Governor Reagan set in
motion a series of actions that resulted in a significant reduction in the number of public hospitals.
In 1960 there were 49 public general hospitals in

California's 58 counties. By 1980 there were only
37 public hospitals operating in 29 counties. Fourteen other counties had experimented with management contracts with private firms in an effort
to reduce the county tax burden of operating a public hospital, but the efforts have not been successful.[41] The management firms did have some success in increasing billings to third-party–payment
sources, but they did not reduce the cost of care.
The basic motivation of the counties was fiscal:
under the Governor's leadership, the property tax
cost of the public hospitals increased rapidly and
the state made every effort to convince the counties
to close their operations and join with the state in
reducing the cost of indigent care rather than to
attempt to operate a public hospital and capture
more Medicaid revenue.

Shonick and Roemer, in their review of the experience,[41] proceed to make a disquieting observation. The evidence suggests that the private sector has clearly recognized the fiscal advantages of
investing in the health care system. With its cost-
based reimbursement support and extensive insurance coverage, the return on an investment in
health care is greater than can be realized in virtually any other segment of the economy. In the
1960s and early 1970s it was hoped that businesses
and labor would begin to recognize the losses they
were incurring through the unique economics of
medical care. The cost of medical insurance began
to represent one of the most expensive commodities
purchased by manufacturing industries—a greater
part of the purchase price of a new car than the
products of U.S. Steel. This reduced profits to the
owners and wages to the workers. There are some
signs in some communities that business and
labor have formed effective coalitions to produce
new and more responsive forms of medical care
such as prepayment systems and health maintenance organizations in which enrollees pay a fixed
premium and are entitled to all covered services
without additional cost.[42] The advantages of such
systems are well known by now, but they are not
widespread. In many communities, the business
leaders seemed to have realized the profitability of
the medical business and have formed new medical-industrial complexes that have the potential for
rivaling the "big three" auto makers in size and
revenue in a few years. Hospital chains have not

only developed management contracts but have bought voluntary hospitals and built new ones, chains have merged and formed still larger corporations, and the owners have begun to move aggressively into the provision of ambulatory care and community-based, free-standing "emergency centers," which are little more than high-priced drop-in clinics. The employed physicians receive a percentage of the gross and are expected to double the billed price of every visit by ordering laboratory and x-ray services, which are provided by the parent hospital corporation. They often receive a bonus for patients admitted to the hospital. The profitability of such enterprises is such that physician incomes have taken another leap upward. Given the ability of the physician to increase revenue for the corporation by ordering tests, medications, operations, hospitalizations, and other ancillary services, physician earnings of $200,000 per year are neither unusual nor a source of concern to the corporation. Lacking federal government support and faced with state legislative bodies that are reluctant to increase the state's vulnerability to pay for medical care costs that they cannot control, public sector enterprises are going to have a very difficult time surviving the 1980s. Given the entrepreneurial instincts of the private sector and their insistence on proof of ability to pay at the outset of any encounter, it is more important than ever to preserve a vigorous public presence in both ambulatory care and hospital care.

It seems likely that the trend toward oligopoly now going on will lead to further corporate concentration of the resources of medical care in the space of the next 5 to 8 years. By the end of the decade it is likely that a few corporations will have effective control over most of the medical care business in the United States and that they will be the principal negotiators with Congress and the White House over the size of the health care budget and the uses to which it can be put. At that point the nation will have moved from a cottage industry through competitive growth to corporate socialism and centralization of control in what may function as a national health service corporation. Public sector strength at the state and local level will then determine whether that corporation can be decentralized to meet the needs of communities or whether it will continue to be treated as a problem in fiscal management at the national level.

REFERENCES

1. Falk, I.S., Rorem, C.R., and Ring, M.D.: The costs of medical care: a summary of investigations of the economic aspects of the prevention and care of illness, Chicago, 1933, University of Chicago Press.
2. Raffel, M.W.: The U.S. health system: origins and functions, New York, 1980, John Wiley & Sons, Inc.
3. Donabedian, A.: Aspects of medical care administration: specifying requirements for health care, Cambridge, Mass., 1973, Harvard University Press.
4. Starr, P.: The social transformation of American Medicine, New York, 1982, Basic Books, Inc., Publishers.
5. Feldstein, M.: Hospital costs and health insurance, Cambridge, Mass., 1981, Harvard University Press.
6. Shryock, R.H.: In Galdston, I., editor: Social medicine, New York, 1949, Commonwealth Fund.
7. Kircher, A.: Scrutinium pestis, Rome, 1658. Noted in Garrison, F.H.: History of medicine, Philadelphia, 1929, W.B. Saunders Co.
8. Snow, J.: On the pathology and mode of communication of cholera, The London Medical Gazette **9:**730, 745, 923, 1849.
9. Lister, J.: On the antiseptic principle in the practice of surgery, Lancet **2:**353, 1867.
10. Koch, R.: Berliner Klinische Wochenschrifte **19:**221, 1882.
11. Osler, W.: Quoted in Ravenal, M.P., editor: Foreward to a half century of public health, New York, 1921, American Public Health Association.
12. Behneman, H.M.F.: Leaves from a doctor's notebook of seventy years ago, Milit. Surgeon **86:**547, June 1940.
13. Scitovsky, A.: Changes in the use of ancillary services for "common" illnesses. In Altman, S.H., and Blendon, R., editors: Medical technology: the culprit behind health care costs? Department of Health, Education, Welfare Pub. No. (PHS) 79-3216, Washington, D.C., 1979.
14. Bureau of the Census: Statistical abstract of the United States, ed. 102, Washington, D.C., 1981, U.S. Government Printing Office.
15. Warren, B.S., and Sydenstricker, E.: Health insurance, the medical profession, and public health, Public Health Rep. **34**(16), April 18, 1919.
16. Gibson, R.M., and Waldo, D.R.: National health care expenditures, 1980. In Health Care Financing Review, U.S. Department of Health and Human Services Pub. No. (HCFA) 03123, Fall 1981.
17. Freeland, M.S., and Schendler, C.E.: National health expenditures: short-term outlook and long-term projections. In Health Care Financing Review, Winter 1981, U.S. Department of Health and Human Services.
18. Gibson, R.M., and Fisher, C.R.: National health expenditures, fiscal year 1977, Soc. Security Bull. **41:**3, July 1978.
19. The problem of rising health care costs; staff report,

Washington, D.C., April 1976, Executive Office of the President, Council on Wage and Price Stability.

20. Sager, A.: Causes and consequences of urban hospital closure, Annual meeting of the American Public Health Association, Los Angeles, November, 1981.

21. Rosen, G.: Provision of medical care—history, sociology, innovation, Public Health Rep. **74**:199, March 1959.

22. Rosen, G. In Galdston, I., editor: Social medicine, New York, 1949, Commonwealth Fund.

23. Glaser, W.R.: Paying the doctor, Baltimore, 1970, The Johns Hopkins University Press.

24. Flexner, A.: Medical education in the United States and Canada, New York, 1910, Carnegie Foundation.

25. Office of Health Research, Statistics and Technology: Health: United States, 1981, U.S. Department of Health and Human Services pub. no. (PHS) 82-1232.

26. Corning, P.A.: The evolution of medicare, Research Report No. 29, Washington, D.C., 1969, U.S. Department of Health, Education, and Welfare, Social Security Administration.

27. Editorial: J.A.M.A. **99**:1952, Dec. 3, 1932.

28. Falk, I.S.: The committee on the costs of medical care—25 years of progress, Am. J. Public Health **48**:979, Aug. 1958.

29. U.S. Department of Health, Education, and Welfare: Trends affecting the U.S. health care system, DHEW Pub. No. (HRA) 76-14503, Washington, D.C., 1975.

30. Graduate Medical Education National Advisory Committee Staff Papers: Physician manpower requirements, DHEW Pub. No. (HRA) 78-10, Hyattsville, Md., 1978, U.S. Department of Health, Education, and Welfare.

31. Graduate Medical Education National Advisory Committee Staff Papers: Supply and distribution of physicians and physician extenders, DHEW Pub. No. (HRA) 78-11, Hyattsville, Md., 1978, U.S. Department of Health, Education, and Welfare.

32. Graduate Medical Education National Advisory Committee Staff Papers: Physician requirements forecasting: need-based versus demand-based methodologies, DHEW Pub. No. (HRA) 78-12, Hyattsville, Md., 1978, U.S. Department of Health, Education, and Welfare.

33. Graduate Medical Education National Advisory Committee Staff Papers: Social and psychological characteristics in medical specialty and geographic decisions, DHEW Pub. No. (HRA) 78-13, Hyattsville, Md., 1978, U.S. Department of Health, Education, and Welfare.

34. Ginzberg, E., and others: The expanding physician supply and health policy: the clouded outlook, Milbank Mem. Fund Q. **59**(4):508, Fall 1981.

35. Enthoven, A.: Health plan: the only practical solution to the soaring costs of medical care, Reading, Mass., 1980, Addison-Wesley Publishing Co., Inc.

36. Jain, S.C., editor: Role of state and local governments in relation to personal health services, Am. J. Public Health **71**(suppl. 1), January 1981.

37. Miller, C.A., and Moos, M.-K.: Local health departments: fifteen case studies, Chapel Hill, N.C., 1981, American Public Health Association.

38. Wagner, D.A.: Constraining the hospital bed supply: state of New Jersey, Annual meeting of the American Public Health Association, Los Angeles, November 1981.

39. Recent and proposed changes in state medicaid programs, Washington, D.C., 1981, Intergovernmental Health Policy Project.

40. Wilensky, G.R., and Walden, D.C.: Minorities, poverty, and the uninsured, Annual meeting of the American Public Health Association, Los Angeles, November 1981.

41. Shonick, W., and Roemer, R.: Private management of public hospitals: the California experience, J. Public Health Policy **3**(2):182, June 1982.

42. HMO promise and performance, Milbank Mem. Fund Q. (special issue) **58**(4), Fall 1980.

CHAPTER 34

Emergency health services

The ancient Chinese word for "crisis" is made up of two characters.
One means "danger" and the second means "opportunity."

BACKGROUND

One of the most visible of the many critical areas in health care is the appalling amount of disability and loss of life from sudden catastrophic illness and accidents. A few years ago, the nation experienced its two millionth traffic fatality, about the same number as the total population of the American colonies when they achieved their independence, 200 years before. About 50,000 such deaths occur each year, accompanied by more than 4.6 million highway injuries. The toll from nonhighway accidents in the home, at work, and at play is no less alarming. It totals over 57,000 deaths each year plus 67 million nonfatal injuries, resulting in 650 million restricted activity days. Twenty-one and a half million injuries affect children under the age of 16.[1] Currently accidents kill more people in the age groups up to 39 years than any other single factor and are the fourth largest cause of death after that age. The costs of accidental death, disability, and property damage are phenomenal and are estimated at about $62 billion a year.[2] One of the most distressing facts about this carnage is that studies have demonstrated that 15% to 20% of accidental highway deaths could be avoided if prompt, effective care were available at the scene of the emergency, on the way to the hospital, and within it.[3,4]

The situation with regard to sudden medical emergencies is no less disconcerting. Included in this category are coronary occlusions, cerebrovascular strokes, diabetic crises, precipitous miscarriages or deliveries, and various other sudden critical events.

Although there are many assertions about the number of lives that could be saved if a completely developed emergency medical system were universally in place, reliable estimates are simply not available. As will be discussed later, it seems likely that the potential salvage rate for heart attack victims is about 10% to 30% when considering what is realistically feasible rather than what the most optimistic entrepreneurs of emergency services have suggested. In all, Huntley[5] has estimated that prompt and proper emergency care could save about 60,000 lives annually, as shown in Table 34-1.

The amount of suffering, disability, lost income, and the like that could be avoided is impossible to estimate. Then there is perhaps the most ignored component of emergencies—the sociopsychiatric emergency, which includes suicidal and homicidal attempts, battered children and spouses, destructive manic states, drug and alcohol crises—all of which cry for attention and help. This necessitates a broad definition of an emergency as an unforeseen event that affects an individual in such a manner as to require immediate care (physical, psychologic, or social).

Individuals in need of emergency assistance usually have a difficult time finding the appropriate service in most communities and lose vital time in

TABLE 34-1. Deaths preventable annually by proper emergency care, United States, 1970

Medical emergency	Number of deaths
Myocardial infarction	35,000
Vehicular accidents	12,000
Other trauma	6,000
Stroke	2,500
Poisonings, drownings	2,500
Other	2,000
TOTAL	60,000

obtaining care. In many communities emergency patients are transported past an appropriate emergency facility to another hospital because of poor planning and coordination. The patient is thereby denied prompt access to the needed service. For the patient with a heart attack, severe respiratory distress, or extensive bleeding, the difference in time may be a life or death matter. Careful studies in the Seattle area have shown that an immediate response to cardiac arrest must be made within 4 minutes and definitive care initiated within 10 minutes to reap the benefits of modern emergency medical care.[6] In addition, many patients with nonmedical emergency problems are taken inappropriately to a hospital emergency room, where they are not properly attended and where they add to the confusion of a trauma center. Most hospital emergency rooms are poorly equipped with personnel, equipment, or inclination to effectively help the drunk, the addict, the confused, and the abused.

In a description of emergency health services, two phenomena become apparent: (1) considering the attention paid to the development of emergency health services systems in recent years, the data available at the national level are remarkably poor; and (2) the planning that has been done has been accepted as an appropriate involvement of the public in what was until recently considered to be the private practice of medicine. That planning has resulted in an assessment of need, design of systems, work force analysis, training programs, and evaluative methodology that could be readily applied to health care generally with great benefit.

THE PROBLEM

The status of all aspects of emergency health care resources in general leaves much to be desired. In spite of rapid improvements in the past 10 years, there are inadequacies in planning, training, equipment, and especially coordination. To approach the problem perhaps backward, there has been a duplicative and often wasteful proliferation of emergency rooms (not necessarily emergency departments) in most hospitals regardless of need, essentially to meet hospital accreditation standards and also as a means of providing a base of inpatients.

By the end of World War II, many general hospitals had what could only be called "accident rooms"—a crude space used for sewing up minor lacerations and applying casts to simple fractures. Emergency rooms presumably had more equipment and were better able to meet the needs of trauma victims, but it was not until the late 1960s that organized emergency departments were established with personnel specially trained for the work. The mere existence of an emergency room with the familiar blue and white sign does not assure that needed services can be found. In 1971 only 10% of the 5,130 hospitals that had some sort of emergency room were considered equipped to handle all medical and surgical emergencies.[7] In a later study, less than 20% of New Jersey hospitals met all of the criteria for adequacy as specified by the Committee on Trauma of the American College of Surgeons.[8] While the annual statistical report of the American Hospital Association[9] indicates that slightly more than 80% of the 6,321 reporting hospitals have emergency departments, it is clear that the Association's definition (which only requires 24-hour staffing) does not touch on the issue of adequacy or competency. Ten years ago very few hospitals could communicate with ambulances or ambulance workers while they were in the field. Unfortunately, there is surprisingly little reliable information presently available about the current situation. Empirically it has improved considerably, although there are still major gaps, particularly at the boundary between two geographic regions.

Most of the improvement in recent years has been in the management of physical trauma and heart attacks. Hospitals have done relatively little to improve their ability to respond to psychiatric emergencies. The typical pattern a decade ago involved a voluntary rotation of physicians on the medical staff of the hospital through an emergency room duty assignment. This usually did not involve full-time presence in the emergency room, but on-call status, and it did not involve a review of individual capabilities. In recent years, residents in training programs have staffed emergency rooms as a way of earning extra money, but this sometimes left a heart attack patient in the care of an ear, nose, and throat resident. Another common practice has involved the "importation" of graduates of foreign medical schools who were employed to work in hospital emergency rooms. They often provided nighttime coverage for inpatient problems as well as emergency room staffing, but, once again, their training, qualifications, and interest in the work were rarely examined. Since the early 1970s the situation has improved considerably through better training, regional planning, improved communications, and the grading of hospital emergency facilities to indicate their capability for responding to different kinds of emergencies. Overall it appears likely that about one third of the total U.S. population is adequately served by either a basic or advanced life-support system.[10] (A definition of advanced and basic life support is discussed later.)

In 1976 there were more than 72 million patient visits to hospital emergency facilities in the United States. The number has been increasing at the rate of 10% a year. One third of all such visits are not actually emergencies; rather, they occur because of the convenience of a known location where health care is accessible 24 hours a day or because those who come have limited funds or nowhere else to go. This problem is increasing as the costs of health care go up, access to private physicians becomes more difficult, home visits become more rare, and the transiency of family residence increases. There is a serious need, therefore, to sort those who come to emergency departments into at least four groups: (1) those who have true medical emergencies and require the paraphernalia of an emergency room to preserve life or prevent irreversible harm, (2) patients who have urgent medical problems and need care sooner than could otherwise be scheduled but who would not be harmed by a delay of a few hours, (3) patients who have nonemergent medical problems but who are using the emergency room for their source of ambulatory care, and (4) the large and troubled group of people who have nonmedical emergencies. Special attention needs to be given to the last two groups, since they represent a major and growing public health problem that has not been responded to effectively by most hospitals and physicians.

The first group—those with true medical emergencies—requires the services of a well-equipped emergency center, a trained and coordinated prehospital response capability, and a good communications system. This is the area that has received most of the attention and money in recent years in the United States, and progress has been rapid. The second group—nonemergent medical patients—needs better access to primary care, either through private or public clinics or through a hospital-based "drop in" clinic. The third group—those without a family physician—needs the services of a system of primary care as well as better information about available services and how to use them.

The fourth group—those with nonmedical emergency problems—presents the most difficult challenge to health planners. The precipitating event may be an attempted suicide, an episode of child abuse, an acute emotional crisis, acute or chronic alcoholism, or the death of a parent. There may be an acute medical problem complicating the analysis of the situation, but, more often than not, the problem is nonmedical and requires the knowledge and skills of professionals who are not often found in hospital-based emergency rooms—community workers, mental health counselors, alcoholism workers, social workers, and others. Not only are hospitals not equipped to react to such problems effectively but those requiring help can be harmed by the inherently trauma-oriented climate of the emergency room. Then too, such individuals are a source of frustration to the trauma-oriented staff, since they demand time and services the staff cannot supply and use space the staff would rather have for other purposes. The result is often an exacerbation of the individual's problem and a sense of anger and frustration on the part of the professional staff, who may stereotype such individuals as "crocks," "drunks," or "psychos," thus leading to an even worse confrontation when the next episode occurs. Although such episodes are common and serious, it is difficult to organize a planned and systematic response since there is no established income or profit-earning group involved. Laboratory and x-ray equipment is not needed, and fee-for-service practitioners are rarely to be found. Moreover, such emergency work is held in low esteem by the professions that need to be involved. The nonmedical, community-based crisis response system is one of the most important areas requiring community planning on an interagency level. Most textbooks on emergency medical services do not cover the subject.

The Community Mental Health Services Act of 1963 included emergency mental health services as one of the required elements in a community mental health program. The Joint Commission on the Accreditation of Hospitals accredits community mental health centers and requires crisis stabilization services for accreditation.[11] Jacobson[12] has categorized the services into three types: suicide prevention centers, evaluation and referral systems, and crisis intervention programs. He also describes two separate studies with suggestive results. In one of the studies 12.2% of the patients seen at a community mental health center as emergencies had a prior history of hospitalization for psychiatric problems. In the other study 12.5% of psychiatric patients seen in a hospital emergency room had a prior history of psychiatric hospitalization. The two groups may have been grossly similar, but the community mental health center staff described 16.7% of their patients as psychotic, whereas the hosptial staff labeled 46% of their patients psychotic. Although the two studies were not done for purposes of comparison, the suggestive results have a plausible explanation. The staff of a hospital emergency room is oriented toward quick problem solving and movement of patients as rapidly as possible, either to their homes or into the hospital as inpatients. The quickest way to dispose of a psychiatric patient is to label this person psychotic, thereby enabling the staff to commit the patient, at least for a period of observation, to a psychiatric hospital or ward. The community mental health center is more oriented toward continuing services for the mentally ill. Even such centers, however, have not been able to respond to the whole range of nonmedical emergency problems. Alcoholics and many others in need of emergency help resent the label of mental illness and need other entry doors into a helping system.

In spite of recent progress, a number of deficiencies also exist in the medical emergency service system. These include a lack of ambulance coverage in some locations or at certain times; poor vehicular design; inadequate equipment for extrication of trapped accident victims and for on-the-site and in-transit, life-preserving treatment; and inadequate or, more often, a lack of means of communication with the professional persons and the institution that are to receive the patient. Brown[13] reasonably believes that an ambulance should be like an extension of a well-staffed and equipped hosptial emergency department. According to him, "More important than immediate transportation is the immediate life-saving care—control of hemorrhage, splinting fractures, keeping the breathing passages open. On-the-site care should be by trained emergency technicians and then the transportation should be deliberate and gentle." This is the theory, but what is practice?

Before the initiation of the Emergency Medical Services program by the federal government, there were about 44,000 "ambulances" in operation in the United States with about 19,000 of them under the control of morticians. The vehicles were often station wagons or modified Cadillac hearses with no room for trained attendants to administer either basic or advanced life-support services. As the National Highway Safety Administration began to apply new standards for vehicular design and equipment, the old hearses were relegated to routine transport of nonemergency patients while more appropriately designed, equipped, and staffed units took over the emergency responses. Once again, current data are not available, but National Highway Safety Administration officials believe that, by 1976, there were 25,000 to 27,000 adequately equipped units in operation. The total number is probably in excess of 30,000 by now. This apparent reduction (from 44,000 to 30,000) represents a considerable improvement, since the replacement vehicles are well suited for their work and their time is less frequently taken up by routine transportation jobs, which make the actual availability of an appropriate response vehicle much better.

Placement of the vehicles presents an interesting planning challenge. Geographers have been involved in designing service areas. Within some limits the response time for an emergency vehicle can be reduced to any desired level by adding more units and relocating existing ones so that they remain available for response in the center of their area. When one unit is activated, the others can relocate to minimize the response time for all units if another call occurs while one unit is in action. If the resulting response time is still too great for the community, it can be shortened by adding another unit and redesigning the service areas again. Each unit, if properly equipped and staffed with paid workers, costs about $275,000 to $300,000 per year. Obviously the cost of reducing response time in sparsely settled areas is much greater than in densely populated areas. At some point, the effort to reduce response time to an acceptable level will result in each unit receiving so few calls that the emergency medical technicians do not get enough work to maintain their skill levels. In short, the situation is made to order for a cost-benefit analysis that can be used in a political environment to negotiate the level of care to be purchased.

PERSONNEL

Those 30,000 ambulances require 10 attendants each to cover three shifts 7 days a week, or a total of 300,000 trained emergency medical technicians (EMTs). The professional groups involved in emergency medical services recommend that each unit be staffed with two EMTs who have completed 81 hours of carefully planned and presented instruction. An additional 400 hours of training are usually recommended for more advanced levels. There are currently about 200,000 EMTs and 15,000 paramedics. The latter are qualified to provide advanced life-support services. About 65% of the EMTs are certified by the National Registry of Emergency Medical Technicians as a result of a nationally developed and administered examination. During the 1970s it was assumed that the national certifying examination would become the standard examination that would allow EMTs to obtain license reciprocity between states. This would have meant job mobility but, more importantly, the ability to cross state boundaries when necessary to complete an emergency response run. Unfortunately, the move toward national standardization has become bogged down, and reciprocity has become a very difficult issue, making effective regional planning and interstate cooperation difficult. It is not clear just what has led to a reduction in the momentum of development of and information about emergency medical services in the last few years. Budget cutting at the national level has retarded enthusiasm somewhat, since it is no longer possible for governors to give new ambulances to county supervisors and city mayors with federal grant money, but it seems as if the big national effort that began in 1973 has been replaced with a thirst for regional individuality and local hegemony to the detriment of service effectiveness. In 1980, 49 state health agencies reported that they were involved in the development of emergency medical services.[14] Involvement in the training and certification of personnel was reported by 45 and 43 state health agencies, respectively. (These figures were self-reported by state health officials.)

Consideration of emergency vehicle attendants focuses attention on the broader subject of related personnel. Several years ago it was estimated that there were about 300,000 allied health workers of various types in the emergency health care field. (There are no useful data about the number of nonmedical emergency health workers.) This falls far short of the need for dealing with nonmedical emergencies such as suicide attempts, alcoholism,

and acute schizophrenia. New types of personnel must be tried, legal barriers to their effective use must be removed, roles must be defined, appropriate curricula must be planned and presented, and positions must be established with proper career development opportunities.

One of the most difficult and costly problems to solve is the provision of adequately trained physicians. Many medical graduates have had no formal training in emergency care. A survey in the late 1960s of 108 medical schools in the United States and Canada showed only 33 schools with courses in the subject. At present there are about 20,000 physicians devoting most if not all of their time to emergency medicine. Twice that number is needed. This is not a task for which every physician is qualified. Belatedly it has been realized that a special type of training is needed. The first residency in emergency medicine was established at the University of Cincinnati Medical Center in 1970. Since then, 30 other centers of medical education have followed suit. Several professional organizations deserve special mention for their leadership. Among them are the American College of Surgeons, the American Academy of Orthopaedic Surgeons, the American Association of Anaesthesiologists, the newer University Association of Emergency Medical Services, and the American College of Emergency Physicians (ACEP). The ACEP, now with about 10,000 members, has been working especially to improve specialty training in acute care and to make emergentology a board-certified specialty. Another important effort to improve the quality of care was the formation in 1971 of the Emergency Department Nurses Association (EDNA) with a fast-flying bird as its symbol. The American Public Health Association established a section on Injury Control and Emergency Health Services in 1972.

EMERGENCY HEALTH SERVICES SYSTEM[13,15,16]

There are many problems to be overcome in the development of an effective, community-based, emergency response system. Institutional and political boundaries jeopardize effective solutions to communications problems, dispatching problems, and the problems involved in standardization of training programs and equipment. Significant progress has been made since the passage of the Emergency Medical Services Systems Act of 1973. President Nixon, in his State of the Union address in 1972, directed the Secretary of the Department of Health, Education, and Welfare to develop new ways of organizing and providing comprehensive emergency medical care. This resulted in a number of actions by the Department of Health, Education, and Welfare, including the establishment of a focal point in the Health Services Administration's Bureau of Medical Services to provide technical assistance to states, communities, and professional groups. New information systems were developed to collect data and begin evaluative studies. Various approaches to modeling, system design, equipment standardization, and other aspects of emergency medical service systems were adopted together with a limited number of research and demonstration projects. President Nixon then vetoed the bill passed by Congress in 1973 in an anti-inflationary gesture, but Congress overrode the veto in September of that year.

The Department of Transportation has also played a significant role in system development, particularly in the training of emergency medical technicians and through the provision of funds for the purchase of ambulances and equipment in many localities. All equipment purchased has had to meet the recommended standards of the National Academy of Sciences–National Research Council.

Since July of 1970 the Military Assistance to Safety and Traffic Program (MAST) has used Defense Department medical corpsmen and helicopters to supplement local efforts when necessary. The combined military effort is coordinated by a civilian committee according to local plans and has helped transport patients, human organs, blood, special medications, premature infants, and medical personnel and equipment.

At about the same time as the first initiatives of the Department of Health, Education, and Welfare, the Robert Wood Johnson Foundation announced a grant program to develop model comprehensive emergency medical service systems. This coalescing of interest and activities did much to rectify many of the deficiencies that had characterized the emergency medical response system in the United States up until the 1970s. Unfortunately almost all of the activity has been devoted to improvements in medical services; little emphasis has been placed on the equally important but less attractive problem of the nonmedical emergency.

An emergency health services system is an organized procedure for receiving and acting on requests for assistance when there is a likelihood of either trauma requiring rapid medical attention or an illness that poses conditions threatening to life or requiring immediate resuscitation to sustain life. It usually requires a communications system to receive requests for help, a defined procedure for acting on the requests, including central dispatch; and availability of an appropriately staffed transportation system or systems by land, air, or water, and with a capability for immediate on-site treatment and in-transit life support. There must also be available 24-hour, 7-day-a-week emergency care centers prepared to receive emergency patients from within a defined service area and staffed with appropriately trained professional and technical medical and surgical personnel and with supportive laboratory, diagnostic, and treatment facilities. Such centers may be either in large general hospitals as part of their emergency service function or in independent and free-standing specialized institutions for trauma care. Under certain circumstances mobile intensive care units have been found useful. The emergency medical services system should be regarded as an integral part of the total health care system to assure proper medical, rehabilitative, and other follow-up services and assistance so that patients receive maximum opportunity for recovery of personal function after survival from a true emergency situation. Fig. 34-1 presents the elements of an emergency medical system and their interrelationships.

Service levels have been stratified into basic life support and advanced life support services. Generally, EMTs are trained to function at the basic life support level and paramedics are trained for work at the advanced life support level. Basic life support services are defined as "an emergency first-aid procedure that consists of recognizing respiratory and cardiac arrest and starting proper application of cardiopulmonary resuscitation to maintain life until a victim recovers sufficiently to be transported or until Advanced Life Support is available." Advanced life support consists of (1) basic life support, (2) adjunctive equipment and special techniques such as endotracheal intubation and cardiac compression, (3) cardiac monitoring for dysrhythmia recognition and control, (4) defibrillation, (5) establishment and maintenance of an intravenous line, (6) employment of definitive therapy including drug administration, and (7) stabilization of the patient's condition.[17] The special emphasis on heart

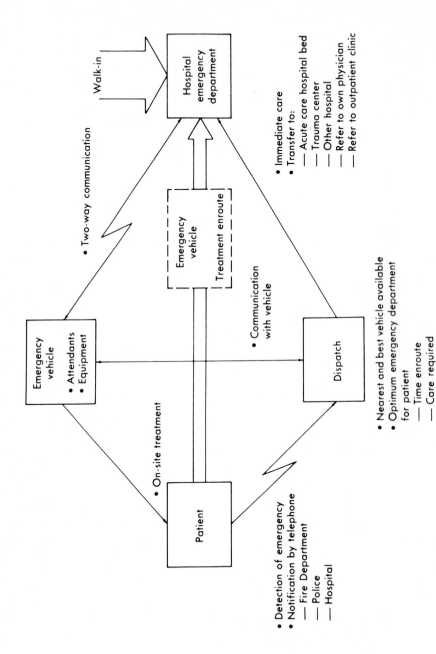

FIG. 34-1. Elements of an emergency medical system.

attacks has characterized almost all of the emergency medical services systems design work in recent years and is attributable to the interest of the American Heart Association and to the high incidence of death caused by sudden ischemic cardiac episodes in the United States.

PHASES OF AN EMERGENCY MEDICAL SERVICES (EMS) SYSTEM

The following outline presents in sequence some of the events that can follow occurrence of a damaging incident that produces emergency medical patients. It provides a reasonable enumeration of points where emergency system failures may exaggerate rather than prevent losses from damaging incidents.

Pretreatment phase
1. Occurrence
2. Detection
3. Notification
4. Dispatch of mobile emergency medical services
5. Travel to site

Preliminary care phase
6. On-site problem analysis
7. On-site treatment
8. On-site extrication
9. On-site stabilization
10. On-site loading
11. Selection of definitive care facility
12. Transport (continuing patient maintenance)
13. En route notification of receiving facility
14. In-transit transmission of patient's condition and receipt of necessary life maintenance instructions and their application
15. Facility preparation for receiving patient
16. Delivery to definitive care facility

Definitive care phase at receiving facility
17. Patient transfer
18. Information transfer
19. Patient evaluation (by facility staff)
20. Triage
21. Continuation of treatment
22. Second stage diagnosis
23. Emergency room treatment
24. Intensive care
25. Definitive diagnosis
26. Definitive treatment

Recuperation phase
27. Recuperative care

Rehabilitation phase
28. Transfer to extended care facility or home
29. Rehabilitative treatment
30. Discharge
31. Return to normal function

CRITERIA, STANDARDS, AND REGULATIONS

Until recently, one of the basic problems in the delivery of emergency medical services in the United States was the absence or inconsistency of personnel qualification requirements or of criteria, standards, guidelines, and regulations for emergency medical services systems. To achieve maximum efficiency, local systems must be compatible with those adjacent to them. To achieve these objectives, uniform standards must be adopted. The Public Health Service and others have provided several recommended standards for reference and guidance.[18] Some of them are summarized as follows:

State legislation[19]
1. Should establish divisions of emergency medical services
2. Should specify duties and qualifications of personnel
3. Should require establishment of a system to supervise and regulate ambulance services and personnel
4. Should assist in establishment of a coordinated central communications and dispatch system

Ambulances[20]
1. Should meet the vehicle design specifications as recommended by the National Academy of Engineering and the National Research Council
2. Should have as minimal equipment those items recommended as essential equipment by the American College of Surgeons
3. Should exist in sufficient numbers and be so placed as to provide maximum utilization and effectiveness in the shortest possible response time

Ambulance personnel[21,22]
1. Should have basic training of at least 70 hours' instruction, plus 10 or more additional hours of emergency room training
2. Should routinely maintain skills by observation and instruction in a hospital emergency department under the supervision of a physician, including regular critique by emergency room physicians with ambulance personnel of care administered to the patient prior to arrival at the emergency room
3. Should meet or exceed requirements of the Registry of Emergency Medical Technicians-Ambulance
4. Should include two emergency medical technicians, one of whom may be the driver, for each emergency ambulance.

Hospital emergency facilities[23,24]

1. Should promote the development of satisfactory plans for regionalization of services
2. Should be categorized according to the National Academy of Sciences' recommended criteria
3. Should provide for ongoing self-improvement training for all emergency department staff, both clinical and administrative
4. Should meet or exceed the emergency department standards recommended by the Joint Commission on Accreditation of Hospitals
5. Should accept a leadership role in providing training for emergency medical technologists
6. Should base ambulance services at the hospital, wherever and whenever feasible

Communications[25]

1. A single telephone number for emergency medical services, that is, "911," instituted throughout the nation
2. Central dispatch provided for all emergency ambulances
3. Radio or environmentally secure communications established between
   a. Central dispatch center
   b. Ambulance
   c. Hospitals
   d. Law enforcement and fire units
   e. Emergency operating centers

Supportive actions

1. Toll-free public telephone service available for all emergency calls from pay telephones
2. Emergency medical identification—to be carried by all persons with conditions or medical histories that should be known to anyone rendering emergency medical care
3. Medical self-help—at least one member of every family trained in medical self-help and/or Red Cross first aid
4. Highway signs (*coordinated with hospital categorization*) placed in adequate numbers and locations to identify emergency medical care facilities

PLANNING

To introduce effective planning, a data collection and analysis system must be implemented. As a minimum, the following information should be collected and analyzed before implementation of large-scale emergency medical services system efforts:

1. Epidemiologic data concerning medical emergencies
2. Geographic, demographic, and topographic data
3. Patient-flow patterns
4. Patient-demand patterns
5. Road networks
6. Travel times (ground and air)
7. Population densities
8. Distances from health care resources
9. Health care resources should be analyzed as follows:
   a. Type
      (1) Personnel—physicians and allied professionals and technicians
      (2) Emergency centers, hospitals, and related facilities
      (3) Ambulance services (ground and air)
      (4) Communications networks
   b. Category
   c. Location
   d. Distribution
   e. Services provided
   f. Capacity
   g. Capability
   h. Availability
   i. Personnel
      (1) Quantity
      (2) Training
      (3) Staffing patterns
   j. Equipment
   k. Administration and control
      (1) Government
      (2) Public
      (3) Private enterprise
      (4) Volunteers
   l. Response times
10. Needs
11. Priorities

All of this information should be used to design local and regional systems tailored to the unique requirements of the area. No two solutions need be exactly the same. In some areas it may be desirable to use the fire department to provide the first and second response units, including advanced life support services, and rely on ambulance companies for transport. In other areas, depending on geography and population density, it may be preferable to develop a combined rescue, advanced life support, and transport system. The number of mobile units and their staffing will also vary, depending on geography and population density. In one system plan it was found that most of the calls came during the working day because the hospital was located in an area of New York City largely populated by persons who commuted into the area for work each day. In this system, one of the four ambulances was replaced with a mobile intensive care unit, which sufficed to give advanced life support capability to the entire system during the peak hours. The additional cost for this change was only 11%.[26] Variations in management structure may depend on who has the initial interest and the resources to take a lead role in planning. Romano and associates[27] found 310 paramedic services to be in existence, of which 102 were operated by fire departments, 97 by municipalities, 5 by police departments, 64 by hospitals, and 42 by commercial firms. Some of the latter may have been developed to respond to specific requests for bids by cities or counties.

The education of the general public is essential to any successful emergency medical services system. The public must continually be made aware of what is being done, who is doing it, and for what purpose. In addition, the public must be informed of the services available, steps to take when a medical emergency is encountered or recognized, as well as who and how to call for assistance. Extensive experiments using a common emergency telephone number have been conducted in the United States. In places where such a number is available, the necessary assistance can be dispatched immediately because the central dispatcher knows current service load levels and the location of the closest appropriate and available medical facility and response vehicle. The common emergency telephone number can be distributed to the public in many ways, including labels to attach to private telephones and mass mailings in utility and other bills.

EMERGENCY MEDICAL SERVICES COUNCILS

Until recently there has been little coordination among providers of emergency medical services in the United States. Ambulance services have operated independently, often without direct communications to hospitals. Hence the possibility has existed for patients to be delivered to hospitals that have not been advised of their pending arrival, condition, or need for emergency treatment. Training of emergency medical services personnel at all levels has differed greatly from community to community. Communications and medical equipment have differed considerably from vehicle to vehicle, and few procedures have been established for exchange of equipment on delivery of a patient to a hospital, thus enabling ambulances to return promptly to further service. Many communities have not established interhospital radio communications systems or interhospital agreements for systematic continuation of care in case of patient transfer.

Many of these problems are in the process of being overcome by the establishment of community emergency medical services councils. Typically these councils are composed of representatives from the community working with representatives from the various elements of the emergency medical services system, such as hospital administrators, public health agencies, medical societies, law-enforcement and fire-protection personnel, private ambulance operators, disaster preparedness personnel, elected officials, and others. The councils have the authority and responsibility for searching out the resources, bringing them together, and coordinating the services provided by all elements of the system by virtue of new laws or local ordinances. In other words, emergency medical services councils offer the potential of establishing and implementing an orderly, efficient, and well-coordinated system for delivering emergency medical care. It is important to begin broadening the interest and memebership of the councils to develop better systems of nonmedical emergency care.

CONCLUSION

In many respects recent developments in emergency medical services systems have been a singular triumph of health planning. Beginning with national and state legislation and specific financing mechanisms, many communities have been able to develop highly sophisticated and efficient emergency medical care systems, overcoming the fractionation and duplication, the territorial rivalries, and the bureaucratic obstacles in the way. Sophisticated needs assessments involving geography, patient flow patterns, road networks, population densities, and other factors, have been performed. Work force analyses have been conducted and curricula developed to produce trained personnel to fill prescribed and carefully planned roles. Continuing inservice training programs have been developed, and interagency communications systems have solved many of the problems of patient continuity. Yet a number of questions remain.

How beneficial are such sophisticated systems?

Public health and health care services

Even when all of the parts work together as planned, are the results worth the effort? Many studies of survival have been used to justify the investments in the systems. As an example, Pozen and associates[28] reported that 778 electrocardiograms were transmitted from the field to the hospital during a period in which 7,654 patients were transported. Ischemic heart disease was apparent in 179 of those transmissions. Prehospital intervention was warranted in 28 of the cases, and 12 of the victims survived through their hospital admission; 6 of them were still alive 3 months later. It cannot be known whether those 6 would have survived without such sophisticated intervention. It would be unwise to make generalizations from one such study, but it would be equally unwise to ignore the obvious questions raised about costs and benefits.

Journal articles purporting to evaluate emergency medical services are a useful lesson in advocacy by health workers. The principal journals are the *Annals of Emergency Medicine,* a publication of the American College of Emergency Physicians and the University Association for Emergency Medicine, and *Emergency Medicine*—both published by those who make their living providing the services. In one review Terrel Hicks and his associates[29] examined 100 consecutive transfers from smaller hospitals to the trauma unit at the University of Louisville, Kentucky, and concluded that the first-line intervenors at the local level, who did not have specialty training in emergency medicine, were woefully deficient. Not only was the result predictable, but they labeled it a "prospective study"—a mistake that any objective, trained evaluator would not have made. Such results are not limited to trade journals: in an article in the *New England Journal of Medicine,* a state health department official claimed that in a city of 500,000, an EMS squad would handle 220 out-of-hospital cardiac arrests per year with 30 to 40 "saves."[30] One of his sources for that assertion was an article in the *Journal of the American College of Emergency Physicians,* which classified 147 out-of-hospital cardiac arrests as "dead-on-arrival," "died in the emergency room," "died in the hospital" or "discharged alive."[31] The only patients counted were those who had a resuscitation attempt by a paramedic, and they called the 22 patients who were discharged alive (15% of that highly selected group) "long-term saves" in spite of the well-known fact that many of them will die during the first year after discharge.

The general conclusion is that a well-trained, well-equipped, and well-designed emergency medical system can save lives but at high cost. Most people seem willing to pay that price, even though considerably less is invested in preventing accidents and heart disease. The investments, within some limits that most communities seem to work out on their own, may be reasonable, but the art and science of health services evaluation is not seen at its best in the study of emergency medical services. The reports from the Seattle–King County program are noteworthy exceptions.[6,32]

What can be done about the nonmedical emergency? As noted repeatedly, almost all of the emphasis, interest, and money has been devoted to medical emergency systems and most of that has been in the area of heart disease. Responding to the medical and surgical emergency is popular, rewarding, and glamorous. It can also be profitable. But what about alcoholism, mental illness, child abuse, and social dislocation emergencies that occur with at least equal frequency and equally disastrous results? Little attention has been paid to the less glamorous and more frustrating social emergencies. This is an area that must receive the attention of public health agencies in conjunction with other involved and responsible organizations.

If it can be done for emergencies, why not for health care generally? The development of emergency medical services systems has involved government agencies and planners working with private physicians and hospitals to produce a sophisticated system of medical care. The development of these systems has required detailed analysis of needs, resources, barriers, work force roles, equipment, and facilities. It has involved the development of communications networks, training programs, and diagnostic and treatment protocols to be followed by nonphysician health care technicians. It has involved the establishment of linkages between various parts of the health care system to assure continuity of care. It has involved, in short, all of the steps that would be required to develop a comprehensive system of primary health care. Why is this possible for emergency care and, to a lesser extent, for continuing care and rehabilitation but not for the vast, important, and costly area in between—acute medical care itself? It is possible that some of the emergency medical care systems that have been developed in recent years can be used as a skeleton for the development of a more comprehensive primary health care system.

REFERENCES

1. U.S. Public Health Service: Current estimates from the health interview survey, United States—1978, PHS Pub. No. 80-1551, Washington, D.C., 1979.
2. Accident facts, Chicago, 1978, National Safety Council.
3. Frey, C.F., and others: Resuscitation and survival in motor accidents, J. Trauma **9:**292, Feb. 1969.
4. Where minutes count, U.S. News and World Report, June 26, 1972.
5. Huntley, H.C.: National status of emergency health services. In Proceedings of Second National Conference on Emergency Health Services, DEHS Pub. No. 16, Rockville, Md., 1972, U.S. Department of Health, Education, and Welfare.
6. Eisenberg, M.S., Bergner, L., and Hallstrom, A.: Cardiac resuscitation in the community: importance of rapid provision and implications for planning, J.A.M.A. **241**(18):1905, May 4, 1979.
7. U.S. Department of Health, Education, and Welfare: Ambulance services and hospital emergency departments: digest of surveys conducted 1965 to March 1971, DEHS Pub. No. 11, Rockville, Md., 1971.
8. Donabedian, A., Axelrod, S.J., and Wyszewianski, L.: Medical care chartbook, ed. 7, Ann Arbor, Mich. 1980, Health Administration Press.
9. Hospital statistics, 1979: data from the 1978 annual survey, Chicago, Ill., 1979, American Hospital Association.
10. Havlick, R.J., and Feinlein, M., editors: Proceedings of the conference on the decline in coronary heart disease mortality, Session II, NIH Pub. No. 79-1610, Bethesda, Md., 1979.
11. Accreditation Council for Psychiatric Facilities: Principles for accreditation of community mental health service programs, Chicago, 1976, Joint Commission on Accreditation of Hospitals.
12. Jacobson, G.F.: Emergency services in community mental health, Am. J. Public Health **64:**124, Feb. 1974.
13. U.S. Department of Health, Education, and Welfare: Emergency medical services communications systems, DHEW Pub. No. (HSM) 73-2003, Rockville, Md., 1972.
14. National Public Health Program reporting system: Public health agencies, 1980: a report on their expenditures and activities, Washington, D.C., 1981, Association of State and Territorial Health Officials.
15. American Medical Association: Developing emergency medical services: guidelines for community councils, Chicago, 1971, The Association.
16. Flashner, B.A., and Boyd, D.R.: The critically injured patient: a plan for organization of statewide system of trauma facilities, Ill. Med. J. **39:**256, March 1971.
17. Standards for cardiopulmonary resuscitation and emergency cardiac care, J.A.M.A. (suppl.) **227:**7, Feb. 1974.
18. U.S. Department of Health, Education, and Welfare: Recommended standards for development of emergency medical services systems, DEHS Pub. No. 4, Rockville, Md., 1971.
19. U.S. Department of Health, Education, and Welfare: Model act for emergency medical services, DHEW Pub. No. (HSM) 72-2016, Rockville, Md., 1972.
20. National Highway Bureau: Ambulance design criteria: report prepared by National Academy of Engineering and National Research Council, Washington, D.C., 1970, U.S. Department of Transportation.
21. American Academy of Orthopaedic Surgeons: Emergency care and transportation of the sick and injured, ed. 3, Menasha, Wis., 1981, George Banta Co., Inc.
22. American Heart Association: Textbook on advanced cardiac life support, Dallas, Tex. 1981, National Center.
23. Commission of Emergency Medical Services: Categorization of hospital emergency capabilities, Chicago, 1971, American Medical Association.
24. Hospital emergency services; and Hospital disaster plan: an Association manual for hospitals, Chicago, 1971, Joint Commission on Accreditation of Hospitals.
25. U.S. Department of Health, Education, and Welfare: Emergency medical services communications systems, DHEW Pub. No. (HSM) 73-2003, Rockville, Md., 1973.
26. Pascarelli, E.F., and Katz, I.B.: Planning and developing a prehospital mobile intensive care system in an urban setting, Am. J. Public Health **68:**389, April 1978.
27. Romano, T.L., and others: Paramedic services: nationwide distribution and management structure, J. Am. Coll. Emergency Physicians **7:**99, March 1978.
28. Pozen, M.W., and others: Studies of ambulance patients with ischemic heart disease. I. The outcome of pre-hospital life-threatening arrythmias in patients receiving electrocardiographic telemetry and therapeutic interventions, Am. J. Public Health **67:**527, June 1977.
29. Hicks, T.C., and others: Resuscitation and transfer of trauma patients: a prospective study, Ann. Emerg. Med. **11**(6):296, June 1982.
30. Hoffer, E.R.: Emergency medical services, 1979, N. Engl. J. Med. **301**(20):1119, Nov. 15, 1979.
31. Lauterbach, S.A., Spadafora, M., and Levy, R.: Evaluation of cardiac arrests managed by paramedics, J.A.C.E.P. **7**(10):355, Oct. 1978.
32. Urban, N., Bergner, L., and Eisenberg, M.S.: The costs of a suburban paramedic program in reducing deaths due to cardiac arrest, Med. Care **19**(4):379, April 1981.

Index